Respiratory Injury: Smoke Inhalation and Burns

NOTICE

Respiratory Injury: Smoke Inhalation and Burns

Edward F. Haponik, M.D., F.A.C.P.

Professor of Medicine
Clinical Director, Section on Pulmonary and Critical Care Medicine
Department of Medicine
The Bowman Gray School of Medicine
Wake Forest University
Winston-Salem, North Carolina

Andrew M. Munster, M.D., F.R.C.S., F.A.C.S.

Professor of Surgery
Johns Hopkins University School of Medicine
Director, Baltimore Regional Burn Center
Francis Scott Key Medical Center
Baltimore, Maryland

McGraw-Hill, Inc.

HEALTH PROFESSIONS DIVISION

New York St. Louis San Francisco
Colorado Springs Auckland Bogotá Caracas
Hamburg Lisbon London Madrid Mexico Milan
Montreal New Delhi Paris San Juan
São Paulo Singapore Sydney Tokyo Toronto

RESPIRATORY INJURY:
SMOKE INHALATION AND BURNS

1234567890 HALHAL 9876543210

ISBN 0-07-026018-4

This book was set in Times Roman by Compset, Inc.; camera and film preparation was done by Jay's Publishers Services. The editors were J. Dereck Jeffers and Muza Navrozov; the production supervisor was Annette Mayeski; the cover was designed by José Fonfrias. The index was prepared by Alexandra Nickerson. Arcata Graphics/Halliday was printer and binder.

Library of Congress Cataloging-in-Publication Data

Respiratory injury: smoke inhalation and burns / [edited by] Edward F. Haponik, Andrew M. Munster.
p. cm.
Includes bibliographies and index.
ISBN 0-07-026018-4 :
1. Respiratory organs — Diseases. 2. Burns and scalds—Complications and sequelae. 3. Respiratory organs — Wounds and injuries. I. Haponik, Edward F. II. Munster, Andrew M., date.
[DNLM: 1. Burns — complications. 2. Respiratory Tract Diseases. WF 140 R4341005]
RC732.R463 1990
616.2′4 — dc20
DNLM/DLC
for Library of Congress 89-2632
CIP

Contents

Contributors*

Caroline Chiles, M.D. [8]
Assistant Professor of Radiology
Duke University Medical Center
Durham, North Carolina

William G. Cioffi, Jr., M.D. [10]
Chief, Burn Study Branch
U.S. Army Institute of Surgical Research
Assistant Professor of Surgery
University of Texas Health Sciences Center
San Antonio, Texas

William R. Clark, Jr., M.D. [18]
Associate Professor of Surgery
Department of Surgery
State University of New York
Health Science Center
Syracuse, New York

Craig L. Coblentz [8]
Assistant Professor of Radiology
McMaster University Medical Center
Hamilton, Ontario, Canada

*The numbers in brackets following the contributor name refer to chapter(s) authored or co-authored by the contributor.

Gene L. Colice, M.D. [17]
Assistant Professor of Medicine
Dartmouth University
Medical and Regional Office Center
Veterans Administration
White River Junction, Vermont

Robert O. Crapo, M.D. [3]
Medical Director
Pulmonary Function Laboratory
Pulmonary Division, LDS Hospital
Associate Professor of Medicine
University of Utah
Salt Lake City, Utah

John W. L. Davies, D.Sc. [19]
Editor
Burns
Department of Surgery
Royal Infirmary
Glasgow, Scotland

William R. Furman, M.D. [13]
Assistant Professor of Anesthesiology
and Critical Care Medicine
Johns Hopkins University School of Medicine
Associate Director, Department of Anesthesiology
Francis Scott Key Medical Center
Baltimore, Maryland

Edward F. Haponik, M.D., F.A.C.P. [2,7]
Professor of Medicine
Clinical Director, Section on Pulmonary and Critical Care Medicine
Department of Medicine
The Bowman Gray School of Medicine
Wake Forest University
Winston-Salem, North Carolina

David M. Heimbach, M.D., F.A.C.S. [9]
Director
University of Washington Burn Center
Professor of Surgery
University of Washington
Seattle, Washington

David N. Herndon, M.D. [4]
Chief of Staff, Professor of Surgery
Shriners Burns Institute
Galveston, Texas

Leonard D. Hudson, M.D. [9]
Professor of Medicine, Head
Division of Pulmonary and Critical Care Medicine
University of Washington
Seattle, Washington

J. A. Jeevendra Martyn, M.D. [14]
Associate Professor of Anesthesia
Department of Anesthesia
Massachusetts General Hospital
Harvard Medical School
Boston, Massachusetts

Francis D. Moore, M.D., F.A.C.S. [1]
Moseley Professor of Surgery, Emeritus
Harvard Medical School
Surgeon-in-Chief, Emeritus
Peter Bent Brigham Hospital
Boston, Massachusetts

Andrew M. Munster, M.D., F.R.C.S., F.A.C.S. [2,12,16]
Professor of Surgery
Johns Hopkins University School of Medicine
Director, Baltimore Regional Burn Center
Francis Scott Key Medical Center
Baltimore, Maryland

Steve Nelson, M.D. [6]
Associate Professor of Medicine
Pulmonary/Critical Care Medicine
LSU Medical Center
New Orleans, Louisiana

James A. O'Neill, Jr., M.D., F.A.C.S. [15]
Professor of Surgery
University of Pennsylvania
Surgeon-in-Chief
Children's Hospital
Philadelphia, Pennsylvania

Basil A. Pruitt, Jr., M.D., F.A.C.S. [10]
Clinical Professor of Surgery
University of Texas Health Sciences Center
Professor of Surgery
Uniformed Services University of the Health Sciences
Commander and Director
U.S. Army Institute of Surgical Research
San Antonio, Texas

Charles E. Putman, M.D. [8]
James B. Duke Professor of Radiology
Vice Provost of Research and Development
Duke University
Durham, North Carolina

Stephen D. Sears, M.D., M.P.H. [11]
Vice-President for Medical Affairs
Kennebec Valleys Medical Center
Augusta, Maine

Michael J. Sendak, M.D. [13]
Assistant Professor
Department of Anesthesiology and Critical Care Medicine
Johns Hopkins University
Chief, Department of Anesthesiology and Critical Care Medicine
The Homewood Hospital Center, Inc.
Baltimore, Maryland

Sam R. Sharar, M.D. [9]
Chief Resident of Anesthesiology
University of Washington School of Medicine
Seattle, Washington

Warren R. Summer, M.D. [5]
Chief, Pulmonary/Critical Care Medicine
Howard Buechner Professor of Medicine
LSU Medical Center
New Orleans, Louisiana

Daniel L. Traber, Ph.D. [4]
Professor of Anesthesiology, Physiology, and Biophysics
University of Texas
Galveston, Texas

Leslie A. Wong, M.D. [16]
Senior Clinical Fellow
Johns Hopkins University School of Medicine
Baltimore Regional Burn Center
Francis Scott Key Medical Center
Baltimore, Maryland

Preface

This volume originates from unique clinical interactions of the Surgery and Pulmonary/Critical Care Services at Johns Hopkins in the daily management of patients hospitalized at the Baltimore Regional Burn Center. During a six-year period, we worked together in the evaluation and care of patients with acute respiratory injuries due to smoke inhalation, cutaneous burns, and their combinations. From these activities it became apparent that this population epitomized the diverse forms of catastrophic respiratory injury, that aspects of the pathophysiology and clinical management of acute lung injuries encountered in other settings were remarkably similar to events in burned patients, that the multisystemic responses unique to burn injury and its treatment modified both the respiratory injury and therapeutic priorities, and that many clinicians were unfamiliar with these issues. Despite the widely acknowledged importance of such problems to physicians having a variety of specialty orientations, no single text synthesizing current information was available.

In this effort to provide a comprehensive, yet practically oriented review, we have sought multidisciplinary, multiinstitutional perspectives. We are privileged that our invited authors include pioneers in the care of burned patients, highly esteemed clinical and basic scientists, and expert clinicians. Their enthusiastically written, authoritative contributions have been organized in major sections that address the background of smoke inhalation injury (Chaps. 1 and 2), its pathogenesis (Chaps. 3 to 6), clinical recognition (Chaps. 7 and 8), and nuances of management (Chaps. 9 to 17). Finally, priorities for future clinically relevant basic science and clinical research are reviewed (Chaps. 18 and 19). We have purposefully chosen to retain mild degrees of overlap and differing opinions. We believe that the text accurately reflects the current state of the art, addressing controversies and uncertainties as well as well-established principles. We hope that it will serve not only to contribute to clinicians' management of patients with these respiratory problems, but also to stimulate future investigation.

We appreciate the superb efforts of all contributors to this volume and the outstanding support provided by the editorial staff at McGraw-Hill, notably J. Dereck Jeffers, Avé McCracken, Bruce Williams, and Muza Navrozov. We are thankful for the tireless secretarial efforts of Debbie McNamara, Millie Drumgoole, and Donald Noel. Most of all, we are indebted to the patients and dedicated staff of the Baltimore Regional Burn Center who inspired this project: the translation of improved understanding of the pathogenesis of smoke inhalation injury to the enhanced care of patients with this problem represents the ultimate goal of this book.

Edward F. Haponik, M.D.
Andrew M. Munster, M.D.

Chapter 1

The Respiratory Tract Injury of Burns: Lessons from the Past

Francis D. Moore

> Some persons with extensive cutaneous burning show little or no evidence of respiratory injury, where others with little or no cutaneous burning may show severe injuries to the respiratory tract.
>
> *Alan R. Moritz*
> *National Research Council*
> *Symposium on Burns, 1950*

In the treatment of respiratory tract injury in burns, the principal lesson from the past has been that in the respiratory tract lies a major site of injury and a continuing cause of death. Although several authorities clearly recognized this 50 years ago it was not generally included in standard surgical teaching texts for another 20 years.

Prior to 1940 respiratory tract injury was little appreciated. In late 1942 a single disaster in a Boston nightclub became the pivot point of our understanding of pulmonary injury in burns. Between 1945 and 1975 many innovations came about, the better to recognize and treat these patients. In the past decade treatment modes have changed somewhat less rapidly but survival becomes still more likely. The pathophysiology of increased lung water in such injury is better appreciated, yet the problem remains pressing. It is the purpose of this paper briefly to review this historic sequence.

There is a broad spectrum of pathology in this field. In some cases, the respiratory tract injury is clearly distinct from any thermal burn of the skin and is more properly termed inhalation injury, often occurring quite aside from any fire, explosion, or burn epidemiology. Even in the absence of any thermal burn of the skin, death from a general conflagration or explosion may occur because of lung injury due to inhalation of ash particles in smoke or of toxic gases. Because of this fact, the treatment of pure inhalation injury has become a part of the responsibility of the surgeon and the respiratory therapist in the burn unit.

In other cases, an extensive thermal burn of the skin is clearly predominant, extensive, and potentially lethal with no evident pulmonary component at the outset. Yet the death of the patient may be traceable to a progressive and refractory pulmonary lesion.

Between these two ends of the spectrum — pure inhalation and pure burn — there is a continuum of lesions and pathophysiologic relations between respiratory tract injury and cutaneous burn. In a curious middle position are those instances where the patient succumbs to the toxicity of inhaled substances (carbon monoxide, cyanide, or phenol and certain phenolic derivatives) that leave no pulmonary footprints even though the lung is the lethal pathway to systemic injury.

All of these are challenging to the surgeon on first examining the patient; in continuing care, they may become the cause of major difficulty leading to death.

ANCIENT HISTORY

Surgical antiquarians would be fascinated could they uncover any studies or reports of burn patients suffering pulmonary deterioration prior to the reports of war gas injury in World War I. People have died in the neighborhood of house fires over the course of centuries. After a fire was put out, bodies were often found nearby, totally unburned but very dead; "smoke inhalation" was often the diagnosis. Every person has had the frightening experience of choking or gasping upon inhaling windblown smoke from a nearby fire, even if only a campfire. When this irritating stimulus to the respiratory tract persists only a few moments longer, the result may be a severe pulmonary injury and, in a person prone to asthma or with emphysema, serious anoxia. Smoke inhaled only a few minutes longer causes suffocation (due to oxygen lack, carbon dioxide excess, alveolar edema, or all three) and death. If life persists after severe exposure there is a massive bronchiolar and alveolar edema with an outpouring of fluid into the airway, nose, and mouth; bronchospasm often plays a role (especially marked in, but not confined to, asthmatics); special treatment is required if the individual is to survive.

Recognition of these facts is absent from early textbook accounts of burns, surgery, trauma, or pulmonary disease prior to World War I.

In the preparation of this manuscript we have conducted an extensive library search in the English-language literature of pathology, surgery, and pulmonary disease from 1900 to 1960. This survey covered articles and texts. Many journal sets and a total of 27 full-length, standard textbooks of surgery, pathology, trauma, and pulmonary disease were reviewed for the years prior to 1940. Most of these made no mention whatsoever of the pulmonary component of burn injury beyond the statement that some of the patients, at death, showed evidences of pneumonia. Representative findings in those few early texts or articles that did recognize or discuss this problem are referred to appropriately below.

Analyzing this curious blank in the literature in medicine and surgery, such a blockade to growing knowledge seems traceable to three states of mind in the bioscientific community. First, there is a tyranny of words. The time-honored term *pneumonia* was invariably used to describe the familiar endemic and epidemic cause of death later proven to be pulmonary infection by pneumococcus, or streptococcus, or the virus of influenza (1918). This word dominated thinking on all forms of pulmonary disease. Second, the first etiologic sequence of Koch's postulates diverted the natural curiosity of medical thinking: if a bacterium were found in a disease process, it was assumed without further question to have been the cause thereof. The pneumonia in burns was considered as due wholly to the subsequent but inevitable microbiologic process despite the lack of the final, or proof, component of Koch's postulates. Third, advances in treatment are often required to set the stage for advances in basic understanding. In this case, patients must remain alive (often under respiratory assistance and metabolic management for several days or weeks) to show some of the fully developed pulmonary changes now regarded as characteristic of respiratory tract injury in burns. Before the advent of machine-driven respiratory assistance, arterial blood gas analyses, and segregated intensive care, the definition of this pulmonary component was unlikely.

WORLD WAR I, WAR GASES, AND INDUSTRIAL TOXICITY

By 1914 there was increasing awareness of pulmonary injury in miners and other workers in hazardous industries. The account of Glaister and Logan[1] in 1914 epitomizes the literature of this period. Inadequate chemical analyses of gas mixtures and a sparsity of autopsy material left many blanks, but choking, hemorrhage, and frothing due to pulmonary exudative edema were described. From this base, later came the knowledge of the anthracoses, pneumoconioses, silicosis, and asbestosis. This literature is not reviewed here, although some reports are pertinent to the pathology of smoke inhalation in burns. The tendency of some particles (asbestos) to cause pulmonary fibrosis and later malignant tumors has never been a feature characteristic of respiratory tract injury in burns.

During World War I (1914–18) the use of chlorine gas was introduced by the Germans at the Battle of Ypres, in 1915. Molecular chlorine (Cl_2) was released from large tanks in a favoring wind toward the Allied trenches. Its effects on those who inhaled it were acute bronchopulmonary irritation with coughing and choking, and edema fluid emitted from the mouth and nose, progressing to severe pulmonary damage and death. Fortunately, activated charcoal could be placed in an inhaling filter device so that virtually all of the chlorine was adsorbed. Thus the gas mask was developed, as used extensively by both armies, and became a sort of symbol of the horrors of trench warfare on the western front. Phosgene gas was also used, as well as mustard gas. Both of these also produced skin injury (not so evident with chlorine), but their most hazardous effects were on the lungs.

There were pathology reports at that time of the effect in the lungs of inhalation of pulmonary irritants of this type. These were the first recorded evidences of the nature of inhalation injury (see below). Many of these patients were not "burned" in the sense of thermal injury; yet the study and care of such patients has become a part of the responsibility of burn teams ever since that time, and in several recent disasters (Bhopal was an example), the pulmonary injury was treated as a "pulmonary burn."

THE COCOANUT GROVE FIRE (1942) AND WORLD WAR II

Two civilian disasters focused attention on the respiratory tract injury of fires and burns.

In 1929 a fire at the Cleveland Clinic involved the combustion of stored x-ray film. Severe and lethal pulmonary injuries were produced.

In 1942 the Cocoanut Grove fire in Boston brought about a sudden appreciation of the respiratory tract injury of burns and stimulated inquiry into its genesis and pathophysiology.

This fire occurred at a Boston nightclub of that name in late November 1942. Many patients (initially, hundreds) were examined and cared for in major teaching hospitals whose staffs had already made a wartime commitment to intensive research on the treatment of burns. The event was clearly a milestone in the pulmonary pathophysiology and care of the lung injury of burns in the western world.

Within minutes of the arrival of the first casualties at the hospitals, it was evident that the injured were affected by something other than skin burns. Many were dead on admission or died shortly after admission with no skin burns. Some of these showed the cherry pink discoloration of lips and mucous membranes which bespoke carbon monoxide poisoning; this was soon recognized and corroborated chemically. Others had no such distinguishing external sign or showed frothing from mouth and nose. Still others had a slowly progressive pulmonary lesion; once the inevitable infection had supervened, it was at first termed "pneumonia." It is to the everlasting credit of Dr. Oliver Cope and his colleagues from surgery, medicine, and pathology at the Massachusetts General Hospital that they looked beyond "pneumonia" to determine what was really going on in these lungs; the same spirit of inquiry was notable under Dr. Charles Lund at the Boston City Hospital.

All patients at the Massachusetts General Hospital had received liberal doses of morphine shortly after admission. Respirations were severely slowed, and in some instances, this was thought to be a sequella of the pulmonary injury*; periodic anal dilatation had to be used for several patients during the night to maintain respiration; morphine overdose was a possibility at this early stage. In others, there was a sort of crowing respiration and obvious evidence of difficulty in the upper airway. Direct examination of the oropharynx and the vocal cords showed what appeared to be blackening or darkening due to either direct thermal injury or inhalation of charred material. This crowing respiration soon became recognized as an urgent sign for direct laryngoscopy and early tracheostomy.

Tracheostomy was carried out in several of these patients; oxygen was administered via the tracheostomy tube, without added pressure. These tubes were then later replaced with cuffed tubes; manual or semiautomated "bag pressure" was used in many instances. The potential for fluid overload, particularly with sodium-containing fluids, was appreciated as exacerbating this pulmonary injury by increasing the extent of pulmonary edema. Suitable precautions were taken.

The description of these patients in the literature constituted the first abundant and integrated set of pathological observations, together with clinical measurements and blood chemical measurements, in the history of our knowledge of pulmonary injury in burns.†[2,3]

Four hundred ninety-one people were killed immediately or died later. One hundred eighty-one survivors and nearly 300 bodies were taken to the hospitals, although there was uncertainty as to whether some individuals were alive or dead at the time of admission. During the first 2 weeks, 39 patients died in hospitals.

Thirty of the 39 patients admitted to the Massachusetts General Hospital had extensive surface burns, and many showed evidences of damage to the respiratory tract. In some this was very severe. In some cases the pulmonary disorder developed 24 hours later. Five cases required tracheostomy, and in one or two, tracheal intubation was performed.

The antibiotic initially available was sulfadiazine, which was given initially to all patients. Penicillin in tiny amounts became available very late (2 or 3 months later) in this episode. Oxygen was given by catheter or by the use of oxygen tents. Deep venous thrombosis and pulmonary embolism were a problem in some instances.

A summarizing description of this episode was prepared by Cope,[3] who points out the prior experience on which some understanding of these pulmonary lesions could be based. "As the hours passed after the disaster, the succession of pulmonary signs in the patients recalled those encountered in the soldiers of World War I poisoned by phosgene, and were also similar to those seen in the victims of the Cleveland Clinic disaster of 1929." Cope clearly recognized the possible role of morphine in some of the early respiratory depressions seen during the first night.

> Morphine in large doses is a universal recommendation in the treatment of burns, and we employed it routinely, and without proper consideration, on the vic-

*It is a rarity for lung injury alone to cause respiratory slowing and failure; anoxia traceable to shunting or diffusion defects is usually the cause of the central nervous system (CNS) changes.

†Volume 117 of the *Annals of Surgery* (June 1943) was given over entirely to a description of the care of these burned patients at the Massachusetts General Hospital.[2]

> tims of the disaster. Each patient received 1/4 gr. immediately on entry. If this did not have a quieting effect, often a second, and occasionally a third, dose was administered. It is probable that the initial dose did not materially depress respiration but did presumably bring comfort by relieving pain. An overdose, however, was certainly given in two or three cases. Respiration ceased in one patient; she was intubated and given artificial respiration with oxygen for a period of five hours, and survived.

Carbon monoxide poisoning, assumed to be present in most patients and possibly a cause of death in several, was treated with a mixture of oxygen and 5 to 7 percent carbon dioxide.

Most of the patients who died at the hospital succumbed to the pulmonary pathology. Cope states that none showed progressive pulmonary signs in the first 12 hours. Then, "beginning twelve hours after the disaster, the clinical picture of the respiratory-tract complication assumed an ominous form. Obstruction of the bronchi and large airways menaced life. Seven patients died, all within a period of thirteen to sixty-two hours after the fire and all as a result of anoxia. No patient died after the third day."

The pathological studies of Winternitz on casualties of poison gas in World War I provided a background for the pathological reports from the Cocoanut Grove fire.[4] There was evidence of pulmonary edema and alveolar wall thickening and, in some instances, suggestive evidence of early pulmonary fibrosis. At this time, it was observed (and later extensively confirmed by other investigators) that very severe and life-threatening respiratory tract injury in burns is capable of such complete recovery that a year later there is no discernable evidence of pulmonary dysfunction. Whatever hint there was of pulmonary fibrosis in the early deaths did not eventuate in the survivors.

World War II was already 3 years along at the time of the Cocoanut Grove fire, and the Pearl Harbor attack had taken place 1 year previously. Under the stimulus of war, additional research on the pulmonary component of burn injuries, explosions, and toxic chemicals was expanded both in the United Kingdom and the United States. The hazard of fire in closed spaces posed an especial hazard in the air force and navy. At the same time the roles of smoke inhalation, carbon monoxide inhalation, and such irritants as phosgene or the mixed toxins that result from incomplete combustion of organic materials in a closed space were investigated in animal models. Apprehension of the widespread use of poison gas in World War II led to many publications at this time reviewing the World War I experience but adding little new. The *NATO Handbook* and the Merck's *Treatment of War Injuries*[5,6] clearly display the almost total ignorance of respiratory assistance and blood gas monitoring introduced less than a decade later.

PATHOLOGY OF THE LUNG INJURY TO 1960

Although the first poison gas attack took place in 1915 using chlorine, as mentioned above, it was not until 1918 that connected accounts of clinical findings, treatment, and pathology became available. These accounts, based on autopsy findings in soldiers of the Allied Armies, form the basis, repeated over and over, for most of the accounts of inhalation injury, even as late as 1958. One of the remarkable features of military history of this century is that war gases were rarely, if ever, used by either side in World War II.

The clinical changes induced by most of the war gases involved early lacrimation with coughing and a choking sensation. This went on to two rather contrasting clinical pictures: The first was of severe plethora with deep flushed cyanosis, sometimes helped by phlebotomy and evidently due to acute right heart failure. The latter is possibly traceable to obstruction of the pulmonary circulation and elevated right atrial pressure (although this was not documented). The other picture was of extreme pallor with some cyanosis, not treated effectively even with oxygen, as major airways were obstructed. These changes are well summarized in the *Atlas of Gas Poisoning* (1918)[7] and the extensive work of

Warthin and Weller (1919)[8] including for the first time extensive illustration of the evolution of vesicant lesions in the bronchopulmonary tissues both in man in experimental animals.

The pathological pictures fell into two groups. For the pulmonary irritants (phosgene and chlorine were the prototypes) pulmonary edema was noted, often very massive, and involving all of the alveolar spaces with frothy transudate in the major bronchi, larynx, and trachea, and in the mouth and nose.

If a vesicant (mustard gas and lewisite were the prototypes), the primary pathology was direct slough of the tracheal bronchial mucous membrane extending even down to the tiny bronchioles of the terminal bronchiolar tree. Pulmonary edema, again, was widespread.

None of these patients in whom an autopsy was performed had lived more than a few days after gassing. The clinical phenomenon was noted that in both chlorine and phosgene exposure, there might be a "free interval" of several hours and even up to a day before the pulmonary edema was manifest.[8] None of these patients had received prolonged oxygen treatment at high oxygen tensions. None of these writers described the findings later so characteristic of inhalation burns treated for long periods on respirators and first described in the period 1955–65. These consisted of alveolar cell hypertrophy, alveolar cell desquamation, widening of the alveolar lining membrane, hyaline membrane formation within the alveoli, and in some cases, changes of early fibrosis. These early descriptions included one article (Moorehead[9]) on smoke inhalation and several accounts of pulmonary blast injury.

During the decade immediately following World War I, there was research on "chemical pneumonia" and the relation of pathogenic bacteria to pulmonary injury caused by chemicals. Representative references are those by Wollstein and Meltzer[10] and by Koontz and Allen.[11] These workers showed that treatment of bacterial pneumonia with strong antiseptic chemicals injured the lung rather than assisted the healing process; they also showed that chemical injury was followed by bacterial infection if the animal lived long enough. The relationship between the injury and the infection seemed controversial at the time, although it seems perfectly clear now that inhalation alone could cause severe injury and a bacterial process was almost always secondary.

In 1916 Karsner and in 1917 Karsner and Ash had sounded a warning on oxygen toxicity, little heeded for another 50 years. They documented oxygen toxicity in the rabbit, the resultant pathology, and what appeared to be the dangerous threshold (about 75 percent oxygen).[12,13]

In 1919, Delafield and Prudden published a textbook of pathology in which they classified pulmonary injury as including "inspiration of smoke and flame" as distinct from inhalation of irritating gases such as those used in the war.[14] This text is remarkable in including a further reference to oxygen toxicity based largely on Karsner's work.

> The inhalation of atmospheres rich in oxygen incites, in twenty-four to forty-eight hours, congestion and edema of the lungs with desquamation of the alveolar epithelium, fibrinous exudate into the alveoli, and, finally, a fibrinous pneumonia.

Pulmonary contusion, blast injury of the airways, and pulmonary damage from fractured ribs and pneumothorax were occasionally lumped together with other traumatic forms of pulmonary injury and thus found their way into textbooks on trauma and burns.

The Cleveland Clinic fire occurred on May 15, 1929. The disaster consisted largely in combustion of a large store of x-ray film and the permeation of the volatile products through several floors of the building. The clinical findings were discussed in several publications. Nichols (1930)[15] discusses the pulmonary effect of the inhalation of nitrogen dioxide, assumed to be the major toxic gas arising from the combustion of x-ray film. This was considered to be the major cause of injury and death. Doub (1933)[16] further describes the x-ray changes seen.

In 1930 Pack and Davis published a monograph on burns in which "autointoxication" (producing minute capillary thrombosis in many organs) was considered to be the agent that produced damage in the lungs as well as the nervous system and kidneys, after skin burns.[17] In this text the authors include war gas injury as part of the pathology of "burns" and refer to them as pulmonary burns. The illustrations of cutaneous and pulmonary pathology from mustard gas and inhalation injury rank this publication as a conscientious summary of the World War I experience, published approximately a decade after the initial reports.

By 1934, Bell, in his *Text-Book of Pathology,* clearly recognized that the term *pneumonia* was inadequate to describe the various pulmonary changes seen in trauma of many types, most particularly burns. He pointed out that severe trauma to any part of the body may be followed by pulmonary disease and consolidation. He emphasized the importance of aspiration of gastric contents.[18]

The pathology described in the postmortem cases from the Cocoanut Grove fire was a mixture of early acute upper respiratory tract damage involving desquamation of tracheobronchial epithelium and replacement by a hyaline membrane on the trachea and large bronchi. There was evidence of pulmonary edema in many cases, occlusion of small bronchioles, and early superimposed infection.

The changes that have come to be regarded as so characteristic of pulmonary burns 25 years later were not described. These included hyaline membrane within the alveoli, widening of the interalveolar septum, and enlargement and desquamation of alveolar lining cells. In retrospect, it appears that prolongation of life with effective respiratory assistance and the control of early superimposed infection by antibiotics to be developed during the next decade were essential preliminaries to the observation of these changes.

The x-ray changes in the Cocoanut Grove patients were particularly remarkable, and in this series of burn patients, early and repeated x-rays were taken of each patient, a preview of critical care unit roentgen management to become current 20 years later. These x-rays were interpreted as showing alternating areas of atelectasis and emphysema, and indeed the pathology at post mortem in some cases did show considerable emphysema due to trapped gas beyond occluded bronchi.[2]

Harkins, in his 1942 textbook on the treatment of burns, does not segregate pulmonary injury in burned patients in whom inhalation has played a major role in the initial event.[19] However, Harkins's book is remarkable in being one of the first to advance a semiquantitative formula for the treatment of burned patients based on changes in the hemoglobin and the blood volume. He also clearly recognized that overtreatment with fluids would exacerbate any pulmonary injury present and wrote, "In few instances is it necessary to give much plasma beyond the second day, as the danger of shock has then become less than the likelihood of pneumonia, which may be aggravated by any possible therapeutically induced pulmonary edema."

Donaldson, in a 1947 textbook on surgery of the chest,[20] clearly emphasized the importance of blast injury and inhalation injury, referring to military service in both world wars as furnishing a prototype for these injuries. No comment was made on pulmonary lesions peculiar to skin burns without direct inhalation or of the Cocoanut Grove experience.

The work of John Moritz was of remarkable interest during World War II and was described briefly in the National Research Council (NRC) symposium on burns conducted in 1950.[21] Moritz was interested in the variable pathology of the inhalation of hot gases, the inhalation of actual flame, and the inhalation of steam.

He showed, in an elegant series of experiments in dogs, that with inhalation of open flame the necrotizing injury is almost confined to the upper respiratory tract. The larynx and vocal cords are charred, but there is frequently no injury below this, suggesting that closure of the glottis and vocal cords is an immediate and effective protective response. He showed, by contrast, that with inhalation of steam, the injury extends to the full anatomic extent of the airway, down to the terminal bronchioles and alveoli. The heat of condensation of the steam is responsible for a widespread and quickly lethal burn of the total pulmonary parenchyma.

Representative texts on pathology in the middle 1950s are those by Karsner[22] and Herbut.[23] Neither of these refers either to inhalation pulmonary injury or to the experience at the Cocoanut Grove almost 10 years before. Indeed, failure to recognize the pulmonary component of large conflagrations and/or extensive skin burns remains notable as late as 1957. In the text by Artz and Reiss (1957)[24] there is only a brief discussion of respiratory tract injury, but no mention of the pathology or the toxicology experience of the Cleveland Clinic or Cocoanut Grove fires. Tracheostomy is recommended, but no mention is made of blood gas analyses or respiratory assistance devices.

Before 1960, the pulmonary injury of burns is notably absent from the literature on burns and from textbooks on surgery, pathology, and pulmonary disease. Although by that time there was a small literature (as reviewed briefly above), there was a rapidly widening clinical experience with the pulmonary component of burns. By 1950, it was frequently stated in clinical teaching and in symposia that pulmonary complications were among the most common causes of death in burns after the first 96 hours. This common teaching was slow to enter published textbooks.

PATHOPHYSIOLOGY AND THEORIES OF CAUSATION

Various theories were advanced as to the cause of the airway injury in burns.

Direct airway injury was evoked for such things as smoke, phosgene, chlorine, and steam. Bloodstream passage of toxic gases from the lung, without direct lung damage, was most obvious in the case of carbon monoxide but might have played a role in other injuries and systemic responses. Ether and nitrous oxide anesthesia bore ancient witness to the effectiveness of the alveolar membrane as a route for drugs and toxins to the bloodstream without pulmonary injury.

Although knowledge of asbestos injury lay far in the future, there was concern about the role of particle size and shape in the respiratory injury of smoke inhalation. Were persons who died of "smoke inhalation" actually dying of suffocation in an atmosphere where the respiratory gas mixture was taken up with combustion products and carbon dioxide? Or were small amounts of smoke very irritating to the lungs because of the chemistry or particle size of the ash? Although no single categorical answer was ever given, it is clear that both components played a role in early death from smoke inhalation.

Thus, by 1945, the nature of the respiratory tract spectrum in the inhalation injury of burns (or as a result of pulmonary complication of burns without evident inhalation injury) was becoming defined even though rarely covered in standard textbooks. Certainly burn units throughout the western world became sensitive to this problem; fluid overloads were reevaluated and avoided whenever possible because of their contribution to increased pulmonary edema. Early physical examination of burned patients now came to include both direct and indirect examination of the airway and early and continuing study of arterial blood gases.

The role of the bloodstream was also emphasized as a source of lung injury by pulmonary artery passage to the lung capillary and parenchyma of products from the burn or venous thrombi. Some years previously Churchill, a pioneer in pulmonary and thoracic surgery, had described the three clinical categories of pulmonary embolization. His observations were based on elegant experiments in the dog, confirmed and corroborated by clinical observation.[25,26] He described the clinical and metabolic differences between multiple small emboli, a few mid-sized emboli, and massive occlusive pulmonary embolization. While the latter picture has been associated for some centuries with sudden death due to a huge snakelike embolus occupying the pulmonary artery, the first picture with its gradual change in blood gases and a gradual occlusion of pulmonary circulation (producing what was later to be called a ventilation/perfusion imbalance) was not so well understood. Nor was the picture of multiple mid-sized emboli with changes in respiratory and pulse rate even though, in the absence of continuation of the process, there were few deleterious results. The greatest importance of this picture lay in its anticipation of things to come; evidences of small emboli were later found to precede massive embolization in many cases and became an indication either for venous ligation or anticoagulant therapy.

These concepts were now transferred to the study of burned patients. Deep venous thrombosis was a frequent observation in burns. Superficial femoral vein ligation was sometimes carried out to prevent pulmonary embolus especially in patients where anticoagulants were contraindicated.[27] Although the use of the leg veins for infusion or sampling sites played a clear etiologic role, it was to be several years before most burn units began assiduously to avoid leg vein manipulation because of the hazard of embolization.

Gastric aspiration was a hazard to the lungs if food and fluids were forced by mouth before the gastrointestinal tract was ready for them. The development of a Curling's ulcer could, later on, threaten obstruction, vomiting, and gastric aspiration.

Other components coming from the burn that might damage the lung included fat embolism. While presumably rare in a florid form, there was the suspicion that some degree of fat liquefaction, capillary passage, and pulmonary embolization might occur beneath severe skin burns and that fat embolism might be more important than was generally realized.

Of other substances originating in the burn that might damage the circulation of the lung, endotoxin occupied an increasingly important role in the view of many workers and is still regarded as an important factor in many burned patients. A growing interest in the systemic effects of endotoxin from trauma and burns resulted from the work particularly of Fine et al., who demonstrated in dogs that all of the clinical and circulatory dynamic changes of hemorrhagic shock could be produced by the injection of endotoxin.[28] This concept originating about 1940 was easily transferred into the burn field as it became understood that coliform infection with gram-negative bacteremia was a terminal event in many severe surface burns with early and late pulmonary changes appropriate to that sequence of events. One of the important observations of Fine et al. was that endotoxemia could produce widespread cardiovascular and pulmonary changes without a positive blood culture for coliform bacteria. This determination depended in turn on a precise assay for endotoxin in the blood; the use of the *Limulus* assay was begun at that time and still plays a role in endotoxin studies. It was demonstrated in several burned patients that endotoxemia was indeed a component of their systemic deterioration and of the pulmonary change that accompanied it.

1950–60: BLOOD GASES, DEMAND RESPIRATORS, INTENSIVE CARE, AND OXYGEN TOXICITY

During the years 1950–60, knowledge in this field began to mature and assume its modern shape. Arterial blood gas analyses (oxygen, carbon dioxide, and pH) moved from a research rarity to clinical availability, even if not yet routine, in larger urban or teaching hospitals. This was soon followed by their availability in larger community referral centers. Such samples had to be obtained expertly, under oil, the samples quickly refrigerated, and the analyses carried out within minutes. The ready availability of blood gas analysis was increased by the use of indwelling arterial lines for simultaneous cathode ray tube (CRT) display of pressures and arterial pulse contours. By 1965 these methods were widely available and, by 1970–75, were becoming miniaturized, technically simplified, computerized, and the subject of much wider understanding by those recently graduated from medical school, if not by the older generation.

The period 1950–60 was also marked by the development of critical care units or "intensive care units." In many instances, as in the case of the Bartlett Unit (established at the Peter Bent Brigham Hospital in 1954), these units were a direct outgrowth of the need to segregate the care of certain patients. These early intensive care units were often centered around two sets of problems: respiratory compromise and severe burns; the two often went together. These units were also based on the easy availability of assisted ventilation using demand-triggered and gas-operated equipment independent of the electrical supply. By 1975 it was estimated that future hospital construction would increasingly move simpler patients to a motel or outpatient setting, and might comprise as many as 35 to 65 percent "critical care" beds in the main unit. The early care of the critically burned patient lay at the genesis of this change in management and architecture of the modern hospital.

By the middle 1960s a stable routine of arterial monitoring, frequent blood gas sampling, daily x-rays, and endotracheal intubation was routine for serious burns that involved airway injury of whatever sort. The availability of demand-triggered assisted ventilation using positive pressures with a cuffed endotracheal tube introduced the phenomenon of patients on positive pressure–assisted ventilation at high oxygen tensions, high pressures, and high flows for very prolonged periods of time. By the late 1960s it was evident that this might have adverse effects due in part to upper airway invasion, drying, and oxygen toxicity. Oxygen toxicity had often been a by-product of efforts to oxygenate individuals whose hypoxemia was insensitive to modest increases in inhaled oxygen tension, later appreciated as due to venoarterial shunting (see below). Work done in several centers showed that animals exposed to high oxygen tensions for prolonged periods of time would develop severe pulmonary injury and death. It was evident that in human beings this was a risk that could not be afforded even though the human threshold for damage was ill-defined.

During this period tracheostomy had been replaced by endotracheal intubation ideally by the nasal route, alternatively by an oral tube. Using pressure cuffs on the tubes it was possible to close the airway to control respiration completely. Many mistakes were made at this time by inexperienced attendants dealing with totally controlled mechanical ventilation. Overventilation was commonplace, with the production of severe hypocarbia (PCO_2 values as low as 8 to 10 mmHg) and very severe acute respiratory alkalosis with irritability, convulsions, and in some cases lethal cardiac arrhythmias. This was due to faulty setting of the apparatus and inadequate blood gas monitoring. Overinflation of endotracheal tube balloons produced damage to the trachea and its cartilaginous rings requiring subsequent repair.[29] As these faults were corrected, expertise in total respiratory control spread to other clinical areas; in degenerative neurologic diseases intubation with total control was maintained for 1 or 2 months with complete respiratory rehabilitation. The body-vacuum "iron lung" of Drinker, a standard lifesaving item in hospitals as late as the polio epidemics of 1954 and 1955, was now a dusty object in the back hall or the museum save for those very particular cases in which intubation was inadvisable and a Drinker respirator (or its cuirass modification) was used.

By 1965 controlled pressure/flow/volume respirators (Engstrom type) had largely replaced the old pulsed high-pressure demand type (Bird).

VENOARTERIAL ADMIXTURE OR PULMONARY SHUNTING

The years after 1960 saw another major turning point in the understanding and management of respiratory tract injury in burns. Venoarterial shunting and ventilation/perfusion disorders emerged as prominent features of the disordered physiology of burns during that period, not only because of the close monitoring mentioned above but also based on increasingly sophisticated physiologic work in pulmonary blood flow and ventilation/perfusion anomalies using isotopic methods. The work of West was of great significance in demonstrating that variations in pulmonary vascular resistance and anomalous distribution of blood flow relative to ventilation could produce remarkable changes in blood gas chemistry with little or no bronchoalveolar pathology.[30,31] As a result of West's work the pulmonary circulation came into its own as a factor in the pathophysiologic sequence after lung injury.

Prior to this time inadequate arterial oxygenation had been considered as due to inadequate diffusion of oxygen across the alveolar membrane and had been treated by the administration of very high concentrations of oxygen. It gradually became evident that there were some patients in which this was not only ineffective but injurious. Arterial anoxemia refractory to high oxygen tensions (the latter often damaging to the respiratory epithelium) was the telltale clinical sign of shunting. This term was used to denote the passage of desaturated venous blood across a nonventilated pulmonary segment, admixing venous blood with oxygenated blood in the pulmonary outflow to the left atrium, thus lowering the mixed arterial PO_2 and saturation in aortic outflow and peripheral arteries. This could occur with only a minor pathologic change in the lung tissue itself.

At that time a classic experiment demonstrated the meaning of venoarterial shunting as a source of anoxemia in the absence of bronchoalveolar (airway) pathology. In this experiment, a dog is ventilated with a branched (Carlins) endotracheal tube. After a time of stabilization one branch of the tube is occluded so that one lung, though normal, is perfused but not ventilated. The arterial oxygen tension, saturation, and content then fall. That lung is then surgically removed, a step intuitively expected to diminish arterial oxygenation. With no other change, the animal's arterial oxygen tension rises immediately to its previous normal high levels. This is merely a spectacular demonstration of the fact that when a large area of functioning pulmonary tissue is perfused but not ventilated and the unsaturated right-heart blood of the pulmonary artery is shunted across unventilated lung to pulmonary veins and the left heart, arterial oxygen tension falls. This does not require the opening up of any new circulatory channels, anatomic blood vessels, or "shunts"; it requires no airway pathology; and it is not dependent on low oxygen tension at the tracheal level. Such anoxemia is of course refractory to increased oxygen tensions in the airway. Not only was venoarterial admixture a cause of deterioration per se but it often led to prolonged use of high airway oxygen tensions, in themselves hazardous to the lung. Shunting can only be rectified by ventilating the offending segments, to be achieved by addressing the specific problem, be it alveolar edema, atelectases, or airway obstruction.

Surgeons carrying out pulmonary extirpative surgery had previously recorded their observation that when one lung that had contained certain types of pathology (collapse, alveolar edema, bronchial obstruction) was removed, arterial oxygenation was restored to normal, rather than being reduced as one might have suspected through loss of pulmonary tissue.

Clearly all these phenomena were related and were often observed in the lungs of burned patients. The passage of venous blood from the right heart across the lungs to the left heart without suitable ventilation would produce venoarterial admixture, a decline in oxygen saturation, and cyanosis. Raising the oxygen content of inspired gas mixture had very little effect. In later stages there was loss of consciousness or death, even though ventilation appeared to be normal, and the added oxygen in the ventilatory mixture had been maintained for many days.

Improved understanding of the pathophysiology of pulmonary ventilation and perfusion and the bedside estimate of their relation added immensely to the security of the burned patient in critical care units. Excessive prolonged oxygen administration was avoided. Efforts to improve ventilation by positive pressure or diminish edema by diuretics and to remove obstruction by bronchoscopy or lavage were often more effective than the prolonged use of 100 percent oxygen, obviously dangerous. Even in smaller hospitals far from the teaching center, the simplistic diagnosis of "pneumonia" for any burn patient who died with pulmonary insufficiency was being replaced by a terminology that included consideration of ventilation/perfusion ratios and venoarterial shunting.

In encircling thoracic burns, escharotomy was increasingly used to release the constricting ventilatory defect. The long-standing, still-smoldering controversy over the use of colloid versus crystalloid solutions in early treatment was resolved by common sense in most units; colloid was used to maintain circulatory blood volume when fluid loss was far advanced, while crystalloid was used to meet early requirements and maintain body water later on. Endotracheal intubation became widely preferred over tracheostomy for many reasons, especially sepsis and problems of closure and/or removal. The use of humidifiers in the ventilatory circuit decreased the insensible water loss and drying of respiratory tract secretions and membranes.

1965–75: PTPI, ARDS, SURFACTANT, HYALINE MEMBRANE, LUNG WATER, AND IMMUNE DAMAGE

The prolonged use of assisted respiration in patients who later died enabled the pathologist to observe the lungs after many days of progressive pulmonary injury. These changes were first observed in detail in the pulmonary injury of burns and included the description of the presence of hyaline membrane (reminiscent of respiratory distress and oxygen toxicity in the newborn), alveolar cell hypertrophy and desquamation, septal widening with interstitial edema, occasional evidence of early fibrosis, and a number of other changes.

The description of a surface-active alveolar secretion, surfactant[32,33] as an important factor in the maintenance of the patency of alveoli was quickly followed by demonstration of its relative absence from the lung of many burned patients. These changes were not confined to burns but could be seen in other forms of trauma and acquired the clinical term *posttraumatic pulmonary insufficiency* (PTPI). Because hyaline membrane was seen in these lungs this was also called adult respiratory distress syndrome (ARDS), a term derived from the syndrome observed in premature infants, especially those treated with high oxygen tension, in which hyaline membrane and surfactant reduction are prominent.

Initially there was the suspicion that this lesion resulted from the prolonged assisted respiration itself or from oxygen toxicity alone. Many patients were removed from respiratory assistance devices for fear of development of this syndrome, when in fact the entire clinicopathologic complex can be produced by the injury itself; if respiratory assistance is given at low oxygen tensions, and with reasonable pressures, the lesion is totally recoverable.

Several burn units at this time again demonstrated what common knowledge had held for several years, that while this pulmonary burn injury (whether or not due to inhalation) could be potentially fatal, total recovery was possible, and certain therapeutic errors made it much worse. These errors included fluid overload, multiple shifting antibiotics (leading to fungus disease, *Serratia,* and *Pseudomonas* infection), oxygen toxicity, careless tracheal toilet, airway contamination by careless nursing, ankle-vein infusion, and premature feeding (with gastric aspiration).

In a book published in 1969, Moore et al. described posttraumatic pulmonary insufficiency as seen in a variety of patients, none of them with severe burns.[34] In this monograph, the phenomenon of venoarterial admixture with anomalous low arterial oxygen tensions totally refractory to increases of the inhaled oxygen tension was clearly described and in the form so often observed in burns. Calculation of shunt fraction from physiologic data was described, as well as the effect of mixed venous oxygen tension and cardiac output on the calculated shunt fraction at a constant arterial oxygen tension. Photomicrographs from these patients clearly showed hyaline membrane, the proliferation of alveolar lining cells, interstitial edema, early fibrosis, and focal hemorrhage. Although none of the patients whose care is detailed in Moore's monograph was admitted to the intensive care unit because of burn, the changes observed and the physiologic and chemical observations made, were characteristic of severe burns, with or without inhalation of noxious gases. This point is emphasized, since in the unburned patients described in this monograph inhalation of noxious substances was never identified as a possible pathogenic mechanism. Surfactant assays were made in some cases by A. P. Morgan, and an attempt was made to relate pulmonary pathology to alterations in surface active materials in the lung, pursuant to the work of Avery.

There was an interesting analogy with posttraumatic renal insufficiency. The disorder of the renal parenchyma associated with severe injury, shock, and renal hemoglobinopathies of various types, while potentially fatal, could recover so that a year or two later no detectable abnormality of renal function remained. The same thing was now shown to be true with the lung: some burned patients with extremely severe pulmonary injury who had been in coma or on assisted respiration for many weeks were found, a year or so later, to have perfectly normal pulmonary function. By contrast, local chemical injury (e.g., certain types of industrial smoke inhalation) can lead to a very disabling chronic bronchiolitis obliterans. During the period 1965–75, as a result of this improved understanding, there was greatly improved management based on integration of all the findings and concepts mentioned in the foregoing paragraphs. With severe pulmonary injury in burns, recovery was now much more frequent.

The source of the hyaline membrane lining the alveoli remained unclear. If a protein-containing fluid is dried by evaporation, a protein crust or membrane is left behind. Two questions were unresolved regarding the hyaline membrane observed in the lungs of patients who died after prolonged ventilatory support. First was this question of whether the membrane observed was merely due to the evaporative effect of mechanical ventilation on protein-rich alveolar transudate or, alternatively, whether it was a secretory or exudative anomaly. Second was the question of whether the membrane (often only 1 to 2 μm in thickness) impaired oxygen diffusion. Although both questions remain moot, I believe that in most cases evidence favors the membrane as an evaporative protein residue providing only minor impairment to oxygen diffusion. Alveolar lining cell desquamation is a much more severe impairment to alveolar function as it denotes surfactant loss. Alveolar cell hypertrophy and desquamation appear to be direct evidence of pulmonary injury. While complete healing is possible, such alveolar wall disintegration is clearly adverse to pulmonary function.

The use of antibiotics played a double role here as it did in so many other aspects of surgical care during the middle years of this century. Although an infectious process often follows the initial injury, pulmonary injury in burns could not be prevented or treated by antibiotics alone, since it is not of bacterial or viral etiology. Antibiotics were often overused for the early pulmonary lesion during this period. At the same time, it was clear that, properly used, antibiotics could be of immense benefit. The constant changing of antibiotic dosage schedules and drug selection on the basis of random laboratory-tested bacterial sensitivities often led to the overgrowth of fungi and the production in the lung of opportunistic infections with organisms of otherwise low virulence. Again, improvement came through a much more restrained and intelligent use of antibiotics. Based only on my own experiences as a visitor to many burn units at that time, I would estimate that antibiotics were being used with much greater wisdom and restraint by 1975 to 1980. Ironically, it is often the infectious disease consultant unfamiliar with burn microbiology who pushes antibiotic overuse with its attendant hazard of immunosuppression, floral conversion, and fungus superinfection.

The role of fresh blood transfusion acquired importance in this era. It had been clearly appreciated as long ago as 1935 to 1940 that fluid overload would make the pulmonary injury in burns much worse. It became evident in the 1960s and 1970s that blood transfusion might play a deleterious role, particularly if this blood was exposed to a blood-gas interface prior to infusion. It was also shown at this time that very fresh blood would be injurious to the lung, and there was some suggestion that this was a graft-versus-host reaction, the lymphocytes and other immunologically competent cells of the blood being exposed to foreign tissue antigens in the lung on their first circulation from the right heart. The extent to which these transfusion-induced components of pulmonary injury were clinically important was never clear. Certainly in the last 10 years, with the decline in the use of fresh blood, these components may have become unimportant, far surpassed by the hazards of human immunodeficiency virus (HIV) infection or other transfusion-borne contamination. Recent evidence corroborates a component of immune damage to the lung as based on sequestration or margination of leukocytes in the lung; deposition of activated neutrophils in the lung, arising from the patient's own immune apparatus, has emerged as an etiologic factor in posttraumatic pulmonary insufficiency.[35]

Infusions into the ankle veins or other tributaries of the saphenous and femoral systems, indwelling arterial monitoring lines in the femoral artery, and repeated femoral venesection for blood sampling have all been avoided in recent years. It became appreciated that these were an invitation to deep venous thrombosis and pulmonary embolism; septic thrombophlebitis of the saphenous system from contaminated infusion sites could become a focus for potentially fatal generalized sepsis.

The nutritional component of burn care was far better managed after 1970 as substrates for protein synthesis were given orally or by vein, particularly pure (crystalline) amino acids. But the unbridled enthusiasm of the nutritionist could also overload the circulation or force-feed burned patients to the point of gastric overloading, vomiting, and aspiration. Like the infectious-disease consultant with a single-minded concern for antibiotics, or the respiratory consultant who wants to push pressure and oxygen, the nutritionist can also be hazardous in thinking only of nitrogen intake.

There is no place in burn care for unbridled zeal in any one direction. It is always the job of the surgeon in charge of the patient to hold in check these sometimes hazardous enthusiasts and zealots and maintain balance among the recommendations of narrow specialists. A few days off all antibiotics may clear the air for diagnosis and the patient's own immune process, diuresis may be worth its weight in oxygen, and the human frame does beautifully for several days on no nitrogen intake whatsoever. Moderation in all things serves burned patients very well, especially their lungs. In my opinion a severe burn is among the most complex of human illnesses or injuries and is very demanding of the broadest kind of clinical wisdom in its management.

Clear differentiation between low pressure and high pressure pulmonary edema was helpful as a guide to treatment. In low-pressure edema the cardiac chamber pressure and pulmonary capillary pressures are normal; irritative transudate of fluid and inflammatory exudate are examples. Such measures as diuresis and antibiotics may be most effective. In some cases prolonged end-expiratory pressure (PEEP) is useful. In high-pressure pulmonary edema, cardiac decompensation with elevated chamber and capillary pressures, in some form, are the causative sequence. Fluid restriction, digitalis, and other inotropic agents, or vasoactive drugs such as dopamine may be helpful.

In either case, the quantification of the extent of pulmonary overhydration could now be estimated chemically by isotope or tracer dilution methods or thermal dilution, applying compositional formulation to a first-pass cardiac output curve. Useful as a research tool, these "lung water" measurements provided a guide to treatment and a monitor of results.[36]

SUMMARY

This history of a 70-year period (approximately 1910–80) constitutes a brief sketch of the background of recent understanding of the respiratory tract injury in burns. The remainder of this book is devoted to a description of current diagnosis and management.

Of special interest in this history are one constraining concept and one remarkable event. The constraining concept was the use of the term "pneumonia" as a diagnostic catch-all for any pulmonary process in an injured patient. Still today, otherwise sophisticated physicians and surgeons will use this term for lung injury even though it fails completely to describe the pathologic process involved and its use blinds the physician or surgeon to the need for more discriminating diagnosis and treatment.

The remarkable event was the nightclub fire in Boston about 1 year after Pearl Harbor and with 3 years of war still ahead that opened new lines of both research and management in the respiratory tract injury of burns under the leadership of Dr. Oliver Cope.

ACKNOWLEDGEMENTS

The author is indebted to Dr. Robert Demling, Dr. Philip Drinker, Dr. Vladimir Fencl, Dr. Francis D. Moore, Jr., and Dr. Leroy Vandam for many helpful suggestions.

REFERENCES

1. Glaister J, Logan DD: *Gas Poisoning in Mining and Other Industries*. New York, William Wood, 1914.
2. Management of the Cocoanut Grove burns at the Massachusetts General Hospital. *Ann Surg*. 117:801, 1943.
3. Cope O: Care of the victims of the Cocoanut Grove fire at the Massachusetts General Hospital. *N Engl J Med* 229:138, 1943.
4. Winternitz MC: *Pathology of War Gas Poisoning*. Princeton, NJ: Yale University Press, 1920.
5. *Emergency War Surgery: US Armed Forces Issue of NATO Handbook Prepared for Use by the Medical Services of NATO Nations*. US Department of Defense. US Government Printing Office, Washington, D.C., 1958.
6. *Treatment of War Injuries*. Rahway, NJ, Merck, November 1941.
7. *An Atlas of Gas Poisoning*. Medical Research Committee. Provided for the American Expeditionary Force by the American Red Cross. 1918.
8. Warthin AS, Weller CV: *The Medical Aspects of Mustard Gas Poisoning*. St. Louis, Mosby, 1919.
9. Moorehead JJ: *Clinical Traumatic Surgery*. Philadelphia, Saunders, 1945.
10. Wollstein M, Meltzer SJ: Experimental chemical pneumonia. *J Exp Med* 28:547, 1918.
11. Koontz AR, Allen MS: On the relation of bacteria to so-called "chemical pneumonia." *J Exp Med* 50:67, 1929.
12. Karsner HT: The pathological effects of atmospheres rich in oxygen. *J Exp Med* 23:149, 1916.
13. Karsner HT, Ash JE: A further study of the pathological effects of atmospheres rich in oxygen. *J Lab Clin Med* 2:259, 1917.
14. Delafield F, Prudden TM: *A Text-Book of Pathology,* 11th ed. New York, William Wood, 1919.
15. Nichols BH: The clinical effects of the inhalation of nitrogen dioxide. *AJR* 23:516, 1930.
16. Doub HP: Pulmonary changes from inhalation of noxious gases. *Radiology* 21:105, 1933.
17. Pack GT, Davis AH: *Burns: Types, Pathology, and Management*. Philadelphia, Lippincott, 1930.
18. Bell ET: *A Text-Book of Pathology,* 2d ed. Philadelphia, Lea & Febiger, 1934.
19. Harkins HN: *The Treatment of Burns*. Springfield, Ill., Thomas, 1942.
20. Donaldson JK: *Surgical Disorders of the Chest: Diagnosis and Treatment,* 2d ed. Philadelphia, Lea & Febiger, 1947.
21. Moritz AR: Pulmonary Injury — Experimental, in National Academy of Sciences, National Research Council: Symposium on Burns, Washington, D.C., 1951, p 86.
22. Karsner HR: *Human Pathology,* 8th ed. Philadelphia, Lippincott, 1955.
23. Herbut PA: *Surgical Pathology,* 2d ed. Philadelphia, Lea & Febiger, 1954.
24. Artz CP, Reiss E: *The Treatment of Burns*. Philadelphia, Saunders, 1957.
25. Churchill ED, Gibbon JH, Hopkinson M: Changes in the circulation produced by gradual occlusion of the pulmonary artery. *J Clin Invest,* 11:543, 1932.
26. Churchill ED: Mechanism of death in massive pulmonary embolism. *Surg Gynecol Obstet* 59:513, 1934.
27. Moore FD: A note on the thrombophlebitis encountered: Management of the Cocoanut Grove burns at the Massachusetts General Hospital. *Ann Surg* 117:931, 1943.
28. Fine J, Frank ED, Ravin HA, Rutenberg SH, Schweinburg FB: The bacterial factor in traumatic shock. *N Engl J Med* 260:214, 1959.
29. Grillo HC: Circumferential resection and reconstruction of the mediastinal and cervical trachea. *Ann Surg* 162:374, 1965.
30. West JB: Topographical distribution of blood flow in the lung, in Field J (ed): *Handbook of Physiology,* Section 3: *Respiration*. Washington, D.C., Americal Physiological Society, 1965, vol 2, p 1437.
31. West JB: Aspects of the pulmonary microcirculaton, in Shepro D, Fulton GP (eds): *Microcirculation as Related to Shock*. New York, Academic Press, 1968, p 23.
32. Avery ME: *The Lung and its Disorders in the Newborn Infant, Major Problems in Clinical Pediatrics,* vol 1. Philadelphia, Saunders 1964.
33. Avery ME, Said S: Surface phenomena in lungs in health and disease. *Medicine* (Baltimore) 44:503, 1965.
34. Moore FD, Lyons JH, Pierce EC, et al: *Post-Traumatic Pulmonary Insufficiency: Pathophysiology of Respiratory Failure and Principles of Respiratory Care after Surgical Operations, Trauma, Hemorrhage, Burns, and Shock*. Philadelphia, Saunders, 1969.
35. Dodeck P, Thommasen HV, Russell JA, et al: Neutrophil margination in the lung in adult respiratory distress syndrome. *J Crit Care* 3:172, 1988.
36. Clark WR, Neiman GF, Goyette D, Gryzboski D: Effects of crystalloid on lung fluid balance after smoke inhalation. *Ann Surg* 208:56, 1988.

Chapter 2

Diagnosis, Impact, and Classification of Inhalation Injury

Edward F. Haponik
Andrew M. Munster

Respiratory problems caused by smoke inhalation and cutaneous burns have been well recognized to have a high morbidity and mortality. As noted in Chap. 1, the ominous effects of these problems have been underscored through careful documentation of experiences from mass disasters, numerous case reports, clinicopathologic correlations, and probit analyses of large populations cared for at burn centers.[1–25] The adverse impact of inhalation injury has not been limited to excess mortality alone; the prolonged exposure to the hospital environment itself predisposes the patient to additional hazards and a spectrum of nosocomial problems. There is little quantitative information about many aspects of the acute hospitalization, convalescence, and social recovery of individuals with inhalation injury, but the personal tragedies of these devastating injuries to patients and their families are immeasurable. Other, yet-unappreciated effects of inhalation injury undoubtedly occur. The extension of hospital stay by a mean of approximately 2 weeks or more, together with intensive and costly technologic resources for patient care, imposes major financial burdens upon individual patients, medical institutions, and society at large.[26–29] Estimates of costs of this care have recently exceeded $300 million, and thus far these costs are funded incompletely by prospective payment programs; none of the five current diagnostic related groups concerned with burns addresses inhalation injury, despite widespread acknowledgments of its importance. The failure to equitably distribute resources according to the severity of illness effectively penalizes those referral institutions providing care to the most critically ill patients.

Recent correlative basic science and clinical investigations of respiratory and cutaneous injuries have resulted in improved understanding of each of these problems, their interactions, and the evolution of technologic tools used to detect and treat them.[28–58] Extensive efforts to design appropriate models of the multifactorial injuries encountered in patients have provided unprecedented insights into the mechanisms of injury. Despite some limitations of these experimental models, there is optimism that future clinically relevant therapeutic innovations will follow. At present, however, although effective fluid resuscitation and application of topical antimicrobial therapy have lowered mortality due to burn shock and wound infection, the respiratory problems that develop in this clinical setting have remained, for the most part, unresolved and are leading causes of death.[59]

The mortality attributed to fire-related inhalation injury has ranged from 30 to 90 percent, depending upon the patient populations analyzed and the characteristics of the reporting center.[9] The frequencies cited for inhalation injury are typically higher in urban institutions (20 to 35 percent) compared with those in more rural communities (10 to 15 percent). Clinical impressions of more hazardous fire environments in which combinations of increasingly toxic inhalants are generated may account for apparent increases in the frequency of inhalation injury during recent years. In addition, however, the enhanced awareness of smoke inhalation among both health care workers and lay persons, the increased availability and application of objective diagnostic tests, and the greater sensitivity of these tools in the detection of earlier, more subtle manifestations of respiratory dysfunction have been contributing factors. As in other clinical situations, reporting biases have tended to skew objective information toward those patients with the more severe respiratory injuries. Surprisingly little is known about the respiratory effects of mild, transient smoke inhalation, burns, and their combinations.

In this chapter we shall provide an overview of the respiratory complications associated with smoke inhalation and burns. Details about the pathogenesis, diagnosis, and management of these problems will be presented subsequently. For the practitioner who is responsible for the highly individualized care of these catastrophically ill patients, a practically oriented system for classification of these complex injuries is essential. Not surprisingly, the principles which underlie timely, systematic diagnosis and therapy are based upon a thorough general understanding of the interaction of smoke inhalation and burns and their impact in the diverse situations in which they are encountered.

DIAGNOSIS OF BURN-RELATED RESPIRATORY PROBLEMS

The popular collective term *inhalation injury* encompasses a broad spectrum of respiratory problems which have diverse clinical, physiologic, and pathologic manifestations.[9] Despite the absence of any universally accepted and applied criteria for the diagnosis of inhalation injury, this term powerfully communicates the high acuity of illness, the setting in which it evolves, and its ominous prognosis. As noted by Clark et al., the terms *smoke inhalation* and *inhalation injury* are often used interchangeably in reference to smoke-induced injury to the proximal airway and/or pulmonary parenchyma that is "severe enough to result in detectable clinical consequences which are significant for the individual."[22–24] Use of the term in reports of extensive clinical experiences has led to the general appreciation that patients with respiratory injury will have poorer outcomes than those without, will require far more extensive clinical and technologic resources during the management of their more complex courses, and will require unique skills for the timely diagnosis and therapy of a number of complications to which they are exceedingly vulnerable. Furthermore, the presence of inhalation injury will influence the primary surgical management of the patient significantly.[60,61]

Definitions of Inhalation Injury

Although *inhalation injury* effectively conveys qualitative messages, is generally used, and for lack of a better alternative will be retained in this volume, the term remains unsatisfactory because of a number of limitations. Just as the historic, "generic" classification of catastrophic respiratory injuries as "pneumonia" is insufficient for current clinical needs (Chap. 1), *inhalation injury* lacks the specificity necessary for effective communication. Respiratory complications differ considerably in their anatomic locations, clinical presentations, severity, and temporal evolution. Smoke inhalation alone may cause minor or life-threatening respiratory dysfunction, and typically its effects are merged imperceptibly with those physiologic changes due to burns and their management. Moreover, definitions of primary inhalation injury vary considerably. Historically important reports defining the problem have relied nearly entirely upon descriptive criteria, outlining the clinical characteristics of patient populations at risk. The recent availability of an array of objective diagnostic tests, each with its own sensitivities and specificities, has altered these definitions still further.

Thus, it should not be surprising that impressions of the degree of inhalational injury have varied according to the ways in which numerous criteria have been applied. The frequency of inhalation injury may range from 2.5 to 15 percent when diagnosis relies completely upon classic clinical characteristics (e.g., closed-space setting, carbonaceous sputum, singed nasal vibrissae, facial burns), to approximately 20 to 30 percent when it is based upon objective tests such as fiberoptic bronchoscopy, radionuclide scanning, or physiologic studies.[58] In some reports, diagnostic criteria are not described. Moreover, institutional differences in the ways in which even objective tests results are used introduce additional uncertainties. Inhalation injury has been defined not only on the basis of clinical findings but also in terms of the supportive care employed during management, such as the requirement for endotracheal intubation and/or mechanical ventilatory support. As a result, some clinical reports have tended to aggregate all of the respiratory problems developing in burned patients as sequelae of inhalation damage. Not only does this approach reflect some of the difficulties inherent to diagnosis, but it also fails to acknowledge the heterogeneity of these problems.

As will be discussed, fire scenarios and, consequently, the settings of individual patient injuries vary considerably, and the host responses to these exposures differ in innumerable ways.[22,24] The term *inhalation injury* implies a uniformity among patients that does not truly exist. The salient characteristic of inhalation injury—its clinical heterogeneity—confounds attempts at comprehensive definitions and classifications that are simultaneously broad and clinically meaningful. Because each of the myriad of respiratory problems differs in its clinical presentations, prognoses, and management, clinical considerations require that these must be specified as precisely as possible. Defining each component of respiratory injury in burned patients requires consideration of the general relationships between smoke inhalation and burns, the spectrum of problems encountered clinically, and the temporal sequence in which they develop. Each of these factors has direct implications for effective patient care.

Smoke Inhalation and Burns: Some General Relationships

Smoke inhalation and burns have a unique relationship that includes the common environments in which these injuries are sustained and shared cellular pathways and physiologic responses through which their clinical manifestations are ultimately expressed. In the early nineteenth century, Hayward alluded to a "sympathy between the skin surface and lungs," suggesting that one site would increase its function following injury to the other.[4] According to this notion, the lungs would become overworked following large surface burns, becoming "exhausted and inflamed." Typically, some time would be expected to elapse after burns for the effects of such respiratory dysfunction to become evident. Improved understanding of lung injury and its course in humans has confirmed this basic concept.

Potential respiratory effects of smoke inhalation, cutaneous burns, and the major infections which complicate these injuries are shown schematically in Fig. 2-1 and Table 2-1. These interactions are fundamental to clinical approaches to diagnosis and management. This model accommodates a spectrum of pulmonary responses and variations in the individual components of smoke inhalation, burns, and their combinations in any single patient. The relative contributions of each injury range considerably, exemplified by individuals with severe smoke inhalation without cutaneous burns, massive burns without smoke inhalation–mediated respiratory damage, and all combinations between these extremes. Predictably, there are institutional differences in the relative mix of patients within these stages. Clark et al. have noted that, depending upon the diagnostic criteria employed and the proportion of patients who have sustained flame burns, the proportion of individuals in a burn unit who have both burns and smoke inhalation ranges from 5 to 35 percent.[22,23]

In many respects, smoke inhalation injury, burns, and their combinations represent prototypic examples of direct and indirect respiratory damage, as varying levels of the respiratory tract respond in near-stereotypic fashion to components of injury which vary with each exposure scenario. The respiratory dysfunction reflects not only the obvious direct effects of inhaled toxins but also the systemic responses to burns. The individual respiratory effects of each component of injury may not be differentiated clinically. The net clinical expression of

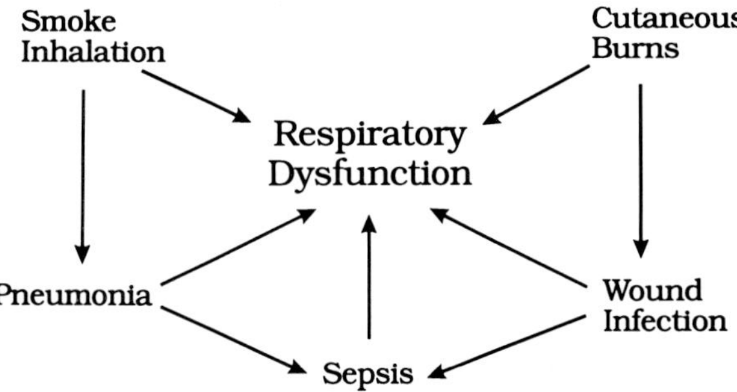

Figure 2-1 Major interactions of smoke inhalation injury and burns. Smoke inhalation and cutaneous burns each can induce respiratory dysfunction, and superimposed infections of the lung and skin lead to further respiratory compromise.

these events often far exceeds that which might be predicted on the basis of either injury alone and results in a spectrum of clinical manifestations (Table 2-2).

Primary Respiratory Effects of Smoke Toxic products of incomplete combustion induce a predominantly oxidant-mediated chemical injury to the upper airway, tracheobronchial tree, and lung pa-

Table 2-1 Some Cardiopulmonary Responses to Isolated Smoke Inhalation, Cutaneous Burns, or Sepsis

	Smoke inhalation	Cutaneous burns	Sepsis
Pulmonary PMN leukocyte sequestration	+	+	+
PMN activation	+	+	+
Lung free radical injury	+	+	+
Pulmonary vasoconstriction*	+	+	+
Microvascular alterations			
Increased lung lymph	+	+	+
Increased lymph protein (increased permeability)	+	−	+
Endothelial injury	+	+	+
Epithelial injury	+	−	−
Decreased thoracic compliance*	+	+	+
Increased bronchial blood flow	+	?	?
Increased airway resistance*	+	+	+
Increased dead space*	+	?	+
Surfactant inactivation*	+	−	+
Hypoxemia*	+	+	+
Increased work of breathing*	+	+	+
Generalized increased permeability	+	+	+
Systemic complement activation*	−	+	+
Myocardial depression*	+	+	+

*Documented in both experimental models and smoke/burn victims.

Table 2-2 Major Respiratory Complications of Burned Patients[9,10]

- I. Inhalation injury*
  - A. Asphyxia
    - 1. Hypoxia
    - 2. Carbon monoxide, cyanide intoxication
  - B. Direct respiratory injury
    - 1. Airway responses
      - a. Upper airway obstruction
      - b. Tracheobronchitis
      - c. Bronchiolitis
      - d. Atelectasis
    - 2. Alveolar-capillary membrane injury (permeability pulmonary edema)
- II. Effects of cutaneous burns
  - A. Pulmonary dysfunction
  - B. Chest wall restriction (e.g., circumferential thoracic burns, soft tissue edema)
  - C. Upper airway compression (e.g., circumferential cervical burns)
- III. Combined smoke inhalation with cutaneous burn
- IV. Concomitant chest trauma
- V. Nosocomial/iatrogenic problems
  - A. Hydrostatic pulmonary edema (overresuscitation)
  - B. Pneumonia (aerogenous, hematogenous)
  - C. Sepsis-related permeability edema
  - D. Drug-induced
    - 1. Hypoventilation (e.g., morphine)
    - 2. Hyperventilation (e.g., topical mafenide)
  - E. Pneumothorax
    - 1. Ventilator-induced barotrauma
    - 2. Central venous access procedures
  - F. Pulmonary embolism
  - G. Complications of artificial airways
  - H. Aspiration
- VI. Exacerbation of preexisting cardiopulmonary disease
  - A. Cardiogenic pulmonary edema
  - B. Chronic obstructive pulmonary disease

*Predominately due to smoke but, in selected circumstances, due to direct thermal injury (e.g., steam inhalation, free-basing explosions).

renchyma that is manifested by inflammation and increased permeability.[13,30,44–48,59,60,61a] The pathogenesis of these lesions is discussed in detail in Chaps. 3 and 4 and has reproducible anatomic and physiologic features. The influx of polymorphonuclear leukocytes, recruitment of macrophages, and liberation of an array of humoral factors by these cell populations appear important in mediating, modulating, or accentuating this primary injury and may serve to "prime" the lung for accentuated responses to secondary insults. The extent of such responses will vary from patient to patient, as well as with the characteristics of each individual smoke exposure. Increased epithelial and endothelial membrane permeability, surfactant inactivation with near-immediate microatelectasis, major airway obstruction by desquamated epithelial casts, and dynamic bronchoconstriction due to neurologic and humoral factors are some of the primary responses to acute smoke inhalation.[30, 61-63] Concurrently, localized airway and/or lung parenchymal injury due to smoke alters host defenses profoundly (Chap. 6).[64,65] Mechanical and physiologic airway obstruction, denudation of airway epithelium with loss of its barrier and mucociliary clearance functions, and compromise of local and systemic host cellular defenses by surface burns[66–73] predispose to aerogenous pneumonia caused by a variety of pathogens. Despite the best of preventative efforts, the environment in which these patients are managed leads to their infection by preselected, virulent, multiple drug-resistant organisms. Once established, nosocomial pneumonia, in turn, not only directly induces additional mechanical respiratory dysfunction but also may represent a primary source of systemic sepsis,[47] a problem which exerts its own adverse effects upon pulmonary function. Recently, inhalation injury has been documented as an independent risk factor for sepsis.[74]

Other systemic responses, not noted in Fig. 2-1 also may occur. For example, cardiac dysfunction mediated by smoke (e.g., due to carbon monoxide, cyanide and/or other inhaled toxins) or myocardial depression related to burns, sepsis, or systemic complement activation may cause respiratory dysfunction in the absence of significant primary respiratory injury.

Primary Respiratory Effects of Burns Independent of the effects of smoke, otherwise uncomplicated cutaneous burns can also cause respiratory dysfunction (Fig. 2-1 and Tables 2-1 and 2-2). The potential for adverse mechanical effects of circumferential chest wall burns (e.g., leading to reduced thoracic compliance and/or alveolar hypoventilation) has been well recognized.[75–82] Limitation of thoracoabdominal excursion by unyielding eschar and burn wound edema, potentially improved by escharotomy and/or excision of full thickness thoracic burn, has straightforward, obvious relationships to respiratory dysfunction. Restrictive ventilatory defects due to respiratory muscle injury, splinting from pain, or soft tissue edema of uninvolved thoracoabdominal areas frequently occur. More subtle has been the recent appreciation that the burn wound has an array of dynamic metabolic functions and represents a source of humoral mediators with potent effects upon the lung.[83–86] Demling and coworkers have observed lung lipid peroxidation, vascular congestion, polymorphonuclear (PMN) sequestration, and mildly reduced lung compliance in their well-established ovine model.[87] While these relatively minor physiologic changes associated with uninfected burn wounds might not account for clinically important respiratory dysfunction, they might serve to "prime" the lung so that an accentuated pulmonary response occurs when burn wound infection and/or sepsis have supervened.[87] Systemic PMN activation, demonstrated by increased expression of complement receptors, occurs in burned patients.[88] Till et al. have observed pulmonary endothelial injury, increased permeability, and interstitial and alveolar edema and hemorrhage in scalded rats.[89,90] These changes were associated with lipid peroxidation products (conjugated dienes) and could be prevented by PMN or complement depletion prior to burn, its burn excision, or treatment with free radical scavengers such as catalase, superoxide dismutase, vitamin E, dimethyl sulfoxide (DMSO), and iron chelators.

The infected burn wound has been associated with exaggerations in the usual diphasic pulmonary response to endotoxin.[76,78,83,91] Typically, an initial phase of pulmonary hypertension is followed by increased microvascular permeability. In animal models, burns (without inhalation injury) are associated with more severe pulmonary hypertension, hypoxia, and higher mortality due to respiratory failure. It has been shown that such enhanced sensitivity of the lung to endotoxin following burn injury relates to products of arachidonic metabolism and PMN activation. The clinical relationship of burn-related sepsis[92,93] to respiratory dysfunction is well-established: in one large series, sepsis accounted for 15.7 percent of episodes of acute respiratory failure which required mechanical ventilatory support.[22]

Secondary Respiratory Effects of Management The supportive measures which, as part of standard care, are employed widely in the treatment of either smoke inhalation or cutaneous burns, exact an added toll. Such commonly encountered respiratory problems are summarized in Fig. 2-2. Management of acute respiratory failure due to smoke inhalation or sepsis in this setting often requires artificial airways and mechanical ventilation, either of which may directly injure the respiratory tract, predispose to nosocomial pneumonia, and extend hospitalization. Recent observations suggest that superimposition of mechanical "tube trauma" upon an airway already injured by toxic combustion products may cause additive or even synergistic damage.[94–96] Positive pressure ventilation may worsen already disrupted ventilation perfusion relationships, or produce barotrauma. As in other patients with respiratory failure, aspects of routine nursing care (e.g., suctioning and turning) can aggravate hypoxemia due to accentuated ventilation perfusion mismatch. Burn wound debridement may add further respiratory stresses, or even unique dangers (e.g., loss of airway control and drowning in Hubbard tank). Major nonspecific complications also result from the prolonged hospitalizations associated with these complex illnesses and the critical care environments in which these patients are managed. Patient immobility and compromised host defenses are major predispositions to pneumonia, sepsis, atelectasis, and pulmonary embolism. Real or perceived needs for invasive monitoring present yet additional hazards related to the trauma of these procedures or misinterpretations of the data they provide.

Vigorous fluid resuscitation, essential to modern

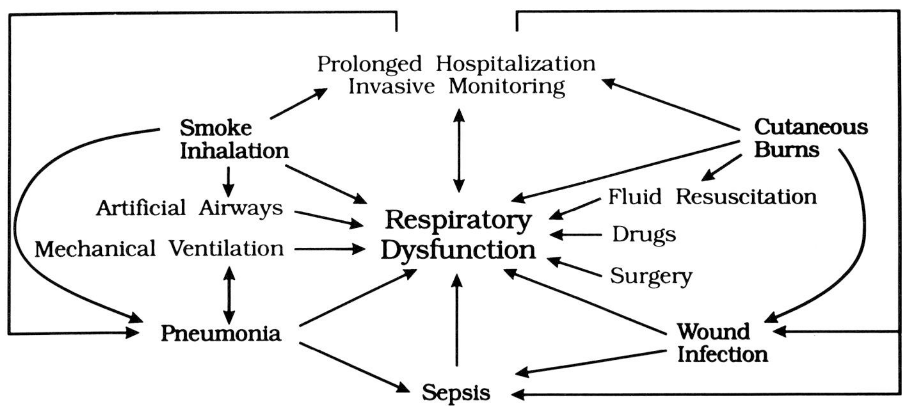

Figure 2-2 Interactions of smoke and inhalation injury, burns, and nosocomial problems. Standard treatments of patients with smoke inhalation and/or burns also may have adverse effects upon respiratory function, and the prolonged hospitalizations associated with severe injuries represents another formidable hazard.

care of cutaneous burns, can alter respiratory function not only through the obvious development of pulmonary edema but also through the restrictive effects of chest wall edema and reduced oncotic pressure. The excessive administration of volume, the underestimation of intraoperative blood and fluid requirements, or changes in the composition of intravenous fluid may have added adverse respiratory effects.[97–106] Ringer's lactate might, by introducing a metabolic alkalemia, influence approaches to mechanical ventilation (requiring increased efforts to avoid severe combined metabolic and respiratory alkalosis). Increased oxygen consumption and carbon dioxide production associated with burns have important influences on patients' ventilatory requirements. Appropriate responses to patients' increased nutritional needs may paradoxically worsen respiratory problems. Carbohydrate loading may increase $\dot{V}_{CO_2}$, augmenting needs for mechanical ventilation. Specific aspects of fluid resuscitation in the setting of inhalation injury are addressed in Chaps. 5 and 10.

Adverse effects of drugs upon respiratory function are of special concern in this clinical situation. Respiratory depression is often induced by morphine, other analgesics, and sedative-hypnotic agents, and we suspect that this impact is underestimated. In patients already receiving mechanical ventilation, this effect is usually of minor consequence, as the airway is already controlled and the effects of the drug may be readily compensated for by minor adjustments of mechanical ventilation. In patients in whom the airway has not been secured, however, and in those with marginal respiratory mechanics, seemingly low doses of drugs might induce abrupt apnea. The timing of drugs with respect to resuscitation is also a factor: in children, sudden, central respiratory arrest has occurred between 24 and 48 hours after narcotic administration following the delayed initiation of fluid resuscitation.[9] Altered pharmacokinetics of a number of medications may also influence respiratory function. Use of depolarizing muscle relaxants (e.g., during preparations for endotracheal intubation or in relation to anesthesia) requires particular caution.[107,108] These and other problems are reviewed in Chap. 14.

Even some medications without obvious respiratory suppressant effects might alter function. Huang and coworkers have noted that haloperidol, a widely used agent, might induce muscular rigidity, which in turn leads to a thoracic compliance change influencing mechanical ventilatory requirements.[109]

Other drugs used in standard, topical burn wound care may contribute to difficulties in differential diagnosis of apparent respiratory distress. Mafenide (Sulfamylon), a carbonic anhydrase inhibitor, has been associated with a marked increase in minute ventilation ($\dot{V}_E$) occurring between the third and fifth postburn days in patients with large burns (>35% BSA).[110] Although increased metabolic demands typically cause alveolar hyperventilation (e.g., up to twice normal) following uncomplicated burns, mafenide may induce an additional 50 percent increase. The degree of this response must be appreciated: investigators have noted that for extreme elevations of $\dot{V}_E$ (e.g., >25 L/min), other conditions such as sepsis, fluid overload, or an acute abdomen must be excluded.

As in other critically ill patients, changes in the environment in which patients are managed might pose unique threats. Transportation of the patient out of the burn center or intensive care unit for diagnostic procedures (e.g., roentgenographic studies, radionuclide scans) or for specialized treatment (e.g., "diving" in a hyperbaric chamber) presents major logistic demands for an environment appropriate for that patient's needs for monitoring and support.[111,112] Even the prepared operating room setting may be associated with untoward effects: Demling has documented episodes of transient alveolar hypoventilation due to the underestimation of patients' intraoperative ventilatory requirements and needs during transport to the operating room.[111] Discontinuation of positive end-expiratory pressure (PEEP) during burn excision surgery resulted in lowered lung compliance and worsened oxygenation, a change that could be minimized by the appropriate intraoperative maintenance of PEEP.

Wound debridement, excisional surgery, and grafting are central to burn care; any of these necessary modalities may represent a life-threatening stress in the patient with compromised respiratory function. Such deteriorations during excisional therapy has been especially important in elderly patients and those with already established inhalation injury. In experimental models, the timing of surgery influences the severity of pulmonary responses; bronchial and pulmonary vasoconstriction associated with high circulating thromboxane levels, is accentuated when excision of an inflammatory wound is delayed. These aspects of burn care are reviewed in Chap. 12.

Clinical Presentations and Diagnosis

Because the clinical manifestations of these diverse problems often overlap or are nonspecific, each, in one series or another, has been purposely or inadvertently classified as inhalation injury. Thus, the approach to the burned patient who either presents with respiratory distress, hypoxemia, and nonspecific chest roentgenographic abnormalities or develops such problems during hospitalization is a major dilemma. On clinical grounds it is often not possible to distinguish the precise contributions of individual components of respiratory dysfunction during prospective assessment and management. Because specific therapy for many of these problems is available, however, they must be differentiated from one another if the ominous prognosis of inhalation injury is to be improved. This ambitious goal requires an especially systematic approach, with an awareness of the spectrum, presentations, and temporal evolution of respiratory complications.

Spectrum of Acute Respiratory Complications The major acute respiratory problems encountered clinically in burned patients with smoke inhalation are summarized in Tables 2-2 and 2-3 and Fig. 2-3, and their relative frequencies in reviews of large populations are outlined in Table 2-4.[113,114] Asphyxia caused primarily by carbon monoxide and/or cyanide intoxication, upper airway and tracheobronchial obstruction due to the irritant effects of smoke, and pulmonary edema which may have multifactorial origins are principal concerns for the clinician. The relative frequencies of these problems vary not only with the clinical settings in which they develop but also with the criteria used for their detection and the effort expended in seeking them. Thus, the exact frequencies of these problems and

Table 2-3 General Impact of Clinical Respiratory Complications* in Burn Victims(9,10)

	Smoke inhalation only	Cutaneous burn only	Both smoke inhalation and burns present
Asphyxia	+ + +	+	+ + + +
Upper airway obstruction	+	0	+ + + +
Tracheobronchitis	+ +	0	+ + + +
Permeability edema			
Toxic	+	+ +	+ + + +
Septic	+	+ + +	+ + + +
Hydrostatic edema	0	+ + +	+ + + +
Pneumonia	+	+ + +	+ + + +
Pulmonary embolism	0	+	+
Mortality	+	+ +	+ + + +
Likelihood of residual respiratory impairment	+	+	+
Need for intubation, mechanical ventilation	+	+ +	+ + + +
Relative duration, cost of hospitalization	+	+ +	+ + + +

*Scale from 0–4+ in increasing severity.

their effects upon outcome are still unclear and necessarily reflect a variety of selection factors.

General relationships of these problems to one another in large referral populations are summarized in Fig. 2-3.[9,10] Importantly, although patients with smoke inhalation in the absence of burns primarily experience asphyxiant and airway injuries, the likelihood of all complications increases when cutaneous burns are present. The higher frequency of injuries at multiple anatomic levels undoubtedly reflects more intense exposures leading to combined injuries. In addition, it is likely that manifestations of respiratory damage are, at each anatomic level, amplified by the burn itself. These acute injuries interact with patients' preexisting cardiopulmonary status and the effects of therapeutic efforts. As noted previously, these patients become predisposed to an array of iatrogenic illness or complications of prolonged hospitalization. Vulnerability to these problems relates to their condition prior to the injury, the severity of their combined respiratory and cutaneous insults, and the effectiveness of measures taken by the managing team to avoid nosocomial disease. The morbidity of these problems also seems to be additive, but precise quantitative data are incomplete because the individual components of inhalation injury are not routinely specified in clinical reports. The relative risks presented by each of these respiratory problems vary with their amenability to therapy: upper airway and tracheobronchial obstruction are usually the most readily treated, while pneumonia and septic adult respiratory distress syndrome (ARDS) have the poorest prognoses. The likelihood of respiratory failure and death are lower in patients with smoke inhalation injury uncomplicated by surface burns.[9,10]

Common Clinical Presentations Medical personnel must be prepared to evaluate patients in diverse settings, including the fire/smoke scene, during transport, the emergency room, the community hospital, the referral burn center, or the intensive care unit. Depending upon local triage practices, referral patterns, and transportation services, patients receive initial treatment at variable times after injury. As noted by Clark and others, several fundamental presentations are often seen (Table 2-5).[22–24] Each of these differs with regard to the acuity of illness, the severity of already established respiratory injury, immediate therapeutic priorities, potential for abrupt deterioration, and needs for diagnostic testing. Despite increased appreciation of the importance of inhalation injury, the relative proportions of patients within each of these general categories is not clear. Such distributions would be expected to vary among institutions, communities, and with referral patterns.

Survivors of the initial exposure may have either obvious respiratory dysfunction of varying degrees or have no overt respiratory problems. An unknown proportion of these latter individuals have sustained

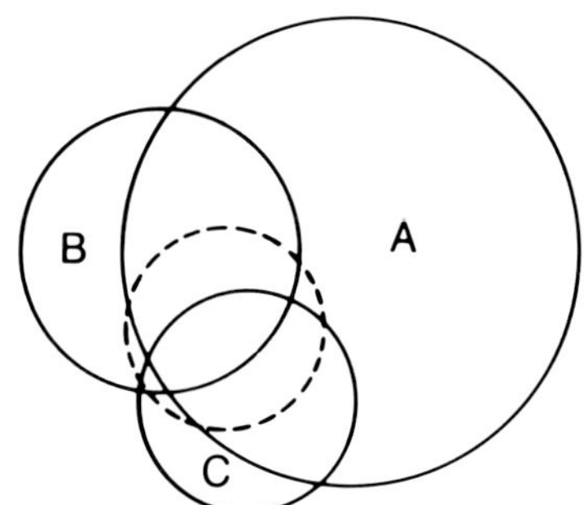

Figure 2-3 Respiratory complications of smoke inhalation. The major respiratory problems associated with smoke inhalation include asphyxia, injury to the airways and parenchyma, and late-onset problems related to infection and prolonged hospitalization. The frequency and adverse clinical impact of these problems are accentuated in patients with cutaneous burns. (*Reprinted with permission from J Crit Care 2:49, 1987.*[9])

Table 2-4 Relative Frequencies of Respiratory Problems Complicating Burns

	Pruitt et al.[15–18] 1962–63 (n = 308)	Pruitt et al.[15–18] 1967 (n = 389)	Venus et al.[113] 1976–77 (n = 998)	Dimick et al.[114] 1972–81 (n = 1271)
Pulmonary edema	27 (8.8%)	21 (5.4%)	45 (4.5%)	—
Pneumonia	70 (23.0%)	56 (14.4%)	29 (2.9%)	204 (16.0%)
Atelectasis	8 (2.6%)	10 (2.6%)	11 (11.0%)	—
Respiratory burn	—	—	—	160 (12.6%)
Pleural effusion	—	7 (2.0%)	—	—
Smoke inhalation injury	3 (1.0%)	1	—	—
Aspiration with asphyxia	—	2	—	—
Analgesia-related respiratory depression	1	1	—	—
Pulmonary embolism	2	3 (1.0%)	—	28 (2.2%)
Chest wall defects, fractured ribs	1	2	—	—
Tracheostomy complications	47 (15.0%)	26 (7.0%)	—	—
Subglottic stenosis	—	—	2 (2.0%)	—
Pneumothorax	1	0	5 (5.0%)	17 (1.3%)
Exacerbation of chronic bronchitis	—	1	—	—

Table 2-5 Early Respiratory Problems in Burned Patients: Common Clinical Presentations

Smoke exposure without overt respiratory dysfunction
No respiratory injury (normal objective tests)
Subclinical injury (abnormal objective tests; ? normal tests)
Clinically overt respiratory dysfunction (respiratory symptoms, signs, +/− abnormalities of objective tests)
Cardiopulmonary arrest at scene, successful resuscitation
Asphyxiant death at scene of exposure

SOURCE: Modified after *J Burn Care Rehabil* 10:52, 1989, and *Burns* 14:473, 1988.

subclinical injury that will either clear spontaneously or progress. Deterioration of respiratory function is more likely to occur when multiple insults are combined (e.g., cutaneous burns, fluid challenges with resuscitation). The lung injured by smoke is more likely to leak during intravenous fluid administration.[115] Thus, even when smoke inhalation injury is itself nonlethal, the threshold for further deterioration of respiratory function is lowered substantially. Superimposition of diverse secondary insults (e.g., burns, pneumonia, sepsis) often converts a subclinical or otherwise tolerable mild respiratory injury to one that is associated with considerably higher morbidity or even death. One especially important group of patients is that composed of individuals with no overt respiratory dysfunction and who truly have no respiratory injury. Because of the delayed onset of some smoke-related problems, accurate identification of persons who are not destined to develop progressive dysfunction and will not require treatment is an important triage issue that has not yet been resolved satisfactorily. As will be addressed in other chapters, whenever there is significant doubt regarding the patient's respiratory status, the high risk associated with undiagnosed and untreated problems strongly favors careful observation and in many instances empiric supportive treatment.

Temporal Evolution of Respiratory Problems Although considerable individual variability exists, the onset of specific respiratory problems has been related to the time which has elapsed after initial exposure and injury.[10,116–122] The sequence of respiratory problems is useful in organizing management priorities and reflects improved understanding about their etiology and pathogenesis. Zawacki et al. have characterized clinically distinct presentations, noting that acute respiratory distress predominates after minor burns with smoke inhalation, while delayed-onset respiratory distress is predominantly a sequela of major burns.[122] These observations, consistent with the large descriptive experiences of Stone and others,[9] have led to a classification system that has immediate therapeutic relevance. In patients who do not succumb immediately to asphyxia, respiratory problems may be regarded as having an early (0 to 48 hours), intermediate or delayed onset (24 hours to 5 days), and late onset (longer than 5 days) after the initial exposure to smoke. These arbitrarily defined stages do not describe a discrete progression that is seen in all injured individuals. Rather, they encompass a continuum of events that occur from the time of initial injury to its repair. These manifestations are modified further by therapeutic interventions in each patient.[116]

This relative timing of respiratory complications is outlined schematically in Fig. 2-4.[9,10] The systemic manifestations of asphyxiants, most notably carbon monoxide and cyanide, are present initially and usually clear rapidly once appropriate treatment with oxygen and antidotes is begun. Upper airway obstruction, typically due to pharyngeal injury by heat and water-soluble combustion products, is another early problem that can also be expected to peak rapidly in its severity and to clear rapidly (generally within 3 days). Concurrently, tracheobronchial obstruction is a hallmark of smoke inhalation injury, resulting in clinical presentations which range from subclinical airflow obstruction detectable only by physiologic testing to a fulminant episode indistinguishable from status asthmaticus. Recognition that these asphyxiant, upper, and lower airway problems develop early in the course

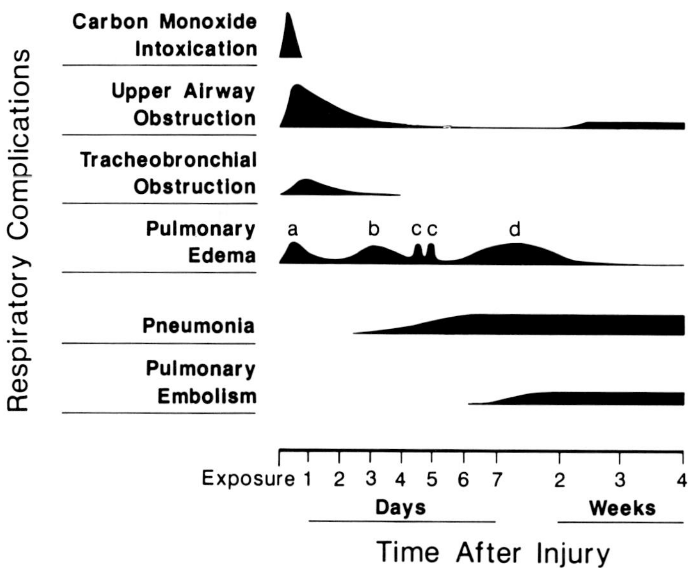

Figure 2-4 Relative timing of respiratory complications in burn victims (Baltimore Regional Burn Center, 1978–1982). Although considerable variability occurs in any individual patient, the relative likelihood and nature of respiratory complications relates to the time elapsed after exposure. Carbon monoxide intoxication, cyanide toxicity, acute upper airway obstruction by pharyngeal edema, and tracheobronchial obstruction are usually early complications. Upper airway obstruction may, less often, complicate the later course (here arbitrarily indicated at 2 weeks), usually as a sequela of airway management or cervical contractures. Pulmonary edema may occur at any time, but its causes can vary substantially. ARDS from toxic gas inhalation, cardiogenic edema, and hypervolemia from fluid resuscitation may occur early (a), while hypervolemia occurring during burn edema remobilization (b) or induced iatrogenically during overhydration (c) has later onset. ARDS due to sepsis (d) may appear at any time but more often develops later in the course. Pneumonia of aerogenous (mean onset, 10 to 14 days) or hematogenous (18 to 21 days) origin and pulmonary embolism are usually later-onset problems in patients with large burns who require long-term hospitalization. (*Reprinted with permission from J Crit Care 2:121, 1987.*[10])

allows the clinician to focus both diagnostic evaluations and early management priorities. Moreover, so long as these problems are recognized in a timely manner, they are perhaps the most treatable sequelae of significant inhalation injury, especially when uncomplicated by large surface burns. As noted previously, late-onset respiratory problems typically occur in persons who have large burns requiring long-term hospitalizations. Pulmonary edema due to ARDS and often developing as a component of multisystem failure, pneumonia, and pulmonary embolism have similar clinical presentations to those of other critically ill patients, but diagnosis and therapy are often more difficult in the burned patient.

The pace of respiratory distress also varies among individuals, ranging from the explosive onset of upper airway occlusion to the more insidious development of atelectasis, interstitial edema, and alveolar flooding. Clark has commented upon the rapid deterioration of patients who sustain combined smoke inhalation injury and cutaneous burns: not only is mortality high but death usually occurs quickly—within 10 days.[22] Individuals without smoke inhalation tend to have a more gradually paced respiratory illness with longer survival; their respiratory failure then punctuates the late hospital course, typically developing as an acute complication of pulmonary or systemic infection.

General Diagnostic Approaches and Pitfalls Major considerations in the clinical diagnosis of smoke inhalation injury are outlined in Table 2-6. The clinician must integrate knowledge about the spectrum and time course of respiratory problems with the presence of classic clinical predictors identified in an individual patient.[123–132] The characteristics of the exposure, objective signs and symptoms referable to the respiratory tract, and markers (facial burn, carbonaceous sputum) associated with respiratory injury have been used historically for this purpose. It must then be determined whether supplemental information from objective diagnostic tests is essential to formulating a management plan. When such additional data are necessary, a realistic diagnostic strategy most consistent with the needs of the patient and the resources at hand must be formulated. Many of the currently used diagnostic criteria are indirect and do not necessarily reflect the degree of pulmonary injury accurately. Abnormalities on one or another objective test documenting respiratory injury have shown only variable relationships to outcome. However, the recent observation that patients with abnormal bronchoscopic findings were more likely to develop pneumonia and have a higher mortality than individuals with abnormal lung scans alone supports the notion that there are clinically detectable gradations in severity of inhalation injury.[73] The roles and limitations of an increasingly available number of diagnostic tests must be appreciated and are considered in detail in Chaps. 7 and 8. It should be obvious that the patient's mode of presentation is central to appropriate focusing of these individualized diagnostic efforts.

Table 2-6 Major Considerations in Clinical Diagnosis of Smoke Inhalation Injury*(9,10)

I. Spectrum and time course of respiratory problems
II. Classic clinical predictors
  A. Exposure characteristics
    Closed-space setting, entrapment
    Unconsciousness
    Known inhaled toxin
  B. Respiratory signs, symptoms
  C. Facial, cervical burns
  D. Carbonaceous sputum
III. Objective diagnostic tests
  A. Measurement of asphyxiants (carboxyhemoglobin, cyanide)
  B. Arterial blood gases
  C. Chest roentgenogram
  D. Direct airway observation (laryngoscopy or nasopharyngoscopy, bronchoscopy)
  E. Radionuclide scanning
  F. Pulmonary function testing (spirometry, complete flow volume curves)

*Reviewed in detail in Chap. 7.

Definitive diagnosis is potentially confounded by the heterogeneity of injuries, their varying severity, the delayed onset of clinical manifestations of resairatory dysfunction, limitations of presently available diagnostic techniques, and the very nonspecificity of respiratory symptoms and physiologic abnormalities. Patients presenting with volume overload, pneumonia, aspiration, sepsis, and pulmonary embolism may have similar acute symptoms. While it is facile to state that more precise categorization of respiratory problems is needed, realizing this goal in the real-world management of patients is intrinsically difficult. In any given patient, respiratory dysfunction may truly be multifactorial, and its precise categorization impossible. Even when concerted efforts to achieve this have been made, identification of patients with significant airway or parenchymal injuries has not always been possible. Some authors have based the diagnosis of inhalation injury on the need for airway support and/or mechanical ventilation. Clearly, total reliance on these criteria will inevitably exclude an uncertain number of individuals with less severe degrees of injury and erroneously include patients with respiratory failure due to other etiologies.

In addition to differential sites and degrees of injury, little is known about the differential rates of resolution of the components of respiratory injury and how each is modified by therapeutic efforts. In many instances, the cause of inhalation injury is appreciated retrospectively, as other potential causes of the patient's respiratory problems are systematically excluded. The inherent difficulties of timely, prospective diagnosis hinder efforts to initiate early therapy. Any diagnostic approach must also take into consideration the fact that timely management of inhalation injury must often precede definitive diagnosis. This is particularly noteworthy in those patients who have the most severe respiratory and cutaneous injuries.

IMPACT OF RESPIRATORY DYSFUNCTION IN BURNED PATIENTS

The adverse impact of the interactions of smoke inhalation and cutaneous burns upon the outcome of patients has long been appreciated; evolution of these perspectives and the appreciation of their implications for management have been reviewed in detail in Chap. 1. Reports of mass exposures and documentation of the extensive experiences accrued at burn centers form the basis of our improving understanding of these problems.

Historical Accounts

Pliny the Elder has been credited with reporting the lethal effects of smoke inhalation in his account of the execution of Roman prisoners during the second Punic War by suspending them in cages above smoldering greenwood fires.[38] Classic, comprehensive descriptions of fires at the Cocoanut Grove, Delwood Nursery, Stardust Night Club, and Las Vegas Hotels, together with the recurrent personal tragedies of residential fires, have presented stark reminders of the lethal potential of smoke inhalation.[133–135] Such mass disasters and the ways they have influenced societal views and public policies related to fire-induced injury have been catalogued recently.[136] In 1822, Coates described respiratory injury accompanying burns in his report of the autopsy findings in a patient who died suddenly 4 days after burns localized to the thorax and face. The lips and nostrils were covered by crusts, and blackening of the tracheobronchial mucosa was attributed to "breathing flames."[4] Long also reported pulmonary injury at an autopsy of a burned patient in 1840,[4] and classic postmortem reports over a century later have documented the importance of respiratory damage.[137–141] Such series have identified respiratory complications as the primary cause of death in from 18 to 24 percent of patients with burns; smoke inhalation injury, pneumonia, and sepsis-related respiratory failure have assumed a dominant role.

Analyses from Burn Centers

General reviews of the improved survival of patients with major burns have consistently underscored the lethal impact of inhalation injury. At the Baltimore Regional Center (Fig. 2-5), burned patients requiring endotracheal intubation for smoke inhalation–related respiratory failure had a mortality of 42.3 percent, in contrast to the very low mortality (2.2 percent) observed in individuals without such clinically diagnosed inhalation injury.[9] In a recent review of 1458 patients by Merrell et al., regression analysis showed that burn size, the presence of inhalation injury, and advancing patient age (in a descending order of relative importance) were significant predictors of death.[142] In the study of burn mortality of Curreri et al., smoke inhalation injury was the principal cause of death in 13 percent of 937 patients; septic complications (54 percent), irreversible burn shock (15 percent), and cardiovascular complications (11 percent) were other lethal problems.[143] When two periods (1978 to 1981 and 1982 to 1986) were compared, it was noteworthy that the mortality rate for individuals with inhalation injury had decreased less than that for patients without inhalation injury. This observation supports some authorities' clinical impressions that despite major progress resulting in overall improvement in burn mortality and reduction of the LA 50 (the surface area of burn associated with a 50 percent mor-

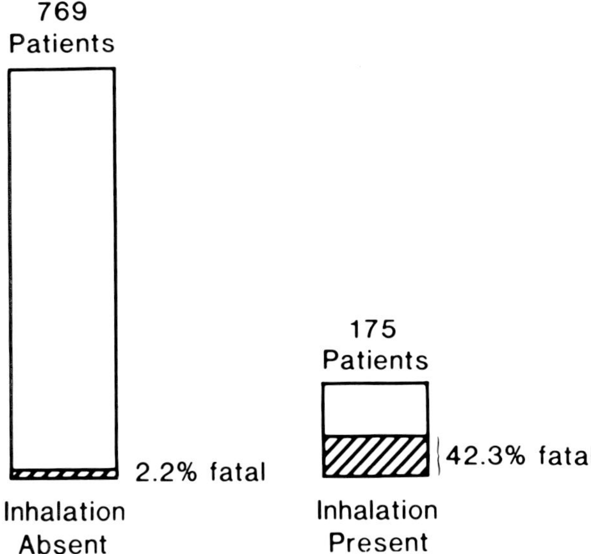

Figure 2-5 Inhalation injury and burn mortality. The presence of inhalation injury, defined by a requirement for endotracheal intubation in patients with clinical risk factors for respiratory damage, is associated with increased mortality in burned patients. This experience at the Baltimore Regional Burn Center (1978–82) has been documented consistently at other burn centers. (*Reprinted with permission from J Crit Care 2:49, 1987.*[9])

tality), deaths due to respiratory complications have remained less influenced by recent therapeutic innovations.

Several authors have found that the presence of inhalation injury independently reduces survival following burn injury and that prognostications about outcome should be adjusted downward whenever this complicating factor is present. When inhalation injury accompanies surface burns, mortality is disportionately higher than that which would be predicted on the basis of the extent of cutaneous injury alone. Herndon et al. have noted that inhalation injury increases mortality by approximately 30 to 40 percent.[144,145] He and others observed that the apparently synergistic lethal impact of inhalation injury is most striking in patients with minimal burns and severe respiratory injury and with burns that would otherwise be associated with a 40 to 60 percent mortality. In their comprehensive analysis of 1018 consecutive admissions to the Shriner's Burns Institute in Galveston, Tex., Thompson et al. reported that the incidence of and mortality from inhalation injury rose with increasing body surface area (BSA) of burn.[145] Moreover, the impact of inhalation injury rose with advancing age, having its lowest mortality in the 5- to 14-year-old age group and highest in patients greater than 59 years old. Diagnosis of inhalation injury was based upon the presence of abnormal bronchoscopic findings (airway edema, inflammation, mucosa necrosis, soot, and charring) and the need for ventilatory support for 7 days or more following hospitalization. With application of these criteria, inhalation injury was present in 8.6 percent of patients. Their overall mortality of 56 percent contrasted with that of persons without inhalation injury (4.1 percent). Although mortality was associated significantly with increasing age and BSA burn, both classic predictors of burn survival, the presence of objectively documented inhalation injury was found to be the most important determinant of mortality. Moreover, the relationship with burn size to death appeared to be more than merely an additive effect. Data from this important study are shown in Tables 2-7 and 2-8.

The lethal impact of inhalation injury has been

Table 2-7 Incidence and Mortality of Inhalation Injury: Relationships to Age

			Mortality	
Age	n	% With inhalation injury (n)	% Without inhalation injury (n)	% With inhalation injury (n)
≤4	317	5 (16)	2 (5)	44* (7)
5–14	195	7 (13)	1 (2)	38* (5)
15–44	394	9 (35)	5 (17)	54* (19)
45–59	67	18 (12)	15 (8)	58* (7)
≥59	45	27 (12)	24 (8)	92* (11)
Totals	1018	9 (88)	4 (38)	56* (49)

*$p < 0.01$ for increase in mortality with inhalation injury.

SOURCE: Reprinted with permission from *J Trauma* 26:163, 1986.[145]

Table 2-8 Incidence and Mortality of Inhalation Injury: Relationships to TBSA Burn

			Mortality	
Age	n	% With inhalation injury (n)	% Without inhalation injury (n)	% With Inhalation injury (n)
0–20	627	2 (11)	1 (6)	36* (4)
21–40	200	11 (21)	2 (4)	38* (8)
41–60	102	20 (20)	18 (15)	50* (10)
61–80	56	32 (18)	24 (9)	67* (12)
81–100	33	55 (18)	47 (7)	83* (15)
Totals	1018	9 (88)	4 (38)	56* (49)

*p value <0.01 for increase in mortality with inhalation injury.

SOURCE: Reprinted with permission from *J Trauma* 26:163, 1986.[145]

confirmed in other probit analyses of large groups of patients managed in fairly consistent ways at burn centers (Table 2-9). Although these reviews were performed at institutions that are widely separated geographically (with anticipated regional differences in referral populations, settings of injury, admission criteria, and nuances of management), objectively diagnosed inhalation injury was found consistently to decrease survival. In Zawacki's multifactorial analysis, even further insight into the impact of respiratory involvement was feasible.[146] At his institution, three of the six independent factors which best differentiated survivors from nonsurvivors were related to respiratory injury: nearly one-third of individuals with preexisting bronchopulmonary disease, half of patients who were hypoxemic at the time of admission to the hospital (Pa_{O_2} less than 70 mmHg), and two-thirds of those who had airway edema documented at bronchoscopy died. Combinations of each of these respiratory factors would, in this analysis, progressively increase the likelihood of death. These relative effects in a prototypic patient, a 42-year-old man with 50% BSA burns (20 percent third-degree injury), are outlined in Table 2-10.[146] In other reviews, inclusion of major clinical characteristics of the fire setting (e.g., closed-space environment) or of scores assigned to the presence or absence of symptoms classically associated with respiratory injury have

Table 2-9 Impact of Inhalation Injury on Burn Mortality: Some Quantitative Estimates

Author, year	Prediction equation
Zawacki et al., 1979*[(146)]	0.036 (age) + 0.037 (BSA) + 0.52 (if Pa_{O_2} < 70 mmHg) + 0.56 (if airway edema) + 0.028 (3° BSA) + 0.4 (if prior bronchopulmonary disease)
Clark et al., 1986†[(21)]	−7.9 + 0.78 (In +) + 0.094 (BSA) + 0.034 (age)
Shirani et al., 1987†[(73)]	−3.4953 + 0.09589 (BSA) − 0.1988 (age) + 9.9944788 $(age)^2$ − 0.000020314 $(age)^3$ + 0.59056 (In +) + 0.92530 (Pn)
Clark and Fromm, 1987†[(23)]	−4.26 + 0.976 (FTB) − 0.0454 (age) + 0.000919 $(age)^2$ + 1.43 (In +)

*Calculation provides Z number.

†Calculation of exponent x, with the probability of mortality $P = \frac{e^x}{1 + e^x}$

ABBREVIATIONS: BSA = Body surface area of burn; FTB = full thickness burn; In + = inhalation injury present (1), absent (0); Pn = pneumonia present (1), absent (0).

also predicted poorer outcomes (Chap. 7).[21] Although one might question the clinical usefulness of application of these relationships to an individual patient, such insights about large populations have provided important general perspectives that, hopefully, can be translated to improvements in patient care.

Inhalation injury diagnosed objectively by bronchoscopy and/or ventilation/perfusion scanning was present in 35 percent of patients managed at the Brooke Center and reported by Shirani et al.[73] Its presence alone increased mortality by a maximum of 20 percent. Furthermore, although pneumonia subsequently complicated the course of only 8.8 percent of individuals without inhalation injury, this life-threatening problem developed in 38 percent of these with inhalation injury. Pneumonia alone increased the likelihood of death by a maximum of 40 percent, and its combination with inhalation injury resulted in a maximum increase of mortality of 60 percent. These investigators concluded that inhalation injury and pneumonia had significant independent, additive effects on burn mortality which varied predictably with age and burn size, confirming bedside observations that many clinicians have made regarding this ominous lethal interaction.

In addition to these reports in which a focus is placed upon smoke inhalation injury, other studies have more broadly addressed the effects of respiratory dysfunction upon survival and have included those problems not specifically related to inhalation injury in their analyses. One recent major review provides special insights into the impact of such respiratory dysfunction. Clark and coworkers profiled patients according to their burns, smoke exposures, objectively diagnosed smoke inhalation injury, and the development of respiratory failure as indicated by the requirement for endotracheal intubation and/or mechanical ventilation during management.[22–24] Intubation was performed for anticipated or impending airway obstruction and airway insufficiency, criteria that are widely observed. Because this experience included both unburned individuals with inhalation injury and burned patients without smoke exposure who required endotracheal intubation, the full spectrum of the interactions of these injuries is represented. These data are summarized in Table 2-11; they support the notion that there is a gradation of the impact of respiratory problems. One-fourth of Clark's patients had respiratory dysfunction: approximately 80 percent of them had smoke inhalation, while the remaining individuals had sepsis-related respiratory failure. Patients who had experienced only smoke exposure without accompanying burns tended to be younger and had a relatively low mortality comparable to that of burned patients without either smoke exposure or respiratory injury. Relatively few of these individuals required intubation, hospital stay was relatively brief, and mortality low. As in other series, patients who sustained both burns and inhalation injuries were older, had larger burns, extended hospitaliza-

Table 2-10 Additive Impact of Respiratory Problems on Burn Mortality

42-year-old man, 50% BSA burn, 20% full thickness burn

Respiratory status	Likelihood of death, %
No respiratory disease	50
Previous bronchopulmonary disease (BPD)	70
BPD + admission Pa_{O_2} < 70 mmHg	80
BPD + hypoxemia + airway edema (bronchoscopy)	90

SOURCE: Reprinted with permission from *Ann Surg* 189:1, 1979.[146]

Table 2-11 Interactive Effects of Respiratory Injury and Cutaneous Burn*

	n (%)	Age*	BSA%* (% degree)* third	LOS* survivors, days	Endotracheal intubation, %	Mortality, %
Burn only	607 (75)	27	12 (7)	16	0	2
Smoke injury, inhalation injury, no burn	41 (5)	29	0	2	12	7
Smoke exposure, inhalation injury, burn	119 (15)	36	33 (18)	45	61	29
No smoke exposure, endotracheal intubation, burn	38 (5)	43	41 (22)	70	100	47

*Mean data indicated.

ABBREVIATIONS: BSA = body surface area; LOS = length of stay.

SOURCE: Reprinted with permission from *J Burn Care Rehabil* 10:52, 1989,[22] and *Acta Chir Scand* [*suppl*] 537, 1987.[23]

tions, and higher mortality. The timing and degree of respiratory failure was a key determinant of the overall severity of the injury. Interestingly, survival time for patients with inhalation injury was short and appeared to be the same whether burns were present or absent. Importantly, nearly 5 percent of older patients with larger burns had respiratory failure in the absence of smoke exposure, and this latter group accounted for approximately one-fourth of deaths. Their respiratory failure was ordinarily a sequela of sepsis, with its progression to multisystem organ failure. The longer duration of hospital stay in individuals without inhalation injury is consistent with the usual timing for the onset of nosocomial sepsis and multiple organ failure. These observations were in agreement with Curreri's findings that "fulminant respiratory failure" due to severe inhalation injury was a major cause of early deaths occurring during the initial 72 hours after burn injury.[143] Respiratory failure or ARDS (10 percent) were important causes of late mortality, and the predominant etiology of late mortality was sepsis (49 percent).

Marshall and Dimick also emphasized the importance of multiple subsystem failure in 168 patients with second- and third-degree burns (≥40 percent).[147] Pulmonary failure, defined by the requirement for mechanical ventilatory assistance, developed in 89 patients (53 percent) and had a 92 percent mortality. While inhalation injury accounted for most of the patients with respiratory failure, sepsis (16 percent) and other unspecified respiratory problems also occurred. Isolated respiratory failure, seen in 8.9 percent of individuals, had a mortality of 67 percent; most of these patients had inhalation injury. The vast majority (83 percent) of patients with respiratory failure, however, experienced this dysfunction as a component of multisubsystem failure. As documented in other series of patients with (and without) cutaneous burns, mortality increased as a function of the number of failed subsystems, reaching 98 percent for two or more systems. Overall, sepsis was the most common cause of death in this population, and three-fourths of individuals with multisystem failure due to sepsis died. Interestingly, subsystem failure correlated more strongly with mortality than either age or BSA burn.

These experiences document not only the heterogeneity of patients with smoke inhalation with regard to their clinical presentations but also the importance of acute respiratory failure unrelated to inhalation injury in burn victims. When mechanical ventilation is necessary within 12 hours of a burn, this requirement is especially ominous in adults with less than 40% BSA burns and children with less than 60% BSA.[144] It has been suggested that the extremely high mortality of more extensive burns is associated with a lesser contribution to outcome from inhalation injury. Nevertheless, many such patients with lethal burns have died of inhalation injury (e.g., manifest by acute upper airway obstruction, pulmonary edema), while others have succumbed to pneumonia or sepsis-related hypoxemic respiratory failure (ARDS) ensuing later during their complex hospital courses.[148]

Outcomes in High Risk Groups

Elderly patients (≥60 years old) are particularly vulnerable to the development of inhalation injury.[149–151] In one recent review two-thirds of such elderly persons with inhalation injury died; moreover, the LA 50, 25 percent for the total population, was less than 5 percent in elderly individuals with inhalation injury.[149] No patients with inhalation injury and burns exceeding 30% BSA survived. The increased frequency of inhalation injury in older individuals is probably multifactorial in origin. Contributing factors include the higher likelihood of flame burns sustained in closed-space settings and the lower likelihood of scalding (generally unassociated with inhalation injury). In addition, immobility, cigarette smoking, alcohol, and drug ingestion, all important risk factors for inhalation injury, are more often implicated in adults. Other predispositions probably relate to combined effects of slower reaction times; limited mobility; or impaired vision, smell, or hearing, all hindering escape from the fire/

smoke scene. This acute insult is often superimposed upon otherwise compromised cardiopulmonary function. In Anous and Heimbach's recent experience, elderly burned patients (>60 years old) were markedly sensitive to intravenous fluid administration.[150] Although a relationship to congestive heart failure might seem to be most obvious, these authors found that fluid loads in individuals developing pneumonia were higher than in those who died without pulmonary sepsis (205 vs. 156 percent of volumes predicted from Baxter formula). Bacterial pneumonia associated with major burns was invariably fatal. Young children, as well, appear particularly vulnerable to effects of inhalation injury.[152–154] Reasons underlying this predisposition, together with the important modifications in the approach to children are summarized in Chap. 15.

Other groups of patients may also have an increased susceptibility to respiratory problems following burn injury. Purdue and coworkers have documented a high prevalence of respiratory and cardiovascular complications among obese individuals with burns.[155] These included pneumonia (18 percent); atelectasis (6 percent); cardiac arrhythmias (10 percent); unexpected cardiac arrests (2.4 percent); and unanticipated, life-threatening airway complications (2 percent). In our experience, the latter problem can be especially difficult in the obese: not only is the already narrowed upper airway of such patients more susceptible to compromise by edema (i.e., due to less "upper airway reserve") but also the placement of endotracheal tubes is technically more difficult. The accentuated risks of atelectasis, hypostatic pneumonia, and pulmonary embolism have been well recognized in other clinical studies and mandate early preventative measures.

The obese patient also has an increased risk for development (or exacerbation) of alveolar hypoventilation, with the increased mechanical loads posed by thoracoabdominal edema or with splinting. Less often, obstructive sleep apnea has been documented in obese adults and children following burns.[156] Because this latter problem can be worsened by pharyngeal edema and/or the narcotic analgesics required for pain relief, simple periodic bedside observations by nursing staff of breathing are diagnostically informative.

CLASSIFICATIONS OF ACUTE RESPIRATORY INJURY

The devastating impact of inhalation injury demands a systematic strategy for its diagnosis and management. Although a universally accepted approach to classification is not presently in use, several similar systems have been derived from present concepts of the pathogenesis of inhalation injury.[8–10,132,157–159] Consideration of the anatomic level of involvement, the principal mechanism of injury (e.g., thermal vs. chemical), and the time of onset of respiratory distress (early vs. late) all have important implications for management and can be incorporated within a clinically relevant classification system. One practical categorization of problems related to smoke inhalation in burn victims is outlined in Table 2-12. This approach, modified from that promulgated by a consensus committee a decade ago, is, with local variations, applied at a number of centers.[7,147]

Anatomic Classifications

In this text we shall consider asphyxia, upper and lower airway obstruction, and parenchymal injury (pulmonary edema) occurring either alone or in combination as the primary effects of inhalation injury. Although the term *inhalation injury* has been retained in this text, we believe that the type of respiratory problem (when it can be delineated) should be characterized as precisely as possible in such anatomic terms. This approach has more direct relevance in the day-to-day evaluation and management of patients. Furthermore, such an approach is desirable for the more comprehensive reporting of data to better assess prognosis and the worth of new therapeutic regimens. Because these problems do not occur in isolation and are necessarily influenced by systemic responses to accom-

Table 2-12 Anatomic Classification of Smoke Inhalation Injury

Anatomic level of injury	Predominant clinical presentation	Usual timing of onset	Primary mechanism of injury	Principal physiologic presentation(s)
Systemic/neurologic	Obtundation	Early	Chemical	Tissue asphyxia
Conducting airways	Respiratory distress			
Upper		Early	Thermal	Airway obstruction +/− Alveolar hypoventilation
Tracheobronchial		Early	Chemical	Airway obstruction +/− Alveolar hypoventilation; Mild hypoxemia, atelectasis
Parenchymal	Respiratory distress	Delayed	Chemical	Hypoxemic respiratory failure; pulmonary edema

panying cutaneous burns, the presence of preexisting diseases, and the cardiopulmonary effects of therapeutic efforts, other, superimposed problems are commonly present. These, too, should be specified as clearly as possible.

Upper Airway Obstruction As in experimental models, massive pharyngeal edema with airway occlusion accounts for asphyxia in some burn victims dying at the scene of exposure.[160,161] Upper airway obstruction (UAO) on an acute "reflex" basis (e.g., with laryngospasm) also occurs. Less often, the upper airway may be occluded mechanically by soot or aspirated material. Endoscopically confirmed pharyngeal edema is present in approximately 20 to 30 percent of burn victims with clinically diagnosed inhalation injury and has correlated with the severity of smoke exposure (inferred from carboxyhemoglobin levels) and the rate of fluid resuscitation.[162,163] Physiologic evidence of upper airway obstruction occurs even more often, lending support to the bedside notion that dynamic, as well as strictly anatomic, elements of UAO are present. The exact frequency of death due to acute UAO following smoke exposure and burns is unknown. The devastating, rapid progression of upper airway edema to complete occlusion is a classically recognized lethal event, but appropriately low clinical thresholds for elective, prophylactic intubation of individuals at risk seems responsible for the apparently low mortality due to this problem. When fatal UAO occurs, underestimation of the severity of pharyngeal edema, preexisting structural abnormalities of the upper airway, delays in the patient's clinical presentation to medical care, and iatrogenic injuries related to unsuccessful intubation attempts (often performed by the least-experienced member of the managing team) contribute to this catastrophe.

Tracheobronchial Obstruction Histologic observations in a variety of experimental models of smoke inhalation and bronchoscopic findings in acutely injured patients have consistently demonstrated a chemically induced tracheobronchitis that is concentrated in large and medium-sized airways.[164,165] We have found that over half of individuals with clinical risk factors for smoke inhalation injury develop physiologic abnormalities during the initial hours after the exposure indistinguishable from those seen in patients with chronic obstructive pulmonary disease. The pathophysiology of these injuries and their relationships to mechanical obstruction by inspissated secretions, mucosal edema, and bronchospasm are reviewed in Chap. 4. While a commonly observed problem, intractable lower airway obstruction is seldom documented as the cause of death in burned patients with smoke inhalation. We suspect that this relates to the efficacy of mechanical ventilation for hypoventilatory respiratory failure and the reversibility of this inflammatory, reactive problem with time rather than to the documented effectiveness of pharmacologic adjuncts (e.g., bronchodilators). The presence of preexisting airflow obstruction, ranging from asthma or nonspecific airways hyperactivity in younger individuals, to bronchitis and emphysema in older patients, is an important predisposition to severe lower airway responses following smoke inhalation. Systemic humoral responses to burn (e.g., histamine, thromboxane release), as well as direct airway irritation, may also occur in patients with combined injuries. The clinical roles of these responses require clarification.

Atelectasis is another major lower airway problem related to acute smoke inhalation. Inspissated viscid secretions, soot, and cinders may cause radiologically apparent lobar, segmental, and subsegmental atelectasis, resulting in varying degrees of hypoxemia. Roentgenographic documentation of either postobstructive emphysema or volume loss with focal infiltrates was seen in Cocoanut Grove fire victims,[166,167] and the frequency of such often subtle findings has varied among more recent series.[168,169] More often, such changes are detected clinically by the bronchoscopic visualization of airway inflammation, segmental retention of radionuclides, or physiologic measurements of reduced airflow. It has been observed recently that focal pulmonary infiltrates occurring early during the course more often represent atelectasis, while those developing later are more likely due to bacterial pneumonia and often precede frank sepsis.[170] When atelectasis is severe, shunt-related hypoxemia typically occurs. As will be discussed later, radiologically inapparent microatelectasis is a common, instantaneous effect of exposure to smoke. Preexisting impairment of airway clearance and/or chest wall mechanics (e.g., as by COPD), the supine posture (effectively resulting in closure of dependent lung units), impaired cough, and local effects of thoracoabdominal burn are other important predispositions to atelectasis.

Parenchymal (Alveolar) Injury Damage to the alveolar-capillary membrane occurs on the basis of cellular events discussed in Chap. 4. Documentation of physiologic shunt, together with radiologic evidence of pulmonary edema are hallmarks of this form of hypoxemic respiratory failure, described by the general term *adult respiratory distress syndrome* (ARDS). Clinical differentiation of such "permeability" or noncardiogenic edema from congestive heart failure and intravascular fluid overload are major practical considerations. Although pulmonary edema can occur early during the course, generally following exposures to high concentrations of irritants or in relation to catastrophic cardiac injuries, this problem more often has a delayed onset that relates to sepsis. Major factors in its development vary in a predictable manner according to the phases of burn injury, recovery, and treatment[9,10] and are addressed in detail in Chap. 5.

Combined Anatomic/Physiologic Classification

The simple partitioning of the anatomic levels of airway involvement in this manner is useful clinically and has direct implications for the diagnostic and management priorities which must be addressed systematically in each patient. Clinical experience, however, suggests that primary respiratory injury presents a continuum in most patients. Several investigators have observed that proximal airway damage is generally more severe than peripheral injury;[126,128] significant distal lung involvement is less likely to occur in the absence of proximal airway damage. Although occasional patients can present with an isolated parenchymal injury, evidence of more proximal involvement of conducting airways generally precedes the onset of pulmonary edema. Ordinarily such individuals will also have significant upper airway and tracheobronchial injuries with signs, symptoms, and physiologic findings referable to these areas. As a result, diagnostic procedures which focus upon the exclusion of proximal airway injury can, when negative, substantially lower the likelihood that major parenchymal damage due to smoke is present. While this does not exclude delayed-onset ARDS due to combustion products, when signs of parenchymal disease develop in a patient without previous evidence of inhalation injury involvement at other levels, other diagnostic considerations (e.g., cardiogenic edema, fluid overload, septic-related ARDS, pneumonia) would be more likely causes of pulmonary infiltrates.

Current classification approaches do not provide either for the tendencies of patients to present with combinations of anatomic injuries or for gradations in the physiologic severity of the damage occurring at each site. We believe that clinically useful classification of patients with smoke inhalation injury should incorporate these factors. One example of a classification system that takes into account the anatomic level of injury, the propensity for respiratory damage to develop at multiple sites, and the physiologic impact of these injuries is suggested in Table 2-13. With this approach, the grade of respiratory injury is classified according to the anatomic location of damage and whether or not certain arbitrary physiologic indices of severity are present. As with any classification of a dynamic event, it must be appreciated that changes may occur rapidly, and serial reassessment of the patient is essential. Moreover, the rates of deterioration should be expected to differ with the initial clinical grade of injury and with specific sites of involvement. The overall clinical evaluation of the patient's respiratory status must reflect the net effect of multiple lesions, each of which may progress and/or resolve at varying rates.

Patients with Grade 0 injury include individuals who are at risk for respiratory injury—those having smoke exposure (0_S), cutaneous burns (0_B), or their combination (0_{S+B})—but who have no apparent respiratory dysfunction on the basis of widely available parameters listed in Table 2-11. Individuals with any suggestion of respiratory abnormalities would be stratified in grades I to V, in order of increasing severity. Patients at risk who have objectively documented clinical abnormalities but in whom severe evidence of dysfunction is not yet established constitute grade I. As stated earlier, the type of injury should be specified as precisely as possible (i.e., that due to asphyxiant toxicity (I_{Asph}), upper airway dysfunction (I_{UA}), lower airway dysfunction (I_{LA}), or parenchymal dysfunction ($I_{Parench}$),

Table 2-13 Combined Anatomic/Physiologic Classification of Acute Respiratory Injuries following Smoke Inhalation and/or Burns

Grade	Criteria
0	Smoke exposure (0_S), cutaneous burns (0_B), or their combination (0_{S+B}), without clinical evidence of respiratory injury
I	Evidence of either *isolated* asphyxiant exposure (I_{Asph}), upper airway (I_{UA}), lower airway (I_{LA}), or parenchymal ($I_{Parench}$) dysfunction, not meeting criteria for grade II or III
II	Evidence of *combined* respiratory injuries (IIa–IIe), but with no individual component meeting criteria for grade III
	IIa Asph + UA
	IIb UA + LA
	IIc Asph + UA + LA
	IId UA + LA + Parench
	IIe Asph + UA + LA + Parench
III	Any isolated or combined injury in which one of the following is present
	IIIa COHb ≥ 20%, CN >0.2 mg/L, or any elevation of COHb and/or CN with neurologic dysfunction
	IIIb Stridor, physiologic or endoscopic evidence of UAO
	IIIc Alveolar hypoventilation ($Pa_{CO_2} \geq 45$ mmHg) present
	IIId Major shunt-related hypoxemia ($Pa_{O_2}/FI_{O_2} \leq 250$) present
IV	Combined injuries (as in grade II) in which two or more criteria in III are present
V	Injuries with which respiratory arrest has occurred

ABBREVIATIONS: Asph = Asphyxiant, UA = upper airway dysfunction, LA = lower airway dysfunction, Parench = parenchymal dysfunction.

and only one of these sites should be involved. Patients with carbon monoxide or cyanide intoxication should have relatively low levels (COHb < 20 percent, CN <0.2 mg/L), with no evidence of neurologic dysfunction. Patients with upper airway injury should not have either stridor, endoscopic evidence of UAO, or physiologic signs of UAO (flow volume curves demonstrating reduced inspiratory flow rates; see Chap. 7). Alveolar hypoventilation should not be present (i.e., arterial blood gas analyses should demonstrate a normal or low Pa_{CO_2} [less than 45 mmHg]) and measurements of oxygenation demonstrate a Pa_{O_2}/FI_{O_2} ratio exceeding 250. (For example, for a patient inspiring 50% oxygen, a Pa_{O_2} would be expected to exceed 300 mmHg.) When injuries at multiple anatomic levels of injury are identified but these physiologic limits suggesting severe dysfunction at any one level have not been exceeded, the patient is categorized as having grade II injury.

Patients with grade III injuries are commonly encountered, and increased hazards are apparent from their many abnormal objective findings. Thus, elevated carboxyhemoglobin levels $\geq$20 percent, CN $\geq$0.2 mg/L, or the presence of neurologic dysfunction with documentation of these asphyxiants constitute a high risk situation. Similarly, the presence of objectively diagnosed UAO in this clinical setting is an immediate life-threatening problem that demands prompt recognition and response. The presence of *any* acute alveolar hypoventilation is inappropriate for these circumstances, and identifies patients who will require mechanical ventilatory support or, at the very least, cautious monitoring. The documentation of shunt-related hypoxemia, suggested arbitrarily by a reduced Pa_{O_2}/FI_{O_2} ($\leq$250), implies that major airspace disease (i.e., pulmonary edema) or high-grade, proximal airway obstruction with atelectasis is already established. When two or more physiologic limits of severity are present, or when frank respiratory arrest has occurred, patients are classified in grades IV and V, respectively. The gravity of the situation and ominous prognosis are usually obvious in these latter groups.

We believe that for the practicing clinician, such a system that combines historic concepts of the anatomic levels of respiratory involvement with objective, widely available physiologic information is highly desirable. More complete specification of the severity of injury using such a system should enhance the communication of research investigations of these patient populations. Although the limits suggested as indicators of physiologic severity are arbitrary, clinical experience suggests that these are reasonable markers of gross injury. Further prospective investigation should assess the optimum "cutoff points" of each of these parameters, to more accurately identify patients with special risks. As with any classification attempt, this approach to acute respiratory injuries following smoke inhalation and burns requires critical reevaluation and refinement. Alternative approaches can and should be designed and investigated, and it must be documented whether such an approach leads to improved patient outcomes.

Furthermore, any classification approach must be reappraised and modified to accommodate inevitable clinical changes that will occur in the future. The currently appreciated respiratory problems in burn victims cannot be expected to remain static but will change with time. Alterations of the fire environment (and combinations of toxic products) will have an impact on the likelihood of inhalation injury; the success of ongoing efforts to prevent exposures will influence the risks confronted by burn victims. Current problems may be alleviated, and in all likelihood new problems will be introduced by further innovations in care. Some entirely new clinical dilemmas might be expected to surface. For example, it has recently been recognized that approximately 10 percent of burned patients admitted to one urban center were found to have serologic confirmation of human immunodeficiency virus (HIV) infection, an observation consistent with an increased prevalence of HIV disease in trauma victims.[171] The diverse pulmonary problems seen in this compromised population in other settings might be expected to occur when these patients are hospitalized for management of burns.

Implications for Therapy

The relationship of major therapeutic priorities to anatomic and physiologic grades of injury are outlined in Table 2-14.[132,172–178] The individual components of respiratory injury and their management are reviewed in detail in other chapters. Early therapy focuses on maintaining a patent upper airway by means of elective endotracheal intubation. Mechanical clearance and pharmacologic dilatation of

Table 2-14 Basic Therapeutic Priorities in Patients with Inhalation Injury*

Respiratory problem	Response(s)
Asphyxia	Oxygenation, antidotes
Upper airway obstruction	Early, elective endotracheal intubation (rarely, tracheostomy)
Lower airway obstruction	
Mild	Pulmonary toilet
	Bronchodilators
	Occasional therapeutic bronchoscopy
Severe (with hypoventilatory failure)	Mechanical ventilation
Parenchymal injury	
Mild	Supplemental oxygen (e.g., low FI_{O_2} achievable by nasal prongs/mask delivery systems)
Severe (with hypoxemic respiratory failure)	Oxygenate (High FI_{O_2} [O_2 via ET tube])
	Increase lung volume (CPAP, PEEP)
	Minimize ongoing leak (e.g., experimental use of antioxidants)
	? Adjustments of resuscitative fluid volumes, composition, and infusion rates

*Reviewed in detail in Chap. 9.

obstructed lower airways is also part of standard care although based upon somewhat scanty documentation of the efficacy of particular maneuvers. When severe lower airway obstruction is present (usually with associated combined hypoxemic and hypoventilatory respiratory failure), mechanical ventilation is a well-established, life-saving modality. While some individuals with mild parenchymal injury may be managed entirely with supplemental oxygen concentrations achievable by mask delivery, patients with severe alveolar capillary membrane damage require combinations of oxygen and continuous positive airway pressure delivered by mechanical ventilator. Efforts to minimize the ongoing leak, both by limiting hydrostatic pressures and by addressing the basic causes of increased permeability, are desirable, but optimum approaches in these areas remain problematic.

Because of the gradations of severity of inhalation injury, not all patients with respiratory distress following burns will require either intubation or mechanical ventilation. In Clark's large series, 38 percent of individuals with smoke inhalation or smoke exposure and burns did not require endotracheal intubation, while the remaining 62 percent did.[22] Patients without apparent inhalation injury accounted for only 5 percent of intubations at this busy burn center. Because most patients who experience smoke inhalation alone either experience self-limited sequelae that require little, if any, medical attention or, following severe exposures, die at the scene of exposure, precise information about these individuals is sparse. On the other hand, epidemiologic studies of fire fighters with either acute or chronic exposures have shown broad variations in individual responses to smoke.

As can be seen in Table 2-13, grade III severity represents a critical level at which the need for major interventions (endotracheal intubation, mechanical ventilation, PEEP) is already established. Grades I and II represent earlier, transitional stages at which less intensive immediate care may be required but from which progressive deterioration should be anticipated. The combination of these respiratory injuries with major burns heightens the risk for the patient: for example, grade II patients who have large burns are at great risk to deteriorate. The elective, prophylactic respiratory support of such individuals *before* they evolve to grades III through V is generally preferred.

COMMENTS

The most salient feature of smoke inhalation injury in burned patients is its heterogeneity: individual variations in exposure scenarios and host responses, differences in the relative contributions of primary pulmonary damage or secondary effects of burns, and diverse clinical responses to therapy present major limitations and challenges for clinicians. Fortunately, the recuperative powers of the lung result in favorable outcomes in those patients whose physiologic reserves are not prohibitively limited and in whom timely, albeit nonspecific, supportive therapy is begun.

Smoke inhalation and cutaneous burns can each cause respiratory dysfunction, and each of these injuries predisposes to yet other problems. There has been compelling support for roles of polymorphonuclear leukocytes and toxic free oxygen radicals in the pathogenesis of smoke inhalation, burns, and sepsis. Such similarities in the cellular and physiologic responses to these disparate injuries (Table 2-2) suggest that the response to any one stimulus might be augmented by the others, but the precise clinical differentiation of the contributions of these events in individual patients is not yet feasible. The similarities of the experimental and clinically observed responses to each of these insults also suggest that they represent stereotypic, nonspecific pulmonary responses to a variety of stimuli. Optimistically, future clarification of cellular and molecular events will provide a basis for improved clinical classification systems and will lead to more specific and effective therapeutic interventions. Until more precise information about such cellular mechanisms is available in humans, however, clinicians remain limited to the recognition and nonspecific treatment of the respiratory dysfunction that ensues. In this effort, familiarity with the anatomic and physiologic manifestations of inhalation injury is essential to management.

REFERENCES

1. Cope O: Management of the Cocoanut Grove burns at the Massachusetts General Hospital. *Ann Surg* 117:801, 1943.
2. Cope O, Rhinelander FW: The problem of burn shock complicated by pulmonary damage. *Ann Surg* 117:915, 1943.
3. Finland M, Davidson CS, Levenson SM: Clinical and therapeutic aspects of conflagration injuries to respiratory tract sustained by victims of Cocoanut Grove disaster. *Medicine* 25:215, 1946.
4. Thomsen M: It all began with Aristotle—the history of the treatment of burns. *Burns* 14 (suppl 1), 1988.
5. Aub JC, Pittman H, Brues AM: The pulmonary complications: A clinical description. *Ann Surg* 117:834, 1943.
6. Phillips AW, Tanner JW, Cope O: Burn Therapy. IV. Respiratory tract damage (an account of the clinical, x-ray and postmortem findings) and the meaning of restlessness. *Ann Surg* 158:799, 1963.
7. Powers SR: Consensus summary on smoke inhalation. *J Trauma* 19:921, 1979.
8. Achauer BM, Allyn PA, Furnas DW, Bartlett RH: Pulmonary complications of burns: The major threat to the burn patient. *Ann Surg* 177:311, 1972.
9. Haponik EF, Summer WR: Respiratory complications in burned patients: pathogenesis and spectrum of inhalation injury. *J Crit Care* 2:49, 1987.
10. Haponik EF, Summer WR: Respiratory complications in burned patients: diagnosis and management of inhalational injury. *J Crit Care* 2:121, 1987.
11. Haponik EF, Crapo RO, Traber DL, et al: Smoke inhalation. *Am Rev Respir Dis* 138:1060, 1988.
12. Loke J, Matthay RA, Smith GJW: The toxic environment and its medical implications with special emphasis on smoke inhalation, in Loke J (ed): *Pathophysiology and Treatment of Inhalation Injuries*, New York, Marcel Dekker, 1988, p 453.
13. Davies JWL: Toxic chemicals versus lung tissue—an aspect of inhalation injury revisited. *J Burn Care Rehabil* 7:213, 1986.
14. Demling RH: Burns. *N Engl J Med* 313:1389, 1985.
15. DiVincenti FC, Pruitt BA, Reckler JM: Inhalation injuries. *J Trauma* 11:109, 1971.
16. Pruitt BA, Flemma RJ, DiVincenti FC, et al: Pulmonary complications in burn patients. *J Thorac Cardiovasc Surg* 59:7, 1970.
17. Pruitt BA, DiVincenti FC, Mason AD, et al. The occurrence and significance of pneumonia and other pulmonary complications in burned patients: Comparison of

conventional and topical treatments. *J Trauma* 10:519, 1970.

18. Pruitt BA, Erickson DR, Morris A: Progressive pulmonary insufficiency and other pulmonary complications of thermal injury. *J Trauma* 15:369, 1975.
19. Heimbach DM, Waeckerle JF: Inhalation injuries. *Ann Emerg Med* 17:1316, 1988.
20. Cahalane M, Demling RH: Early respiratory abnormalities from smoke inhalation. *JAMA* 251:771, 1984.
21. Clark CJ, Reid WH, Gilmour WH, Campbell D: Mortality probability in victims of fire trauma: Revised equation to include inhalation injury. *Br Med J* 292:1303, 1986.
22. Clark WR, Bonaventurea M, Myers W: Smoke inhalation and airway management at a regional burn unit, 1974–1983, Part I: Diagnosis and consequences of smoke inhalation. *J Burn Care Rehabil* 10:52, 1989.
23. Clark WR, Fromm BS: Burn mortality: Experience at a regional burn unit, Literature review. *Acta Chir Scand* 537[suppl]:1, 1987.
24. Clark WR, Nieman, GF: Smoke inhalation. *Burns* 14:473, 1988.
25. Fein A, Leff A, Hopewell PC: Pathophysiology and management of the complications resulting from fire and the inhaled products of combustion: Review of the literature. *Crit Care Med* 8:94, 1980.
26. Silverman P: The advent of prospective payment: How DRGs could affect burn centers. *J Burn Care Rehabil* 5:301, 1984.
27. Hunt JL, Purdue GF: Cost containment/cost reduction: The economic impact of burn DRGs. *J Burn Care Rehabil* 6:417, 1986.
28. Markley K: Burn care: Infection and smoke inhalation. *Ann Intern Med* 90:269, 1979.
29. Sanderson LM, Buffler PA, Pery RR, Blackwell SJ: A multivariate evaluation of determinants of length of stay in a hospital burn unit. *J Burn Care Rehabil* 2:142, 1981.
30. Kinsella J: Smoke inhalation. *Burns* 14:269, 1988.
31. Witten ML, Quan SF, Sobonya RE, Lemen RJ: New developments in the pathogenesis of smoke inhalation induced pulmonary edema. *West J Med* 148:33, 1988.
32. Herndon DN, Barrow RE, Traber DL, et al: Extravascular lung water changes following smoke inhalation and massive burn injury. *Surgery* 102:341, 1987.
33. Herndon DN, Thompson PB, Linares HA, Traber DL: Postgraduate course: Respiratory injury Part I: Incidence, mortality, pathogenesis and treatment of pulmonary injury. *J Burn Care Rehabil* 7:184, 1986.
34. Demling RH, Wong C, Jin L, et al: Early lung dysfunction after major burns: Role of edema and vasoactive mediators. *J Trauma* 25:959, 1985.
35. Demling RH, Will JA, Belzer FO: Effect of major thermal injury on the pulmonary microcirculation. *Surgery* 83:746, 1978.
36. Grosso MA, Viders DE, Brown JM, et al: Local skin burn causes systemic (lung and kidney) endothelial cell injury, reflected by increased circulating and decreased tissue factor VIII–related antigen. *Surgery* 106:310, 1989.
37. Demling RH, Manohar M, Will JA: Relation between pulmonary transvascular fluid filtration rate and measured Starling's forces after major burn. *Chest* 76:448, 1979.
38. Stephenson SF, Esrig BC, Polk HC, Fulton RL: The pathophysiology of smoke inhalation injury. *Ann Surg* 182:652, 1975.
39. Zikria BA, Sturner WQ, Astarjian NK, et al: Respiratory tract damage in burns: Pathophysiology and therapy. *Ann New York Acad Sci* 150:618, 1968.
40. Robinson NB, Hudson LD, Robertson HT, et al: Ventilation and perfusion alterations after smoke inhalation injury. *Surgery* 90:352, 1981.
41. Burke JF: The sequence of events following smoke inhalation. *J Trauma* 21:721, 1981.
42. Ward PA: The role of complement system in smoke inhalation. *J Trauma* 21:722, 1981.
43. Dressler DP: Laboratory background on smoke inhalation. *J Trauma* 19:913, 1979.
44. Nieman GF, Clark WR, Goyette BS, et al: Wood smoke inhalation increases pulmonary microvascular permeability. *Surgery* 98:481, 1989.
45. Traber DL, Linares HA, Herndon DN: The pathophysiology of inhalation injury—a review. *Burns* 14:357, 1988.
46. Kramer GC, Herndon, DN, Linares HA, Traber DL: Effects of inhalation injury on airway blood flow and edema formation. *JCBR,* 10:45, 1989.
47. Dehring DJ, Doty S, Kimura R, et al: Effect of preexisting inhalation injury on response to bacteremia in sheep. *J Burn Care Rehabil* 9:467, 1988.
48. Linares HA, Herndon DN, Traber DL: Sequence of morphologic events in experiemental smoke inhalation. *J Burn Care Rehabil* 10:27, 1989.
49. Traber DL, Schlag G, Redl H, Traber LD: Pulmonary edema and compliance changes following smoke inhalation. *J Burn Care Rehabil* 6:490, 1985.
50. Harms BA, Kramer GC, Bodai BI, Demling RH: Effect of hypoproteinemia on pulmonary and soft tissue edema formation. *Crit Care Med* 9:503, 1981.
51. Demling RH, Niehaus G, Perea A, Will J: Effect of burn-induced hypoproteinemia on pulmonary transvascular fluid filtration rate. *Surgery* 85:339, 1979.
52. Harms BA, Bodai BI, Kramer GC, Demling RH: Microvascular fluid and protein flux in pulmonary and systemic circulation after thermal injury. *Microvasc Res* 23:77, 1982.
53. Harms BA, Bodai BI, Smith M, et al: Prostaglandin release and altered microvascular integrity after burn injury. *J Surg Res* 31:274, 1981.
54. Demling RH, Kramer GC, Gunther R, Nerlich M: Effect of non-protein colloid on postburn edema formation in soft tissues and lung. *Surgery* 95:593, 1984.
55. Demling RH, Kramer G, Harms B: Role of thermal injury–induced hypoproteinemia on fluid flux and protein permeability in burned and nonburned tissue. *Surgery* 95:136, 1984.
56. Meredith JW, Martin MB, Poole GV, et al: Measurement of extravascular lung water in sheep during colloid and crystalloid resuscitation from smoke inhalation. *Am Surg* 49:637, 1983.

57. Thorning DR, Howard ML, Hudson LD, Schumacher RL: Pulmonary responses to smoke inhalation: Morphologic changes in rabbits exposed to pine wood smoke. *Hum Pathol* 13:355, 1982.
58. Herndon DN, Thompson PB, Brown M, Traber DL: Diagnosis, pathophysiology, and treatment of inhalation injury, in Boswick JA (ed): *The Art and Science of Burn Care*. Rockville, MD, Aspen Publishers, 1987.
59. Moylan JA: Inhalation injury—A primary determinant of survival following major burns. *J Burn Care Rehabil* 1:81, 1979.
60. Thompson P, Herndon DN, Abston S, Rutan T: Effect of early excision on patients with major thermal injury. *J Trauma* 27:205, 1987.
61. Herndon DH, Barrow RE, Rutan RL, et al: A comparison of conservative versus early excision therapies in severely burned patients. *Ann Surg* 209:547, 1989.
61a. Nieman GF, Clark WR, Wax SD, Webb WR: The effect of smoke inhalation on pulmonary surfactant. *Ann Surg* 191:171, 1980.
62. Herndon DH, Traber DL, Nichaus GD, et al: The pathophysiology of smoke inhalation in a sheep model. *J Trauma* 24:1044, 1981.
63. Herndon DH, Barrow RE, Linares HA, et al: Inhalation-injury in burned patients: Effects and treatment. *Burns* 14:349, 1988.
64. Demarest GB, Hudson LD, Altman LC: Impaired alveolar macrophage chemotaxis in patients with acute smoke inhalation. *Am Rev Respir Dis* 119:279, 1979.
65. Fick RB, Paul ES, Merill WW, et al: Alternations in the antibacterial properties of rabbit pulmonary macrophages exposed to wood smoke. *Am Rev Respir Dis* 129:76, 1984.
66. Alexander JW, Ogle CK, Stinnett JD, MacMillan BG: A sequential, prospective analysis of immunologic abnormalities and infection following severe thermal injury. *Ann Surg* 188:809, 1978.
67. Skornik WA, Dressler DP: Lung bacterial clearance in the burned rat. *Ann Surg* 172:837, 1979.
68. Heiderman M: The effect of thermal injury on hemodynamic, respiratory, and hematologic variables in relation to complement activation. *J Trauma* 19:239, 1979.
69. Gelfand JA, Donelan M, Burke JF: Preferential activation and depletion of the alternative complement pathway by burn injury. *Ann Surg* 198:58, 1983.
70. Munster AM, Winchurch RA: Infection and immunology. *Crit Care Clin* 1:119, 1985.
71. Moran K, Munster AM: Alterations of the host defense mechanism in burned patients. *Surg Clin North Am* 67(1): 47, 1987.
72. Heideman M: The effect of thermal injury on hemodynamic, respiratory, and hematologic variables in relation to complement activation. *J Trauma* 19:239, 1979.
73. Shirani KZ, Pruitt BA, Mason AD: The influence of inhalation injury and pneumonia on burn mortality. *Ann Surg* 205:82, 1987.
74. Merrell SW, Saffle JR, Larson CM, Sullivan JJ: The declining incidence of fatal sepsis following thermal injury. *J Trauma* 29:1362, 1989.
75. Demling R: Postgraduate course: Respiratory Injury Part III: Pulmonary dysfunction in the burn patient. *J Burn Care Rehabil* 7:277, 1986.
76. Wenger H, Wong C, Demling RH: Pulmonary dysfunction secondary to soft-tissue endotoxin. *Arch Surg* 120:159, 1985.
77. Katz A, Ryan P, Lalonde C, et al: Topical ibuprofen decreases thromboxane release from endotoxin-stimulated burn wound. *J Trauma* 26:157, 1986.
78. Demling RH, Wenger H, Lalonde CC, et al: Endotoxin-induced prostanoid production by the burn wound can cause distant lung dysfunction. *Surgery* 99:421, 1986.
79. Demling RH, Smith M, Bodai B: Comparison of postburn capillary permeability in soft tissue and lung. *J Burn Care Rehabil* 1:86, 1981.
80. Demling RH, Crawford G, Lind L, Read T: Restrictive pulmonary dysfunction caused by the grafted chest and abdominal burn. *Crit Care Med* 16:743, 1988.
81. Quinby WC: Restrictive effects of thoracic burns in children. *J Trauma* 12:646, 1972.
82. Whitener DR, Whitener LM, Robertson J, et al: Pulmonary function measurements in patients with thermal injury and smoke inhalation. *Am Rev Respir Dis* 122:731, 1980.
83. Wong C, Wenger H, Demling RH: Effect of a body burn on the lung response to endotoxin. *J Trauma* 25:53, 1985.
84. Demling RH: Effect of early burn excision and grafting on pulmonary function. *J Trauma* 24:830, 1984.
85. Demling RH, Wenger H, Lalonde CC, et al: Endotoxin-induced prostanoid production by the burn wound can cause distant lung dysfunction. *Surgery* 99:421, 1986.
86. Demling RH, Katz A, Lalonde C: The effect of immediate and delayed burn wound excision on pulmonary function. *J Crit Care* 1:54, 1986.
87. Demling RH, LaLonde C, Lio Y, Zhu D: The lung inflammatory response to thermal injury: Relationship between physiologic and histologic changes. *Surgery* 106:42, 1989.
88. Moore FD, Davis C, Rodrick M, et al: Neutrophil activation in thermal injury as assessed by increased expression of complement receptors. *N Engl J Med* 314:948, 1986.
89. Till GO, Beauchamp C, Menapace D, et al: Oxygen radical dependent lung damage following thermal injury of rat skin. *J Trauma* 23:269, 1983.
90. Till GO, Hatherill JR, Tourtellet WW, et al: Lipid peroxidation and acute lung injury after thermal trauma to skin: Evidence of a role for hydroxyl radical. *Am J Pathol* 119:376, 1985.
91. Nerlich M, Flynn J, Demling RH: Effect of thermal injury on endotoxin-induced lung injury. *Surgery* 93:289, 1983.
92. Pruitt BA Jr: Sepsis and survival in burn patients. *J Intensive Care Med* 2:294, 1987.
93. Hansbrough JF: Burn wound sepsis. *J Intensive Care Med* 2:313, 1987.
94. Colice GL, Munster AM, Haponik EF: Tracheal stenosis complicating cutaneous burns: An understanding problem. *Am Rev Respir Dis* 134:1315, 1986.
95. Lund T, Goodwin CW, McManus WF, et al: Upper air-

way sequelae in burn patients requiring endotracheal intubation or tracheostomy. *Ann Surg* 201:374, 1985.

96. Jones WG, Madden M, Finkelstein J, et al: Tracheostomies in burn patients. *Ann Surg* 209:471, 1989.
97. Demling RH: Fluid and electrolyte management. *Crit Care Clin* 1:27, 1985.
98. Demling RH: Fluid replacement in burned patients. *Surg Clin North Am* 67:15, 1987.
99. Goodwin CW, Dorethy J, Lam V, Pruitt BA: Randomized trial of efficacy of crystalloid and colloid resuscitation on hemodynamic response and lung water following thermal injury. *Ann Surg* 197:250, 1983.
100. Rubin WD, Mani MM, Hiebert JM: Fluid resuscitation of the thermally injured patient: Current concepts with definition of clinical subsets and their specialized treatment. *Clin Plast Surg* 13:9, 1986.
101. Baxter CR: Fluid volume and electrolyte changes of the early postburn period. *Clin Plast Surg* 1:693, 1974.
102. Martyn JAJ, Burke JF: Is there a selective increase in pulmonary capillary permeability following cutaneous burns? *Chest* 76:374, 1979.
103. Scheulen JJ, Munster AM: The Parkland formula in patients with burns and inhalation injury. *J Trauma* 22:869, 1982.
104. Navar PD, Saffle JR, Warden GD: Effect of inhalation injury on fluid resuscitation requirements after thermal injury. *Am J Surg* 150:716, 1985.
105. Baxter CR: Guidelines for fluid resuscitation. *J Trauma* 21:687, 1981.
106. Carlson RG, Miller SF, Finley RK, et al: Fluid retention and burn survival. *J Trauma* 27:127, 1987.
107. Tolmie JD, Joyce TH, Mitchell GD: Succinylcholine danger in the burned patient. *Anesthesiology* 28:467, 1967.
108. Bush GH, Graham HAP, Littlewood AHM, et al: Danger of suxamethonium and endotracheal intubation in anaesthesia for burns. *Br Med J* 2:1081, 1962.
109. Huang V, Figge H, Demling R: Haloperidol complications in burn patients. *J Burn Care Rehabil* 8:269, 1987.
110. Petroff PA, Hander EW, Mason AD: Ventilatory patterns following burn injury and effect of sulfamylon. *J Trauma* 15:650, 1975.
111. Jin LJ, Lalonde C, Demling RH: Effect of anesthesia and positive pressure ventilation on early postburn hemodynamic instability. *J Trauma* 26:26, 1986.
112. Grube BJ, Marvin JA, Heimbach DM: Therapeutic hyperbaric oxygen: Help or hindrance in burn patients with carbon monoxide poisoning? *J Burn Care Rehabil* 9:249, 1988.
113. Dimick AR, Potts LH, Shaw SE, et al: Ten-year profile of 1,271 burn patients. *J Burn Care Rehabil* 6:341, 1985.
114. Venus B, Matsuda T, Copiozo JB, et al: Prophylactic intubation and continuous positive airway pressure in the management of inhalation injury in burn victims. *Crit Care Med* 9:519, 1981.
115. Clark WR, Nieman GF, Goyette D, Gryzboski D: Effects of crystalloid on lung fluid balance after smoke inhalation. *Ann Surg* 208:56, 1988.
116. Summer WR, Haponik EF: Inhalation of irritant gases. *Clin Chest Med* 2:273, 1981.
117. Moylan JA, Alexander G: Diagnosis and treatment of inhalation injury. *World J Surg* 2:185, 1978.
118. Moylan JA: Inhalation injury. *J Trauma* 21:720, 1981.
119. Boutros AR, Hoyt JL, Boyd WC, Hartford CE: Algorithm for management of pulmonary complications in burn patients. *Crit Care Med* 5:89, 1977.
120. Trunkey DD: Inhalation injury. *Surg Clin North Am* 58:1133, 1978.
121. Inhalation injury: No mere puff of smoke. *Lancet* 2:849, 1984.
122. Zawacki BE, Jung RC, Joyce J, et al: Smoke, burns, and the natural history of inhalation injury in fire victims: A correlation of experimental and clinical data. *Ann Surg* 185:100, 1977.
123. Horovitz JH: Diagnostic tools for use in smoke inhalation. *J Trauma* 21:717, 1981.
124. Bingham HG, Gallagher TJ, Powerll MD: Early bronchoscopy as a predictor of ventilatory support for burned patients. *J Trauma* 27:1286, 1987.
125. Moylan JA, Wilmore DW, Mouton DE, Pruitt BA: Early diagnosis of inhalation injury using 133 xenon lung scan. *Ann Surg* 176:477, 1972.
126. Head JM: Inhalation injury in burns. *Am J Surg* 139:508, 1980.
127. Moylan JA, Chan CK: Inhalation injury—an increasing problem. *Ann Surg* 188:34, 1977.
128. Hunt JL, Agee RN, Pruitt BA: Fiberoptic bronchoscopy in acute inhalation injury. *J Trauma* 15:641, 1975.
129. Agee RN, Long JM, Hunt JL, et al: Use of ^{133}Xenon in early diagnosis of inhalation injury. *J Trauma* 16:216, 1976.
130. Schall GL, McDonald HD, Carr LB, et al: Xenon ventilation-perfusion lung scans: The early diagnosis of inhalation injury. *JAMA* 240:2441, 1978.
131. Wroblewski DA, Bower GC: The significance of facial burns in acute smoke inhalation. *Crit Care Med* 7:335, 1979.
132. Artz CP, Moncrief JA, Pruitt BA: *Burns: A Team Approach*. Philadelphia, Saunders, 1979.
133. Cox ME, Heslop BF, Kempton JJ, et al: The Dellwood fire. *Br J Med* 942, 1955.
134. Robinson NB, Hudson LD, Riem M, et al: Steroid therapy following isolated smoke inhalation injury. *J Trauma* 22:876, 1982.
135. Miller EJ: Management of patients with smoke inhalation: The Las Vegas experience, in O'Donohue WJ (ed): *Current Advantages in Respiratory Care*. Park Ridge, IL, American College of Chest Physicians, 1984.
136. Layton TR, Elhauge ER: U.S. fire catastrophes of the 20th century. *J Burn Care Rehabil* 3:21, 1982.
137. Mallory TN, Brickley WJ: Pathology: With special reference to the pulmonary lesions. *Ann Surg* 117:865, 1943.
138. Sochor FM, Mallory GK: Lung lesions in patients dying of burns. *Arch Pathol* 75:303, 1963.
139. Foley FD, Moncrief JA, Mason AD: Pathology of the lung in fatally burned patients. *Ann Surg* 167:251, 1968.
140. Nash G, Foley FD, Langlinais PC: Pulmonary interstitial edema and hyaline membranes in adult burn patients:

Electron microscopic observations. *Hum Pathol* 5:149, 1974.
141. Foley FD: The burn autopsy: Fatal complications of burns. *Am J Clin Pathol* 52:1, 1985.
142. Merrell SW, Saffle JR, Sullivan JJ, et al: Increased survival after major thermal injury: A nine year review. *Am J Surg* 154:623, 1987.
143. Curreri PW, Luterman A, Braun DW, Shires GT: Burn injury: Analysis of survival and hospitalization time for 937 patients. *Ann Surg* 192:472, 1980.
144. Herndon DN, Thompson PB, Traber DL: Pulmonary injury in burned patients. *Crit Care Clin* 1:79, 1985.
145. Thompson PB, Herndon DN, Traber DL, Abstron S: Effect on mortality of inhalation injury. *J Trauma* 26:163, 1986.
146. Zawacki BE, Azen SP, Imbus SH, Chang YTC: Multifactorial probit analysis of mortality in burned patients. *Ann Surg* 189:1, 1979.
147. Marshall WG Jr, Dimick AR: The natural history of major burns with multiple subsystem failure. *J Trauma* 23(2):102, 1983.
148. Monafo WW, Robinson HN, Yoshioka T, Ayvazian VH: Lethal burns: A progress report. *Arch Surg* 113:397, 1978.
149. Manktelow A, Meyer AA, Herzog SR, Peterson HD: Analysis of life expectancy and living status of elderly patients surviving a burn injury. *J Trauma* 29:203, 1989.
150. Anous MM, Heimbach DM: Causes of death and predictors in burned patients more than 60 years of age. *J Trauma* 26:135, 1986.
151. Baux S, Mimoun M, Saade H, Lioret M, et al: Burns in the elderly. *Burns* 15:239, 1989.
152. Vivori E, Cudmore RE: Management of airway complications of burns in children. *Br Med J* 2:1462, 1977.
153. Stone HH: Pulmonary burns in children. *J Ped Surg* 14:48, 1979.
154. Cudmore RE, Vivori E: Inhalation injury to the respiratory tract of children. *Prog Pediatr Surg* 14:173, 1981.
155. Purdue GF, Hunt JL, Lang ED: Obesity: A risk factor in the burn patient. Proceedings of American Burn Association, 1989, p. 115.
156. Robertson CF, Zuker R, Dabrowski MSc, Levison H: Obstructive sleep apnea: A complication of burns to the head and neck in children. *J Burn Care Rehabil* 6:353, 1985.
157. Stone HH, Reame DW, Corbitt JD, et al: Respiratory burns: A correlation of clinical and laboratory results. *Am Surg* 165:157, 1967.
158. Bartlett RH: Types of respiratory injury. *J Trauma* 19:918, 1979.
159. Chi-Shing C: New concepts of pulmonary burn injury. *J Trauma* 21:958, 1981.
160. Bartlett RH, Niccole M, Tavis MJ, et al: Acute management of the upper airway in facial burns and smoke inhalation. *Arch Surg* 111:744, 1976.
161. Waymack JP, Law E, Park R, et al: Acute upper airway obstruction in the postburn period. *Arch Surg* 120:1042, 1985.
162. Haponik EF, Munster AM, Wise RA, et al: Upper airway function in burn patients: Correlation of flow-volume curves and nasopharyngoscopy. *Am Rev Respir Dis* 129:251, 1984.
163. Haponik EF, Meyers DA, Munster AM, et al: Acute upper airway injury in burn patients: Serial changes of flow-volume curves and nasopharyngoscopy. *Am Rev Respir Dis* 135:360, 1987.
164. Thorning DR, Howard ML, Hudson LD, et al: Pulmonary responses to smoke inhalation: Morphologic changes in rabbits exposed to pine wood smoke. *Hum Pathol* 13:355, 1982.
165. Weil RB, Capozi A, Falces E, et al: Smoke inhalation study. *Ann Plast Surg* 4:121, 1980.
166. Schatzki R: Roentgenologic report of the pulmonary lesions. *Ann Surg* 117:841, 1943.
167. Finland M, Rivto M, Davidson CS, Levenson SM: Roentgenologic findings in the lungs of victims of the Cocoanut Grove disaster. *Am J Roentgenol* 55:1, 1946.
168. Teixidor HS, Rubin E, Novick GS, Alonso DR: Smoke inhalation: Radiologic manifestations. *Radiology* 149:383, 1983.
169. Peitzman AB, Shires GT, Teixidor HS, et al: Smoke inhalation injury: Evaluation of radiographic manifestations an pulmonary dysfunction. *J Trauma* 29:1232, 1989.
170. Kundel KR, Barrow RE, Rubin SA, et al: Early densities in chest x-rays in pure thermal injuries are not due to increased extravascular lung water. Proceedings of American Burn Association, 1989, p. 189.
171. Hammong J, Ward CG: The occurrence of acquired immunodeficiency syndrome and unsuspected human immunodeficiency virus in burn patients. *J Burn Care Rehabil* 1:156, 1989.
172. Munster AM: The early management of thermal burns. *Surgery* 87:29, 1980.
173. Wachtel TL: Epidemiology, classification, initial care, and administrative considerations for critically burned patients. *Crit Care Clin* 1:3, 1985.
174. Wachtel TL, Frank DH, Frank HA: Management of burns of the head and neck. *Head Neck Surg* 3:458, 1981.
175. Boutros AR, Hoyt JL: Management of carbon monoxide posioning in the absence of hyperbaric oxygenation chamber. *Crit Care Med* 4:144, 1976.
176. Wald PH, Balmes JR. Respiratory effects of short-term, high-intensity toxic inhalations: Smoke, gases, and fumes. *J Intensive Care Med* 2:260, 1987.
177. Wallfisch HK: Part IV: Bedside management and weaning of the burn patient on mechanical ventilation. *J Burn Care Rehabil* 7:285, 1986.
178. Madden MR, Finkelstein JL, Goodwin CW: Respiratory care of the burn patient. *Clin Plast Surg* 13:29, 1986.

Chapter 3

Causes of Respiratory Injury

Robert O. Crapo

DEFINITION

Smoke is a generic term used to describe the gases and suspended particulate matter associated with fires. It includes all noxious materials that can result in inhalation injuries in fires. Such materials may be produced by combustion or by pyrolysis (chemical decomposition as a result of heat).[1] As technology advances, the number and kinds of materials — and thus the components of smoke — continue to increase. The exact composition of smoke (gases and particulate matter) is determined by the materials being burned, the temperature, the rate at which temperature rises, the humidity, the duration of the exposure to the heat, and the amount of oxygen present (Table 3-1).[2–4]

The extraordinary and lethal nature of smoke inhalation is graphically presented by Davies in a summary of 24 papers, many of which reported studies of the 1981 Stardust Nightclub fire that killed 48 people in Dublin.[5] The portion of the night club where the fire started was reconstructed and burned, this time with numerous monitors in place. The results were staggering. Within minutes, the temperature close to the fire reached 1160°C, and smoke production exceeded 1000 m^3/min. Visibility dropped to less than a meter within 1 minute. In the area close to the fire, oxygen concentrations sank to less than 2 percent, carbon monoxide concentrations rose to more than 3 percent (>30,000 ppm), hydrogen cyanide concentrations of about 250 ppm, and hydrogen chloride concentrations of 3000 to 8500 ppm were reached. Near the exit, oxygen concentrations were found to be 10 to 15 percent; the other chemical concentrations were reduced but remained in highly toxic ranges.[5] Figures 3-1 and 3-2 illustrate the gas concentrations close to the origin of the fire and close to the exit in the first few minutes of the fire.[6]

Toxicology studies on the blood of victims of other fires have shown more than 50 chemicals, only about half of which have been identified.[5] Similar studies in nonfire fatalities show only a fraction of these chemicals. Of necessity the discussion here will touch upon only a fraction of the smoke contents that have been identified and studied. Readers

Table 3-1 Factors Affecting Smoke Composition

Fuel composition
Oxygen concentration
Temperature
Rate of temperature rise
Duration of exposure to heat
Distance from fire
Location of fire in open or closed space

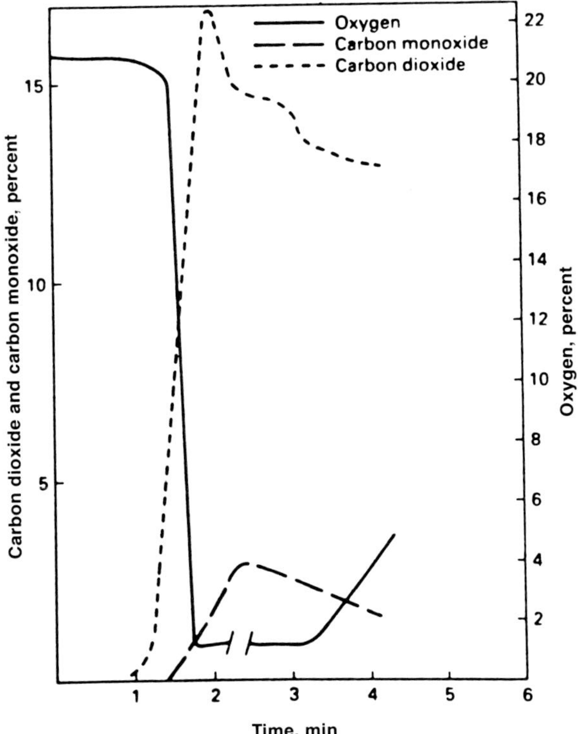

Figure 3-1 Data from the simulation of the Stardust Nightclub fire. Concentrations of oxygen and the oxides of carbon close to the origin of the fire. (*Reproduced with permission from Woolley et al, Fire Safety J, 1984.*[6])

can, therefore, expect information on smoke injury to change with time.

THERMAL INJURY

Direct thermal injury occurs when the heat energy of smoke is transferred to airway mucosal or lung

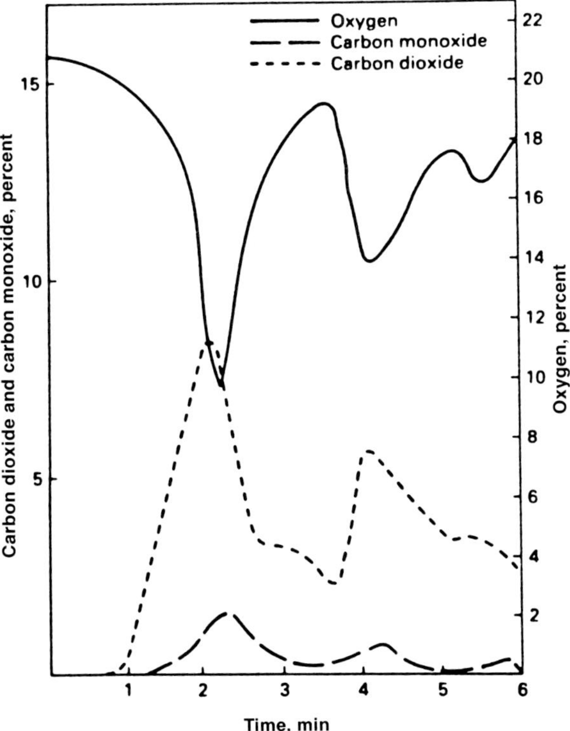

Figure 3-2 Data from the simulation of the Stardust Nightclub fire. Concentrations of oxygen and oxides of carbon at the structure exit. (*Reproduced with permission from Woolley et al, Fire Safety J, 1984.*[6])

parenchymal tissue. Mucosa is injured at air temperatures above 150°C.[7,8] Smoke temperatures of 260 to 280°C are commonly encountered in fires, and temperatures exceeding 1000°C are recorded.[5,9,10] The severity and location of thermal burns in the respiratory tract are related to the temperature and heat capacity of the material inhaled and to the efficiency of the natural protective mechanisms.

Heat or *thermal capacity* is defined as the quantity of heat necessary to raise a gram of substance 1°C.[11] The units are commonly given as calories per gram per degree centigrade. Dry air, even hot dry air, has a low heat capacity, about 0.24 cal/g/°C compared to 1.0 cal/g/°C for water. At an air density of about 0.0013 g/mL, cooling of a half liter of hot dry air 100°C would release only about 16 calories.

Though the heat capacity of steam (0.48 cal/g/°C) is about twice that of dry air and the density not much different, the potential for injury is much higher. As steam cools, it is transformed from vapor to liquid, releasing 539 cal/g of vapor (heat of condensation or transformation). Compared to air, this energy is likely to be released over a smaller area, which also increases the potential for injury. As the water continues to cool to body temperature, the heat capacity is 1.0 cal/g/°C.

Smoke may also contain considerable quantities of soot and other particulate matter. Particles as small as 1 to 10 μm have been recorded so that while most particles are filtered by the upper airway, some may reach the lower airway.[10,12] Particulate matter will, in general, have higher specific heats and densities than air, and some may be superheated and may therefore contribute to heat injury in both the upper and lower airways.

If the combustion of inhaled gases is not complete, further oxidation may occur within the respiratory tract. This further oxidation has the potential for releasing large quantities of heat energy, which may also contribute to injury in the lower airways.[13,14]

Thermal injury is usually immediate. Direct heat injury causes edema, erythema, hemorrhage, and ulceration.[7] Fortunately, there are mechanisms in place to protect the lower airway and lung parenchyma. The efficiency of the upper airway as a heat exchanger is well known and has been described in some detail.[15] The same principles that allow the upper airways to perform their normal function of heating and humidifying cool dry inhaled air serve to protect the respiratory system from extreme heat. Water lining the mucosa acts as a "heat reservoir".[15] The 16 calories liberated in the 100°C cooling of 500 mL of hot dry air would raise the temperature of 1 mL of mucosal water only 16°C. The number of calories released from the mucosa in the heat of transformation as water evaporates to humidify the air is about the same as occurs when steam condenses.[16] Air turbulence in the upper airway improves heat exchange from air to mucosa, while the transfer of heat energy from air to mucosa by convection reduces the amount of energy absorbed at any given point. Sudden exposure to hot air may also trigger reflex closure of the vocal cords further reducing the potential for lower airway injury.[17,18]

Moritz[16] tested the efficiency of this heat exchanger in a series of experiments. The experiments deserve to be briefly recounted here because they are so often quoted and the journal is not readily available. In the experiments, dogs were anesthetized and their skin protected from thermal injury with asbestos shielding. Hot air was introduced just below the larynx through an insulated transoral cannula, and an auxiliary heat source was provided to reduce heat loss as air was transferred from the heat source to the larynx. The heat sources were an oven with dry air heated to 350°C and a combustion oven with air at 500°C. The 500°C air was delivered with a pump. Thermocouples recorded temperature at the distal end of the cannula and near the bifurcation of the trachea.

In a second series of experiments the dogs breathed air from a glass blower's blast burner through a funnel-shaped transoral cannula. The temperature at the source was unknown, but the flame was adjusted to reach the distal end of the cannula at the level of the larynx.

In the final series of experiments the animals inhaled steam at temperatures above 100°C. Multiple inhalations were given for each experiment. Oven air originated at 350°C, was about 180°C at the distal end of the larynx, and was not recorded at the tracheal bifurcation. The air from the combustion oven originated at 500°C, was 267 to 327°C at the distal end of the cannula, and was 50°C at the tracheal bifurcation. The temperature of the flame at the distal end of the cannula was over 500°C, with tracheal bifurcation temperatures of 64 to 100°C. The steam temperatures were about 100°C at the distal end of the cannula and 53 to 94°C at the level of the tracheal bifurcation.

At autopsy, all animals had upper tracheal thermal injury: mild for the hot dry air inhalations and moderate to severe for the flame and steam inhalations. Lower tracheal injury was not observed with hot dry air, was mild with flame inhalation, and was severe with steam inhalation. None of the hot dry air inhalations was associated with parenchymal injury. One of four dogs with flame inhalation had parenchymal injury, while four of six of those exposed to steam had parenchymal lung injury.[16]

The efficiency of respiratory heat exchange was not completely tested in this experiment because, in preliminary experiments, delivering several breaths of hot (300°C) dry air into the pharynx caused such severe local edema of the laryngopharynx and larynx that the dogs died of asphyxia. The experiments clearly showed the resistance of the airways to injury with hot dry air and just as clearly that steam has enough heat energy to damage lung parenchyma.

Clinical evidence supports the suggestion that hot air is an uncommon source of lower airway and lung parenchyma injury. In cases involving only smoke exposure (no steam), lower airway injury is frequently delayed in contrast to the immediate injury patterns seen with direct thermal injury. In a study of 697 patients, Pruitt[19] found convincing evidence of lower airway injury in only one patient. The injured patient was exposed in a 100 percent oxygen environment in a hyperbaric chamber and, even then, the injury extended only a few centimeters below the glottis.[19,20] Others have similarly found that convincing evidence of thermal injury to the lower airways is not commonly encountered.[21–23] Estimates for the frequency of thermal burns below the larynx range from 0.1 to 5 percent.[19,24] When victims are exposed to enough heat to cause significant lower airway injury, they are likely to die at the scene of the fire.[25] Dressler expressed it graphically[1]:

> . . . I think that we have come to believe that heat is not a factor in the lower airway in the sense that one cannot actually burn the alveoli without incinerating the victim.

Direct thermal injury is usually limited to the upper airway including the larynx and is uncommon below the vocal cords except when the exposure has been to steam. In steam exposures, lower airway thermal injury should be considered. Thermal injury of the face and upper airway should serve as a marker for significant exposure of the lower airway and lung parenchyma to smoke.[9] In experimental settings, smoke toxicity is increased when the inhaled smoke is hot.[1,26]

The role of thermal injury in smoke inhalations is not settled. Particulate matter and continued combustion of incompletely oxidized gases may cause lower airway injury. Hot smoke also potentiates the injury from other inhaled gases.[27]

INHALATION INJURIES

Anoxic Injury

In his review of the 1981 Stardust Nightclub fire, Davies[5] pointed out that the oxygen (O_2) concentration in the environment close to the point of ignition decreased to less than 2 percent within 2 minutes of ignition. It remained at that level for a just over 1 minute and then fluctuated somewhat. At the exit, 14 m away from the point of ignition, the O_2 concentration averaged about 16 percent but fluctuated considerably with a transient fall to about 8 percent. The carbon dioxide (CO_2) concentrations adjacent to the fire reached 17 percent and were about 8 percent at the exit. Dressler[1] pointed out that in closed environments and in flashover fires, O_2 concentrations can be less than 5 percent. In a closed environment simulation, Chu[23] reported O_2 concentrations of 15.6 percent and CO_2 concentrations of 4.94 percent. Zawacki[28] reported O_2 concentrations of 17.7 percent. These and other reports demonstrate that the O_2 and CO_2 concentrations vary widely and transiently in fire environments. The lowest concentrations are associated with flash fires and closed spaces.

The low levels of oxygen concentration reported with fires, even though they are transient, can be associated with anoxic injury. More than a minute of exposure to the 2 percent concentrations reported in the Dublin simulation could be associated with severe anoxic injury and death. In addition, an anoxic environment could potentiate injuries from other chemicals which may be present.[26,29] For example, injury from exposure to toxic carbon monoxide (CO) concentrations is thought to be potentiated in a hypoxic environment. The hypoxic environment causes an injury of its own and may increase the competitive binding advantage of the CO molecules. High concentrations of CO_2 may be lethal in and of themselves and are observed in smoke inhalation victims.[29] In lower concentrations, CO_2 may potentiate other smoke inhalation injuries by stimulating respiratory drive.

Chemical Injuries

While direct thermal and anoxic injuries are possible, the greatest threat from smoke inhalation comes from the toxic chemical constituents of the smoke. Analyses in the laboratory and from simulations of fires provide some insight into the chemical contents. Table 3-2 illustrates the complexity of smoke from a single type of fuel.[30]

The actual chemical contents of any fire are a function of several variables centering around oxygen, heat, and fuel. The composition of the fuels is the first major variable in determining the chemicals produced by combustion or pyrolysis. Table 3-3 lists some of the chemicals associated with combustion or heat degradation of commonly encountered materials. The products of combustion may vary according to whether they are being decomposed in a high-, medium-, or low-oxygen environment. The third major constituent is the heat present. Some of the important heat-associated variables are the absolute temperatures encountered, the duration of exposure to the heat, and the rate at which the temperature rises.[4] For example, production of CO from the combustion of polyvinyl chloride (PVC) increases from 20 mg/g at temperatures from 280 to 350°C to 181 mg/g at temperatures of 510 to 580°C.[4] If the temperature rise is 3°C/min, the CO production is 429 mg/g, and if the rise is 50°C/min, the CO production is 269 mg/g.[4]

Other factors that may affect the toxicity of an exposure include duration of exposure and impaired consciousness. The importance of duration of exposure is illustrated by carbon monoxide poisoning, where the final carboxyhemoglobin concentration is a function of both concentration and the length of exposure. As concentration increases, the length of time required to reach dangerous carboxyhemoglobin levels decreases.

Whether the injury occurs in a closed or open space affects gas concentrations and duration of exposure. In a closed-space environment, concentrations of chemicals are increased, the level of oxygen

Table 3-2 Compounds in 1 L of Cotton Smoke

Identification	Concentration ng/L air
Methylacetylene or propadiene	3,817
Acetaldehyde	10,969
Butadiene and butylene	1,355
Ethanol	235
Methyl nitrile	173
Acrolein	5,210
Acetone	1,787
Furan	5,210
Cyclopentadiene	311
Allyl alcohol	545
2,5-Dihydrofuran or methacrolein	1,005
Unknown	2,270
Methyl ethyl ketone hydroperoxide	321
α-Methylfuran	1,493
α-Methylfuran	195
Crotonaldehyde	735
Dimethylkentene	423
Benzene	1,326
α-Heptane	214
α-Hexane	290
Furfural	535
Phenol	228
α-Methylfuran	747
C_6 alcohol	2,307
Toluene trichloride	839
α-Furaldehyde	832
α-Furaldehyde	11,363
m-Cresol	246
Ethylbenzene or xylene	272
Styrene	373
Furylmethylketone or dimethylhexadiene	408
5-methyl-2-furaldehyde	1,097

SOURCE: Reproduced with permission from Kimura et al, *J Appl Physiol* 64(3):1107, 1988.[30]

Table 3-3 Common Toxic Products of Incomplete Combustion

Material burned	Chemical products
Wood, cotton, paper, polyvinyl chloride, polystyrene	Carbon monoxide
Polyurethane, nylon, melamine resins, upholstery, silk, wool	Cyanide
Polyvinyl chloride, fire-retardant materials	Aldehydes
Polyvinyl chloride, rubber	Hydrochloric acid
Polyvinyl chloride	Chlorine
Cellulose nitrate, celluloid, wall paper fabrics, melamine resins	Phosgene
Nylon, rubber, silk, wool, petroleum products	Ammonia
Compounds containing sulfur	Sulfur dioxide
Petroleum products, nitrocellulose products wallpaper, wood, cotton, paper	Acetic acid

SOURCE: Compiled from Refs. 4, 7, and 9.

decreased, and the level of carbon dioxide increased. Smoke density in a closed space is generally higher and may lead to reductions in visibility, impairing the ability of the victim to escape. These factors increase the intensity and the duration of exposure.

An impairment in consciousness from whatever cause also increases the risk of chemical injury to the lungs. One of the chemicals most commonly associated with inhalation injuries — ethanol — is not inhaled in smoke. Drinking alcohol is also associated with an increase in the mortality in smoke exposures.[31] Barillo et al.[31] examined 39 fire victims and found that increased alcohol concentrations were present in 21 of 26 adults and 0 of 12 children. Eighteen of the 26 adult victims had ethanol levels about 100 mg/dL. Those victims who had made no evident attempt at escape had blood ethanol levels that averaged 268 mg/dL, while blood alcohol levels in those with evidence of an escape attempt averaged 88 mg/dL. The presumption was that ethanol intoxication impaired the ability of the fire victims to escape and therefore contributed to their mortality.

In addition to the products of combustion or pyrolysis in smoke, industrial chemical leakage may also increase the danger of industrial fires. While these are not specifically products of combustion, they are available to be inhaled in the smoke environment and should be considered part of the potential smoke constituents in those special circumstances.

The type and concentration of chemical exposures associated with fires can also be gathered from forensic materials.[5,32] Anderson[32] constructed a "fingerprint" from gas chromatograph and mass spectrographic studies of the chemical constituents in blood from 130 fire fatalities. That "fingerprint" showed at least 50 different compounds, only about half of which have been identified, in fire fatalities. Of course, the chemical compounds present in the blood of fire victims can come from cigarette smoke and other exposures as well as the gases inhaled in the fire, but in similar "fingerprint" constructions from nonfire deaths, only about one-fifth of the number of compounds were found.[5] In addition to the compounds obviously associated with burning, the blood of fire victims shows significant concentrations of antimony, bromine, cadmium, chromium, cobalt, gold, iron, lead, and zinc.[5] The smoke environment may also contain significant reactive free radicals.[5]

Chemical exposures can be divided into three categories: asphyxiants, irritants, and systemic toxins. The two major asphyxiants are carbon monoxide and hydrogen cyanide.

Asphyxiants

Carbon Monoxide Carbon monoxide (CO) is a combustible, nonirritating, colorless, tasteless, odorless gas of about the same density as air.[33,34] It is produced by the incomplete combustion of organic material and is sparingly soluble in water.[34] CO is produced endogenously in human beings from the alpha methane carbon atom of the protoporphyrin ring during the metabolism of hemoglobin.[35] Produced at a rate of about 0.42 mL/h, this endogenous production results in a background carboxyhemoglobin (COHb) of about 0.4 percent in humans.[36] Concentrations of about 7 percent CO are common in automobile exhaust, and concentrations as high as 30 percent may be reached. CO may also be produced in the absence of combustion. For example, PVC does not ignite until it reaches a temperature of 475°C.[3] At temperatures between 225 and 475°C, PVC will lose approximately 60 percent of its weight by thermal degradation; CO is one of the principal products of this decomposition.[3,37] The exposures to CO in fire environments can be extraordinary. Chu and Chan[38] reported CO concentrations of 35,700 ppm in an open-space environment and 571,400 ppm in a closed space. Stewart et al.[39] reported CO concentrations in fires to vary from 0.1 percent (1000 ppm) to 10 percent (100,000 ppm). The CO concentration that results from a given concentration of CO in the atmosphere is a function of the duration of exposure.[40] For example, exposure to a CO concentration of 0.02–0.03 percent (200–300 ppm) would lead to COHb concentrations of 20–30 percent after 5–6 hours. Exposure to CO concentrations of 0.07–0.1 percent (700–1000 ppm) would lead to COHb concentrations of 40–50 percent in 3–4 hours, and exposures to a CO concentration of 0.5–1.0 percent would lead to COHb concentrations of 70–80 percent in 1–2 minutes. At the moment, CO is probably still the most serious chemical compound in smoke. In a study of fire-related deaths in Maryland and New York, CO was thought to have made a significant contribution to the deaths of 80 percent of the victims.[3,41] The toxicity of CO is increased with increasing exertion, ventilation, air and smoke temperature, and air and smoke humidity.[3,26,42]

The primary mechanism of CO poisoning is secondary to its displacement of oxygen and its effect on the hemoglobin molecule. CO binds avidly with hemoglobin (its affinity for hemoglobin is 200 to 250 times that of oxygen). It therefore displaces oxygen from the hemoglobin molecule and proportionally reduces oxygen content. In addition to the displacement of oxygen molecules from hemoglobin, CO also shifts the oxyhemoglobin dissociation curve to the left. This impairs the ability of hemoglobin to release oxygen molecules and may increase tissue injury.[7,9] The brain and heart are the organs most sensitive to CO poisoning. In addition, CO blocks oxidative phosphorylation by binding to cytochrome oxidase and may alter muscle activity by binding to myoglobin, thus interfering with oxidative metabolism at the cellular level. This cellular activity may account for some of the injury seen in special circumstances[7,9] though the clinical significance of the effect of CO on the cytochrome system is not well understood.[36] CO also impairs mucociliary clearance, increases bronchial gland secretions, and interferes with oxidative reduction reactions in type II cells.[8] Whatever other toxic effects are involved, current opinion suggests that the primary toxic effect of CO stems from its effect on the hemoglobin molecule in displacing oxygen and shifting the oxyhemoglobin curve to the left.

Hydrogen Cyanide Hydrogen cyanide (HCN) is a colorless combustible gas, slightly less dense than air, with a characteristic odor of burnt almonds.[34] However, 20 to 40 percent of individuals are congenitally unable to detect it.[33] Cyanide (CN) is released from the combustion or incomplete combustion of nitrogen-containing materials, especially plastics and polyurethanes. Once polyurethane foam is ignited, atmospheric oxygen is no longer required for its continued combustion and HCN production; polyurethanes will "produce as much HCN in a pure nitrogen atmosphere as in air".[5] In his discussion of the simulation of the Stardust Nightclub fire in Dublin, Davies reported that at the temperatures encountered in the simulation, all of the nitrogen-containing materials would have been converted primarily to HCN gas but with some traces of organic nitriles, another extremely toxic material.

The toxic effects of HCN occur in seconds when the exposure is by inhalation; toxicity as a result of oral exposure may be delayed for up to 40 minutes. As expected, toxicity is related to the concentration of the gas and the length of the exposure. Inhalational exposures of 45 to 54 ppm can be tolerated for an hour without serious difficulty. Exposures to 110 to 135 ppm will cause death in one-half to 1 hour; exposures to 181 ppm cause death in about 10 minutes, and exposures to 280 ppm cause immediate death.[5] Cyanide toxicity also increases the ventilatory rate, which will increase the exposure to both cyanide and the other toxic components of smoke.[5]

Cyanide blocks oxidative metabolism at the cellular level by competitively binding to cytochrome a-a_3.[7,43] This essentially blocks a step in oxidative phosphorylation and thereby prevents the mitochondria from utilizing oxygen. The tricarboxylic acid cycle is arrested, shifting cellular metabolism to anaerobic pathways, and resulting in lactic acid production. The lactic acid production and its associated metabolic acidosis also stimulates respiratory drive.[7,9]

Carbon monoxide has been considered the primary poison in smoke, but the increasing use of plastics and other polymers in building materials and textiles raises concern about new toxic products of which cyanide is the most common and one of the most dangerous. Cyanide and carbon monoxide poisoning may be additive.[44] Pitt et al. demonstrated that cyanide and carbon monoxide act synergistically to reduce cerebral oxygen consumption.[45] Symington[46] reported cyanide levels in fatal and nonfatal fire casualties and in firemen. They found that fire-associated fatalities in a small number of individuals were associated with toxic concentrations of cyanide. In a 1986 study, Jones reported on six fatalities in Ohio; four of the six had toxic cyanide serum levels.[44]

Irritant Gases

Irritant gases have direct cytotoxic effects. The location and severity of the injury are, in large part, determined by the degree of water solubility of the chemical and the duration of the exposure.[9] Table 3-4 lists relative water solubilities for some common smoke-associated chemicals.

Table 3-4 Relative Water Solubilities of Common Chemical Components of Smoke

Chemical	Solubility in water
Aldehyde (acrolein)	High
Ammonia	High
Chlorine	High
Hydrogen chloride	High
Sulfur dioxide	High
Oxides of nitrogen (nitrogen dioxide)	Low
Phosgene	Low

Irritant Gases with High Solubility Highly soluble toxic gases dissolve rapidly into the first water-covered surfaces they contact and therefore tend to injure the upper airway mucosa.[7,9] The onset of injury is rapid. Reflex laryngeal spasm caused by these soluble irritant gases may also reduce distal exposure (although the spasm can cause injury or death in itself). In lower concentrations soluble irritant gases cause conjunctivitis, rhinitis, and pharyngitis impelling the victim to flee the environment. In higher concentrations, these same symptoms may become so intense that they incapacitate the victim, making escape less likely and thereby increasing the duration of exposure and the extent of the injury.

Lower airway injury is possible when the ventilatory rate is increased, driven by such factors as increased CO_2 levels, metabolic acidosis, or exertion. At higher ventilatory rates, the total amount of chemical delivered is increased, and the higher flows increase delivery to the lower airway. Impaired consciousness increases the duration of exposure and the likelihood of distal airway or parenchymal injury. Water-soluble chemicals may also be absorbed on particulate matter in smoke and reach the lower respiratory tract.[7] In pathologic examinations of fire victims, Chu[23] found that "erosive chemical toxicants, together with soot, adhere firmly to the mucosal layer of air passages." Hours later, mild but extensive edema and scattered submucosal hemorrhages were found beneath the soot particles. No ulceration was observed.

Aldehydes The principal aldehydes are formaldehyde, acetaldehyde, butyaldehyde, and acrolein. All are used in the manufacture of resins, plastics, rubber, and disinfectants[7]; all are highly soluble and hence irritating to the upper respiratory tract, though lower airway injury is also observed. Many consider the aldehydes the most toxic of the irritant gases, and acrolein is the most common of them.[47]

Acrolein (2-propenal, C_3H_4O) has a pungent odor.[34] Acrolein is produced in the combustion of wood, cotton, paper, and petroleum products. The concentrations of aldehydes in wood smoke are 15 to 20 times those found in kerosene smoke.[47] Zikria reported total aldehyde concentrations of 200 ppm in smoke from common household materials.[47] In experimental animals, exposure to 5.5 ppm caused severe upper respiratory tract and conjunctival irritation. Pulmonary edema occurs with exposures to 10 ppm.[23] In humans, an exposure of 30 to 100 ppm is estimated to cause death in 10 minutes.[4] Acrolein is a weak sensitizer and may cause mild asthmatic reactions.[34] It may also impair antibacterial defenses.[7,24]

Ammonia Ammonia (NH_3) is a colorless, highly soluble, alkaline, irritant gas about half as dense as air and with an extremely pungent odor.[34] It is thought to be nonflammable, but in the proper environment, mixtures of NH_3 and air can explode. Ammonia is used in the manufacture of explosives, synthetic fibers, fertilizers, chemicals, and pharmaceuticals; it is used extensively in refrigeration. In fires, ammonia is produced by the combustion of wool, silk, nylon, melamine resins, and plastics. When NH_3 contacts the water in the airway mucosa, it reacts to form ammonium hydroxide (NH_4OH), a strong alkali which may dissociate to hydroxyl ions.[7,9] The result is liquefaction necrosis with edema and sloughing of the mucosa.[9]

As with other soluble gases, the location and the extent of the injury depend upon the concentration of the gas, the duration of the exposure, and the depth of inspiration. All of these can be intensified if the gas binds to soot and is carried to the lower airways. Edema and bronchoconstriction of the airways occurs. Ammonia is intensely irritating to the conjunctiva and nasopharynx. In severe exposures, asphyxia can occur as a result of severe laryngeal edema.[48] Injuries include sloughing of respiratory mucosa, edema, airway obstruction, pneumonitis, pulmonary edema, adult respiratory distress syndrome, laryngeal edema, tracheitis, bronchitis, and bronchiectasis.[9] The onset of pulmonary edema may be delayed over 6 hours after the exposure.[33] The olfactory perception threshold is about 5 ppm and 20 ppm is quite irritating.[3] Higher exposures can result in incapacitating irritation; acute blindness due to ammonia exposure may prevent escape, leading to fatal inhalation injury. Concentrations above 1000 ppm are estimated to be lethal in 10 minutes.[4]

Chlorine Chlorine (Cl_2) is a green-yellow gas with a density about 2.5 times that of air.[34] It has a pungent odor and is intensely irritating. In water it forms hydrochloric acid (HCl) and hypochlorous acid (HOCl),[9,49] which is 20 times more toxic than HCl alone.[7] Oxygen free radicals are also released.[9] Its solubility is intermediate between that of ammonia and phosgene. Chlorine is used widely in industry, and exposures in industrial fires are often increased because of chemical leaks in storage equipment. However, it is also an important product of combustion. Chlorine is used in the manufacture of many chemicals including plastics and resins,[7] and employed extensively as a bleaching agent and a germicide. Its odor threshold is 0.2 to 0.4 ppm.[34] Individuals can tolerate exposures to 1 to 2 ppm, while 3 to 6 ppm is irritating, 5 to 8 ppm causes mild illness, concentrations greater than 40 to 50 ppm are dangerous and can cause pulmonary edema, and 1000 ppm is rapidly fatal.[7,40,48,49] The toxicity of chlorine is thought to be due to its powerful oxidizing properties. It is intensely irritating to the eyes and mucous membranes of the upper airway. In higher concentrations, chlorine is associated with intense laryngospasm, bronchospasm, and pulmonary edema. In occasional cases, pulmonary edema can be delayed.[48]

Hydrogen Chloride Hydrogen chloride (HCl) is a colorless, corrosive, nonflammable, irritating gas slightly more dense than air (1.2 times) with a pungent odor.[34] It is produced in the combustion or pyrolysis of polyvinyl chloride, chlorinated acrylics, olefins, and fabrics treated with fire-retardant materials.[4,37] HCl is produced from the pyrolysis of polyvinyl chloride (without ignition) once temperatures reach 250°C.[3,17] HCl is used in the manufacture of dyes, fertilizers, and textiles and in the rubber and ore industries.[48] Particulate matter coated with HCl is potentially more toxic than the gas alone.[4] HCl causes irritation of the throat and conjunctiva at concentrations of 5 to 10 ppm.[9] Fifty to 100 ppm concentrations can be tolerated for barely 1 hour.[9] The concentration thought to be fatal with a 10-minute exposure is >500 ppm.[4] Concentrations of 1000 to 2000 ppm are immediately life-threatening.[5] HCl toxicity is said to include acute bronchitis, laryngospasm, glottal edema, and pulmonary edema.[9,48] However, Schwartz found no convincing reports that laryngospasm and pulmonary edema occurred as a result of acute exposures to HCl.[9]

Sulfur Dioxide Sulfur dioxide (SO_2) is the primary oxidation product of sulfur-containing materials in fires.[4] It is a colorless, soluble, nonflammable gas with a strong "suffocating" odor. It is twice as dense as air.[34,48] It is widely used in the chemical, paper, and smelting industries. SO_2 is hydrated rapidly on the mucosal surface and then oxidized to produce sulfurous acid (H_2SO_3) and sulfuric acid (H_2SO_4).[2,9,48] It is an extremely intense irritant in concentrations below those which are fatal.[4] SO_2 causes coagulation necrosis of mucosal membranes, especially of the upper airway. It is estimated that in 1 to 50 ppm concentrations, 99 percent is deposited in the naso- and hypopharynx.[9] If SO_2 or its resultant acids are absorbed on soot, their toxicity may be increased.[3] In higher concentrations or with prolonged exposures, it is associated with lower airway injury and pulmonary edema.[7,9] In addition to direct cellular injury which causes pulmonary edema, SO_2 has been noted to cause vasoconstriction which could increase pulmonary capillary hydrostatic pressure and increase the severity of the pulmonary edema.[9] In lower doses it may cause bronchoconstriction.[7] The odor is detectable at 0.5 ppm, and irritation of the conjunctiva and nasopharynx is noted at 6 to 10 ppm.[9] The estimated lethal concentration for a 10-minute exposure is >500 ppm.[4]

Irritant Gases with Low Water Solubility Gases with low solubility in water, such as the oxides of nitrogen, are more likely to cause lower respiratory tract and parenchymal injury. Since there is little conjunctival, nasal, or pharyngeal irritation, there is little warning. Injury onset is slower. These two factors tend to prolong the duration of exposure, increase the extent of injury and partially account for the clinically observed delay between exposure and symptoms seen in some victims.

Oxides of Nitrogen The oxides of nitrogen include nitrous oxide (N_2O), nitric oxide (NO), nitrogen dioxide (NO_2), nitrogen trioxide (N_2O_3), nitrogen tetroxide (N_2O_4) and nitrogen pentoxide (N_2O_5).[7,9,33,48] Nitrogen dioxide polymerizes to nitrogen tetroxide, which rapidly dissociates back to nitrogen dioxide. The equilibrium of this reaction is dependent largely upon temperature. Nitric oxide is oxidized slowly in air to NO_2. Nitrogen dioxide is the most important of these oxides from the viewpoint of medical injury.[7,48] Nitrogen dioxide is a reddish-brown gas of limited solubility. It is used in the manufacture of explosives and in the chemical, welding, and cleaning industries. It is produced by the combustion of fabrics, cellulose nitrate, and celluloid products. Its relative insolubility makes its injury more insidious. There are few, if any, immediate symptoms and virtually no upper respiratory or conjunctival warning symptoms. Exposure may therefore be somewhat unknown.[9] The acute injury commonly becomes evident 5 to 72 hours later.[33] The initial injury may, therefore, pass unnoticed but result in death several days later.[34] Nitrogen dioxide reacts slowly with water to form HNO_2 and HNO_3. These acids are thought to reach maximal concentrations in the distal airways and to be the principal mediators of the injury.[48] Others have suggested that part of the injury is caused by its lipid solubility with resultant alterations of the lipid fraction of the cell membranes and cell death.[50,51] Pathologic examination of victims of nitrogen dioxide inhalation shows extensive damage to the respiratory epithelium and hemorrhagic pulmonary edema.[48] NO_2 also reacts with blood to form methemoglobin.[9,48] Although methemoglobinemia occurs with exposures to high concentrations of NO_2, it is thought to play a minor role in the fatal NO_2 exposures.[9] Exposure to concentrations as low as 5 ppm has been associated with increases in airway resistance in humans.[48] Concentrations of 50 ppm may be associated with respiratory injury; injury can occur in minutes at concentrations of 200 ppm or more.[4,5,9]

Phosgene Phosgene (carbonyl chloride, $COCl_2$) is a strong pulmonary irritant that has been used as a chemical weapon. It is a colorless, relatively water insoluble gas that is three times as dense as air.[2,34,48] In concentrations of 1 to 1.5 ppm it is reported to have a sweet, pungent smell, similar to new-mown hay or green silage.[9,48,49] Phosgene is used in the chemical industry in the synthesis of organic compounds and in the metallurgical industry for the separation of metals. It is produced in fires by the combustion or pyrolysis of chlorinated hydrocarbons, most commonly polyvinyl chloride. The quantities are, however, small and, in the usual fire setting, are thought to contribute little to the toxicity of smoke.[48] It is hydrolyzed slowly in the lung to HCl and CO_2.[9] Phosgene is considerably more toxic than chlorine.[48] In high concentrations it may cause cough and chest tightness, but symptoms may also be mild or absent. The primary sites of injury are the small airways and the alveoli, where phosgene causes necrosis of the epithelium and pulmonary edema and pneumonia.[7,34,48]

Systemic Toxins

Systemic toxins refer to the effects of metal oxides and degraded fluorocarbons[9] but may also be used to describe the toxic effects observed in experimental smoke exposures that are not explained by other known toxic chemicals. The presumption is that a chemical in the smoke is directly responsible for the toxic effect observed. Petajan, for example, observed seizures in rats exposed to a polymeric material that were not explained by carbon monoxide levels or other exposures.[52,53] Such materials may constitute an additional hazard in smoke inhalation injuries.

OTHER SOURCES OF SMOKE INHALATION INJURIES

Volcanic Dusts and Gases (Pyroclastic Flow Injury)

The eruptions of Mount Augustine in Alaska in March 1986 and Mount Saint Helens in 1980 raise questions about the potential for inhalational injury as a result of exposure to the effluent from volcanos.[54] Pyroclastic flow is the result of the release from the volcano of high-energy–containing material (gases, ash, and water vapor).[55] The energy released in the Mount Saint Helens eruption was estimated to be about 100 times the generating capacity of all U.S. electric power stations.[56] The energy and heat dissipate as distance from the volcanic vent increases. The ash particle size and content may vary from volcano to volcano and with distance and direction from the vent. Autopsy studies of the first 25 deaths from the Mount Saint Helens eruption showed that the most common cause of death was asphyxia secondary to the inhalation of volcanic ash. Ash was observed to combine with mucus to form plugs that occluded upper airways.[56] Studies of the Mount Saint Helens ash showed that 94 to 99 percent of the particles were less than 10 μm

in size and therefore clearly in the respirable range and capable of reaching the alveoli.[56,57] The free crystalline silica content (the form of silicates with the greatest fibrogenic potential) was estimated to be 3 to 7 percent. A summary of multiple in vitro and animal studies concluded that the cytotoxic and fibrogenic injury potential of volcanic ash is small.[58] Follow-up studies of loggers exposed to the Mount Saint Helens eruption suggest that the risks of chronic bronchitis and pneumoconiosis from inhalation of volcanic ash are negligible given the circumstances of a large initial exposure followed by decreasing exposure with time.[54] The health risk from acute exposures to volcanic ash is dependent upon the volume but appears to be small in otherwise healthy persons. Persons with known asthma or chronic lung disease appear to be at increased risk of experiencing an exacerbation of their disease.[57]

Smoke Bombs

Chemical smoke bombs contain mixtures of solid or liquid particles which become hydrated when exposed to air. The hydrated material then intercepts or diffuses light, creating the smoke.[59] The mixtures in common use contain hexachloroethane (C_2Cl_6) and either powdered zinc or zinc oxide (ZnO) and aluminum.[59,60] On combustion, zinc chloride ($ZnCl_4$) is formed and rapidly absorbs water from the air.[60] Zinc chloride is a known corrosive respiratory tract irritant. In open areas these compounds are relatively harmless, but in closed spaces or when the humidity is too low to allow rapid deliquescence to occur, they may be harmful.[59] Humans and animals exposed to $ZnCl_4$ may develop chemical bronchitis-bronchiolitis and pulmonary edema, and deaths have been reported.[59,60]

Another mixture used contains titanium dioxide (TiO_2) and HCl, which react to form titanium tetrachloride ($TiCl_4$) with a secondary smoke that contains titanium hydroxide ($Ti(OH)_4$), oxychlorides, and HCl.[60] There is no information about human toxicity from $TiCl_4$ smoke exposures, and animal toxicity experiments present conflicting information.[60] Until more is known, $TiCl_4$ should also be considered potentially toxic.

Laser Smoke

The proliferation of laser surgery creates the potential for acute and chronic exposures to the by-products (smoke) generated by the surgery. The particulate matter is small enough to be inhaled easily ($<1.1\ \mu m$).[61,62] Carbon monoxide concentrations of 400 ppm have been recorded.[62] In sheep experiments, exposure to laser smoke resulted in decreases in Pa_{O_2}, impairment of mucociliary clearance, and an inflammatory response diagnosed by bronchoalveolar lavage.[62] Rats exposed to laser smoke developed bronchiolitis, interstitial pneumonia, and emphysema.[61] Little is known about acute or chronic human toxicity, but with evidence of potential injury, the use of proper smoke evacuation equipment is recommended.

REFERENCES

1. Dressler DP: Laboratory background on smoke inhalation. *J Trauma* 19:913, 1979.
2. Dodge RR: Smoke inhalation, in Clark RJ, Taussig LM, Weese WC (eds): *Seminars in Chest Medicine. Ariz Med* 34:749, 1977.
3. Coleman DL: Smoke inhalation — Medical Staff Conference, University of California, San Francisco. *West J Med* 135:300, 1981.
4. Terrill JB, Montgomery RR, Reinhardt CF: Toxic gases from fires. *Science* 200:1343, 1978.
5. Davies JWL: Toxic chemicals versus lung tissue — An aspect of inhalation injury revisited. *J Burn Care Rehabil* 7:213, 1986.
6. Woolley WD, Smith PG, Fardell PJ, et al: The Stardust Disco fire, Dublin 1981: Studies of combustion products during simulation experiments. *Fire Safety J* 7:267, 1984.
7. Wald PH, Balmes JR: Respiratory effects of short-term, high intensity toxic inhalations: Smoke, gases, and fumes.

J Intensive Care Med 2:260, 1987.
8. Herndon DN, Langner F, Thompson P, et al: Pulmonary injury in burned patients. *Surg Clin North Am* 67:31, 1987.
9. Schwartz DA: Acute inhalation injury. *State Art Rev Occup Med* 2:297, 1987.
10. Trunkey DD: Inhalation injury. *Surg Clin North Am* 58:1133, 1978.
11. Weast RC (ed): *CRC Handbook of Chemistry and Physics*, 65th ed. Boca Raton, Fla, CRC Press, 1984.
12. Silverman HM: Smoke inhalation, in Schwartz GR, Safar P, Stone JH, et al (eds): *Principles and Practice of Emergency Medicine*. Philadelphia, WB Saunders Company, 1978, vol 1.
13. Farrow CS: Smoke inhalation in the dog: Current concepts of pathophysiology and management. *VM/SAC* 70:404, 1975.
14. Mellins RB, Park S: Respiratory complications of smoke inhalation in victims of fires. *J Pediatr* 87:1, 1975.
15. Walker JEC, Wells RE, Merrill EW: Heat and water exchange in the respiratory tract. *Am J Med* 30:259, 1961.
16. Moritz AR, Henriques FC, McLean R: The effects of inhaled heat on the air passages and lungs: An experimental investigation. *Am J Pathol* 21:311, 1945.
17. Peters WJ. Review article: Inhalation injury caused by the products of combustion. *CMA J* 125:249, 1981.
18. Achauer BM, Allyn PA, Furnas DW, et al: Pulmonary complications of burns: The major threat to the burn patient. *Ann Surg* 177:311, 1973.
19. Pruitt BA, Flemma RJ, DiVincenti FC, et al: Pulmonary complications in burn patients: A comparative study of 697 patients. *J Thorac Cardiovasc Surg* 59:7, 1970.
20. DiVincenti FC, Pruitt BA, Beckler JM: Inhalation injuries. *J Trauma* 11:109, 1971.
21. Pruitt BA, Erickson DR, Morris A: Progressive pulmonary insufficiency and other pulmonary complications of thermal injury. *J Trauma* 15:369, 1975.
22. Head JM: Inhalation injury in burns. *Am J Surg* 139:508, 1980.
23. Chu, C-S: New concepts of pulmonary burn injury. *J Trauma* 21:958, 1981.
24. Fein A, Leff A, Hopewell PC: Pathophysiology and management of the complications resulting from fire and the inhaled products of combustion: Review of the literature. *Crit Care Med* 8:94, 1980.
25. Madden MR, Finelstein JL, Goodwin CW: Respiratory care of the burn patient. *Clin Plas Surg* 13:29, 1986.
26. Stone HH, Rhame DW, Corbitt JD, et al: Respiratory burns: A correlation of clinical and laboratory results. *Ann Surg* 165:157, 1967.
27. Zikria BA, Sturner WQ, Astarjian NK, et al: Respiratory tract damage in burns: Pathophysiology and therapy. *Ann NY Acad Sci* 150:618, 1968.
28. Zawacki RE, Jung RC, Joyce J, et al: Smoke, burns, and the natural history of inhalation injury in fire victims: Correlation of experimental and clinical data. *Ann Surg* 185:100, 1977.
29. Phillips AW, Tanner JW, Cope O: Burn therapy: IV. Respiratory tract damage (an account of the clinical, x-ray and postmortem findings) and the meaning of restlessness. *Ann Surg* 158:799, 1963.
30. Kimura R, Traber LD, Herndon DN, et al: Increasing duration of smoke exposure induces more severe lung injury in sheep. *J Appl Physiol* 64(3):1107, 1988.
31. Barillo DJ, Rush BF, Goode R, et al: Is ethanol the unknown toxin in smoke inhalation injury? *Ann Surg* 52:641, 1986.
32. Anderson RA, Thomson I, Harland WA: The importance of cyanide and organic nitriles in fire fatalities. *Fire Materials* 3:91, 1979.
33. Gosselin RE, Hodge HC, Smith RP, et al: *Clinical Toxicology of Commercial Products: Acute Poisoning*, 4th ed. Baltimore, Williams & Wilkins Co, 1976.
34. Windholz M (ed): *The Merck Index: An Encyclopedia of Chemicals, Drugs and Biologicals*. Rahway, NJ, Merck & Co., 1983.
35. Myers RAM, Linberg SE, Cowley RA: Carbon monoxide poisoning: The injury and its treatment. *JACEP* 8:479, 1979.
36. Unsworth IP: Acute carbon monoxide poisoning. *Anaesth Intensive Care* 4:329, 1974.
37. Dyer RF, Esch VH: Polyvinyl chloride toxicity in fires: Hydrogen chloride toxicity in fire fighters. *JAMA* 235:393, 1976.
38. Chu C-S, Chan M: Chemical pulmonary burn injury and chemical intoxication. *Burns Incl Therm Inj* 9:111, 1982.
39. Stewart RD, Stewart RS, Stamm W, et al: Rapid estimation of carboxyhemoglobin level in fire fighters. *JAMA* 235:390, 1976.
40. Arena JM. *Poisoning*, 4th ed. Springfield, Ill, Charles C Thomas Publisher, 1979.
41. Zikria BA, Weston CG, Chodoff M, et al: Smoke and carbon monoxide poisoning in fire victims. *J Trauma* 12:641, 1972.
42. Watanabe K, Makino K: The role of carbon monoxide poisoning in the production of inhalation burns. *Ann Plast Surg* 14:284, 1985.
43. Vogel SN, Sultan TR: Cyanide poisoning. *Clin Toxicol* 18:367, 1981.
44. Jones J, McMullen JO, Dougherty J: Toxic smoke inhalation: Cyanide poisoning in fire victims. *Am J Emerg Med* 5:318, 1987.
45. Pitt BR, Radford EP, Gartner GH, et al: Interaction of carbon monoxide and cyanide on cerebral circulation and metabolism. *Arch Environ Health* 34:354, 1979.
46. Symington IS: Cyanide exposure in fires. *Lancet*, July 8, 1978, p 91.
47. Zikria BA, Ferrer JM, Floch HF. The chemical factors contributing to pulmonary damage in "smoke poisoning." *Surgery* 71:704, 1972.
48. Parkes WR: *Occupational Lung Disorders*, 2d ed. London, Butterworths, 1982.
49. Kaye S: *Handbook of Emergency Toxicology*, 4th ed. Springfield, Ill, Charles C Thomas Publisher, 1980.
50. Cahalane M, Demling RH: Early respiratory abnormalities from smoke inhalation. *JAMA* 251:771, 1984.
51. Demling RH: Postgraduate course: Respiratory Injury Part III: Pulmonary dysfunction in the burn patient. *J Burn Care Rehabil* 7:277, 1986.

52. Petajan JH, Voorhees KJ, Packham SC, et al: Extreme toxicity from combustion products of a fire-retarded polyurethane foam. *Science* 187:742, 1975.
53. Petajan JH: An approach to the toxicology of combustion products of materials. *Environ Health Perspect* 17:65, 1976.
54. Cytotoxicity of volcanic ash: Assessing the risk for pneumoconiosis. *MMWR* 35:265, 1986.
55. Parshley PF, Kiessling PJ, Antonius JA, et al: Pyroclastic flow injury: Mount St. Helens, May 18, 1980. *Am J Surg* 143:565, 1982.
56. Buist AS: Are volcanoes hazardous to your health? What have we learned from Mount St Helens? — The Oregon Health Sciences University (specialty conference). *West J Med* 137:294, 1982.
57. Baxter PJ, Ing R, Falk H, et al: Mount St. Helens eruptions: The acute respiratory effects of volcanic ash in a North American community. *Arch Environ Health* 38:138, 1983.
58. Martin TR, Wehner AP, Butler J: Chapter 7: Evaluation of physical health effects due to volcanic hazards: The use of experimental systems to estimate the pulmonary toxicity of volcanic ash. *Am J Public Health* 76 (suppl 3):59, 1986.
59. Matarese SL, Matthews JI: Zinc chloride (smoke bomb) inhalation injury. *Chest* 89:308, 1986.
60. Karlsson N, Cassel G, Fangmark I, et al: A comparative study of the acute inhalation toxicity of smoke from TiO_2-hexachloroethane and Zn-hexachloroethane pyrotechnic mixtures. *Arch Toxicol* 59:160, 1986.
61. Baggish MS, Elbakry M: The effects of laser smoke on the lungs of rats. *Am J Obstet Gynecol* 156:1260, 1987.
62. Freitag L, Chapman GA, Sielczak M, et al: Laser smoke effect on the bronchial system. *Lasers Surg Med* 7:283, 1987.

Chapter 4

Pathophysiology of Smoke Inhalation

Daniel L. Traber
David N. Herndon

The pathophysiology of smoke inhalation injury involves all levels of the respiratory tract and the lung.[1] In addition, there is indirect evidence that an injury to systemic organs also exists, since thermally injured patients with concomitant inhalation injury have greater fluid requirements for resuscitation following injury than individuals with burned skin alone.[2,3] Although the exact mechanisms responsible for the lung damage have as yet to be defined completely, these pulmonary lesions are presently considered to be responsible for a large proportion of the morbidity and mortality found in thermally injured patients.[4–6] For the purposes of this review, we shall discuss smoke inhalation injury in terms of damage to the oropharyngeal, tracheobronchial, pulmonary parenchymal, and systemic areas.

UPPER AIRWAY

The oropharyngeal portion of the respiratory tract normally thermoregulates and humidifies inspired air and can be subjected to direct damage from heat. These soft tissues can swell rapidly from edema formation which may be severe enough to result in obstruction of the upper airway (Fig. 4-1). The mechanisms responsible for initiating the processes causing the transvascular fluid flux apparently relate to the thermal denaturization of plasma proteins,[7] with a subsequent release of free oxygen radicals and products of arachidonic acid metabolism into the microvascular areas.[8,9] The free oxygen radicals damage the capillary beds, and thromboxane A_2, a catabolite of arachidonic acid, causes vascular constriction. This combination of increased

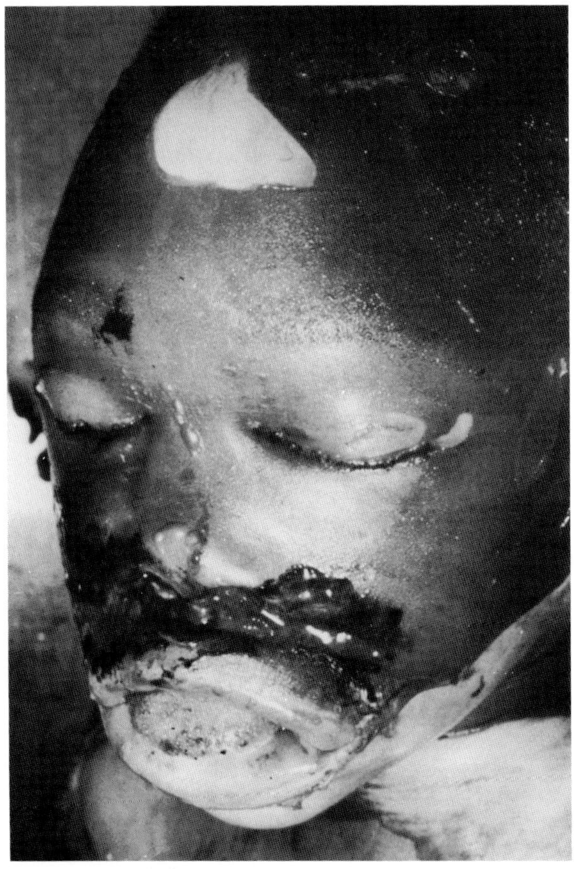

Figure 4-1 The head of a child who has sustained thermal injury. The figure illustrates severe edema of the soft tissues to the extent that there is an upper airway occlusion.

microvascular permeability and increased microvascular pressure leads to a rapid and profound edema.[10] In a period as short as 1 hour, this edema can be so marked as to result in complete upper airway obstruction.

Edema as a result of heat has been of interest from an experimental standpoint for a number of years.[11] The degree of fluid flux can be attenuated using oxygen free-radical scavengers and cyclooxygenase inhibitors. However, neither of these classes of compounds has received a clinical trial in human beings. Nicotinic acid, which blocks the formation of the catabolites of arachidonic acid through an inhibition of phospholipase, has been reported to markedly reduce edema formation and the fluid requirements for resuscitation in severely injured individuals.[12]

The larynx can be injured directly by heat as well as by the products of combustion, namely acids and aldehydes. This injury can lead to permanent damage of this organ with subsequent speech impairment and has been the subject of a report of the dangers of endotracheal intubation in these patients, especially when performed by paramedical personnel.[13]

TRACHEOBRONCHIAL AREA

As noted in Chap. 3, injury to the tracheobronchial area will seldom be the result of thermal damage because of the low heat content of inspired air at this level. In addition, the airways have an intrinsic ability to dissipate heat.[14] The degree of injury to the tracheobronchial area therefore depends more upon the gaseous and particulate content of the inhaled material. The smoke from burning kerosene, which is high in particulate matter, has been shown to produce very little damage to the respiratory tract.[15] This is in marked contrast to injuries caused by smokes containing aldehyde-like materials, apparently a much more toxic component.[15–17] It produces changes similar to those seen after the upper airway is exposed to acid.[16,18–20] However, of these toxic materials, acrolein was found to be present in higher concentrations relative to its toxicity than the other compounds.[21] Acrolein by itself has been shown to produce tracheobronchial injury when vaporized into a canine preparation.[16] Free radicals have been reported to be present in smoke and have been implicated in edema formation.[22] Nebulization of dimethylsulfoxide, an oxygen free-radical scavenger, into sheep at the time of smoke inhalation has been shown to greatly reduce the injury and the associated mortality.[23] Thus, there is strong evidence that O_2 radicals in smoke may be involved in

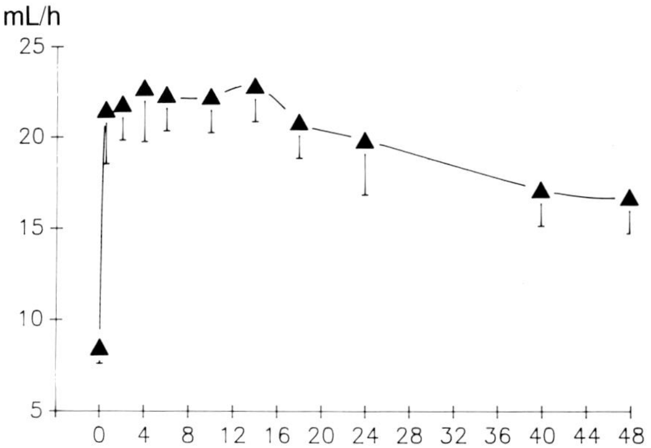

Figure 4-2 The bronchial artery shows an increase in flow which is almost immediate. The animals were subjected to a total of 48 breaths of cotton smoke. The techniques utilized in the study for smoke insufflation are from Kimura et al.[17]

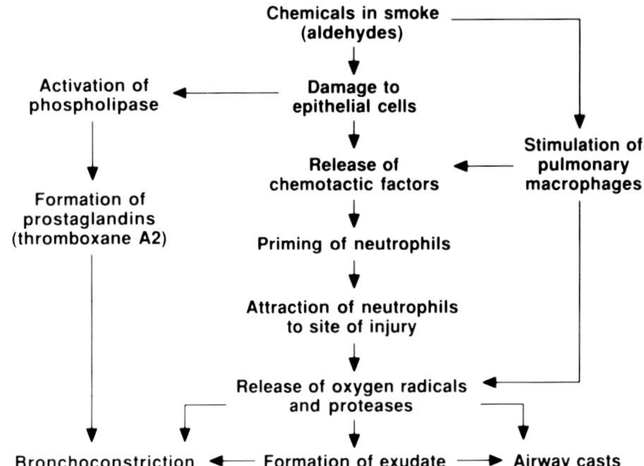

Figure 4-3 Pathophysiology of tracheobronchial damage by smoke inhalation.

the response; however, the role of these materials in initiating the airway injury requires further evaluation.

The caustic materials in smoke produce a localized inflammatory reaction characterized on bronchoscopic examination by erythema and edema.[1] The tracheobronchial area receives its blood supply from the bronchial artery. This vessel supplies some 80 percent of the systemic circulation to the lung in sheep.[24] Figure 4-2 demonstrates the changes in blood flow in this vessel in ewes following inhalation injury. As can be seen, a marked hyperemia occurs almost immediately following inhalation injury and probably plays a very important role in the degree of erythema and edema formation which exists at the time of bronchoscopic diagnosis of smoke inhalation injury.[25] This hyperemic response peaks immediately after injury and is sustained for some 24 hours. At this time the bronchial blood flow begins to return toward baseline, which is attained at 48 hours. These changes in the systemic blood flow were in agreement with those measured utilizing the radioactive microsphere technique.[26] The elevation in blood flow is fairly well distributed throughout the lung after inhalation injury and is about 11 times greater than baseline in the trachea, carina, bronchi, and bronchioles.[26] Although the mediators of this hyperemia have not yet been identified, a similar hyperemia is seen after acid aspiration.[27] Certainly, one would be safe to predict that other mediators of inflammatory hyperemia such as those of the kallikrein-bradykinin system were active.

The pathobiochemical changes in the tracheobronchial areas which result from inhalation injury have been studied serially in sheep,[28,29] and are summarized in Fig. 4-3. After several hours' delay, this localized inflammatory response is followed by a cellular infiltration with exudate formation.[28] This exudative material contains numerous polymorphonuclear neutrophils and lymphocytes and is rich in B-glucuronidase and thromboxane.[29,30] Shortly after the appearance of this exudate, there is a separation of the mucosal areas, leaving behind a naked basement membrane.[28] Perhaps this tissue damage is the result of lysosomal enzymes from the polymorphonuclear cells and macrophages in the area. Between 12 and 36 hours after injury, castlike material may be coughed up, an example of which can be seen in Fig. 4-4. Such casts have been reported to occur both in animal preparations[29] and in human beings.[31] The dissolution of this castlike material is followed by the reparative processes which begin some 48 hours after injury.[28] This process involves the

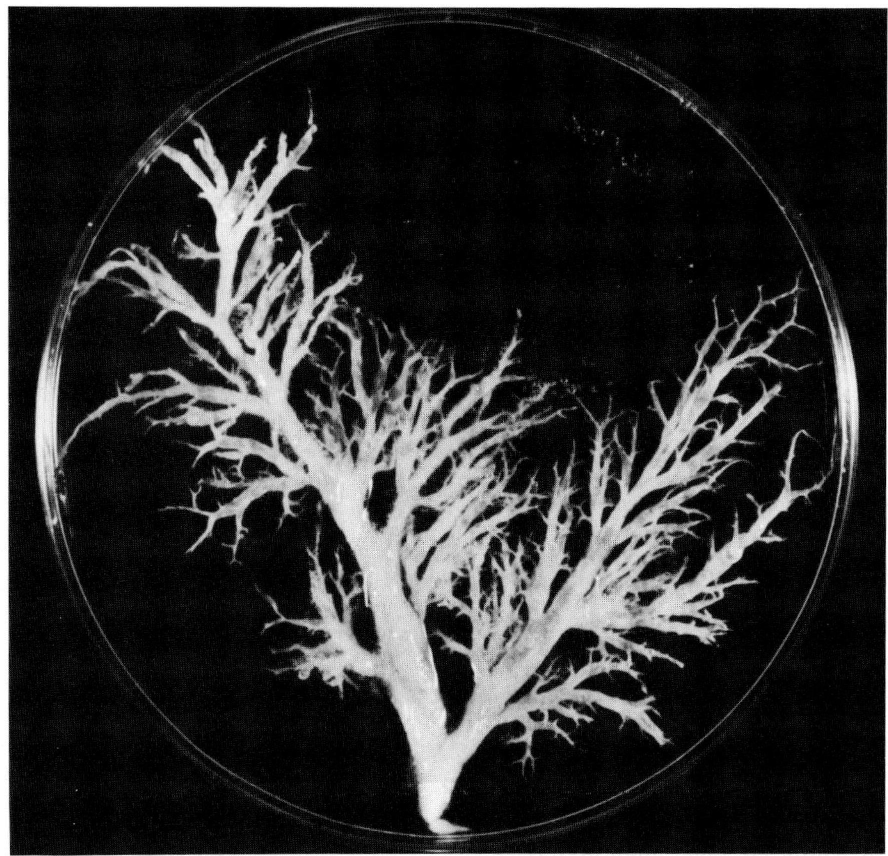

Figure 4-4 This tracheobronchial cast was removed from a sheep at autopsy. It has been shown to contain multiple polymorphonuclear cells as well as cellular debris mainly from the epithelial areas.

spread of epithelial cells to reline the respiratory areas. This may occur initially in a squamous metaplastic fashion.

The factors responsible for attracting the polymorphonuclear cells into the tracheobronchial areas have yet to be identified. Stein et al.[32] have shown that macrophages obtained from the lung following bronchial alveolar lavage produced chemotactic materials, but it is probable that tissue factors released from the injured epithelium result in complement activation and subsequent formation of chemotactic polypeptides.

In association with a smoke inhalation injury to the tracheobronchial area, there is a bronchoconstriction with an increase in respiratory resistance.[33,34] This increase in resistance could be related to the presence of the potent smooth muscle constrictor thromboxane A_2 in the airway. Shinozawa et al.[18] and Kimura et al.[35] have both shown some reduction in lung injury with the use of cyclooxygenase inhibitors. This could be related to the blockade of the synthesis of thromboxane. On the other hand, these elevated airway resistances could be secondary to the presence of mucous plugs and castlike materials.

These changes in bronchial resistance result in a

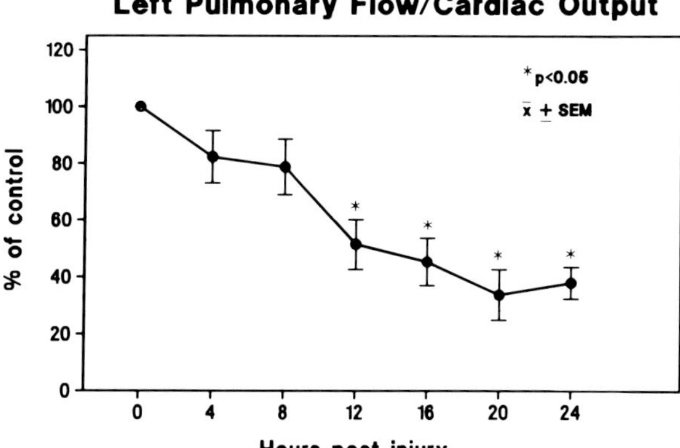

Figure 4-5 Changes in blood flow in the left pulmonary artery following smoke inhalation. The right lung was insufflated with air. The data are means ± the standard error of the mean and were obtained from eight sheep.

probable hypoxic pulmonary vasoconstriction. In studies by Prien et al.[36] in which one lung of sheep was insufflated with smoke and the other with air, there was a marked shunting of blood flow from the injured lung. Figure 4-5 shows the result of experiments in which an ultrasonic flow transit-time measuring device was placed around the left pulmonary artery and the left lung insufflated with smoke. Note the gradual diminution in blood flow to the injured lung. This shunting phenomenon has also been confirmed with radioactive microspheres.[36] These airway reactions may be the causative agents responsible for changes in the ventilation/perfusion ratio that lead to the early fall in arterial oxygenation noted after inhalation injury.[37,38] In support of the eicosanoid mediation of these bronchial changes, Wu et al.[39] have recently reported normalization of acute changes in the ventilation/perfusion ratio following inhalation injury by treatment with cyclooxygenase inhibitors.

PARENCHYMAL AREA

Some controversy exists as to whether damage to the parenchyma is actually seen following inhalation injury. Tranbaugh et al.[40,41] have denied the existence of such an injury, since they were unable to identify increases in extravascular lung water in thermally injured patients who had suffered a concomitant inhalation injury. In these studies they used the double indicator dilution technique to evaluate the presence of extravascular water. Peitzman et al.[42] showed an elevation in extravascular lung water in patients with inhalation injury, utilizing the same technique in burned victims who also sustained inhalation injury as the result of an explosion in a paint factory. Prien et al. have recently reported situations in which there is a significant ventilation/perfusion mismatch, concomitant with severe inhalation injury in a sheep model. In this study the thermal dye technique was used for estimating extravascular lung water. With this method they were unable to detect the edema formation in these animals, although edema was documented at autopsy, both histologically and by gravimetric technique.[36] Consequently, the inability of the Tranbaugh group to identify edema in these patients may be a factor of this technique of measurement. In a recent study, Herndon et al.[2] compared patients with thermal injury, inhalation injury, and a combination of these two. The double indicator dilution technique was likewise used in this clinical study. While they demonstrated an increase in extravascular lung water in both groups with inhalation injury, the group with a combined insult showed a biphasic response, with an elevation in extravascular lung water occurring during the first 24 hours and again during a period 3 to 4 days later. There was no increase in extravascular lung water during the second and third day following injury in the patients with both thermal injury to the cutaneous areas and smoke inhalation damage. During this time there was a marked depression of the ratio of Pa_{O_2}/FI_{O_2}. Since this would be the time one would predict a significant tracheobronchial insult with a ventilation/perfusion mismatch, it is possible that the pulmonary edema was not identified due to a failure of the indicator technique in this situation.[2] Thus, the presence of pulmonary edema following inhalation injury is a definite probability in the clinical setting, in agreement with the finding in the animal models.

Parenchymal injury with a resultant increased microvascular fluid flux has been studied extensively in an ovine model of inhalation injury.[7,37,43,44] Following inhalation injury produced by the insufflation of cotton smoke, there is a marked increase in lung lymph flow. Although these changes are associated with a mild elevation in pulmonary artery pressure and resistance, there is an elevation in the lymph–to–plasma protein concentration ratio, consistent with an elevation in pulmonary microvascular permeability. These changes take place with cardiac outputs and left atrial pressures which have been normalized to baseline level. Consequently, changes in lung lymph protein concentration and flow should not reflect a change in the surface area of the pulmonary microvasculature which is being perfused.

The tracheobronchial interstitial space is continuous with that of the parenchymal areas. Therefore, an elevation in lung lymph flow might result if there were an elevation in transvascular fluid flux across the bronchial microvasculature which would then flood into the parenchymal area. To test this hypothesis, the bronchial artery was occluded in sheep for a period before and at 24 hours after inhalation injury. Interruption of the bronchial circulation by occlusion of the arterial supply will lead to cessations of fluid flux across the pulmonary microvascular bed. The effect of this removal of bronchial fluid flux on the lung lymph flow measurements was determined. The results of these studies are shown in Fig. 4-6. Before inhalation injury, occlusions of bronchial artery had little effect upon lung lymph flow. This is not surprising if one takes into consideration that pulmonary blood flow is the cardiac output and bronchial blood flow is only about 1 percent of this.[24] Twenty-four hours following inhalation injury, when the bronchial artery is occluded, lung lymph flow drops by approximately 25 percent.[45] This demonstrates the probable presence of a significant pulmonary microvascular fluid flux. However, placed into the context of the differences of the perfused surface areas of the two microvasculatures (pulmonary versus bronchial), it also reflects a significant amount of flooding from the bronchial areas.

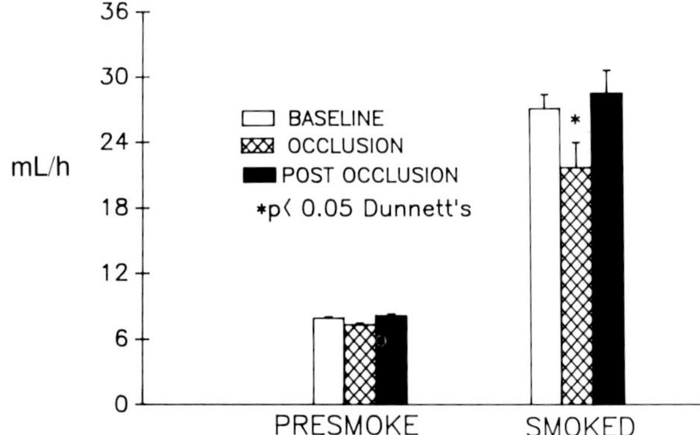

Figure 4-6 This figure shows the changes in pulmonary lymph flow before and 24 hours after inhalation injury and the influence of occlusion of the bronchial artery on this variable during the baseline period before inhalation injury. Occlusion of the bronchial artery produces very little change in pulmonary lymph flow. Twenty-four hours after the sheep was insufflated with smoke there is a marked elevation in pulmonary lymph flow. After occlusion of the bronchial artery there is an approximate 25 percent reduction in this variable. These data were obtained from six sheep which were insufflated with smoke (48 breaths) from burning cotton materials as described by Kimura et al.[17]

The changes in lung lymph flow in the sheep model following inhalation injury are accompanied by elevations in extravascular lung water measured by both the double indicator dilution and gravimetric techniques.[7,30] The changes, however, have a delayed onset, becoming manifest between 12 and 24 hours after injury. These increases in extravascular water correlate with impairment of gas exchange and the increases in lung lymph flow.

Histologically, the parenchymal tissues also show the presence of interstitial edema with increased numbers of polymorphonuclear cells in the tissues.[7,28,30,46] The increased presence of polymorphonuclear cells was seen in the lung lymph of sheep which had been insufflated with smoke and also in lavage fluid obtained from their alveolar areas.[37] When polymorphonuclear cells are activated, they release proteolytic enzymes and oxygen free radicals.[47] These materials can interact with contractile components of endothelial cells to change microvascular permeability, especially in the large surface areas on the venular side of the microvasculature.[49,50] Proteolytic enzymes released from neutrophils can likewise affect the fibronectin materials which join microvascular endothelial cells together, thus opening gaps between them.[48,51] The release of free radicals from these cells, as well as endothelial cells[52] and macrophages[53] which are found in the vascular and airway areas,[54] likewise causes the formation of chemotactic materials which in turn attract additional neutrophils to the area.[55] Oxygen free radicals interact with lipid materials in the tissue to produce conjugated dienes.[56] These materials are elevated in the plasma of animals subjected to inhalation injury.[27] Proteolytic enzymes interact with antiproteases, decreasing their activity.[57] Following inhalation injury there is a reduction of the antiprotease alpha$_2$-macroglobulin as well as the elastase inhibitory capacity.[7,37,57,58] In animals depleted of leukocytes and subjected to inhalation injury, there are only minimal increases in lung lymph flow and plasma conjugated dienes and very little change in alpha$_2$-macroglobulin, thus implicating the polymorphonuclear cell as a primary vector of an injury following smoke inhalation.[27] To confirm the hypothesis that free radicals mediate this response, experiments have been carried out in sheep insufflated with smoke and treated following injury with the oxygen free radical scavenger dimethylsulfoxide. The injury to these animals was much less severe than that to untreated, injured animals.[58,59]

Experiments have also been accomplished in animals treated with antiproteases following smoke inhalation injury. The damage is also less severe in these animals.[60] These studies confirm that there is injury to the parenchyma following inhalation injury and that the injury noted is primarily the result of the release of oxygen free radicals and proteolytic enzymes from polymorphonuclear cells. The pathophysiologic events leading to parenchymal damage are summarized in Fig. 4-7.

Because of the delay between the time of injury and the elevation in lung lymph flow, it is obvious that the injury to the lung parenchymal areas produced by the inhalation of chemicals in smoke is mediated by the hematogenous cells. The mechanisms responsible for the deposition of neutrophils in the parenchymal areas are yet to be determined, and certainly one would predict that the release of chemotactic materials from the tracheobronchial areas would result in priming of polymorphonuclear cells in the circulation. One would also predict that the pulmonary vasoconstriction noted following inhalation injury would entrap these primed cells in the pulmonary microvasculature. Preliminary studies have been accomplished in which the pulmonary artery is occluded for a brief time following inhalation injury. There are additional numbers of polymorphonuclear cells in the tissues of the occluded lung. These lungs have a greater extravascular lung water than their contralateral, unoccluded lungs,[61] providing evidence that there was a more severe injury to the occluded lung. The mechanism by which these entrapped polymorphonuclear cells release oxygen free radicals is unknown but may be related to contact with the endothelial cells of the pulmonary microvasculature.

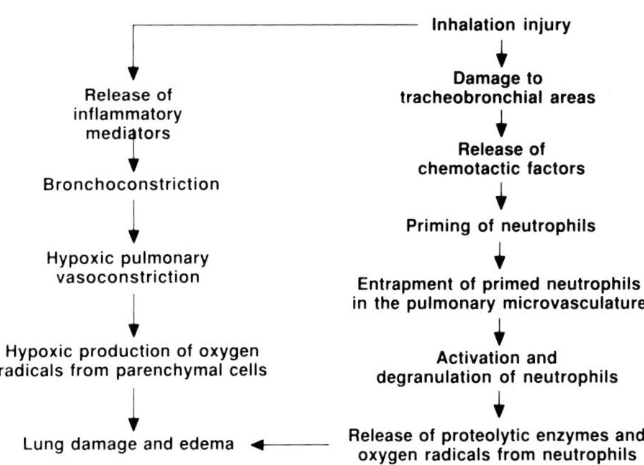

Figure 4-7 Pathophysiology of lung parenchymal damage by smoke inhalation.

Pulmonary compliance has been reported to be decreased following inhalation injury in patients[33,62,63] as well as in animals.[30,62,64] The early changes in compliance are correlated with the accumulation of extravascular lung water.[30] Some controversy exists as to whether changes in surfactant materials are affected by the injury. Studies by Clark et al.[65] have indicated that following the inhalation of smoke, marked atelectasis occurs in the canine model. These changes were associated with reductions in surfactant activities, and the changes in surfactant were seen acutely (i.e., within 4 hours of injury). Examining surfactant materials from the lavage of sheep 24 hours after inhalation injury, Prien et al.[66] were unable to find any significant differences in surfactant compounds between smoked and nonsmoked lungs. Surfactant deficiency has been reported in patients with inhalation injury by Head et al.[67] An interpretation of these data is, however, difficult, since the nutritional status of an individual will also affect his or her surfactant synthesis.[68] This is a problem with burn patients as well as in patients requiring ventilatory support, since feeding is difficult in both situations. One would predict, however, that there should be damage to the epithelial areas in the alveoli, including the alveolar type II cell, which is responsible for the synthesis of surfactant materials, and consequently a deficiency of surface active substances. This is certainly an area which is prime for future investigations.

SYSTEMIC AREAS

There is a higher incidence of multiple organ-system failure in thermally injured patients with inhalation injury than in those with thermal injury alone.[69,70] These patients require larger amounts of fluid for normalization of cardiovascular function.[23] There have been few laboratory investigations of this phenomenon. A recent study found an increase in cutaneous lymph flow in sheep subjected to inhalation injury. This increase in cutaneous lymph flow occurred in both normal and thermally injured sheep (40 percent third-degree flame burn) when the animals were insufflated with smoke.[71] These changes occurred although the plasma-to-lymph oncotic pressure gradient remained unchanged and there were no changes in systemic vascular resistance. Past studies were unable to show any changes in blood flow to the skin following inhalation injury.[26] Thus, the changes in lymph flow may be the result of a change in the microvascular permeability. These changes are isolated to an earlier time period (first 48 hours).

Sugi et al.[72] have also shown that myocardial depression was present following severe inhalation injury in a preliminary report. Figure 4-8 illustrates a comparison of myocardial contractility as evalu-

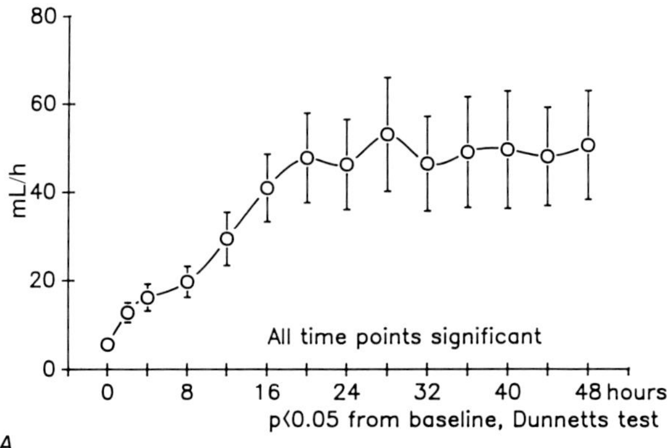

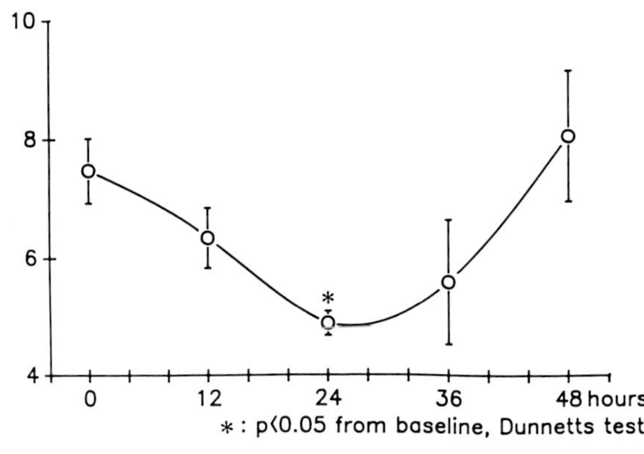

Figure 4-8 A comparison of changes in lung lymph flow (*A*) with the left ventricular end-systolic pressure volume ratio E_{max} (*B*). This ratio was obtained at different loading conditions. These were data obtained from four animals and demonstrate a marked fall in myocardial contractility. The smoking procedure was as described by Kimura et al.,[17] and a total of 64 breaths of cotton smoke were insufflated into these animals.

ated using the index of myocardial contractility, known as E_{max}. (This index is derived from the end systolic pressure/volume ratio and remains relatively constant with changes in preload and after load.) This myocardial depression was correlated with the degree of lung injury as gauged by the changes in lung lymph flow. Smoke exposure is also related to the changes in carbon monoxide levels.[17] With increasing smoke exposure there are increasing levels of carbon monoxide. There are likewise increasing changes in lymph flow.[17] The reduction in myocardial contractility was greater with the higher levels of carbon monoxide. These systemic changes would therefore be the result of ischemia and possibly reperfusion injury. In another experiment in which sheep were exposed to equivalent dosages of carbon monoxide without inhalation injury, myocardial depression was not noted. The mechanisms responsible for these changes in peripheral circulatory function remain to be evaluated. The changes in myocardial contractility did, however, occur in close correlation with the changes in lung lymph.[73] Since the changes in myocardial contractility correlate with the changes in lung damage, it would be tempting to speculate that the damage to the periphery was the result of the release of cytotoxic mediators from the lung.

REFERENCES

1. Moylan JA: Inhalation injury — a primary determinant of survival following major burns. *J Burn Care Rehabil* 3:78, 1981.
2. Herndon DN, Barrow RE, Traber DL, et al: Extravascular lung water changes following smoke inhalation and massive burn injury. *Surgery* 102:341, 1987.
3. Navar PD, Saffle JR, Warden GD: Effect of inhalation injury on fluid resuscitation requirements after thermal injury. *Am J Surg* 150:716, 1985.
4. Thompson PB, Herndon DN, Abston S: Effect on mortality of inhalation injury. *J Trauma* 26:163, 1986.
5. Herndon DN, Thompson PB, Linares HA, et al: Incidence, mortality, pathogenesis and treatment of pulmonary injury. *J Burn Care Rehabil* 71:84, 1986.
6. Shirani KZ, Pruitt BA, Jr, Mason AD, Jr: The influence of inhalation injury and pneumonia on burn mortality. *Ann Surg* 205:82, 1987.
7. Nosaki M, Guest MM, Hirayama T, et al: EDPF: Heat-activated permeability factor derived from erythrocytes and its significance in burns. *J Burn Care Rehabil* 5:30, 1984.
8. Till GO, Ward PA: Oxygen radicals and lipid peroxidation in experimental shock. *Prog Clin Biol Res* 236A:235, 1987.
9. Jin LJ, Lalonde C, Demling RH: Lung dysfunction after thermal injury in relation to prostanoid and oxygen radical release. *J Appl Physiol* 61:103, 1986.
10. Pitt RM, Parker JC, Jurkovich GJ, et al: Analysis of altered capillary pressure and permeability after thermal injury. *J Surg Res* 42:693, 1987.
11. Demling RH: Burn Edema, Part 1: Pathogenesis. *J Burn Care Rehabil* 3:138, 1982.
12. Wells CH, Hilton JG, Larson DL, et al: Effects of nicotinic acid upon postburn edema: A preliminary report of clinical trials. *Burns* 2:152, 1976.
13. Sataloff DM, Sataloff RT: Tracheotomy and inhalation injury. *Head Neck Surg* 6:1024, 1984.
14. Morwitz AR: The effects of inhaled heat on the air passages of the lung: An experimental model. *Arch Intern Med* 126:466, 1970.
15. Zikria BA, Ferrar JM, Floch HF: The chemical factors contributing to pulmonary damage in "smoke poisoning." *Surgery* 71:704, 1972.
16. Hales CA, Barkin PW, Jung W, et al: Synthetic smoke with acrolein but not HCl produces pulmonary edema. *J Appl Physiol* 64:1121, 1988.
17. Kimura R, Traber LD, Herndon DN, et al: Increasing duration of smoke exposure induces more severe lung injury in sheep. *J Appl Physiol* 64:1107, 1988.
18. Shinozawa Y, Hales CA, Jung W, et al: Ibuprofen prevents synthetic smoke-induced pulmonary edema. *Am Rev Respir Dis* 134:1145, 1986.
19. Winn R, Stothert J, Nadir B, et al: Lung mechanics following aspiration of 0.1 N hydrochloric acid. *J Appl Physiol* 55:1051, 1983.
20. Winn R, Stothert J, Nadir B, et al: Lung fluid balance, vascular permeability, and gas exchange after acid aspiration in awake goats. *J Appl Physiol* 46:979, 1984.
21. Treitman RD, Burgess WA, Gold A: Air contaminants encountered by fire fighters. *Am Ind Hyg Assoc J* 41:796, 1980.
22. Crapo JD, Barry BE, Chang L, et al: Alterations in lung structure caused by inhalation of oxidants. *J Toxicol Environ Health* 13:301, 1984.
23. Brown M, Desai M, Traber LD, et al: Dimethylsulfoxide with heparin in the treatment of smoke inhalation injury. *J Burn Care Rehabil* 9:22, 1988.
24. Magno MG, Fishman AP: Origin, distribution, and blood flow of bronchial circulation in anesthetized sheep. *J Appl Physiol* 53:272, 1982.
25. Maguire JP, Traber LD, Sugi K, et al: Bronchial blood

flow in response to inhalation injury. *Am Rev Respir Dis* 137:194, 1988.
26. Kramer GC, Herndon DN, Linares HA, et al: Effects of inhalation injury on airway blood flow and edema formation. *J Burn Care Rehabil* 10:45, 1989.
27. Basadre JO, Sugi K, Traber DL, et al: The effect of leukocyte depletion on smoke inhalation injury in sheep. *Surgery* 104:208, 1988.
28. Linares HA, Herndon DN, Traber DL: Sequence of morphological events in experimental smoke inhalation. *J Burn Care Rehabil* 10:27, 1989.
29. Herndon DN, Traber LD, Linares H, et al: Etiology of the pulmonary pathophysiology associated with inhalation injury. *Resuscitation* 14:43, 1986.
30. Traber DL, Schlag G, Redl H, et al: Pulmonary edema and compliance changes following smoke inhalation. *J Burn Care Rehabil* 6:490, 1985.
31. Pruitt BA, Flemma RJ, DiVincenti FC, et al: Pulmonary complications in burn patients. *J Thorac Cardiovasc Surg* 59:7, 1970.
32. Stein MD, Herndon DN, Stevens JM, et al: Production of chemotactic factors and lung cell changes following smoke inhalation in a sheep model. *J Burn Care Rehabil* 7:117, 1986.
33. Petroff PA, Hander EW, Clayton WH, et al: Pulmonary function studies after smoke inhalation. *Am J Surg* 132:346, 1976.
34. Prien T, Traber DL, Richardson JA, et al: Early effects of inhalation injury on lung mechanics and pulmonary perfusion. *Intensive Care Med* 14:25, 1988.
35. Kimura R, Traber LD, Herndon DN, et al: Ibuprofen reduces the lung lymph flow changes associated with inhalation injury. *Circ Shock* 24:183, 1988.
36. Prien T, Traber DL, Herndon DN, et al: Pulmonary edema with smoke inhalation undetected by indicator dilution technique. *J Appl Physiol* 63:907, 1987.
37. Traber DL, Herndon DN, Stein MD, et al: The pulmonary lesion of smoke inhalation in an ovine model. *Circ Shock* 18:311, 1986.
38. Robinson NB, Hudson LD, Robertson HT, et al: Ventilation and perfusion alterations after smoke inhalation injury. *Surgery* 90:352, 1981.
39. Wu W, Barie P, Halebian P, et al: Attenuation of ventilation-perfusion mismatching with ibuprofen in inhalation lung injury. *Proc Am Burn Assoc* 20:105, 1988.
40. Tranbaugh RF, Elings VB, Christensen JM, et al: Effect of inhalation injury on lung water accumulation. *J Trauma* 23:597, 1983.
41. Tranbaugh RF, Lewis FR, Christensen JM, et al: Lung water changes after thermal injury: The effects of crystalloid resuscitation and sepsis. *Ann Surg* 192:479, 1980.
42. Peitzman AB, Shires GT III, Corbett WA, et al: Measurement of lung water in inhalation injury. *Surgery* 90:305, 1981.
43. Herndon DN, Traber DL, Niehaus GD, et al: The pathophysiology of smoke inhalation injury in a sheep model. *J Trauma* 24:1044, 1984.
44. Herndon DN, Traber DL, Linares HA, et al: Effects of smoke inhalation on airway blood flow and edema formation. *Circ Shock* 16:45, 1985.
45. Walsh JC, Maguire J, Herndon D, et al: The bronchial circulation contributes to lung lymph flow after inhalation injury. *Fed Proc* 2:A953, 1988.
46. Prien T, Linares H, Traber LD, et al: Lack of hematogenous mediated pulmonary injury with smoke inhalation. *J Burn Care Rehabil* 9:462, 1988.
47. Simchowitz L, Mehta J, Spilberg I: Chemotactic factor-induced generation of superoxide radicals by human PMN's. *Arthritis Rheum* 22:755, 1979.
48. McDonald JA, Baum BJ, Rosenberg DM, et al: Destruction of a major extracellular adhesive glycoprotein (fibronectin) of human fibroblasts by neutral proteases from polymorphonuclear leukocyte granules. *Lab Invest* 40:350, 1979.
49. Svensjo E, Grega GJ: Evidence for endothelial cell-mediated regulation of macromolecular permeability by postcapillary venules. *Fed Proc* 45:89, 1986.
50. Miller FN, Sims DE: Contractile elements in the regulation of macromolecular permeability. *Fed Proc* 45:84, 1986.
51. Richards PS, Saba TM, Del-Vecchio PJ, et al: Matrix fibronectin disruption in association with altered endothelial cell adhesion induced by activated polymorphonuclear leukocytes. *Exp Mol Pathol* 45:1, 1986.
52. Brigham KL, Meyrick B, Berry LC Jr, et al: Antioxidants protect cultured bovine lung endothelial cells from injury by endotoxin. *J Appl Physiol* 63:840, 1987.
53. Sibilly Y, Merrill W, Cooper J, et al: Effects of a series of chloromethyl ketone protease inhibitors on superoxide release and the glutathione system in human polymorphonuclear leukocytes and alveolar macrophages. *Am Rev Respir Dis* 130:110, 1984.
54. Warner AE, Brain JD: Intravascular pulmonary macrophages: A novel cell removes particles from blood. *Am J Physiol* 250:R728, 1986.
55. Petrone WF, English DK, Wong K, et al: Free radicals and inflammation: Superoxide-dependent activation of a neutrophil chemotactic factor in plasma. *Proc Natl Acad Sci* 77:1159, 1980.
56. Ward PA, Till GO, Hatherill JR, et al: Systemic complement activation, lung injury, and products of lipid peroxidation. *J Clin Invest* 76:517, 1985.
57. Zaslow M, Clark R, Stone P, et al: Human neutrophil elastase does not bind to alpha-1-proteinase inhibitor that has been exposed to activated human PMN's. *Am Rev Respir Dis* 128:434, 1983.
58. Desai MH, Brown M, Mlcak R, et al: Reduction of smoke lung injury with dimethylsulfoxide (DMSO) and heparin treatment. *Surg Forum* 36:103, 1985.
59. Kimura R, Mlcak R, Richardson J, et al: Treatment of smoke induced pulmonary injury with nebulized dimethylsulfoxide (DMSO). *Proc Am Burn Assoc* 19:133, 1987.
60. Kimura R, Lubbesmeyer H, Traber L, et al: Antiprotease inhibition of smoke induced lung lymph flow elevations. *Fed Proc* 46:1100, 1987.
61. Maguire J, Linares HA, Traber L, et al: Reperfusion injury of the lung following smoke inhalation. *Physiologist* 30:144, 1987.
62. Garzon AA, Seltzer B, Song IC, et al: Respiratory me-

chanics in patients with inhalation burns. *J Trauma* 10:57, 1970.
63. Demling RH: Effect of early burn excision and grafting on pulmonary function. *J Trauma* 24:830, 1984.
64. Esrig BC, Stephenson SF, Fulton RL: Role of pulmonary infection in the pathogenesis of smoke inhalation. *Surg Forum* 26:204, 1975.
65. Clark WR, Webb WR, Wax S, et al: Inhalation injuries: The pathophysiology of acute smoke inhalation. *Surg Forum* 28:177, 1977.
66. Prien T, Strohmaier W, Gasser H, et al: Normal phosphatidylcholine composition of lung surfactant 24 hours after inhalation injury. *J Burn Care Rehabil* 10:38, 1989.
67. Head JM: Inhalation injury in burns. *Am J Surg* 139:508, 1980.
68. Thet LA, Alvarez H: Effect of hyperventilation and starvation of rat lung mechanics and surfactant. *Am Rev Respir Dis* 126:286, 1982.
69. Aikawa N, Shinozawa Y, Ishibiki K, et al: Clinical analysis of multiple organ failure in burned patients. *Burns Incl Therm Inj* 13:103, 1987.
70. Herndon DN, Traber DL, Traber LD: The effect of resuscitation on inhalation injury. *Surgery* 100:248, 1986.
71. Montero K, Lubbesmeyer HJ, Traber DL, et al: Inhalation injury increases systemic microvascular permeability. *Surg Forum* 38:303, 1987.
72. Sugi K, Kimura R, Traber L, et al: Myocardial depression following inhalation injury. *Proc Am Burn Assoc* 20:77, 1988.
73. Sugi K, Newald J, Traber LD, et al: Correlation between lung injury and myocardial depression after endotoxin (LPS) in sheep. *Circ Shock* 24:251, 1988.

Chapter 5

Adult Respiratory Distress Syndrome

Warren R. Summer

Adult respiratory distress syndrome (ARDS) is a condition which was first described in 1967 by Ashbaugh et al. in what is now a benchmark article.[1] These investigators reported a number of patients with unexplained tachypnea, diffuse chest radiographic infiltrates, and profound hypoxemia. A substantial proportion of those patients died, with the pathology reminding the authors of the neonatal respiratory distress syndrome (NRDS). Consequently, they coined the term *adult respiratory distress syndrome,* which is now the general appellation used to describe this acute clinical pulmonary condition. Many other names have been applied, with each reflecting either the circumstances under which lung injury occurred or the place where the problem was identified initially (e.g., shock lung, posttraumatic respiratory insufficiency, DaNang lung, etc.).[2,3]

Currently there seem to be a number of problems with our perceptions of ARDS: we do not have any general consensus on definition, we do not know the possible etiology, and we have no specific treatment. This confusion is aggravated further by our appreciation of an unacceptably high mortality. The timely clinical recognition and effective management of ARDS in patients with smoke inhalation and/or cutaneous burns requires a thorough general understanding of this devastating clinical condition.

GENERAL RECOGNITION AND DIAGNOSIS OF ARDS

Recently, Murray et al.[4] have suggested ways in which we can better recognize and diagnose ARDS. Although the clinical problem is usually acute edema, the process may proceed to pulmonary fibrosis in 5 to 6 days. The mechanism by which rapid fibrosis occurs is not known, but differentiating the two stages of this condition is reasonable since the approach to therapy and outcome differs. Thus, ARDS should be defined as either acute or chronic.

The principal aspects of ARDS recognition include a characteristic clinical presentation[5] and, most of the time, identification of one or more patient risk factors (Table 5-1).[6–8] The list of these predispositions appears somewhat disjointed but is likely to contain a common thread which is yet undefined. It is also convenient to consider risk factors in two groups, according to whether they predominantly and primarily affect the respiratory system or whether they are more systemic in nature. For example, primary local respiratory risk factors include smoke inhalation, gastric acid aspiration, and influenza pneumonia; more commonly, ARDS is seen following a systemic event such as the sepsis syndrome, hemorrhagic shock, nonthoracic traumatic shock, etc. If either the local or systemic risk factors can be associated with mechanisms that injure the lung differently, this characterization will ultimately be helpful. However, at this time we have relatively little insight into the predominant mechanisms producing lung injury. Whether there are significant group differences or distinctions among individual risk factors within any currently devised classification is unknown.

Clinical Presentations

The clinical presentation of ARDS is usually characteristic. The condition is relatively sudden in onset, developing over hours to days.[4,5] This temporal relationship is likely telling us something about its pathogenesis and certainly helps us in differential diagnosis. There is often a recent chest roentgenogram of the patient that is unremarkable. Some hours after an inciting event, the patient suddenly develops severe tachypnea and diffuse radiographic changes. Dyspnea may precede the development of pulmonary infiltrates by several hours. The sudden clinical change, together with the setting, make it highly unlikely the patient is suffering from lymphangitic cancer, tuberculosis, acute idiopathic pulmonary fibrosis, or other more chronic conditions. Even if a previous recent chest radiograph is not available, there is often clinical evidence that the patient was well immediately before the onset of acute respiratory distress. Thus, a woman who had an apparently normal pregnancy now reports difficulty breathing in the postpartum period, or a young man in prior good health who, suddenly, after a motorcycle accident and femoral fracture, experiences an acute respiratory problem, represent common historical vignettes. Either acutely developing or delayed-onset dyspnea in patients with smoke inhalation or the typically late onset of dyspnea and hypoxemia in patients with burn-related sepsis are too-familiar scenarios (Fig. 5-1). Another important aspect to remember about the suddenness of this condition is that we are likely to be dealing with a patient who was basically well before this recent illness. If the patient is salvaged from the acute illness, he or she can often be returned to near normal health with adequately functioning lungs. In general, these patients are not in the twilight of their lives with little chance to be returned to complete health. The presence of such functional reserve is of crucial significance: when ARDS does occur in the elderly or in individuals with severe underlying chronic illnesses, its prognosis is all the more ominous.

Table 5-1 Risk Factors Associated with ARDS

Common
Sepsis syndrome with or without shock
Severe trauma (thoracic, extrathoracic)
Pneumonia (bacterial, viral)
Aspiration of gastric contents
Disseminated intravascular coagulation
Near-drowning
Occasional
Fluid overload
Smoke or toxic gas inhalation
Surface burns
Fat embolization
Anaphylactic reaction to drugs and blood
Neurogenic injury
Toxic drugs and poisons

Roentgenographic Clues

The next important aspect of clinical ARDS recognition is the radiographic pattern.[9,10] Alveolar consolidation, which was described classically as

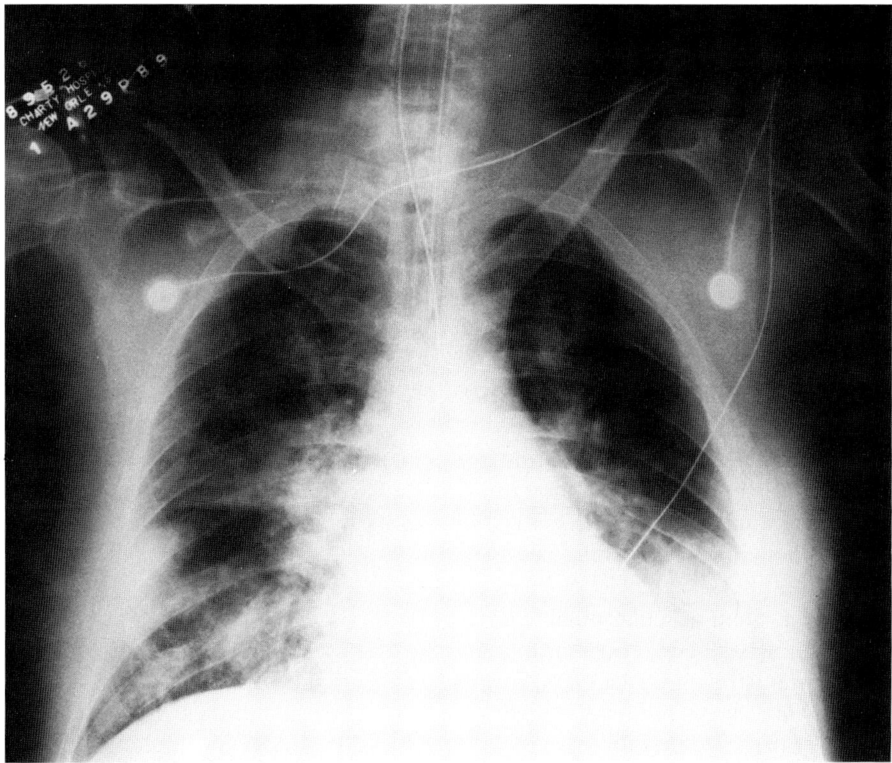

Figure 5-1 A chest roentgenogram obtained 24 hours after massive smoke inhalation during a residential fire. The patient had 10 percent of body surface area burn, with predominant facial involvement, and an admission arterial carboxyhemoglobin level of 50 percent. Progressive hypoxemia developed prior to the onset of patchy, bilateral roentgenographic infiltrates. Note the normal heart size and narrow vascular pedicle. The patient was tachypneic ($R > 30$ breaths/min), with a Pa_{O_2}/FI_{O_2} ratio of less than 60, total thoracic compliance of approximately 22 mL/cmH_2O, and normal pulmonary capillary wedge pressure. Acute treatment included endotracheal intubation, administration of high concentrations of oxygen (including hyperbaric oxygen), and the use of PEEP. The patient improved dramatically, with minimal residual injury, but required prolonged hospitalization.

generalized and diffuse, can appear patchy or multifocal and may initially involve only a few portions of the lung.[11] Air bronchograms and a peripheral distribution of infiltrates are common. Costophrenic angles are often only minimally involved with infiltrates, while interstitial (Kerley's) lines and pleural effusions are usually absent. Lung involvement is generally patchy, even when it appears generalized and diffuse on an anterior/posterior roentgenogram (Fig. 5-1). An inhomogeneous injury has been demonstrated by computed tomography[12] and suggests that there are areas between the infiltrates or densities which are morphologically and physiologically "normal." Theoretically, these areas could be injured by the wrong therapy. Alternatively, the function of these units might be optimized with appropriate treatment. There are several investigations which have generated radiographic scores (e.g., by dividing the x-ray into various quadrants and grading them) in an attempt to quantitate involvement and extent of disease.[4,13,14] To date, there is neither a well-accepted system nor evidence that this form of classification predicts outcome. In general, the relationship between a quantified radiographic scoring and a Pa_{O_2} is also inconsistent.[15]

Certain radiographic features have been reported to distinguish permeability edema from hydrostatic or volume overload pulmonary edema,[13,14] although this is controversial and may depend on who is interpreting the x-ray. In some patients the x-ray is more helpful than in others in distinguishing volume overload. In general, patients with ARDS have a normal-sized heart and a small vascular pedicle. An enlarging vascular pedicle has been reported to precede lung edema in patients being resuscitated from smoke inhalation and large surface burns, presumably as a radiographic correlate of volume overload contributing to vascular leak.[16] The lack of demonstrable Kerley's B lines in permeability pulmonary edema probably results because the peripheral alveolar infiltrates silhouette out intralobular septal edema. Peribronchial edema is usually not observed in roentgenograms of ARDS patients, despite the fact that morphologic observations show that pulmonary edema fluid (ARDS or that due to other causes) initially accumulates in the peribronchial space because of the low absolute pressure of this area.[9]

Studies have generally failed to show a good correlation between lung water as measured by double dye dilution techniques, Pa_{O_2}, percent right to left intrapulmonary shunting, or quantitative radiographic scoring.[15,17,18] This is not a surprise, considering that lung injury is probably patchy and irregular. Moreover, individuals may vasoconstrict to varying degrees due to hypoxemia and/or released mediators, and varied ventilator settings further influence alveolar distention and blood flow through these units. Methods to obtain radiographic scores usually require that patients be taken off positive end-expiratory pressure (PEEP) to produce a more uniform density, a maneuver that is not clinically practical. In one recent study of radiographic findings in burned patients, however, increases of extravascular lung water (EVLW thermal-green dye double indicator technique), decreases of static of thoracic compliance, and increases of shunt fraction ($\dot{Q}_S/\dot{Q}_T$) correlated with increasing radiologic grades of severity. Interestingly, measurements of the plasma colloid osmotic pressure-pulmonary artery wedge pressure gradient (COP-PAW) did not correlate with either radiologic scores or EVLW measurements. More correlative investigations in this area are needed. Roentgenographic manifestations of inhalation injury are reviewed in detail in Chap. 8.

Physiologic Changes

There are a number of characteristic physiologic changes in ARDS which aid in its recognition and diagnosis (Table 5-2).[4,6,14,19] These nonspecific alterations have been encountered with diverse etiologies of lung injury, including smoke inhalation with or without cutaneous burns, and suggest common pathways in their pathogenesis. The first and foremost abnormality is a massive right-to-left intrapulmonary shunt which is responsible for the severe hypoxemia. For years, it has been accepted that the level of shunting was important in defining ARDS.[4] The ratio of arterial Pa_{O_2} to FI_{O_2} is an easy way to characterize this degree of shunting; a Pa_{O_2}/FI_{O_2} of less than 150 to 200 was required for diagnosis of ARDS.[4] It is now known that there are gradations of severity of ARDS from mild to severe, with a ratio below 100 considered to represent very severe disease; a ratio between 100 and 200 is the standard boundary currently best characterized in the literature.[4] A number of cases of acute lung injury may occur with a similar pathogenesis but milder physiologic changes.[20] This presentation has been poorly studied but appears to have an entirely different

Table 5-2 Physiologic Parameters in ARDS

Parameter	Indicator	Normal values	ARDS ranges
Gas Exchange			
A-a gradient	Ventilation/perfusion	<10 mmHg	>300 mmHg
Pa_{O_2}		>90 mmHg	<55 mmHg
$\dot{Q}s/\dot{Q}t$	Shunt	<6%	>20%
Pa_{O_2}/FI_{O_2}		>500	<300
Mechanics			
Peak inspiratory pressure	Airway resistance and lung recoil or stiffness	7 cmH_2O with VT = 600	>40 cmH_2O
Plateau pressure	—	6 cmH_2O with VT = 600	>30 cmH_2O
Compliance	Lung recoil or stiffness	100 mL/cmH_2O	<30 mL/cmH_2O
Hemodynamics			
Pulmonary artery pressure	Cross-section area or resistance of vascular bed	15 mmHg (mean)	>20 mmHg (mean)
Pulmonary artery minus pulmonary capillary wedge	Resistance	1–2 mmHg	>6 mmHg
Cardiac output	Adequacy of blood flow	4–6 L/min	8–12 L/min
Pulmonary vascular resistance	Vasoconstriction ± embolic obstruction, loss of vascular area	1–2 mmHg/L/min	>3 mmHg/L/min

VT = Tidal volume.

prognosis and should be considered separate from ARDS.

Most patients with ARDS have a decreased pulmonary compliance. Interestingly, the reduced compliance correlates very poorly with the chest x-ray and Pa_{O_2}.[4,21] The mechanism for the decrease in compliance is predominantly due to increased lung water and inactivation of surfactant. Surfactant is not reduced in its quantity as much as it is inactivated by proteinaceous pulmonary edema. Effects of smoke inhalation injury upon pulmonary surfactant have suggested its acute inactivation by the particulate component of smoke.[22] Most recently, identification of normal phosphatidylcholine measurements within bronchoalveolar lavage fluid within 24 hours of experimental smoke inhalation have suggested that this is a transitional change.[23] Addition of surfactant to the injured lung may be of some value in improving compliance in ARDS patients, but this has not been studied satisfactorily. In the more chronic ARDS the decrease in pulmonary compliance may be due to fibrosis.[24] Although reduced lung compliance is the major mechanical change associated with ARDS, it has recently been recognized that abnormally increased airflow resistance occurs as well.[25] This change, potentially due to tissue factors, airway hyperactivity, airway inflammation, or their combinations, is consistent with bedside observations in patients with ARDS due to inhalation injury and might ultimately have implications for bronchodilator therapy.

The hallmark of ARDS is permeability pulmonary edema due to injury of the capillary endothelium and/or alveolar epithelium.[26] This injury changes the permeability surface area product of the lung and the reflection coefficient, allowing more fluid to pass through the surface membranes at any hydrostatic pressure, with a loss of selective sieving of larger protein molecules. The ratio of pulmonary edema fluid protein to that in serum is high (>70 percent), and large molecules such as α_2 macroglobulin appear outside the microvascular membranes. Measurements of these protein ratios and large molecules can help differentiate between permeability and hydrostatic pulmonary edema but are seldom used clinically.[27]

For many years clinicians have required hemodynamic measurements demonstrating left atrial filling pressures of less than 14 to 18 mmHg to document the diagnosis of ARDS.[6] This rigid criterion for demonstrating normal pulmonary capillary wedge pressures now relates predominantly to research studies, where subtle distinctions among patients may be necessary. Wedge pressure measurements are not absolutely essential for diagnosis of ARDS, since clinical correlations are often satisfactory and a high wedge pressure does not necessarily exclude increased "capillary leak."[4] In this regard, elderly persons after cardiac bypass surgery are often excluded from reports of permeability pulmonary edema, as are individuals with some combination of permeability and hydrostatic pulmonary edema. This approach overlooks the fact that on some occasions an elevated wedge pressure occurs transiently and is not documented, resulting in a presumed but erroneous diagnosis of nonhydrostatic pulmonary edema. For example, a 93-year-old woman with high fever went into what appeared to be acute pulmonary edema; by the time she was intubated and a balloon flotation catheter inserted, her wedge pressure was only 7 mmHg. She was thought to have ARDS, but 2 days later her infiltrates were markedly improved. There must have been a problem with left ventricular diastolic compliance or papillary muscle dysfunction brought about by stress: respiratory work and fever precipitated transient hydrostatic pulmonary edema, which was diagnosed erroneously as permeability edema because of overreliance on hemodynamic requirements rather than sound clinical judgments. In addition, permeability pulmonary edema may be caused by acute hydrostatic trauma. If the pulmonary vasculature is immediately distended by rapid elevations in left atrial pressures and then the pressures return rapidly back to normal, the measured fluid flux may remain elevated for some time. Thus, hydrostatic changes may alter endothelial gaps; the resultant fluid shift through these vessel walls appears to be that of permeability pulmonary edema, even though the injury was actually hydrostatic. Such clinical dilemmas are apt to be even more complex in burned patients with inhalation injury, particularly when their acute problems are superimposed on preexisting cardiac disease and when transient increases of hydrostatic pressure occur during resuscitation.

Diagnosis of ARDS is made clinically by observing the sudden onset of dyspnea in a patient with certain risk factors who has severe hypoxemia unresponsive to administration of high $F_{I_{O_2}}$ and a radiograph compatible with noncardiogenic pulmonary edema (Table 5-3). Usually, increased permeability can be inferred in the absence of elevated neck veins or peripheral edema and the presence of a normal-sized heart, even without hemodynamic measurements. There has been increasing skepticism about the risk/benefit ratios of pulmonary artery catheterization and the interpretation of hemodynamic data in the presence of marked pleural pressure swings with PEEP; in addition, external stresses are forcing reductions in hospital costs. In the future, documentation of increased permeability may evolve around noninvasive means of demonstrating flux of large molecules in the alveolar space. Loss of selectivity for large molecules defines increased permeability[27–29] and is a better estimation of capillary leak than either measurements of elevated bronchoalveolar lavage (BAL)/plasma total protein ratios[28,29] or reduced wedge pressures.

Table 5-3 Diagnosis of Adult Respiratory Distress Syndrome

High probability	Moderate probability
Tachypnea	Tachypnea
$Pa_{O_2}/FI_{O_2} < 200$	$Pa_{O_2}/FI_{O_2} < 300–350$
Known common risk factors	Uncommon risk factors
Diffuse pulmonary infiltrates	Patchy or multiple segmental infiltrates
Reduced compliance	Near-normal compliance
Pulmonary hypertension	Normal pulmonary resistance
Coagulopathy (thrombocytopenia, DIC)	Normal coagulation or only thrombocytopenia
Multiorgan failure	Only pulmonary involvement
High BAL/serum total protein ratios > 0.8 or large protein molecules found in BAL > 70A	BAL/serum total protein < 0.6; BAL molecular protein radii < 70A
Characteristic pathology	No pathology specimen available

BAL = Bronchoalveolar lavage.

Several aspects of each of these latter parameters make them difficult to interpret currently.[4]

Pathologic Findings

There is a characteristic but nonspecific histologic picture in ARDS.[30,31] The sequential morphologic abnormalities observed in models of smoke inhalation[32] and in burn victims with fatal inhalation injuries[33–35] typify these changes (Fig. 5-2). Cellular infiltration of the lung interstitium, alveolar cell hyperplasia, and hyaline membranes have been associated with the prior treatment with positive pressure ventilation and oxygen in high concentrations.[33] Electron microscopic studies of patients with lethal burn-related respiratory failure have revealed severe interstitial edema involving the thick portion of the alveolar capillary membrane. Despite severe epithelial necrosis, endothelial damage was minimal, and the appearance of cells resembling type II pneumocytes suggested alveolar epithelial regeneration. The hyaline membrane layer seems to correspond to cellular debris from necrotic alveolar epithelium and fibrogen-like material. Changes observed in a carefully standardized sheep model of smoke inhalation injury (Table 5-4) seem consistent with pathophysiologic events in humans.

Unfortunately, routine histology does not help early in differential diagnosis, because by the time the usual pathological pattern develops, the patient has advanced disease. Moreover, lung biopsy procedures are hazardous, nonspecific, and impractical in these patients and are not recommended for routine diagnosis. Electron microscopic studies of a young traumatized patient dying within 24 hours of clinical diagnosis of ARDS may not show damaged endothelial or epithelial membranes.[35] Such sparse early morphologic changes are consistent with the pathophysiologic concept that early permeability in some cases may be a dynamic event rather than a purely morphologic change. ARDS associated with gastric acid aspiration, seizures, and heroin administration may resolve within 24 hours or less. A physiologic increase in permeability, in contrast to irreversible destruction, is supported further by recent evidence that certain mediators implicated in sepsis syndrome and ARDS (e.g., tumor necrosis factor) can produce fluid leak when placed on endothelial monolayers. Although hyaline membranes may indicate increased vascular permeability to large molecules such as fibrinogen, electron micrographs show that these substances may pass into the pulmonary interstitium through apparently intact endothelium.[36] Endothelial cell swelling has been observed within hours of ARDS diagnosis without evidence of widened intercellular junctions or interstitial edema, consistent with an alternative concept that direct damage to endothelial cells occurs early in some circumstances and results in increased permeability through intracellular pores and eventual loss of cell integrity.[37] In the carefully studied sheep model of smoke inhalation, although endothelial damage appears less severe than that to epithelial cells, "loose junctions" or interendothelial gaps with cytoplasmic swelling have been observed. Characteristic histologic findings of ARDS are usually found in patients who succumb after 48 to 72 hours and may reflect combinations of multi-

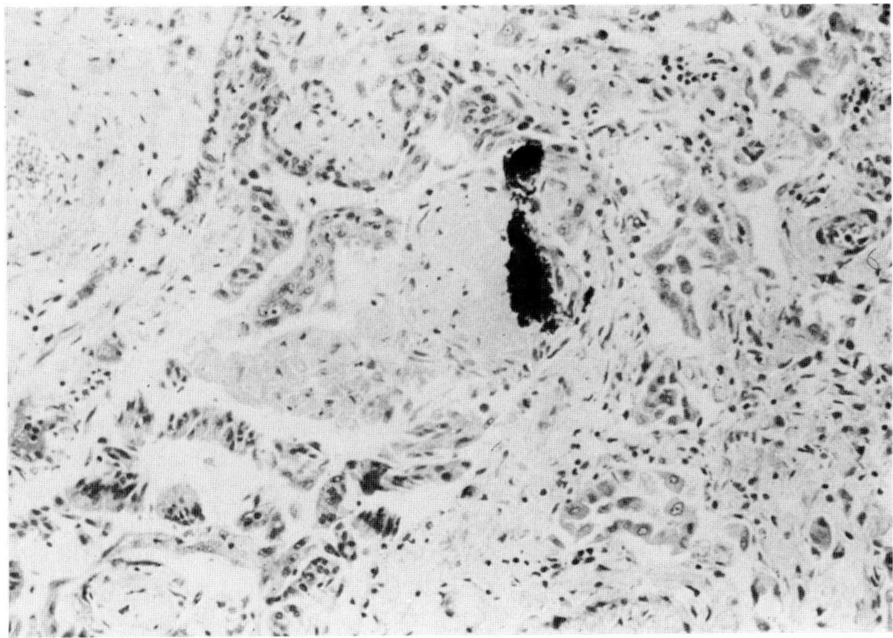

Figure 5-2 Histologic changes in a patient with fatal smoke inhalation injury. Although the presence of inhaled carbonaceous material suggests a specific etiology, the exudative and cellular response is similar to that seen in ARDS due to other etiologies. (*Reprinted with permission from Ref. 35.*)

Table 5-4 Evolution of Parenchymal Responses to Experimental Smoke Inhalation Injury

	Phase	Timing	Predominant histologic characteristics
I.	Exudative	0–48	Interstitial edema; alveolar edema, hemorrhage; PMN influx; variable type I pneumocyte changes
II.	Degenerative	12 h–72 h	Type I pneumocyte injury, denuding basement membrane; necrosis; hyaline membranes
III.	Proliferative	48 h–7 days	Type II pneumocyte hyperplasia, covering basement membrane; mobilization of macrophages
IV.	Reparative	>4 days	Type II pneumocyte transformation (to type I), proceeding to complete repair vs. fibroblast proliferation proceeding to interstitial fibrosis

SOURCE: Modified from Linares HA, Herndon DM, Traber DL (Ref. 32).

ple diseases and iatrogenic insults.[36] Severe pulmonary fibrosis may also develop in 5 to 7 days.[4,21] The mechanism for this rapid scarring is unknown.

PREDISPOSITIONS TO ARDS

Clinical Risk Factors

Knowledge of risk factors can help to identify the probability of ARDS.[6–8,38,39] Several studies have found some definable risk factor in 100 percent of ARDS cases (Table 5-1). However, among patients with designated risk factors, the predictability of these ranges from 6 to 50 percent. In general, about one-fourth of all patients who are identified to have a high risk will develop ARDS. Some predispositions are clearly more injurious than others, with sepsis syndrome and near-drowning having a 40 to 50 percent predictability for ARDS. Similar epidemiologic studies show that ARDS is unlikely to follow cutaneous burns alone (2.3 percent risk).[6] The likelihood of ARDS appears to be substantially higher in women compared to men with burns,[6] but reasons for this difference are unclear. Herndon and coworkers have noted that noncardiogenic pulmonary edema occurs in approximately one-fourth of patients with inhalation injury, typically develops from 6 to 72 hours after burn, and connotes a 60 to 70 percent mortality.[40]

Although knowledge of risk factors is helpful, the incidence of ARDS is not high enough to institute preventive treatment on the basis of this information. Currently, there are no prospective studies demonstrating a therapy capable of preventing ARDS in patients at risk. However, the more risk factors that can be identified, the more the chance that ARDS may develop.[6–8,38] This is not a surprise, since the sicker the patient, the more likely that amplification of factors likely to injure the lung will occur. Although there are large numbers of diseases that have been associated with ARDS, i.e., a large number of potential risk factors, the vast majority of patients suffer from one or more of a few diseases. The major predisposition seen on medical wards is sepsis or sepsis syndrome, while multiple trauma is the major risk factor overall. Aspiration, bacterial, and viral pneumonia are common in some investigations. One risk factor reported in some studies is fluid administration, and probably represents a co-contributor in most instances in which it is implicated. However, fluid administration may under certain extreme circumstances produce vascular overdistention and damage vascular integrity. In most cases patients are developing increased capillary permeability when fluid resuscitation is begun, and excess administration of volume simply amplifies the fluid flux and edema. For example, Clark et al. have demonstrated the increased vulnerability of the smoke-injured lung to fluid challenge.[41]

Markers of Acute Lung Injury

Among patients at risk for ARDS, a number of markers have been identified and reported to increase syndrome predictability. These markers often have an implied link to pathogenesis in the form of a suspected disease mediator.[38,39,42,43] The diverse humoral changes seen in ARDS of other etiologies have been recognized in that associated with smoke and burns, suggesting a common pathway to this lung injury. In the past, a fall in polymorphonuclear leukocytes (PMNs) and Pa_{O_2} with the onset of hemodialysis suggested that activated leukocytes might cause hypoxemia and shunt due to endothelial cell injury and lung leak.[44] It has been recognized that the fall in Pa_{O_2} with routine dialysis results from mild hypoventilation due to the removal of CO_2 by the dialysis machine and probably has nothing to do with the fall in Pa_{O_2} during ARDS. However, this intriguing, chance observation launched 10 to 15 years of vigorous investigation of the roles of complement and neutrophils in the pathogenesis of ARDS.[39] The neutrophil may play a substantial role in this dynamic process and has been implicated in numerous models of smoke inhalation injury and burn-associated pulmonary dysfunction. However, a fall in neutrophil number in patients at risk does not predict lung disease in humans. Of more than a dozen factors that have been suggested as markers for ARDS, none really distinguishes patients who will develop the syndrome from those who will not. In fact, in some cases the converse is true. Although PMN activation may amplify lung injury, the presence of PMNs is not always essential, since leukopenic patients with few (if any) PMNs may experience ARDS.[45,46] Furthermore, chemiluminescence and white cell activation has been noted to be reduced among septic patients who develop ARDS. A fall in platelets, activation of complement, and increase in C5a fragments have been inconsistently associated with lung injury.[47] Although smoke inhalation alone appears to have little effect upon the complement system, reductions of complement and properdin levels, alternate complement pathway activation, elevations of plasma C3a Des ARG and fibrin split products, and thrombocytopenia have been documented in patients with severe burns.[48–51] Elevation of Factor VIII antigen, a substance found in megakaryocytes and endothelial cells, has been reported as a marker of endothelial injury and, therefore, a predictor of altered capillary permeability in sepsis.[4,42,42a] This finding has yet to be well tested; Factor VIII antigen can be elevated in diseases not necessarily associated with ARDS. Moreover, the prolonged time (48 hours) needed for this measurement prevents Factor VIII antigen from being a practical clinical predictor. Increased circulating and decreased tissue Factor VIII–related antigen and increased lung permeability (inferred from ^{126}I-albumin study) suggest that the lung is one site of a systemic vascular injury due to cutaneous burn.[42a] Inhibition of these systemic changes by pretreatment with allopurinol or dimetholthyiourea (DMTU) suggested that xanthine oxidase-derived oxygen metabolites were important in the etiology of this injury. Phospholipase A_2, which is found within endothelial membrane, is being investigated as an endothelial release factor predicting ARDS. To date, however, no practical measurement is available to accurately differentiate which of those patients at risk will develop ARDS.[39]

PATHOGENESIS OF ARDS

It is generally assumed that there must be some correlation between the varied events that are associated with ARDS and ARDS itself, although it would not be a surprise if different mechanisms were more important in some cases than in others. It is unlikely that the mechanism of ARDS following viral pneumonia is identical to that following disseminated intravascular coagulation or even sepsis. Clearly, the most common thread that links most of these conditions is some clinical catastrophe which initiates numerous events including complement, white blood cell, and Hageman factor activation, together with some degree of intravascular coagulation. However, none of these processes is unique to ARDS. It is assumed that one or many factors are released or activated during the initial catastrophic disease, leading to injury of the capillary endothelium and/or alveolar epithelium.[52–57] Clark and Nieman have observed that three major events—increased epithelial permeability, increased endothelial permeability, and surfactant loss or deactivation—contribute to lung water accumulation following smoke inhalation.[58] These events have been associated with ARDS of diverse origins. Whether there is initial endothelial cell constriction and widening of intercellular gaps with increased permeability or direct cell damage may vary from case to case. At present, no single primary etiology can be incriminated in the development of ARDS.

A number of mediators have been associated with ARDS.[57] Recently, tumor necrosis factor (TNF), a macrophage-released cytokine, has been reported to be a prime mediator released during clinical catastrophes such as sepsis syndrome.[59,60] TNF activates endothelial cells and makes them constrict; at high concentrations it may cause direct endothelial cell damage. This cytokine stimulates alveolar macrophages to release numerous other cytokines, leukotrienes, and O_2 free radicals associated with tissue damage. Alveolar macrophages may be activated by TNF originating from either side of the alveolar-capillary membrane. Photomicrographs have shown

PMNs to stick in capillaries when endotoxin or TNF is administrated to animal models. TNF also appears to be chemotactic for PMNs and stimulates their release of O_2 radicals. Pulmonary capillary leak may be induced by injection of TNF.

Increased protease activity has been observed inconsistently in patients with ARDS, while free alpha$_1$-antitrypsin is not present in bronchoalveolar lavage.[61] Even in bacterial pneumonias it is uncommon to find excess proteolytic enzyme activity in the lung. Proteolytic enzymes are usually bound to alpha$_1$-antitrypsin or alpha$_2$-macroglobulin. The fact that alpha$_1$-antitrypsin is inactive in the lung does not establish that proteolytic activity from neutrophils is either increased or important in ARDS injury. Further information in this exciting area is necessary. Interestingly, PMN microvascular sequestration, neutrophilic BAL, increased PMNs within lung lymph, elevated β-glucuronidase concentrations, and reduced antiprotease activity have all been observed following experimental smoke inhalation[58,62–64]; these changes have been attenuated by leukopenia.[63] In addition, pulmonary PMN sequestration and lipid peroxidation products (conjugated dienes) have been demonstrated in models of cutaneous burns without accompanying inhalation injury.[65] Endogenous cationic proteins derived from neutrophil lysosomes during inflammation are released into the lung circulation and may contribute to lung microvascular injury by a charge-dependent mechanism.[56]

Endothelial cells can produce a number of substances that activate or allow neutrophil binding to the endothelial membrane.[66] The lung may contain half of all marginated white cells; thus, a large number of PMNs are always in close proximity to the pulmonary endothelium. Whether endothelial cell or circulating PMN activation is a prominent mechanism in disease initiated from the alveolar side is unknown. Currently, although a great deal of sophisticated research has provided us with information about the potential pathogenesis of acute lung injury, the precise mechanisms causing ARDS remain elusive.[67] Recent data suggest that the recruitment of PMNs into the lung and the generation of xanthine oxidase-derived oxygen metabolites have an important role in the development of burn-associated pulmonary dysfunction.[67a] This series of experiments suggests that cutaneous burns cause release of local wound oxidants, which lead to lipid peroxidation and lung inflammation. In Demling's model, these changes were accompanied by a mild reduction of lung compliance, but neither lung permeability nor water content was increased. Once PMNs were recruited to the lung, these inflammatory cells persisted despite resolution of lipid peroxidation, the absence of either burned tissue or lung infection, or the excision and closure of the burn wound. Such a persistence of burn-induced lung inflammation into the post-resuscitation period might lead to exaggerated responses to injuries originating either from the epithelial (e.g., due to smoke) or endothelial (e.g., due to endotoxin) sides of the alveolar capillary membrane.

PULMONARY EDEMA IN BURNED PATIENTS[35]

These general concepts of ARDS influence clinicians' approaches to the evaluation of patients who develop pulmonary edema following smoke inhalation and/or burns. Pulmonary edema, nonspecific in its clinical and physiologic manifestations, can be caused by a variety of factors that are present alone or in combination in burned patients. Prospective clinical differentiation of the relative contributions of increased epithelial and endothelial permeability due to toxic combustion products, persistent or transient elevations (e.g., "surges") of hydrostatic pressures during fluid resuscitation, cardiac dysfunction, and reductions of oncotic pressure caused by burn-related hypoproteinemia is difficult. The relative contributions of these factors vary according to the phase of injury and recovery (Table 5-5).[35] Low pressure, permeability, or noncardiogenic edema (ARDS) can be caused by smoke inhalation, aspiration, sepsis, transfusion of blood products, or burn shock. High pressure, hydrostatic (cardio-

Table 5-5 Major Causes of Acute Pulmonary Edema in Burned Patients

Hemodynamic classification*	Timing*	Cause(s)
Increased permeability		
ARDS (normal or low pcwp)	Early	Smoke inhalation, burn shock, aspiration, upper airway obstruction
	Late	Sepsis, transfusion
Hydrostatic edema		
Cardiogenic (elevated pcwp)	Early	CO, CN intoxication, acute myocardial infarction
Fluid overload	Late	Mobilization of edema fluid, overhydration

*pcwp = pulmonary capillary wedge pressure.

genic) edema might occur on the basis of overt or occult myocardial infarction, left ventricular dysfunction due to burn or sepsis-related myocardial depression, lactic acidosis, or on the basis of intoxication by carbon monoxide, cyanide, or other combustion products. Preexisting cardiac disease might decompensate during stresses from hypoxemia, asphyxiants, or fluid resuscitation. Intravascular volume overload could complicate excessive administration of resuscitative fluid or the mobilization of burn edema fluid during recovery, especially in the presence of burn-related renal failure. It has been observed that the tendency for fluid retention in individuals who will later develop acute respiratory failure during edema fluid mobilization is often suggested by inappropriate weight gain (e.g., as detected from careful daily measurement of intake/output),[35,68a,b] and appreciation of early radiographic signs of overhydration may contribute to this appraisal.[16] Although pulmonary edema is unlikely to occur on the basis of hypoalbuminemia alone, its presence lowers the critical hydrostatic pressure at which leak occurs.

These and other factors may evolve acutely and typically interact in various combinations. Because of their nonspecific manifestations (e.g., dyspnea, hypoxemic respiratory failure, radiologically obvious pulmonary edema), examination alone is seldom distinguished accurately on the basis of clinical grounds alone and timely diagnosis and management are difficult. Such uncertainties often alter thresholds for the use of invasive hemodynamic monitoring. This objective information confirms that pulmonary edema may have different etiologies even in the same patient, depending on the phase of illness, and suggests that hemodynamic measurements made at one time should not be extrapolated to account for either previous or subsequent episodes. The roles of newer technologies (e.g., use of Swan Ganz catheters, clinical lung water measurements, computed chest tomography) in the more precise categorization of patients with pulmonary edema require clarification, and they are addressed in later chapters. Unfortunately, invasive monitoring predisposes the patient to iatrogenic problems and, in general, has not been documented to improve survival from ARDS. Because of these concerns, few authors have routinely specified the hemodynamic pattern of edema. Venus et al. found that approximately half of their patients with inhalation injury (4.5 percent of their burned patients overall) developed pulmonary edema. Of these 45 individuals, 18 (40 percent) had cardiogenic edema and the remaining 60 percent had noncardiogenic edema (ARDS).[68c]

Just as the overall distribution of respiratory problems differs according to the temporal relationship to injury (Chap. 2), the roles of potential contributing causes of pulmonary edema should be expected to vary. This concept is shown schematically in Fig. 2-4 (Chap. 2) and Table 5-5 and is consistent with recent experimental findings. Demling's benchmark investigations in sheep have shown a reproducible sequence of microvascular changes accompanying large burns (40 to 50% BSA).[68d] Distinctive periods of burn resuscitation (up to 24 hours following injury), fluid mobilization (24 to 48 hours), and early recovery (48 to 72 hours) occur in this model, paralleling clinical stages that are recognized to occur in burned patients. The initial increase of lung fluid flux appears to be caused by systemic hypoproteinemia rather than due to an increase in pulmonary microvascular permeability to protein. Pulmonary vascular resistance and hydrostatic pressure rise as well. During the second phase, fluid flux appears to result from hypervolemia, paralleling the intravascular resorption of soft tissue edema fluid. Elevated hydrostatic pressure seems to be the chief determinant of fluid flux during this period. The later onset of edema in such experimental models typically reflects sepsis-induced ARDS.

In humans with smoke inhalation and burns, when pulmonary edema occurs during the initial few hours after injury, the gravity of this situation is usually obvious. Precise delineation of the etiology of pulmonary edema is perhaps most difficult during this phase because of the number of possible interacting factors. This problem most often complicates especially severe exposures, typically associated with very high concentrations of irritant gases and the patient's unconsciousness and/or entrapment. These circumstances are frequently combined with large body surface area burns and shock. Because of the importance of carbon monoxide and cyanide intoxication during the first few hours after exposure, myocardial dysfunction and true hydrostatic edema may also represent an early complication, particularly when significant underlying cardiac disease is present. Carbon monoxide might also cause a permeability edema. Another important mechanical factors in the early development of pulmonary edema may go unrecognized by many clinicians: alveolar flooding may accompany severe upper airway obstruction, often developing immediately following the relief of acute UAO. While we suspect that in many instances the simultaneous onset of UAO and pulmonary edema represents a global respiratory damage due to severe inhalation injury, in some patients acute noncardiogenic pulmonary edema appears to have truly occurred on this mechanical basis. Although the exact frequency of this problem is unclear, this form of ARDS has been reported in up to 11 percent of burned patients with clinically suspected inhalation injury.[68c,e] Several factors appear to interact in the pathophysiology of this form of pulmonary edema with marked pleural pressure swings resulting in reduced interstitial pressures appearing to be especially important.[68e,f]

Later during the course (e.g., from two to five days after injury), responses to resuscitation resulting in volume overload, together with delayed-onset ARDS due to smoke inhalation or sepsis become more important diagnostic considerations. With increasing emphasis on early excisional therapy, perioperative edema caused by inadvertent, intraoperative overhydration, unappreciated volume losses with resultant myocardial dysfunction and congestive heart failure (including myocardial infarction), or ARDS related to sepsis accompanying burn wound manipulations are important problems to be avoided. Individual stresses or precipitating events temporally linked to the onset of edema seem to be more readily differentiated late in the course, perhaps because a "clinical baseline" of function has been established for the patient, and abrupt deviation from this course is more apparent. As the hospitalization becomes more prolonged, septic ARDS is increasingly likely to be the cause of pulmonary edema. During this late phase, differentiation of ARDS from diffuse involvement by pneumonia is a common clinical dilemma for which there is no obvious current solution. The interpretation of slight variations in the severity and distribution of radiographic infiltrates in patients who have had pulmonary edema earlier during the course is difficult.

Contrary to popular belief, smoke inhalation alone seldom causes pulmonary edema unless the exposure is especially severe.[35] None of 225 persons evaluated after smoke inhalation during the Las Vegas Hotel fires developed ARDS.[69] ARDS is also unlikely to be a sequela of cutaneous burns alone; it was observed only in 2.3 percent of individuals who were at risk in one epidemiologic review. In the comprehensive Brooke experience, pulmonary edema occurred in only 2.7 percent and 3.8 percent of burned patients during two separate periods of data collection (Chap. 2, Table 2-4[68a,b]). Stone found that transudation into the airway prior to the eighth hour after burn was unusual and that such edema typically accompanied fluid administration.[35,69a]

Pruitt observed that pulmonary edema developed from 4.6 to 6.3 days following injury and was associated with larger burns, extremes of patient age, renal failure, and obvious overhydration during surgical procedures.[35;68a,b] These associations are useful in identifying patients at risk. In 191 patients with clinical risk factors for inhalation injury evaluated at the Baltimore Regional Burn Center, pulmonary edema was present at the time of hospitalization only in one patient and developed during the first week in 18 others.[16] These patients were significantly older and had received more resuscitative fluid than those who did not develop this complication. In addition, widening of the vascular pedicle, a noninvasive radiologic sign of increased circulating blood volume, had antedated the development of alveolar flooding, suggesting that excessive intravenous fluid administration during the first 24 hours had predisposed to alveolar flooding during the fluid mobilization phase of the response to burn injury. The relationship of pulmonary edema to older patient age suggests that either a lack of cardiac reserve and/or an increased susceptibility to oxidant injury occurs in elderly individuals; the importance of these and other potential predispositions requires further delineation.

TREATMENT OF ARDS: GENERAL SUPPORTIVE CARE

The basic principles of treatment are to improve oxygen tension and overall oxygen delivery. This must be accomplished without oxygen toxicity, nosocomial infection, or barotrauma. Attempts to avoid malnutrition and multiorgan failure are also important. These are somewhat unusual principles for therapy: one must maintain a physiologic goal and, the rest of the time, attempt to stay out of trouble. Because we do not have any proven specific therapy for ARDS, our primary goal is to support the patient until healing can occur.[52]

Applications of these principles are outlined in Table 5-6 and are reviewed in further detail in Chap. 9. The major supportive measures currently available include oxygen and PEEP. The patient may be hypovolemic and need fluid resuscitation; responding to such needs in the face of large burns and inhalation injury is especially challenging. About 20 to 30 percent of ARDS patients will be hypotensive, and vasoactive drugs are often necessary. A number of investigators believe that heparin is of some help as standard prophylaxis, because ARDS patients have a high incidence of pulmonary emboli, but there is no evidence that full heparinization can alter lung injury by blocking initial or continued activation of the coagulation cascade. A significant number of ARDS patients are found to have multiple small thromboemboli by angiography and postmortem examination. Heparin could theoretically stop or help resolve in situ clots, but there is no evidence that the number of intravascular clots can be reduced by full anticoagulation. Streptokinase has been administered into the pulmonary bed of a few patients with documented microthrombi, but there is no documentation that pulmonary vascular resistance improves following thrombolytic therapy. Moreover, there is no evidence that the number of documented thrombi correlate with outcome in ARDS patients.[69b] Extracorporeal membrane lung support is one means of helping to maintain adequate blood gases without the hazards of excess $F_{I_{O_2}}$ or lung distention.[69c] Recent data have suggested that ventilatory assistance with high peak airway pressure and overinflation can be harmful to the lung, producing increased leak.[70,71] If the lung is

Table 5-6 ARDS: General Approaches to Management

Nonspecific supportive measures
Oxygen therapy*
Positive end-expiratory pressure (PEEP)*
Enhancing oxygen delivery*
Extracorporeal CO_2 removal
Mechanical ventilation*
Fluid administration/resuscitation/diuresis
Vasoactive drugs
Specific treatments (largely investigational)
Avoid iatrogenic/nosocomial complications*

*Standard modality of care.

kept from being overdistended and is actually "rested" by requiring only a few ventilations per minute through use of an extracorporeal device (which eliminates CO_2), patients theoretically could be kept alive while the lung repairs itself.

Other supportive measures that should be mentioned are purposeful positioning and the maintenance of adequate nutrition. There is evidence that turning patients may result in sustained improvement of Pa_{O_2} and lung edema when they are moved from the supine position to the prone position and may reduce length of stay in intensive care units.[72] However, practical difficulties in delivering nursing care may sometimes limit the value of this approach, and the distribution of surface burns may make it unfeasible altogether. The impact of nutritional support on the outcome of critically ill patients remains undefined.[73–76] Despite theoretically advantageous options, there is no specific nutritional supplement that is yet proven to be better than another. However, malnutrition is harmful to both repair processes and host defense and in burn victims is a well-recognized, common problem. The maintenance of physiologic balances is one of the foundations of intensive care therapy. Because of the implication of a role of lipid peroxidation in the pathogenesis of both smoke inhalation injury and burns, there are concerns about potential adverse effects of the administration of lipid infusions in the nutritional support of these patients. Accentuated pulmonary arterial hypertension, bronchoconstriction, reduced lung compliance, and worsened hypoxemia have been documented experimentally following lipid infusion. However, Demling and Tortella found no adverse effect of lipid infusion upon the pulmonary function of burned patients with smoke inhalation injuries.[76a]

Oxygen Therapy

"Some degree of relief" of acute respiratory distress was observed "in a few" of 12 Cocoanut Grove victims treated with 100% oxygen and positive pressure. Clinical improvement was documented by reduction of cyanosis and audible rattles.[77,78] Clearly, the main problem of ARDS patients is that they are severely hypoxemic. The first question necessary to answer is, How low a Pa_{O_2} is detrimental to a human being? Interestingly, mitochondria function at Pa_{O_2}'s in the 1- to 2-torr range. People can go to very high altitudes or run on a treadmill with low FI_{O_2} (i.e., 14%) and are capable of a normal oxygen consumption. Although a normal individual does not develop anoxic lactic acidosis until the Pa_{O_2} is below 30 mmHg, it has been observed clinically that ARDS patients seem to do poorly with acute reductions of their Pa_{O_2} below 55 mmHg. The Pa_{O_2} does not correlate with either tachypnea or the sense of respiratory distress, since dyspnea does not improve tremendously in these patients when their Pa_{O_2} is elevated over 60 mmHg. Therefore, the desired level of Pa_{O_2} must be balanced with the cost of achieving a specific arterial oxygen tension. The desirable level of Pa_{O_2} might be related to the age of the patient or to underlying coronary and cerebral vascular status. There is some evidence that in the presence of ischemic disease, higher driving pressures of oxygen (i.e., Pa_{O_2} as high as 150 mmHg) might be helpful for organ function. Because of the curvilinear nature of the hemoglobin-oxygen dissociation curve (Fig. 5-3),[79] small changes in Pa_{O_2} from 30 to 45 mmHg will produce large changes in oxygen saturation. Individuals with severe ARDS thus benefit a great deal from small increases in O_2 tension up to 45 mmHg. Above 60 mmHg Pa_{O_2} elevations in arterial oxygen tension produce little change in oxygen saturation. However, in order to avoid the steep part of the hemoglobin saturation curve (where small reductions in O_2 tension will result in large drops in oxygen content), it is reasonable to maintain a Pa_{O_2} between 55 to 60 mmHg. Unless there is some reason to suspect that higher arterial oxygen tensions are necessary, this represents a recommended range to seek during initial therapy.

The risk of alveolar O_2 excess is considerable in normals and ARDS patients. Oxygen clearly has been shown to be harmful to the lung.[80] Physiologic changes that occur during hyperoxia in normal animal model and human volunteers have been inves-

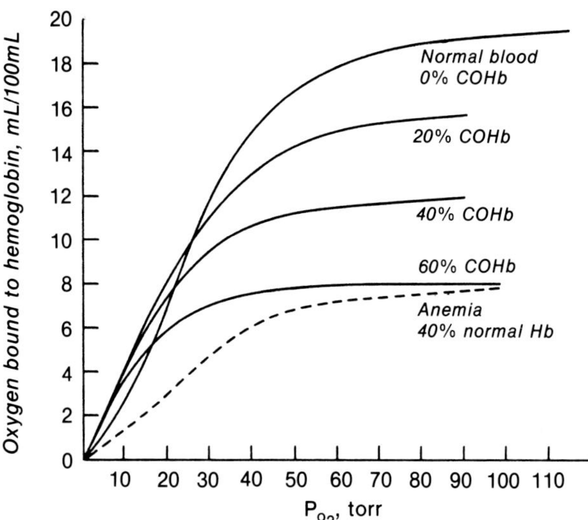

Figure 5-3 Oxyhemoglobin dissociation curves. Note that Pa_{O_2} exceeding 60 mmHg places a patient on the plateau of the curve, with hemoglobin oxygen saturation exceeding 90 percent. Further increments of Pa_{O_2} have relatively little impact upon saturation or delivery but might be achieved with administration of an unacceptably high FI_{O_2}, leading to oxygen toxicity. Also depicted are the effects of progressively increasing levels of carboxyhemoglobin, as typically encountered in patients with smoke inhalation. This effect, similar to that of anemia, is accompanied by a slightly leftward shift of the oxyhemoglobin dissociation curve, further compromising tissue oxygen delivery. (*Reprinted with permission from Ref. 79a.*)

tigated more thoroughly than in injured patients. During the first 6 hours of breathing 100% O_2, mucous flow is reduced. At approximately 6 to 8 hours, alveolar macrophage migration is impaired and chest pain from epithelial injury and tracheobronchitis occurs. After about 17 hours of 100% O_2 breathing, bronchopulmonary lavage demonstrates an increased amount of protein in the alveolar lining fluid. After 24 to 48 hours, the lung begins to show reduced compliance, a widening alveolar-arterial (A-a) gradient, and reduced alveolar macrophage function. Some studies also show a reduced diffusing capacity with loss of functional alveolar capillary bed at 48 hours, indicating that the lung develops major injury after 2 days of high oxygen exposure. After 48 to 72 hours, there is increased pulmonary shunting and definite microscopic lung damage. In human studies, 5 to 7 days of 100% O_2 results in endothelial cell injury and, in baboons, causes pulmonary edema. There are few clinical studies evaluating oxygen toxicity. One investigation was performed in brain dead individuals who received either 100% oxygen or sufficient FI_{O_2} to maintain the P_{O_2} in the 60-mmHg range. The end point of the study was cardiac arrest. In the group on 100% oxygen, there was more pulmonary congestion and more atelectasis than in controls but no morphologic finding distinctive of ARDS. Since every experimental model demonstrates oxygen to be toxic over relatively short periods of time, however, it must be assumed that oxygen is toxic in ARDS patients. What is not known is how much time it takes for high FI_{O_2} concentrations to injure the already-damaged lung. There are a few experiments in which injured lungs are evaluated carefully with and without excess FI_{O_2}. However, sequential elevations of oxygen concentrations over time in such models have shown varying degrees of additional damage. Exposure to 100% oxygen will increase a previously injured lung's weight by 100 percent within 24 hours compared to a similarly injured lung ventilated with room air. While exposure to 80% oxygen produces no injury on the first day, some excess lung weight develops after 40 hours and, by day 6, there is a marked increase in lung leakage (200 percent) compared to control. Comparison of lung leak occurring with lower FI_{O_2} shows a reduction in total edema and a progressive delay in the time it takes to develop leak. Although 50% O_2 at day 6 is associated with only a small increase of excessive lung water, this FI_{O_2} is still injurious to a previously damaged lung. Others have shown that 40% O_2 may be harmful at the subcellular level after a week or two, with injury to mitochondria. Thus, *any* increased concentration of oxygen may be harmful over time; the higher the FI_{O_2}, the shorter the time until injury and the greater amount of damage which occurs. Previously injured lungs are probably more susceptible to O_2 toxicity than normal lungs.[81] The clinical caveat from such experimental data analysis is to administer as little oxygen as is reasonable to maintain an adequate O_2.

Positive End-Expiratory Pressure (PEEP)

The second major component of ARDS therapy is the administration of PEEP.[82–84] It is now well understood that the major role of PEEP is to increase transpulmonary pressure and to open unstable alveoli; when unstable alveoli are recruited, inspired gas can enter and exchange with capillary blood. In the normal alveolus, gas approximates the alveolar surface and rapidly diffuses into the capillary. When the lung is severely injured in ARDS, there is interstitial and alveolar edema with atelectasis. Surfactant is inactivated by proteinaceous material and resulting alveolar instability, contributing to atelectasis. Direct inactivation of surfactant by smoke inhalation has been well documented, and leads to near-immediate atelectasis.[22] Oxygen can no longer enter the collapsed alveolus, and blood flow continues through patent capillaries, producing a right to left shunt. Another common mechanism for failure of O_2 exchange and secondary shunting occurs when an alveolus fills completely with fluid, also preventing oxygen from approximating with a capillary for diffusion.

Therapy attempts to recruit or enlarge atelectatic or edematous air sacs by increasing the pressure within the alveolus relative to the pressure around that alveolus. Since the injury is usually patchy, noninjured alveoli will also increase in size when exposed to higher transpulmonary pressure and are thus subject to barotrauma. It is not uncommon for ARDS patients to have normal lung units which are markedly overexpanded before some of the damaged units open at all. In fact, the initial Pa_{O_2} may actually fall as one begins to apply PEEP because the elevated alveolar pressure, relative to capillary pressure, overdistends these good units, increases the resistance to blood flow through them, and forces more blood through the bad (collapsed or edematous) units. Once a critical transpulmonary pressure is reached in a particular unit relative to the surrounding pressure, it will open. Resting lung volume will be larger, air will enter, and, as blood flows by, gas exchange will occur. In the lung unit which is theoretically filled with fluid, PEEP increases the size of the alveolus, spreading fluid out over a larger surface area and reducing the anatomic barrier to diffusion.

Normal spontaneous breathing is associated with a zero end-expiratory pressure (ZEEP); any end-expiratory pressure above zero barometric pressure can be called PEEP. The amount of end-expiratory pressure necessary to increase alveolar size depends on the stiffness of the alveolus. One needs to recruit a large number of alveoli with varying compliances to reduce the significant amount of shunting seen in ARDS and arrive at a satisfactory oxygen tension, even with supplemental FI_{O_2}. Photomicrographs of lungs that are exposed to PEEP show two interesting things: First, the alveolar spaces are larger because the pressure in them relative to the pressure around them is greater. Second, the microcirculation or capillary bed is markedly diminished, because the pressure in the alveolus relative to the surrounding pressure is transmitted to the small collapsible capillaries and compresses them. Upstream junctional vessels (which are intrapulmonary extraalveolar vessels) appear larger, indicating that the vascular pressure relative to the surrounding interstitial pressure is higher with PEEP. In fact, PEEP can elevate backpressure and simulate left ventricular failure or pulmonary emboli, thus imposing an increased load on the right ventricle. The increased pressure in intrapulmonary extraalveolar vessels may also allow these upstream vessels to leak at an accelerated rate. Thus, by elevating pressure in more proximal, intrapulmonary extraalveolar vessels, PEEP may actually increase pulmonary edema.[82,84]

What is the clinical value of PEEP? First and foremost is PEEP's ability to recruit groups of alveoli, reduce right to left shunt, and allow increased Pa_{O_2} to be achieved at a lower FI_{O_2}. This modality spares or delays the risk of oxygen toxicity as the lung attempts to repair itself. Other inherent values of PEEP have been postulated.[84] By opening alveolar units that would otherwise be closed, PEEP allows surfactant to shift from adjacent undamaged units, improving compliance and stabilizing alveoli. PEEP allows oxygen to reach the alveolar surface, possibly accelerating the rate of repair. Despite these considerations, however, confirmation that PEEP is directly beneficial to the lung is lacking. On the other hand, there are some detrimental aspects of PEEP.[82–85] If ARDS is simulated by HCl acid injury, the lung will gain weight faster during administration of high levels of PEEP. Intrapulmonary shunting may also increase, because with patchy damage there are collapsed units that will not be recruited at any particular transpulmonary pressure. The high pressure transmitted to exposed capillaries diverts additional blood flow through such units, functioning as right to left shunt, and actually lowering the Pa_{O_2}. As PEEP is elevated further and a large number of unstable alveoli are recruited, however, the overall shunt is almost always reduced. In the presence of alveoli filled with cellular exudates (e.g., as observed in bacterial or pneumocystis pneumonia), PEEP may completely fail to improve overall shunt. The increased distending pressure of PEEP may also enlarge dead space ventilation, elevating arterial Pco_2. This effect is usually minor except in the most severely damaged lungs, where PEEP may substantially elevate Pa_{CO_2}.

Since pulmonary edema and adequate gas exchange are the problems that require respiratory assistance, it is wise to keep both peak- and end-expiratory airway pressures as low as possible. Thus, to gain maximum benefit with minimum harm, adjustments of the "dosage" of PEEP should be balanced with the Fi_{O_2} to obtain a satisfactory and safe therapeutic mix. Although it has been claimed that the empiric, prophylactic administration of "an optimum level" of continuous positive airway pressure (CPAP) to burn victims with multiple risks for inhalation injury has prevented pulmonary deaths,[68c] the absence of controls in published reports limits this descriptive experience. These modalities are valuable adjuncts in the treatment of established hypoxemic respiratory failure, but it has not been demonstrated that the prophylactic administration of CPAP or PEEP alters outcome in individuals with smoke inhalation and/or burns.

How do we decide on how much positive end pressure is necessary in a particular patient? The answer is straightforward and simple, i.e., enough! In patients who present with ARDS, functional residual capacity (FRC) is usually diminished to approximately 30 percent of normal. Providing all these patients with the same amount of PEEP is not reasonable, since transpulmonary pressure, increase in lung volume, and extent of alveolar recruitment will depend entirely upon the compliance of the injured lung in that specific individual. If the compliance is very poor, a fixed amount of PEEP may not move the lung at all. In one analogy, the effects of pushing against a door will depend upon how heavy the door is and how hard one pushes. If there is not enough pressure applied across the door, it will not open. Similarly, if the pressure across the alveolus is insufficient, it will not open and lung volume will not increase; if alveoli are not recruited, there will be no improvement in Pa_{O_2}. In an individual patient with different amounts of injury throughout thc lung (as is usually the case), the net increase in lung volume will vary with PEEP, depending on the sum of the compliances of individual units. Thus, the precise amount of PEEP required depends on how much pressure is needed to increase resting lung volume back toward normal, and obviously will vary among individuals. There is no practical measure of FRC or resting lung volume in patients as an indication of how much PEEP is necessary. Such a measure is probably not important, because the goal of therapy is to recruit sufficient lung units until the Pa_{O_2} is improved to some satisfactory level.

In experimental models and in the majority of patients, it usually takes only seconds to improve or change lung volume with with PEEP.[86] In fact, the stiffer the lung, the quicker the response. Occasionally, improvement in Pa_{O_2} takes hours; this is an exception, and it is not clear how this is accomplished sequentially. Therefore, when PEEP adjustments are made clinically, an oximeter provides a real-time, second by second indication of effective change in lung volume as reflected in Pa_{O_2} and increased Pa_{O_2}/FI_{O_2} ratio. It should also be remembered that when PEEP is reduced, it only takes seconds to de-recruit units and to increase shunting. Thus, suctioning, removing patients from the ventilator for hemodynamic measurements, or sending patients off the unit for special x-rays or procedures (with interruption of PEEP) can be extremely dangerous. If suctioning procedures are not productive, it is better to maintain uninterrupted PEEP. Some of the newer suction catheter devices help to maintain PEEP during this maneuver.

A number of investigators have suggested there is a "best" PEEP for an individual patient, based on estimates of tissue oxygen delivery and not on Pa_{O_2} alone.[83] The best PEEP has been correlated with the lung's best compliance. However, lung compliance does not correlate well with lung water, Pa_{O_2}/FI_{O_2} ratio, or chest radiography.[87] As some lung units are recruited, others are more distended and pushed up higher on their individual compliance curves. If at some point increases in resting transpulmonary pressure with PEEP fail to recruit sufficient new units but continue to elevate pleural pressure relative to "mean systemic venous pressure," cardiac output could diminish. This point may coincide with the highest compliance. If cardiac output begins to fall, oxygen delivery may suffer despite increased Pa_{O_2} and O_2 content. However, static compliance in patients with ARDS will be entirely different if the tidal volume is reduced. When tidal volume is small the lung's pressure volume relationship will lie on a steeper portion of the compliance curve, with lower peak or plateau alveolar and pleural pressures. In addition, if oxygen transport and cardiac output should fall with PEEP (because of a combination of elevated pleural and/or alveolar pressure), administering fluids to improve venous return can usually improve oxygen delivery back to baseline. Thus, there is no single optimum PEEP; the "best PEEP" is the least amount necessary to achieve a satisfactory P_{O_2}. If cardiac output falls, a reduction in tidal volume with administration of intravenous fluids or infusion of vasoactive drugs may be necessary to reestablish satisfactory O_2 delivery.[82,83] Although it has been arbitrarily noted that PEEP must be maintained at least 2 weeks in patients with burn-related inhalation injury, the appropriate level of PEEP and the duration of its administration are highly individualized, necessitating the clinician's continuous, careful assessment of benefits of this modality.

Fluid Administration and Resuscitation

There are two major questions concerning fluid administration in patients with ARDS. These relate to the optimum volume and choice of fluid, and represent controversial issues even in the absence of cutaneous burn injury. In general, most authorities recommend administration of maintenance fluids which replace losses and prevent hypervolemia: early clinical practices with ARDS patients in the 1970s centered on keeping individuals as dry as possible in an attempt to pull water from the lung and minimize microvascular pressure. More recently, investigators have been attuned to the problem of multiorgan failure and the importance of maintaining good perfusion to different organs, although prospective randomized studies seeking to achieve this end are not yet available. These concerns are particularly relevant to patients with combined smoke inhalation and burn injuries. Clark and others have observed that the smoke-injured lung loses the ability to protect itself when challenged with fluid.[41]

In retrospective studies of ARDS it has been demonstrated that patients losing or gaining little weight have a better survival.[88] Thus, for groups of individuals with ARDS, those who continue to have fluid intake in excess of output (and continue to gain weight) have higher mortality than those who are not receiving excess fluid. A possibility, of course, is that patients who receive more fluid have more capillary permeability, more third spacing, and are more ill, requiring more fluids to maintain oxygen delivery. Their increased mortality would reflect severity of illness and not necessarily the volume of excess fluids. The other alternative is that excess fluid contributes in some way to poor patient outcome. Recently, Eisenberg et al. prospectively measured lung water by double dilution measurement in intensive care unit (ICU) patients with ARDS and followed a protocol with hemodynamic monitoring that minimized any increases of lung water and pulmonary capillary wedge pressures.[87] Survival in those patients who had lung water carefully monitored and adjusted to prevent increases was better in spite of similar vascular pressures. Although there was not a large difference in survival, and only a relatively small number of patients were examined, this study suggests that paying very careful attention to fluid management may make a difference in ARDS outcome. Carlson and coworkers have shown that the development of fluid retention during the first 48 hours after burn correlated with patients' survival: 95 percent of individuals who retained less than 230 cm^3 of fluid per kilogram of lean body mass during this period survived the burn injury.[88a] These observations were confirmed in a follow-up study in which the net fluid retention during the first 48 hours was corrected for the estimated fluid loss from the burn wound.[88b] This relationship of fluid retention to survival was present in patients with inhalation injury as well as in the total group of patients.

There is some evidence that even transient high intravascular volumes due to overadministration of fluids can actually produce vascular trauma by distending vessels to the point that microvascular junctions separate, leading to increased permeability. The dilemma is accentuated in burn patients with inhalation injury. These individuals are typically overresuscitated, receiving about 30 percent of fluid in excess of their predicted needs.[89,90] While such observations might suggest that administered fluid volumes be limited accordingly, it is also well-recognized that underresuscitation leads to worsened outcome. Herndon and coworkers have noted that animals with experimental smoke inhalation injury develop more extravascular lung water formation when they are resuscitated with less fluid (with resultant lower central venous pressures and cardiac indices) in comparison to animals receiving routine resuscitation.[91] These investigators have speculated that "resuscitation to normal cardiac output and vascular flow rates may increase shear rates," potentially reducing the margination of PMNs within the pulmonary vasculature.[92]

The other major question, "What kind of fluid is best to administer to ARDS patients?" has also produced a great deal of controversy. The critical capillary pressure which produces leak is dependent upon the plasma osmotic pressure. In normal individuals with a plasma osmotic pressure of 25 mmHg, lungs will not become edematous until the rise in capillary pressure approaches 25 mmHg. However, if oncotic pressure is reduced (e.g., by burn-related protein losses and replacement of plasma with saline), the hydrostatic pressure at which a normal lung will leak falls significantly. Protein malnutrition (with a narrow ratio of oncotic to vascular pressure) has been associated with poor clinical outcomes. In models employing isolated lungs injured to simulate ARDS, perfusion with colloid is associated with lower fluid flux compared to similar models perfused with crystalloids. Saline resuscitation of a sheep hemorrhagic shock model has resulted in "wetter lungs" than animals resuscitated with colloid.[93] However, whether maintenance of oncotic pressure is important in steady state situations in patients with increased permeability has produced conflicting results. Both retrospective and prospective clinical studies which have assessed changes in blood gases or right to left shunting following maintenance infusion of colloid, blood, or crystalloid administration have found similar results regardless of what type of fluid is infused.

In critically ill burn patients, colloid resuscitation produces greater increases in cardiac output and oxygen consumption than twice the amount of crystalloid. Crystalloid primarily expands the interstitial space, with only 20 percent remaining within the intravascular compartment after 1 to 2 hours. Despite the few potential theoretical benefits of reducing pulmonary leak by administration of colloid, experience in burn victims has not shown a beneficial effect of plasma oncotic pressure on lung water. Furthermore, in one controlled trial, lung water actually increased in patients treated with colloid. These individuals had a higher mortality and more often developed roentgenographically documented pulmonary edema than did patients receiving crystalloid.[94] These observations suggest that the magnitude of the disruption of alveolar capillary membrane is so great that effective sieving does not occur. Thus, therapeutically administered colloid passes directly into air spaces, potentially drawing further fluid from the vascular component.

Studies suggest that resuscitation with saline usually requires four times as much volume to achieve the same circulatory improvement as with colloid. Thus, to improve intravascular volume by 1 L, one must give 4 L of saline, 10 L of dextrose and water, or 1 or less liters of colloid. Some investigators report that the vascular volume following colloid administration is almost 1.7 times the volume infused because it is more hyperoncotic than plasma. Thus, in the shocked or burned individual or with early ARDS, blood volume and oxygen delivery can be provided more effectively by colloid or packed red blood cells (if hemoglobin is required). Recently, the use of pentastarch in successful burn resuscitation has, in a randomized crossover comparison with 5% albumin, been associated with increased preload, cardiac output, oxygen delivery, and oxygen consumption.[95] Hypertonic saline regimens have been associated with less fluid administration and less burn edema but no clear-cut difference in pulmonary edema or outcome. Avoidance of fluid overload is especially important in management of patients with multisystemic injury. For example, in individuals with shock or sepsis syndrome who often stop urinating soon after resuscitation, it is important not to have 4 or 5 extra liters of increased interstitial volume which cannot easily be diuresed.

The type of resuscitative fluid selected must also be integrated with other aspects of patient care. For example, while alveolar hyperventilation typically accompanies mechanical ventilator care, an especially severe alkalemia might be induced when such hyperventilation occurs during resuscitation with Ringer's lactate.[96] Specific problems related to the effective fluid resuscitation of burn patients with inhalation injury are reviewed in further detail in Chap. 10. Clearly, the general clinical challenges encountered in other patients with ARDS are accentuated in this population with multifactorial injuries. At present, decisions about the best fluid regimen are made on a highly individualized basis.[96]

Enhancing Oxygen Delivery

General Considerations There has been great controversy concerning oxygen delivery in patients with ARDS.[82,97] Oxygen delivery depends on the Pa_{O_2} and pH of the blood (which together determine saturation), the hemoglobin level, and the cardiac output: Oxygen delivery = $(SaO_2)(1.34)(Hgb)(CO)$. A gram of hemoglobin is very important to oxygen content and delivery; without sufficient hemoglobin, even a cardiac output of 100 L might not meet tissue demands for oxygen. The level of hemoglobin is too often neglected in critically ill hypoxemic patients. In cases of increased oxygen demand, elevation of the hemoglobin above 7 to 9 g/dL may be helpful, although exact end points for transfusion in this setting have not been well characterized. In individuals who have increased right to left shunting, the mixed venous oxygen tension also contributes heavily to the Pa_{O_2} level. If the cardiac output or hemoglobin is low then the $a\text{-}\bar{v}_{O_2}$ difference will widen and the mixed venous P_{O_2} will be low. Shunting blood with a low mixed venous O_2 tension produces a major fall in the arterial Pa_{O_2}. The sicker and more hypermetabolic the patient, the more accentuated are the effects of cardiac output and hemoglobin as determinants of mixed venous P_{O_2}. These factors, in turn, significantly lower P_{O_2} and oxygen delivery in ARDS. Patients with ARDS and low cardiac outputs have poorer survival. The remarkable metabolic demands (with increased oxygen consumption), hemodynamic dysfunction, malnutrition, and multisystemic failure seen in burn victims all further compound the problem of ensuring suitable tissue oxygen delivery. These problems are exacerbated by anemia, hemodilution, carbon monoxide poisoning, and cyanide intoxication.

While theoretically attractive, the role of comprehensive metabolic monitoring of patients in this setting has not yet been translated to unequivocally improved outcomes.

Delivery Dependence of Oxygen Consumption Under normal circumstances, tissues have great ability to extract additional oxygen and increase local blood flow by changing their vascular resistances, thus ensuring fulfillment of oxygen demands. Classical physiologic studies have shown stable O_2 consumption over wide ranges of delivery until some critical point is reached at which extraction can no longer increase and consumption falls in a linear fashion as delivery further falls.[97,98] Most of these studies have been performed in anesthetized animal models where the cardiac output is artificially increased or decreased. Recently, a number of diseases (ARDS, sepsis, cor pulmonale, primary pulmonary hypertension) have been reported to demonstrate O_2 supply dependency: changes in either cardiac output or O_2 content may dictate oxygen consumption. Reports on the relationship between $\dot{V}_{O_2}$ and O_2 delivery in humans with respiratory failure are conflicting.[99–102] In normal individuals during exercise, the relationship between O_2 supply dependence occurs in ARDS; it may be present in the majority of patients. The corollary to this concept suggests that higher delivery may increase O_2 consumption further, implying that unmet tissue demands exist. Consequently, a number of investigators have attempted to force oxygen delivery higher, with the view that increased supply will increase O_2 consumption and produce a better patient outcome. This approach is analogous to recent supply-side economic theories: although we all may recognize the extent to which increasing available money has trickled down to those in greatest need, whether "supply-side oxygen delivery" works is not known. Some of the patients with the most measurable supply-dependent oxygen consumptions have the worst outcomes, possibly because they are the most critically ill. There has been little evidence that markedly increasing cardiac output (CO) is helpful, although better patient survival has been correlated with higher CO. It is not a surprise that those patients with ARDS who survive have better hearts and are capable of maintaining higher COs, while individuals with lower CO and bad lungs do worse. The question of whether ARDS patients given fluids until their COs are increased to the 6- to 8-L minimum range have improved outcomes in comparison to concurrent controls (who do not have their CO manipulated to these levels), is unanswered. In addition, there is no evidence that lactic acidosis correlates with either cardiac output or O_2 delivery in ARDS patients. Moreover, persons with normal lactate levels (as a possible indicator of adequate O_2 supply) do not necessarily have a good outcome. Although lactate levels may remain normal in clinically shocked individuals, the presence of lactic acidosis, whatever its genesis, indicates a poor prognosis.

In patients who have sustained burns as well as inhalation injury, these alterations of oxygen delivery associated with ARDS must also be assessed in the context of the hemodynamic response to thermal injury. In their sheep model, Demling and coworkers have recently shown that increasing oxygen delivery after cutaneous burns (15% BSA) resulted in a 32 percent increase of oxygen consumption, suggesting that standard burn resuscitation had not provided oxygen delivery that was satisfactory for tissue oxygen demands.[102a] This relationship between oxygen delivery and oxygen consumption suggests that an otherwise occult oxygen debt, inapparent from conventional hemodynamic measurements, may be present and that tissue oxygen demands are not being met. In an accompanying editorial, it was suggested that conventional approaches to resuscitation after thermal injury may require modification.[102b] The roles of maximizing tissue oxygen consumption soon after injury or modulating local cellular stimuli for increased oxygen consumption require further appraisal.

Vasoactive Agents About 20 percent of ARDS patients will have low COs because of underlying heart disease, ventricular underfilling, or septic shock. Vasoactive drugs may be instituted for resuscitation or for improving CO in such carefully selected individuals.[82] However, increase in CO with fluids and/or vasoactive drugs may increase pulmonary shunting. Depending on the need to correct hypotension, dobutamine increases CO with minimal increase in pulmonary artery pressure, in contrast to dopamine, a mild pulmonary vasoconstrictor.[103] Minimizing pulmonary artery pressure may help to minimize capillary leak.[104] In addition, McFarland et al. have examined the effects of dopamine and dobutamine in either a hypoxic lung ventilated with 95% O_2 or a collapsed lung.[104a] In this model, dobutamine produces less increase in right to left shunting than dopamine for any given CO, due to the lower pulmonary artery pressure achieved. Conversely, for the same degree of shunt, CO is higher and arterial P_{O_2} better with dobutamine. Despite such observations, there is no evidence that ARDS patients with shock respond better to a particular vasoactive strategy. Martyn and coworkers have observed that dopamine administration to burn victims did not improve either right ventricular function or systemic hemodynamics.[105] This agent increased pulmonary artery pressure, particularly in patients with already established pulmonary hypertension.

Extracorporeal Therapy

Supportive therapy with the extracorporeal membrane oxygenator (ECMO) has been used in ARDS patients since the 1970s without proven utility.[106] Recently, ECMO with apneic ventilation has been reported to improve patient outcome. Several investigations have demonstrated that peak inspiratory pressure exceeding 50 cm of water is associated with increased lung leak.[70,71] In an attempt to minimize inflation pressures or overventilation,[107] and, to allow the lung to "rest and repair," ECMO has been reintroduced as a mode of ARDS therapy.[108] A number of series using extracorporeal CO_2 removal (compared to historically treated ARDS patients) have reported a mortality of less than 50 percent.[70] At this time a prospective randomized study using a carefully designed protocol which attempts to make extracorporeal support the only dependent variable is being investigated. This protocol is structured to avoid the usual errors (introduced with any new therapy) that result from the intense attention experimental patients receive, leading to their better outcomes. Although it is too early to predict the results of this extracorporeal CO_2 removal trial, careful attention to clinical detail appears to be a very important determinant of patient outcome. Nonventilatory means of removing CO_2 is not yet an obvious solution to the present high mortality of ARDS.

Mechanical Ventilator Support

Although a number of European investigations have popularized the use of various ventilatory techniques, including high-frequency ventilation, there is no evidence that this mode of assisted respiration is better than standard volume ventilation.[82,109] Recently, Cioffi and coworkers have used high-frequency percussive ventilation as salvage therapy in five burned patients with inhalation injury and were able to achieve levels of oxygenation and ventilation which could not be maintained with conventional techniques.[110] An additional 10 patients were subsequently managed successfully with this approach, with little morbidity. Prospective studies of the optimum ventilator management of patients in this clinical setting remain necessary.

Until they are displaced by proven superior modalities, volume-cycled ventilators (rather than pressure-limited units) are the ventilators of choice in this clinical setting. Principles of artificial ventilation that seem reasonable in ARDS patients are to minimize peak inflation pressure by restricting tidal volume to around 7 mL/kg or less and to not utilize periodic sighs while patients are receiving PEEP. In most cases a rapid inspiratory flow rate of over 60 L/min allows for a minimal elevation in mean intrathoracic pressure and results in less of an impediment to venous return. The high minute volume requirements of these patients are satisfied through increasing respiratory rate. When oxygen consumption in ARDS patients is very high, the assist-control mode of ventilation appears to minimize respiratory work. On rare occasions sedation or paralysis of patients may aid assisted ventilation and improve oxygen saturation by reducing O_2 demand and the a-$\bar{v}_{O_2}$ gradient. Among the currently available volume ventilators, there are no clear preferences other than those dictated by personal familiarity. Although certain precautions can minimize iatrogenic lung damage induced by the ventilator, there is no strong evidence that resting the lung (like a fractured leg or injured heart) is beneficial to patient outcome.

Despite considerable enthusiasm at some centers regarding the superiority of specific modes of weaning patients from ventilatory therapy, there is no established, "best approach" to all ARDS patients. In addition, the benefits on patient outcome of an increasing array of innovative ventilatory techniques (e.g., pressure support or inverse ratio ventilation) have not been established either in ARDS patients at large or in burn victims with respiratory failure. Other aspects of the use of mechanical ventilation in burned patients are reviewed in detail elsewhere.[110a]

Other Respiratory Therapy Modalities

Several other modalities of standard respiratory care are, by convention, administered to patients with ARDS.[77,111] While the benefits of many of them appear intuitively obvious, there is little firm proof of their efficacy in this setting. Nevertheless, they are delivered as part of routine management. Clearing of secretions (often copious in burn victims with inhalation injury and/or superimposed pneumonia) and maneuvers to minimize development of atelectasis are used. Unfortunately, the distribution and extent of cutaneous burn injury often limits the use of chest percussion and postural drainage. Protection of graft sites or escharotomy wounds by sterile foam rubber pads has permitted vibratory therapy in some patients. Although benefits of humidification, surface active agents, and mucolytics have been noted in some animal models, their efficacy in humans with inhalation injury has not been established.

SPECIFIC THERAPY FOR ARDS

There have been a number of specific modalities reported to reduce lung injury to to improve patient outcome in ARDS (Table 5-7). Despite periodic enthusiasm about individual regimens, careful review of the literature fails to validate any specific therapy for ARDS at this time.[67]

Corticosteroids

A number of recent clinical studies which prospectively evaluate the effect of methylprednisolone on the prevention and/or treatment of ARDS have been reported.[112–114] None of these studies has shown an ability of steroids to prevent or improve gas exchange abnormalities, reduce lung water, or increase survival in patients with ARDS. In a large randomized, prospective multicenter study of sepsis and sepsis syndrome, the incidence of ARDS and the mortality of patients who develop ARDS were no different than in controls. In fact, the mortality was slightly worse in the steroid-treated group, while the converse, the reversal of ARDS, was better in the nonsteroid group. Therefore, despite animal experimental evidence of potential prednisone usefulness,[67] corticosteroids are not indicated for acute ARDS prevention or treatment.

Table 5-7 Suggested Specific Treatments for ARDS

Corticosteroids
Cyclooxygenase blockers
Leukotriene inhibitors
Vasodilators
B_2 agonists
Free radical scavengers
Furosemide
Surfactant
Antiproteases
Prostacycline or PGE_1
Pentoxifylline
Monoclonal antibodies

These observations are consistent with the lack of recognized steroid benefit in patients with smoke inhalation[115] and the markedly accentuated mortality and morbidity of this therapy in burned patients with inhalation injury.[116,117]

If ARDS is considered to have both acute and chronic phases,[118] there are a number of anecdotal reports suggesting a beneficial steroid effect in the chronic phase. However, no investigation has carefully evaluated the role of prednisone in either preventing or treating the pulmonary fibrosis associated with ARDS; accurate identification of the subset of patients who might benefit from this therapy is not yet feasible. One of the problems with the recent prospective, negative steroid studies may relate to the fact that high-dose steroids were administered for too prolonged a period (30 mg/kg for four doses). As in the clinical trials of burn patients with inhalation injury, many individuals in the steroid group succumbed to secondary infection.[112,113] Thus, if excessive steroids are given for too long a time they may alter host defense, increasing susceptibility to infection. Steroids have not been shown to improve the outcome of ARDS following near-drowning or smoke inhalation, although there is a report suggesting steroids may help to reduce the acute lung injury seen with fat embolism.[67]

Modifying Mediators

Experimental studies initially reported cyclooxygenase inhibitors to be helpful in ARDS.[119–123] Subsequent investigators demonstrated that with blockade of thromboxane A_2 release, although hydrostatic pressure and initial lung edema were reduced, lung damage and increased permeability were unaltered. A number of studies have shown beneficial effects of ibuprofen.[122–124] Recently, Bernard et al. have reported that ibuprofen may improve Pa_{O_2}, airway resistance, dynamic pulmonary compliance, pulmonary artery pressure, systemic vascular resistance, and survival in models of ARDS and in patients with sepsis-induced lung injury.[125,126] However, a beneficial role for nonsteroidal anti-inflammatory agents is clearly far from proven at this time. A number of leukotriene antagonists have been reported to reduce lung weight gain over time following free radical lung injury in a rabbit model of ARDS.[127,128] The reduction in lung leak was not due to reductions in pulmonary artery pressure. Moreover, other investigators have not found leukotrienes to be beneficial in ARDS models, and no clinical studies are yet available examining these agents for human ARDS.

Effects of Vasodilators on Vascular Pressure and Leak

The development of pulmonary edema is determined by the difference between transvascular fluid flux and lymph flow. Fluid flux, in turn, is determined by the permeability of the vascular membranes and a number of forces described by Starling. The latter include primarily the microvascular pressure and the colloid osmotic pressure.[129] The extent of the surface area exposed to these forces is also important in determining overall fluid flux, i.e., the greater the number of open and perfused vessels, the greater the potential for leak. In the normal lung, as pulmonary capillary pressure is increased there is increased extravascular fluid flux. This is compensated by increased lymph flow until some critical pressure is attained at which the volume of flux is so great that the capacity of clearance mechanisms is exceeded and edema develops. In models of ARDS there is an increased capillary leak at normal hydrostatic pressures. Leak exceeds lymph flow and the relationship between edema and subsequent rises in pressure is much more pronounced.[130] Thus, the lung leaks at low (normal) microvascular pressures, and small additional changes in microvascular pressure can produce very large changes in fluid flux and edema. Many experimental studies of ARDS models have shown that very modest reductions in pulmonary artery pressure can attenuate lung leak compared to controls, often resulting in erroneous presumptions that the particular therapy had reduced permeability.[130] The potential need to minimize pulmonary artery and left atrial pressure is a factor in ARDS management which must be carefully considered whenever one is giving fluid or attempting to increase cardiac output.[61]

It has been well documented that pulmonary artery pressure is often elevated in ARDS patients.[131] This finding may result from released vasoactive substances (e.g., thromboxane), intravascular thrombi, PMN sludging, and platelet plugs, as well as postcapillary extravascular compression from edema. Volume loading, often required during vigorous resuscitation of myocardial injury from sepsis or ischemia, may also elevate left atrial pressure and contribute to increased capillary pressure. The microvascular pressure which determines hydrostatic Starling forces depends upon the left atrial pressure plus 4×1 (pulmonary artery mean minus the left atrial pressure). If elevated pulmonary artery pressure can magnify extravascular leak, then reducing this pressure might be beneficial.[132] Several recent observations suggest that dynamic changes of the pulmonary vasculature might contribute to the genesis of ARDS due to smoke inhalation. In the sheep model, it has been observed that the local effects of unilateral smoke inhalation were associated with reduced pulmonary arterial flow to the smoked lung, and that ibuprofen could attenuate this injury. Furthermore, in preparations in which a band was placed around the pulmonary artery, more severe injury was found in the lung whose direct flow was limited. These observations have suggested that dynamic alterations of perfusion (e.g., that associated with bronchospasm due to smoke), might lead to localized ischemia or eventually lead to a form of reperfusion injury.[63] If established as an important factor in human inhalation injury, such events might provide added support for bronchodilator therapy, vasoactive medications, anti-inflammatory agents, and/or antioxidants. Whether alterations of bronchial arterial flow also contribute to pulmonary edema of inhalation injury is yet another issue to be resolved and has implications for strategies using vasoactive agents. Selective bronchial arterial vasodilation has been well documented in the sheep model of smoke inhalation[133]; relevance of this observation to pulmonary edema encountered clinically has not been established.

A number of studies of hemodynamic changes in ARDS patients following administration of hydralazine or nitroprusside have shown that pulmonary artery pressure and resistance can be reduced substantially.[82,104,134] The Pa_{O_2} also falls, but the cardiac output and oxygen delivery are usually improved. Whether this sequence of events produced by vasoactive drugs is clinically beneficial in reducing pulmonary edema, sustaining right heart performance, or providing better O_2 consumption has not been defined.[104,132,134,135] In one report of a small number of burn victims, hydralazine improved cardiac output and peripheral perfusion during the second postburn day.[136] However, there were no benefits of pulmonary function reported with this therapy.

The usefulness of any vasodilator is dependent upon what vessels are affected and the location of the major site of resistance. If most of the vascular resistance is upstream to the leaky vessels and these upstream vessels are dilated therapeutically, then it is possible to elevate the pressure in the fluid exchanging vessel (capillaries) and make the leak worse. If the resistance is downstream to the leak, as is often the case in sepsis (i.e., the postcapillary venule), venodilation will drop microvascular pressure. If the pressure is fixed in some areas (i.e., as due to thrombi) and dynamic in others (i.e., due to vasoconstriction), dilating the upstream vessels in some areas could theoretically increase regional flow and microvascular pressure even though the mean arterial pressure is improved. In one experimental ARDS model where vasoactive drugs and lung leak were examined, the treated group had lower pulmonary artery pressure, but lung water accumulation and edema were worsened.[135] The Pa_{O_2} and shunt also worsened, suggesting that the opening of vascular units perfusing injured, congested lung with damaged capillaries had occurred.[104,135]

Thus, routine use of vasodilators in ARDS cannot be recommended. At present, these agents should be limited to conventional indications such as achieving afterload reduction in patients with systemic hypertension or left ventricular dysfunction.

In individuals with severe pulmonary hypertension (mean >40 to 50 mmHg) and right heart failure, vasodilators may be administered carefully with improvement in cardiac output,[134] but special attention to monitoring parameters which could indicate worsening pulmonary edema should be instituted. Individuals who have the highest pulmonary artery pressures have the worst outcomes, but there is no clinical evidence that even successful therapeutic attempts to reduce this pressure will improve survival.

Beta Agonists in ARDS Management

Monjo et al., using endotoxin, histamine, and other mediators to produce increased capillary permeability, have shown that reversible postcapillary leaks occur in a number of nonpulmonary tissues.[137] Studies have shown that when the lung leaks, many other tissues in the body leak simultaneously; however, edema is merely recognized as an earlier (and more threatening) clinical problem in the lung. Whether generalized increases in capillary permeability accompany cutaneous burns has been a longstanding issue. Demling has shown that in his model, increased permeability to protein does not account for the lung fluid flux which occurs after surface burns.[138,139]

One of the major reasons for development of pulmonary edema in the injured lung may be physiologic capillary leak and not anatomic destruction. There are cases of ARDS in which the excess lung water seems to clear in hours (e.g., postictal pulmonary edema, heroin pulmonary edema). A number of patients with ARDS following aspiration of gastric contents have been observed to improve within 24 hours. Under such circumstances of rapid clinical clearing it can be postulated that increased capillary leak could be due to a physiologic change in the permeability surface area product and not a purely anatomic alteration of membrane architecture. It has been reported that young individuals who die during the first 24 hours after developing ARDS have little, if any, ultrastructural change in their endothelial membranes at electron microscopy, suggesting that in some circumstances a component of the leak in early ARDS may be dynamic.[36] Functional alterations in permeability may relate to contraction of microfilaments or widening of tight junctions between endothelial cells. The development of gaps between endothelial cells could explain how large molecules such as fibrinogen can appear outside the endothelial basement despite the absence of electron microscopic evidence of anatomic damage.

Constriction of endothelial microfilaments can move endothelial cells apart, leaving wide gaps with increased permeability. These dynamic events can be attenuated by beta agonists, with prevention of the increased fluid flux. A number of isolated ARDS lung models have shown less edema to occur following aminophylline or isoproterenol pretreatment.[137,140] Isoproterenol can even change the rate of fluid flux after HCl-induced lung injury, suggesting that there is a dynamic aspect to increased permeability in some ARDS models.

Currently, there is a poor understanding of how fluid-filled alveoli remove excess water. New research has suggested that fluid is actively pumped out of the lung against a concentration gradient, very similar to mechanisms observed in the kidney. Terbutaline can increase the rate of fluid removal from alveoli experimentally filled with edema fluid, but it is too early to anticipate a clinical role for this beta agonist in removal of lung edema.[141] There have been no clinical trials documenting that either isoproterenol, terbutaline, or aminophylline either modulate or reverse lung leak in humans.

Interestingly, in experimental and clinical studies of sepsis-induced ARDS, there is increased airway resistance associated with lung inflammation. Aerosolized bronchodilators have been reported to improve airway resistance and compliance.[142,143] The improved airway function might result in better ventilation and perfusion matching and gas exchange, but this has not yet been well studied. In the absence of cardiac arrhythmias, it is possible that aerosolized beta agonists might help to mobilize fluid from the lung more rapidly, decrease the rate of early initial leak, lower airway resistance, and increase compliance, thus possibly improving distribution of airflow and reducing peak airway pressures. Although the risks appear to be relatively small, further studies will be necessary to assess the utility of this therapy.

Other Innovative Approaches

A number of experimental studies have demonstrated that the production of free radicals associated with lung injury may cause or amplify pulmonary edema by directly injuring alveolar capillary membranes and/or by increasing microvascular pressure.[144] Several lung injury models have been designed in which either the generation of free radicals or increased free radical scavenging are modified pharmacologically: for example, in one preparation or another, allopurinol, catalase, dimethyl sulfoxide (DMSO), dimethylthiourea (DMTU), deferoxamine, and acetylcysteine have all been associated with reduced lung leak. In various animal models of smoke inhalation and/or cutaneous burn, beneficial physiologic effects of DMSO, cyclooxygenase inhibitors (ibuprofen), vitamin E, dimethylthiourea sodium benzolate, and iron chelators have been noted.[77] Interpretation of these results, however, require special attention to the nuances of each experimental preparation. Although no prospective clinical trials are available which might support this therapeutic strategy in humans, a number of investigators are actively pursuing techniques to remove free radicals from cellular sites where they may be injurious.[144–147]

Lung inflammation documented by histologic findings and elevated white blood cells in bronchoalveolar lavage material has implicated neutrophil elastase in the production and progression of ARDS.[148] Recent studies have demonstrated increased neutrophil elastase and proteolytic activity from the lungs of patients with ARDS and are reminiscent of observations in animal models of smoke inhalation injury.[145,146] However, the level of proteolytic activity has not been shown to correlate with shunt fractions, lung compliance, pulmonary vascular resistance, or patient outcome. With the recent availability of large amounts of alpha$_1$-antitrypsin and synthetic neutralizers of elastase, clinical studies are beginning to evaluate the role of these agents in ARDS therapy.

Inhalation of toxic agents (including smoke) and alveolar flooding itself can inactivate surfactant, resulting in unstable alveolar units and atelectasis; damage to the alveolar epithelium with local metabolic changes also delays production of new surfactant.[149] Hyperventilation may also inactivate surfactant, which might potentially be conserved by administration of PEEP. Whether addition of surfactant will be useful in ARDS is being evaluated further as potential agents for surfactant replacement are being developed through sophisticated molecular biologic and biophysical progress. Surfactant replacement or the aerosolization of surfactant components have been shown to reduce morbidity and mortality in some premature infants, but not all with the respiratory distress syndrome respond.[150] In a recent multicenter trial, single-dose surfactant therapy to infants with the respiratory distress syndrome lowered the severity of respiratory distress during the 72 hours after treatment.[151] However, neither later clinical status nor mortality were altered.

In patients with possible volume overload or heart failure, furosemide administration may have practical and potential benefits in ARDS treatment. Based on the possible therapeutic value of reductions of central blood volume and microvascular pressure, furosemide has been evaluated in lung injury models. Interestingly, this approach has been associated with reductions of lung water and shunt that are apparently unrelated to changes in either capillary pressure or diuresis. These observations suggest that unexplained mechanisms, perhaps related to alteration in vascular reactivity or the scavenging of free radicals, are responsible.

Prostaglandin E_1 has been shown in animal studies to affect the function of platelets and leukocytes, both of which have been implicated in acute lung injury. In addition, prostaglandin E_1 is a strong pulmonary vasodilator and increases pulmonary shunting in ARDS patients.[152] Although one clinical study has reported this agent to improve survival in patients with ARDS, a subsequent multicenter placebo-controlled study has failed to demonstrate a beneficial prostaglandin effect on patient outcome.[153]

Pentoxifylline, a methylxanthine derivative, is reported to decrease the adherence of neutrophils to endothelium and reduce neutrophil superoxide anion production.[154,155] This drug has also been shown to improve survival in a rat fecal peritonitis model and decrease endotoxin-induced pulmonary vascular permeability to protein. This agent is currently available only by oral administration and has not been investigated in patients with sepsis syndrome or ARDS.

Sepsis or sepsis syndrome precedes ARDS in 30 percent of patients,[156] and sepsis, often culture-negative, is a well-recognized cause of ARDS in burned patients. A monoclonal antibody to endotoxin has been associated with improved survival and reduced lung injury in some models challenged by gram-negative organisms, and is currently being tested in humans. Viewed optimistically, realization of such potential benefits in management of burn infections could have a major effect on the frequency and impact of ARDS.

SUMMARY: MANAGEMENT STRATEGY FOR PATIENTS WITH ARDS

Upon recognition and diagnosis of ARDS, the primary goal is to establish adequate systemic blood pressure, cardiac output, and arterial oxygenation and to relieve tissue hypoxia. A sufficient FI_{O_2} to maximize Pa_{O_2} should be administered. Patients with high ventilatory requirements usually require endotracheal intubation to establish a satisfactory Pa_{O_2}, but closed-mask, high-flow systems may suffice in carefully selected individuals. Initial delivery of a 0.9 FI_{O_2} may maximize alveolar oxygen pressure while balancing absorptive atelectasis. In the presence of a Pa_{O_2}/FI_{O_2} ratio of <300, PEEP or CPAP should be instituted. Administration of PEEP >8 to 10 cmH_2O usually requires intubation but not necessarily assisted ventilation. Arterial cannulation is helpful in monitoring therapeutic effects, but initial treatment can be guided by continuous pulse oximetry and periodic arterial blood gas analysis. PEEP should be increased by increments of 2.5 to 5 cmH_2O every 4 to 5 minutes until oximetric saturation reaches 98 percent. As PEEP is increased, tidal volume should be lowered to ensure that peak airway pressure is <50 cmH_2O. Aerosolized beta agonists may help to reduce airway resistance and peak pressure. CPAP, intermittent mandatory ventilation (IMV), or the assist-control modes of ventilatory support are all acceptable and should be individualized according to the needs of each patient.

Once a satisfactory Pa_{O_2} is established, reduction in FI_{O_2} and subsequent incremental elevation in PEEP to effectively titrate the Pa_{O_2} to 55 to 60 torr (or saturation of 90 percent) with an FI_{O_2} of 0.70 or less is the initial goal. Once the Pa_{O_2} is stable at an FI_{O_2} of around 0.70, PEEP should be reduced to the minimal level which prevents significant hypoxemia. Patients having difficulty establishing a satisfactory Pa_{O_2} may improve with assist-control ventilation or sedation to reduce oxygen consumption. Further attempts to alter FI_{O_2} and PEEP can then be made slowly, seeking goals of $FI_{O_2} < 0.5$ and end-expiratory pressures of <10 cm of water. It usually requires more PEEP to open units than to keep them open. Most patients improve their Pa_{O_2}/FI_{O_2} ratio over the first 24 to 48 hours, although this finding has little prognostic value. Fluid replacement should be monitored carefully, with efforts to minimize excess volume administration. In burn victims, this goal must be balanced with the patient's overall requirements for and response to fluid resuscitation. High cardiac outputs are common with ARDS, and attempts to optimize ventricular filling pressure while maintaining satisfactory microvascular pressures are justified. Once these basic goals are established, meticulous attention to detail is necessary to avoid complications. The best outcome is achieved with early extubation, which inevitably will be delayed if untoward events develop.

OUTCOME OF ARDS

There are an estimated 150,000 cases of ARDS in the United States each year. Approximately two-thirds of these patients die.[156,157] This high mortality has been relatively unchanged for 20 years. Varying reports have noted group mortalities to vary as low as 30 percent and as high as 90 percent. Because inhalation injury, nosocomial pneumonia, and respiratory effects of sepsis often overlap (and are not systematically differentiated) in most reports, the precise frequency of ARDS and its outcomes in burn victims are unclear. Despite increased appreciation of the role of hypoxemic respiratory failure as the cause of death in this setting, reduced mortality due to therapeutic innovations has not yet been documented. Many authorities believe that the outcome of ARDS is related to the specific stimulus and intensity of the initial injury, but this notion lacks substantiating evidence. Initial clinical, radiographic, or physiologic measurements do not predict survival with a high degree of certainty. Early predictors of death have been the presence of metabolic acidosis and low percentages of band forms in initial peripheral blood smears.[158] Among survivors, major clinical improvement is usually seen during the first 24 to 48 hours. Among critically ill patients who have similar risk factors and comparable adjusted acute physiologic and chronic health evaluation (APACHE) scores, the absence of ARDS connotes a much better outcome.[159]

Most of the deaths that occur within the first 72 hours after ARDS diagnosis result from the precipitating disease or injury. Interestingly, irreversible respiratory failure is usually responsible for only 15 to 20 percent of ARDS fatalities. The majority of deaths that occur more than 72 hours after the onset of ARDS usually result from some form of complication.[159] It is certainly possible that more widespread use of available therapies contributes to poor outcome (e.g., overhydration, excess PEEP, poor nutrition, etc.), but few studies have carefully evaluated the deleterious effect of therapeutic regimens. The leading cause of mortality in these patients is infection, a problem accentuated by defective systemic host defenses in patients with burn injury, and/or compromise of local pulmonary defenses by smoke inhalation. The development of sepsis syndrome and multiorgan failure markedly increases mortality. Not surprisingly, the presence of one or more organ failures, liver failure, or hemorrhagic complications indicate a poor outcome.

Among ARDS patients who survive to hospital discharge, over 80 percent will subsequently have near-normal pulmonary function studies and chest radiographs.[160] In one recent investigation of ARDS survivors, residual pulmonary symptoms were uncommon (10.5 percent) and related more often to complications of intubation rather than to lung dysfunction.[161] Recently, Ghio et al. have reported that physiologic impairment, mild in most patients, was present in two-thirds of ARDS survivors.[162] The presence of such residual abnormalities correlated with physiologic indices of the severity of ARDS (maximal pulmonary artery pressure, lowest static thoracic compliance, and maximum level of PEEP). The good overall long-term prognosis of patients who survive acute, devastating pulmonary injury underscores the gains to be made from their vigorous (albeit nonspecific) supportive care. These general observations in patients with ARDS of varying etiologies also seem to apply to patients with ARDS following either smoke inhalation injury or burn sepsis, but prospective long term follow-up of the pulmonary function of such patients is not available.

COMPLICATIONS OF ARDS AND ITS MANAGEMENT

Without better understanding of the pathogenesis of ARDS and specific therapy of primary lung injury, our major means of increasing patient survival will be through reducing secondary complications. The most common of these are listed in Table 5-8 and are reviewed further in Chap. 16.

Table 5-8 Complications Seen in ARDS Patients

Infection (primarily pulmonary)
Pulmonary hypertension
Pulmonary emboli
Pulmonary fibrosis
Ventilator-associated complications
Barotrauma
Respiratory alkalosis
Hypoventilation—increased dead-space ventilation
Laryngeal injury
Tracheal injury
Cardiac complications
Reduced output
Interdependence
Related to hemodynamic monitoring
Gastrointestinal complications
Renal complications
Hematologic complications
Central nervous system complications

Infection

The major complication observed in ARDS is infection.[159,160] Infection occurs predominantly in the lung, possibly because of destroyed parenchymal architecture and reduced pulmonary host mechanisms.[82] The presence of endotracheal tubes also clearly alters host defense by irritating the trachea and allowing microbes to colonize the airways and later infect the lung. However, patients intubated for other reasons seem to have a substantially lower incidence of secondary pulmonary infections. Despite widespread appreciation of the rate of nosocomial lung infection, its timely diagnosis remains problematic in these patients with already abnormal chest roentgenograms. Sepsis or sepsis syndrome frequently follows pulmonary infections; this secondary bacterial invasion may represent a major contributor to multiorgan failure in this group of patients.[163] Among patients without evidence of infection, survival is two to three times higher than that of individuals who develop secondary infection.[164,165] Identification of the source of infection has some benefit, but in the majority of patients, infections are exceedingly hard to eradicate. Interestingly, those patients who appear to be treated adequately (i.e., who receive appropriately selected antibiotics) often have similar poor outcomes as those seen in individuals whose antibiotic treatment would be considered to be less than optimum.[165]

A number of prophylactic strategies have been attempted in efforts to reduce infection, but none has received critical evaluation at this time.[166–169] However, reducing the incidence of the colonization which antedates secondary infection, finding better means of recognizing and treating established infection, and/or improving host defense are likely to improve mortality.[170] Strict adherence to aseptic techniques with invasive procedures,observance of handwashing, and meticulous observation of other standard measures in ICU infection control are all the more important in what is fundamentally an immunocompromised population. Whether appropriate antibiotics can be better selected on the basis of diagnostic information obtained through diagnostic bronchoscopic techniques such as protected brush catheterization or lavage has yet to be demonstrated.[171–173] Endotracheal administration of antibiotics for the treatment of documented gram-negative infections has been suggested as a topical means of improving eradication of highly virulent microorganisms.[174] Although there is limited experience with this therapeutic modality, our prejudice favors such additional local antibiotics when possible.

Pulmonary Hypertension and Pulmonary Emboli

Pulmonary hypertension is commonly observed in patients with ARDS and tends to be more severe in those patients with worse outcomes. The mechanism for elevated pressure is unclear.[175] There is no evidence that treatment of pulmonary hypertension with vasodilators improves survival, although this approach may decrease vascular resistance and increase cardiac output.[104,175] Since lung inflation can contribute to the level of pulmonary hypertension, and pulmonary hypertension may exacerbate capillary leak, it is reasonable to minimize pulmonary microvascular pressure. This can be accomplished by maintaining left ventricle pressure at the lowest level consistent with good cardiac output and by using the least amount of PEEP and peak inflation pressure consistent with adequate arterial blood gases.[82] Because pulmonary emboli are commonly seen in postmortem studies of ARDS patients, prophylactic anticoagulation is recommended by some critical care groups. Whether minidose heparin is sufficient to prevent emboli in these patients is not clear, however, and efficacy of this approach in the presence of surface burn is unknown. Microangiograms can often demonstrate small thromboemboli in both antemortem and postmortem cases, but their relationships to either subsequent fibrosis or patient survival are not established.

Pulmonary Fibrosis

Pulmonary fibrosis has been reported in a number of patients with ARDS and may contribute to a poor outcome in up to 20 percent of cases. This problem is uncommonly observed in survivors of smoke inhalation with or without burns. The mechanism for rapid pulmonary fibrosis is unclear, but this process has been related to imbalances of protease and antiprotease activity. Patients who progress to pulmonary fibrosis seem to have lower levels of alpha$_1$-antitrypsin in their bronchoalveolar lavage (BAL) fluid and more persistent elevations in BAL albumin concentrations, but neither reduction in alpha$_1$-antitrypsin nor increase of neutrophil elastase has been shown to correlate with physiologic parameters of lung injury. Although elevated BAL neutrophil elastase has been associated with ARDS, the therapeutic addition of antiprotease has not been shown to prevent fibrosis.[176] The administration of corticosteroids has been reported to improve patients with biopsy-documented early fibrosis, but no prospective randomized control groups have been evaluated.[118] On the basis of anecdotal reports, corticosteroids have been advocated to prevent possible evolution to bronchiolitis obliterans in patients with inhalation injuries caused by oxides of nitrogen. The infrequency of this development in patients with smoke inhalation does not support the routine use of steroids.

Acute Mechanical Problems

Ventilatory Complications Ventilatory complications in ARDS patients are widely prevalent.[82,177–181] The most devastating of these is barotrauma with the development of pneumothorax, subcutaneous emphysema, pneumoperitoneum, and pneumopericardium.[82,178] The incidence of barotrauma appears to be higher in patients with demonstrated high peak inspiratory pressures (e.g., >50 cmH_2O) and mandates careful serial monitoring. Subpleural and interstitial emphysema often precede lung rupture. Reduction in tidal volume or use of high frequency ventilation techniques may help reduce peak airway pressure and extrathoracic air leak in patients with large bronchopleural fistulas.

Minor problems from either over- or underventilation may also result in complications. Excessive tidal volumes or ventilatory rates can produce respiratory alkalosis with the development of cardiac arrhythmias and/or shifts of the oxygen hemoglobin dissociation curve, resulting in less optimum release of oxygen. Overdistention of lung units by high tidal volumes or increased PEEP can augment dead-space ventilation, resulting in minor elevation in Pa_{CO_2}.[175] With severely decreased lung compliance, maintenance of adequate alveolar ventilation may be difficult. Attempts to increase alveolar ventilation with higher tidal volumes are usually unsuccessful; rapidly delivered smaller tidal volumes or high-frequency ventilation may be necessary to overcome alveolar hypoventilation. Lung inflation may also increase the rate of fluid flux contributing to pulmonary edema.[84]

Trauma from Endotracheal Tubes Upper airway and tracheal injury occur with intubation.[82] The extent of vocal cord injury is correlated poorly with the duration of intubation. By contrast, tracheal injury increases with the time of intubation, the cuff pressures needed to achieve an effective seal, and the requirement for PEEP, and is aggravated by avoidable predispositions such as high balloon occlusion pressures (e.g., >25 cmH_2O) or instability of the endotracheal tube. Tracheostomy is often necessary in patients requiring intubation for more than 3 weeks and results in both acute and chronic complications. Jones and coworkers have recently reviewed a 5-year experience with tracheostomies in burn patients and found that late-onset upper airway complications developed in approximately 30 percent of patients.[182] Interestingly, ARDS had been the indication for intubation in only 6 percent of these patients receiving tracheostomy, and five of these individuals died.

Because intubation alters host defense and contributes to infection, early extubation is a major goal of ARDS therapy. Patients with burn injury and smoke inhalation have additional complications from intubation, and there is clinical evidence that there is a synergistic relationship between these insults in the pathogenesis of subglottic stenosis.[183] While the favored approach to intubation (i.e., nasotracheal versus orotracheal route) is generally based on personal expertise rather than objective proof, orotracheal tubes in patients with perioral burns have been associated with lip contractures.

Multisystem Organ Failure

Importantly, many of the mediators which have been implicated in models of isolated ARDS are also prominently incriminated in the development of posttraumatic multisystemic organ failure.[184–189] The development of multisystem failure markedly affects the incidence and outcome of ARDS, particularly when there is involvement of two or more organ systems in addition to the lung, and is a strong predictor of mortality.[6,8,158,163,184] In the presence of liver failure the vast majority of ARDS patients succumb.[185] Marshall and Dimick have reported that 81 of 168 patients with second- and third-degree burns developed multiple subsystem failure and had a higher mortality than those with no organ failure or failure of only a single system (98 percent mortality versus 21 percent).[186] While inhalation injury was the most common cause of death in individuals with isolated system failure, sepsis was the predominant cause of death in individuals with multisystem disease (present in 75 percent of these individuals), providing added support for vigorous diagnosis and therapy of infection. Recently, Aikawa and coworkers have also documented the importance of multiorgan failure in burn patients. The combinations of lung failure, heart failure, and disseminated intravascular coagulation (DIC) were of particular note in this experience.[189]

Cardiovascular Problems A number of cardiac complications have been reported with ARDS and compound both the assessment and management of the hemodynamic responses to thermal injury that occur in the absence of ARDS. A reduced cardiac output has been attributed primarily to elevated pleural pressures and to secondary reduction in venous return.[190] Patients with stiff, noncompliant lungs have less transmission of airway pressure to the pleural space.[191] Individuals who have relatively good pulmonary compliances are more likely to experience elevations in pleural pressure than are patients who have markedly stiff lungs. Because an increase in pleural pressure relates directly to the compliance of the chest wall and the amount of lung inflation, patients who require the highest levels of PEEP usually do not increase their pleural pressures substantially (<30 percent transmitted).[191]

Elevated pulmonary artery pressure may result in a substantial increase in afterload to the right ventricle, with possible right ventricular failure. Reduced right ventricular ejection fractions and increased right ventricular diastolic volumes have been reported in victims of severe multiple trauma and in older, more severely burned patients with pulmonary hypertension.[192] Right ventricular ejection fractions of ARDS nonsurvivors are usually lower than those of survivors. Typically, cardiac performance continues to deteriorate until death. Isolated right ventricular dysfunction usually correlates with significantly higher pulmonary artery pressures. Ventricular dysfunction may occur in patients with sepsis or sepsis syndrome.[190,193–196] Martyn and coworkers have reported that right ventricular dysfunction also occurs in burn victims, particularly in those who are older, with larger burns, mild pulmonary hypertension, and reduced systemic arterial diastolic pressure and vascular resistance. These authors observed that an unusual pressure flow burden was imposed on the right ventricle due to the "requirement for higher than normal blood flow and a hypermetabolic burn state."[197] Increased pulmonary artery pressure and resistance has been observed clinically and in a variety of animal models of burn injury. These changes have been attributed to reductions of blood volume, the embolization of platelet aggregates, and the effects of catecholamines and other humoral mediators.

There are no studies yet demonstrating that early intervention aimed at improving such right ventricular dysfunction can benefit long-term patient survival. Increases in right ventricular diastolic volume may, because of ventricular interdependence, cause reduced diastolic compliance and underfilling of the left heart, thus leading to decreased cardiac output. There is little evidence that PEEP influences myocardial contractility.[198–200] Several cardiopulmonary complications have arisen due to balloon flotation catheter monitoring and the insertion of intravenous lines in patients with ARDS,[199,201] but the incidence of these iatrogenic problems does not seem to be unique to ARDS. On the other hand, central venous thrombosis and line-associated infection are well-documented hazards in burn victims.

Gastrointestinal Problems Upper gastrointestinal bleeding due to acute gastritis or peptic ulcer is seen in 30 percent of all critically ill patients and up to 85 percent of ARDS patients.[82] Acute upper gastrointestinal bleeding has a mortality in critically ill patients of over 50 percent. The use of large amounts of antacids, H_2 blockers, or sucralfate may reduce the frequency of gastrointestinal hemorrhage.[202] Direct titration of gastric pH is effective in reducing significant bleeding but is not achieved easily. There is some recent evidence that elevations in gastric pH increase bacterial colonization, resulting in a higher incidence of nosocomial pneumonia.[170,203] Early enteral feeding appears to confer mucosal protection. Sucralfate may provide satisfactory bleeding prophylaxis with a lower incidence of colonization and nosocomial infection.[204] However, unequivocal advantages of one prophylactic regimen over another as yet are not defined. Thus, combination therapy is often chosen empirically on the basis of personal prejudices.

Gastric overdistention due to swallowing of air leaking from high intrathoracic pressure support can produce bloating, elevation of the diaphragms (with a restrictive ventilatory defect), and actual gastric rupture. This complication, increased with nasotracheal intubation and a closed mouth, can be prevented by insertion of a nasogastric tube and nasogastric suctioning. Reduced perfusion of splanchnic beds may lead not only to other intraabdominal catastrophes but also to shifts of enteric pathogens across bowel mucosa, seeding the bloodstream.

Renal Problems Renal insufficiency is a frequent complication of sepsis-related multiorgan failure.[82,205] Urinary tract infections also occur frequently due to insertion of Foley catheters as monitoring devices, and drug-induced renal dysfunction is commonplace. Patients receiving ventilator assistance often have excess serum antidiuretic hormone and retain free water. This can be corrected by judicious free water restriction and use of diuretics.

Hematologic Problems Anemia is commonly due to phlebotomy and associated stresses which prevent normal red cell production and shorten red cell survival. Disseminated intravascular coagulation has been observed as an associated condition with ARDS in as many as 25 percent of patients, but whether it causes, or is caused by, lung injury is not clear. Thrombocytopenia due to increased consumption or sequestration of platelets has been reported to occur in over half of patients with ARDS and has been associated with an increased mortality.[82]

Central Nervous System Problems Altered levels of consciousness are common in critically ill patients, and often have multifactorial origins. Effects of coincident trauma, cerebral hypoperfusion, alcohol intoxication, therapeutically administered drugs, or inhaled tissue asphyxiants are frequently present in burn victims. Treatment with PEEP can increase intracerebral pressure by secondary elevation of pleural pressure, transmission of pleural or increased alveolar pressure to the right atrium, and resultant elevations of back pressure for central nervous system venous drainage. Patients at greatest risk for increased cerebral pressure with PEEP are those who have major head injury and decreased intracranial compliance.[206]

SUMMARY

The pathogenesis of the adult respiratory distress syndrome is poorly understood. Basic therapeutic goals focus upon treating any precipitating or underlying illness, maintaining tissue oxygenation, and reducing or preventing complications. Despite promising observations in some experimental models, there are no specific interventions available at this time. Because of the high severity of illness in ARDS patients and the frequent presence of multiorgan dysfunction, careful and simultaneous therapeutic adjustments of many variables are required. Invasive monitoring may provide guidance in this regard but offers no substitute for clinical judgment. Currently, even in the best hands, mortality remains high, making favorable patient outcome a goal which is difficult to achieve. The presence of formidable multisystemic problems and multiple predispositions for ARDS in burn victims with and without smoke inhalation accentuates this therapeutic challenge and demands that the respiratory injury be managed within the context of the overall status of the patient.

REFERENCES

1. Ashbaugh DG, Bigelow DB, Petty TL, Levine BE: Acute respiratory distress in adults. *Lancet* 2:319, 1967.
2. Fishman AP: Shock lung: A distinctive nonentity. *Circulation* 47:921, 1973.
3. Fulton RL, Jones CE: The cause of post-traumatic pulmonary insufficiency in man. *Surg Gynecol Obstet* 140:179, 1975.
4. Murray JF, Matthay MA, Luce JM, Flick MR: Pulmonary perspectives: An expanded definition of the adult respiratory distress syndrome. *Am Rev Respir Dis* 138:720, 1988.
5. Petty TL, Ashbaugh DG: The adult respiratory distress syndrome: Clinical features, factors influencing prognosis and principles of management. *Chest* 60:233, 1971.
6. Fowler AA, Hamman RF, Good JT, et al: Adult respiratory distress syndrome: Risk with common predispositions. *Ann Intern Med* 98:593, 1983.
7. Rinaldo JE: Indicators of *risk,* course, and prognosis in adult respiratory distress syndrome, letter. *Am Rev Respir Dis* 133:343, 1986.
8. Pepe PE, Potkin RT, Reus DH, et al: Cllinical predictors of the adult respiratory distress syndrome. *Am J Surg* 144:124, 1982.
9. Milne ENC: A physiological approach to reading critical care unit films. *J Thorac Imaging* 1(3):60, 1986.
10. Heffner JE, Silvers GW, Petty TL: Diagnosis of adult respiratory distress syndrome associated with underlying severe emphysema. *Arch Intern Med* 141:1684, 1981.
11. Mishkin FS: Radiological findings in acute pulmonary edema. *Intern Med* 7(6):127, 1986.
12. Maunder RJ, Shuman WP, McHugh JW, et al: Preservation of normal lung regions in the adult respiratory distress syndrome. *JAMA* 255(18):2463, 1986.
13. Pistolesi M, Miniati M, Milne ENC, et al: The chest roentgenogram in pulmonary edema. *Clin Chest Med* 6:315, 1985.
14. Halperin BD, Feeley TW, Mihm FG, et al: Evaluation of the portable chest roentgenogram for quantitating extravascular lung water in critically ill adults. *Chest* 88:649, 1985.
15. Milne ENC: A physiological approach to reading critical care unit films. *J Thorac Imaging* 1(3):60, 1986.
16. Haponik EF, Adelman M, Munster AM, Bleecker ER: Increased vascular pedicle width preceding burn-related pulmonary edema. *Chest* 90:681, 1986.
17. Brigham KL, Kariman K, Harris T, et al: Correlation of oxygenation with vascular permeability surface area but not with lung water in humans with acute respiratory failure and pulmonary edema. *J Clin Invest* 72:339, 1983.
18. Sibbald WJ, Warshawski FJ, Short AK, et al: Clinical studies of measuring extravascular lung water by the thermal dye technique in critically ill patients. *Chest* 82:725, 1983.

18a. Peitzman AB, Shires GT, Teixidor HS, Curreri BPW, Shires, GT: Smoke inhalation injury: evaluation of radiographic manifestations and pulmonary dysfunction, *J Trauma* 29:1232, 1989.

19. Petty, TL: Adult respiratory distress syndrome: Definition and historical perspective. *Clin Chest Med* 3:3, 1982.
20. Weigelt JA, Norcross JF, Borman KR, Snyder WH:

Early steroid therapy for respiratory failure. *Arch Surg* 120:536, 1985.

21. Ratliff JL, Eberhart RC, Tucker HJ, Hill JD: Pathologic features and mechanisms of hypoxemia in adult respiratory distress syndrome. *Am Rev Respir Dis* 114:267, 1976.
22. Nieman GF, Clark WR, Wax SD, et al: The effect of smoke inhalation on pulmonary surfactant. *Am Surg* 191:171, 1980.
23. Prien T, Strohmaier W, Gasser H, et al: Normal phosphatidylehaline composition of lung surfactant 24 hours after inhalation injury. *J Burn Care Rehabil* 10:38, 1989.
24. Mancebo J, Benito S, Martin M, et al: Value of static pulmonary compliance in predicting mortality in patients with acute respiratory failure. *Intensive Care Med* 14:110, 1988.
25. Wright PE, Bernard G: The role of airflow resistance in patients with the adult respiratory distress syndrome. *Am Rev Respir Dis* 139:1169, 1989.
26. Brigham KL: Fluid and solute transport in the acutely injured lung. *Lung Biol Health Dis* 24:209, 1982.
27. Holter JF, Weiland JE, Pacht ER, et al: Protein permeability in the adult respiratory distress syndrome: Loss of size selectivity of the alveolar epithelium. *J Clin Invest* 78:1513, 1986.
28. Mishkin FS, Niden A, Kumar A, et al: Albumin lung/heart ratio change: A simple clinical means of documenting increased pulmonary endothelial permeability to protein. *JAMA* 257(7):953, 1987.
29. Sprung CL, Long WM, Marcial EH, et al: Distribution of proteins in pulmonary edema. *Am Rev Respir Dis* 136:957, 1987.
30. Pratt PC: Pathology of adult respiratory distress syndrome: Implications regarding therapy. *Semin Respir Med* 4(2):79, 1982.
31. Bachofen M, Weibel ER: Structural alterations of lung parenchyma in the adult respiratory distress syndrome. *Clin Chest Med* 3(1):35, 1982.
32. Linares HA, Herndon DM, Traber DL: Sequence of morphologic events in experimental smoke inhalation. *J Burn Care Rehabil* 10:27, 1989.
33. Foley FD: The burn autopsy: Fatal complications of burns. *Am J Clin Pathol* 52:1, 1969.
34. Nash G, Foley FD, Langlinais PC: Pulmonary interstitial edema and hyaline membranes. *Hum Pathol* 5:149, 1974.
35. Haponik EF, Summer WR: Respiratory complications in burned patients. Pathogenesis and spectrum of inhalation injury. *J Crit Care* 2:49, 1987.
36. Pietra GG, Ruttner JW, Wust W, Glinz W: The lung after trauma and shock: Fine structure of the alveolar-capillary barrier in 23 autopsies. *J Trauma* 21:454, 1981.
37. Schlag G, Redl HR: Morphology of the human lung after traumatic injury. *Lung Biol Health Dis* 24:161, 1982.
38. Petty TL: Indicators of *risk,* course, and *prognosis* in adult respiratory distress syndrome (ARDS), editorial. *Am Rev Respir Dis* 132:471, 1985.
39. Simon RH: Predictors of the adult respiratory distress syndrome, editorial. *J Crit Care* 2(2):81, 1987.
40. Herndon DM, Thompson PB, Brown M, Traber DL: Diagnosis, pathophysiology, and treatment of inhalation injury, in Boswick JA (ed): *The Art and Science of Burn Case*. Rockville, MD, Aspen Publishers, 1987.
41. Clark WR, Nieman GF, Goyette D, Gryzboski D: Effects of crystalloid on lung fluid balance after smoke inhalation. *Ann Surg* 208(1):56, 1988.
42. Carvalho ACA, Bellman SM, Saullo VJ, et al: Altered factor viii in acute respiratory failure. *N Engl J Med* 307:1113, 1982.

42a. Grosso MA, Viders DE, Brown JM, et al: Local skin-burn causes systemic (lung and kidney) endothelial cell injury reflected by increased circulating and decreased tissue Factor VIII-related antigen. *Surgery* 106:310, 1989.

43. Rauvala H, Hallman M: Glycolipid accumulation in bronchoalveolar space in adult respiratory distress syndrome. *J Lipid Res* 25:1257, 1984.
44. Jacob HS, Craddock PR, Hammerschmidt DE, Moldow CF: Complement-induced granulocyte aggregation: An unsuspected mechanism of disease. *N Engl J Med* 302(14):789, 1980.
45. Ognibene FP, Martin SE, Parker MM, et al: Adult respiratory distress syndrome in patients with severe neutropenia. *N Engl J Med* 315(9):547, 1986.
46. Glauser FL, Fairman RP: The uncertain role of the neutrophil in increased permeability pulmonary edema. *Chest* 88(4):601, 1985.
47. Duchateau J, Haas M, Schreyen H, et al: Complement activation in patients at risk of developing the adult respiratory distress syndrome. *Am Rev Respir Dis* 130:1058, 1984.
48. Moore FD, Davis C, Rodrick M, et al: Neutrophil activation in thermal injury as assessed by increased expression of complement receptors. *N Engl J Med* 314:948, 1986.
49. Fjellstrom KE, Arturson G: Changes in the human complement system following burn trauma. *Acta Pathol* 59:257, 1963.
50. Gefland JA, Donelan MB, Hawiger A, et al: Alternative complement pathway activation increases mortality in a model of burn injury in mice. *J Clin Invest* 70:1170, 1982.
51. Gelfand JA, Doneland M, Burke JF: Preferential activation and depletion of the alternative complement pathway by burn injury. *Ann Surg* 198:58, 1983.
52. Hyers TM, Fowler AA: Adult respiratory distress syndrome: Causes, morbidity, and mortality. *Fed Proc* 45:25, 1986.
53. Fowler AA, Fisher BJ, Centor RM, Carchman RA: Development of the adult respiratory distress syndrome: Progress alteration of neutrophil chemotactic and secretory processes. *Am J Pathol* 116:427, 1984.
54. Harlan JM, Schwartz BR, Reidy MA, et al: Activated neutrophils disrupt endothelial monolayer integrity by an oxygen radical-independent mechanism. *Lab Invest* 52(2):141, 1985.
55. Rubanyi GM: Vascular effects of oxygen-derived free radicals. *Free Radic Biol Med* 4:107, 1988.
56. Chang SW, Voelkel NF: Charge-related lung microvascular injury. *Am Rev Respir Dis* 139(2):534, 1989.

57. Demling RH: The role of mediators in human ARDS. *J Crit Care* 3(1):56, 1988.
58. Clark WR, Nieman GF: Smoke inhalation. *Burns* 14:473, 1988.
59. Tracey KJ, Lowry SF, Cerami A: Cachectin/TNF-a in septic shock and septic adult respiratory distress syndrome. *Am Rev Respir Dis* 38(6):1377, 1988.
60. Tracey KJ, Beutler B, Lowry SF, et al: Shock and tissue injury induced by recombinant tissue cachectin. *Science* 234:470, 1986.
61. Weiland JE, Davis WB, Holter JF, et al: Lung neutrophils in the adult respiratory distress syndrome: Clinical and pathophysiologic significance. *Am Rev Respir Dis* 133:218, 1986.
62. Herndon DN, Traber DL, Nichaus GD, et al: The pathophysiology of smoke inhalation in a sheep model. *J Trauma* 24:1044, 1981.
63. Traber DL, Linares HA, Herndon DM: The pathophysiology of inhalation injury: A review. *Burns* 14:357, 1988.
64. Kinsella J: Smoke inhalation. *Burns* 14:269, 1988.
65. Till GO, Hatherill JR, Tourtellotte WW, et al: Lipid peroxidation and acute lung injury after thermal trauma to skin: Evidence of a role for hydroxyl radical. *Am J Pathol* 119:376, 1985.
66. Strieter RM, Kunkel SL, Showell HJ, Marks RM: Monokine-induced gene expression of a human endothelial cell-derived neutrophil chemotactic factor. *Biochem Biophys Res Commun* 156(3):1340, 1988.
67. Adult respiratory distress syndrome, editorial. *Lancet* 1:301, 1986.
67a. Demling RH, LaLonde C, Liu Y, Zhu D: The lung inflammatory response to thermal injury: Relationship between physiologic and histologic changes. *Surgery* 106:52, 1989.
68a. Pruitt BA, Flemma RJ, DiVincenti FC, et al.: Pulmonary complications in burn patients. *J Thorac Cardiovas Surg* 59:7, 1970.
68b. Pruitt BA, DiVincenti FC, Mason AD, et al.: The occurrence and significance of pneumonia and other pulmonary complications in burned patients: Comparison of conventional and topical treatments. *J Trauma* 10:519, 1970.
68c. Venus B, Matsuda T, Copiozo JB, Mathru M: Prophylactic intubation and continuous positive airway pressure in the management of inhalation injury in burn victims. *Crit Care Med* 9:519, 1981.
68d. Demling RH, Wong C, Jin LJ, et al.: Early lung dysfunction after major burns: Role of edema and vasoactive mediators. *J Trauma* 25:959, 1985.
68e. Mathru M, Venus B, Tadikonda L, et al.: Noncardiac pulmonary edema precipitated by tracheal intubation in patients with inhalation injury. *Crit Care Med* 11:804, 1983.
68f. Willms D, Shure D: Pulmonary edema due to upper airway obstruction in adults. *Chest* 94:1090, 1988.
69. Miller EJ: Management of patients with smoke inhalation. The Las Vegas experience, in O'Donohue WJ (ed): *Current Advances in Respiratory Care*. Park Ridge, IL, American College of Chest Physicians, 1984.
69a. Stone HH, Reame DW, Corbitt JD, et al: Respiratory burns: A correlation of clinical and laboratory results. *Ann Surg* 165:157, 1967.
69b. Vesconi S, Rossi GP, Pesenti A, et al: Pulmonary microthrombosis in severe adult respiratory distress syndrome. *Crit Care Med* 16(2):111, 1988.
69c. Gattinoni L, Pesenti A, Mascheroni D, et al: Low-frequency positive-pressure ventilation with extracorporeal CO_2 removal in severe acute respiratory failure. *JAMA* 256:881, 1986.
70. Kolobow T, Moretti MP, Fumagalli R, et al: Severe impairment in lung function induced by high peak airway pressure during mechanical ventilation. *Am Rev Respir Dis* 135:312, 1987.
71. Dreyfuss D, Basset G, Soler P, Saumon G: Intermittent positive-pressure hyperventilation with high inflation pressures produces pulmonary microvascular injury in rats. *Am Rev Respir Dis* 132:880, 1985.
72. Summer WR, Curry P, Haponik EF, et al: Continuous mechanical turning of intensive care unit patients shortens length of stay in some diagnostic-related groups. *J Crit Care* 4(1):45, 1989.
73. Koretz RL: Breathing and feeding: Can you have one without the other? *Chest* 8:298, 1984.
74. Rochester DF, Esau SA: Malnutrition and the respiratory system. *Chest* 85:411, 1984.
75. Koretz RL: Nutritional support: Whether or not some is good, more is not better. *Chest* 88:2, 1985.
76. Pingleton SK, Harmon GS: Nutritional management in acute respiratory failure. *JAMA* 257(22):3094, 1987.
76a. Demling RH, Tortella B: The effect of lipid infusion on pulmonary function in burn patients with inhalation injury. *J Burn Care Rehab* 6:222, 1985.
77. Haponik EF, Summer WR: Respiratory complications in burned patients: Diagnosis and management of inhalation injury. *J Crit Care* 2(2):121, 1987.
78. Finland M, Davidson CS, Levenson SM: Clinical and therapeutic aspects of the conflagration injuries to the respiratory tract sustained by victims of the Cocoanut Grove disaster. *Medicine* 25:215, 1946.
79. Fein A, Leff A, Hopewell PC: Pathophysiology and management of the complications resulting from fire and the inhaled products of combustion: Review of the literature. *Crit Care Med* 8:94, 1980.
79a. Roughton FJW, Darling RC: The effect of carbon monoxide on the oxyhemoglobin dissociation curve. *Am J Physiol* 141:17, 1944.
80. Jenkinson SG: Oxygen toxicity. *J Intensive Care Med* 3:137, 1988.
81. Witschi HR, Haschek WM, Klein-Szanto AJP, Hakkinen PJ: Potentiation of diffuse lung damage by oxygen: Determining variables. *Am Rev Respir Dis* 123:98, 1981.
82. McCaffree DR: Adult respiratory distress syndrome. In Dantzker DR (ed). *Cardiopulmonary Critical Care*. Grune & Stratton, Inc., New York, 1986, p. 613.
83. Weisman IM, Rinaldo JE, Rogers RM: Current concepts: Positive end-expiratory pressure in adult respiratory failure. *N Engl J Med* 307(22):1381, 1982.

84. Rizk NW, Murray JF: Peep and pulmonary edema. *Am J Med* 72:381, 1982.
85. Wise RA: Effect of circulatory mechanics on hydrostatic forces producing pulmonary edema. *J Crit Care* 1:247, 1986.
86. Rose DM, Downs JB, Heenan TJ: Temporal responses of functional residual capacity and oxygen tension to changes in positive end-expiratory pressure. *Crit Care Med* 9(2):79, 1981.
87. Eisenberg PR, Hansbrough JR, Anderson D, Schuster DP: A prospective study of lung water measurements during patient management in an intensive care unit. *Am Rev Respir Dis* 136:662, 1987.
88. Simmons RS, Berdine GG, Seidenfeld JJ, et al: Fluid balance and the adult respiratory distress syndrome. *Am Rev Respir Dis* 135:924, 1987.
88a. Carlson RG, Miller SF, Finley RK, Billett JM, Fegelman E, Jones LM, Alkire S: Fluid retention and burn survival. *J Trauma* 27:127, 1987.
88b. Carlson RG, FInley RK, Miller SF, et al.: FLuid retention during the first 48 hours as an indicator of burn survival. *J Trauma* 26:840, 1986.
89. Navaro PD, Saffle JR, Warden GD: Effect of inhalation injury on fluid resuscitation requirements after thermal injury. *Am J Surg* 150:716, 1985.
90. Scheulen JJ, Munster AM: The Parkland formula in patients with burns and inhalation injury. *J Trauma* 22:869, 1982.
91. Herndon DM, Traber DL, Traber LD: Effect of resuscitation on inhalation injury. *Surgery* 100:248, 1986.
92. Herndon DM, Barrow RE, Linares HA, et al: Inhalation injury in burned patients: Effects and treatment. *Burns* 14:349, 1988.
93. McKeen CR, Bowers RE, Harris TR, et al: Saline compared to plasma volume replacement after volume depletion in sheep: lung fluid balance. *J Crit Care* 1(3):133, 1986.
94. Goodwin CW, Dorothy J, Lam V, et al: Randomized trial of efficacy of crystalloid and colloid resuscitation on hemodynamic response and lung water following thermal injury. *Ann Surg* 197:520, 1983.
95. Waxman K, Holness R, Tominga G, et al.: Hemodynamic and oxygen transport effects of pentastarch in burn resuscitation.
96. Demling RH: Fluid and electrolyte management. *Crit Care Clin* 1:27, 1985.
97. Gutierrez G: Peripheral delivery and utilization of oxygen. In Dantzker DR (ed): *Cardiopulmonary Critical Care*. Grune & Stratton, Inc., New York, 1986, p. 169.
98. Dantzker DR: Pulmonary gas exchange. In Dantzker DR (ed): *Cardiopulmonary Critical Care*. Grune & Stratton, Inc., New York, 1986, p. 25.
99. Lutch JC, Murray JF: Continuous positive-pressure ventilation: Effects on systemic oxygen transport and tissue oxygenation. *Ann Intern Med* 76:193, 1972.
100. Powers SR, Mannal R, Neclerio M, et al.: Physiologic consequences of positive end-expiratory pressure (PEEP) ventilation. *Ann Surg* 178:265, 1973.
101. Danek SJ, Lynch JP, Weg JG, Dantzker DR: The dependence of oxygen uptake on oxygen delivery with adult respiratory distress syndrome. *Am Rev Respir Dis* 122:387, 1980.
102. Mohsenifar Z, Goldbach P, Tashkin DP, Campisi DJ: Relationship between O_2 delivery and O_2 consumption in the adult respiratory distress syndrome. *Intensive Crit Care Digest* 3(2):36, 1984.
102a. Demling RH, Lalonde C, Fogt F, Zhu D, Liu Y: Effect of increasing oxygen delivery post-burn on oxygen consumption and oxidant-induced lipid peroxidation in the adult sheep. *Crit Care Med* 17:1025, 1989.
102b. Waxman K: Toward a re-evaluation of burn resuscitation. *Crit Care Med* 17:1077, 1989.
103. Fuhrman W, Summer W, Kennedy T, Sylvester J: Comparison of the effects of dobutamine, dopamine and isoproterenol on hypoxic pulmonary vasoconstriction in the pig. *Crit Care Med* 10:371, 1982.
104. Melot C, Naeije R, Mols P, et al: Pulmonary vascular tone improves pulmonary gas exchange in the adult respiratory distress syndrome. *Am Rev Respir Dis* 136:1232, 1987.
104a. McFarland PA, Mortimer AJ, Ryder WA, et al: Effects of dopamine and dobutamine on the distribution of pulmonary blood flow during lobar ventilation hypoxia and lobar collapse in dogs. *Eur J Clin Invest* 15:53, 1985.
105. Martyn J, Wilson RS, Burke JF: Right ventricular function and pulmonary hemodynamic during dopamine infusion in burned patients. *Chest* 89:357, 1986.
106. Zapol WM, Snider MT, Hill JD, et al: Extracorporeal membrane oxygenation in severe acute respiratory failure. *JAMA* 242:2193, 1979.
107. Wyszogrodski I, Kyei-Aboagye K, Taensch HW Jr, et al: Surfactant inactivation by hyperventilation: Conservation by end-expiratory pressure. *J Appl Physiol* 38:461, 1975.
108. Hickling KG, Downward G, Davis FM, et al: Management of severe ARDS with low frequency positive pressure ventilation and extracorporeal CO_2 removal. *Anaesth Intens Care* 14:79, 1986.
109. Tobin MJ, Dantzker DR: Mechanical ventilation and weaning. In Dantzker DR (ed): *Cardiopulmonary Critical Care*. Grune & Stratton, Inc., New York, 1986, p. 203.
110. Cioffi WG, Graves TA, McManus WF, Pruitt BA: High-frequency percussive ventilation in patients with inhalation injury. *J Trauma* 29:350, 1989.
110a. Wallfisch HK: Bedside management and weaning of the burn patient on mechanical ventilation. *J Burn Care Rehab* 7:285, 1986.
111. Wootton R, Hodgson E: Physiotherapy in treatment of burns with inhalation involvement. *Physiotherapy* 63:153, 1977.
112. Bone RC, Fisher C, Clemmer TP, et al: A controlled clinical trial of high-dose methylprednisolone in the treatment of severe sepsis and septic shock. *N Engl J Med* 317:653, 1987.
113. The Veterans Administration Systemic Sepsis Cooperative Study Group (multiple institutions): Effect of high-

dose glucocorticoid therapy on mortality in patients with clinical signs of systemic sepsis. *N Engl J Med* 317:659, 1987.
114. Bernard GR, Harris T, Luce JE, et al: High dose corticosteroids in patients with the adult respiratory distress syndrome: A randomized double-blind trial. *N Engl J Med* 317(25):1565, 1987.
115. Robinson NB, Hudson LD, Riem M, et al: Steroid therapy following isolated smoke inhalation injury. *J Trauma* 22:876, 1982.
116. Levine BA, Petroff PA, Slade CL, et al: Prospective trials of dexamethasone and aerosolized gentamicin in the treatment of inhalation injury in the burned patient. *J Trauma* 18:188, 1978.
117. Moylan JA, Chan CK: Inhalation injury: An increasing problem. *Ann Surg* 188:34, 1977.
118. Ashbaugh DG, Maier RV: Idiopathic pulmonary fibrosis in adult respiratory distress syndrome. Diagnosis and treatment. *Arch Surg* 120:530, 1985.
119. Fuhrman TM, Hollon MF, Reines HD, et al.: Beneficial effects of ibuprofen in oleic acid induced lung injury. *J Surg Res* 42:284, 1987.
120. Kopolovic R, Thrailkill KM, Martin DT, et al: Effects of ibuprofen on a porcine model of acute respiratory failure. *J Surg Res* 36:300, 1984.
121. Snapper Jr, Hutchinson AA, Ogletree ML, Brigham KL. Effects of cyclooxygenase inhibitors on the alterations in lung mechanics caused by endotoxemia in the unanesthetized sheep. *J Clin Invest* 72:63, 1983.
122. Mizus I, Michael J, Summer W, Gurtner G. Acid aspiration induced pulmonary artery pressure rise is attenuated by hypoxia or ibuprofen. *Crit Care Med* 11:241, 1983.
123. Sielaff TD, Sugerman HJ, Tatum JL, Blocher CR. Successful treatment of adult respiratory distress syndrome by histamine and prostaglandin blockade in a porcine pseudomonas model. *Surgery* 102:350, 1987.
124. Perkowski SZ, Havill AM, Flynn JT, Gee MH. Role of intrapulmonary release of eicosanoids and superoxide anion as mediators of pulmonary dysfunction and endothelial injury in sheep with intermittent complement activation. *Circ Res* 53:574, 1983.
125. Bernard GR, Reines HD, Metz CA, et al: Effects of a short course of ibuprofen in patients with severe sepsis. *Am Rev Respir Dis* 137(4):138, 1988.
126. Bernard GR, Brigham KL: Increased lung vascular permeability: Mediators and therapies, in Shoemaker W (ed): *Textbook of Critical Care Medicine*. Philadelphia, Saunders, 1989, pp. 1049–1054.
127. Burghuber OC, Strife RJ, Zirrolli J, et al: Leukotriene inhibitors attenuate rat lung injury induced by hydrogen peroxide. *Am Rev Respir Dis* 131:778, 1985.
128. Farrukh IS, Michael JR, Spannhake EW, et al: The role of cyclooxygenase and lipoxygenase mediators in oxidant-induced lung injury. *Am Rev Respir Dis* 137:1343, 1988.
129. Brigham KL: Primary (high permeability) pulmonary edema. *Sem Respir Med* 4(4):285, 1983.
130. Demling RH. Role of prostaglandins in acute pulmonary microvascular injury. *Ann New York Acad Sci* 384:517, 1982.
131. Zapol WM, Snider MT, Rie MA, et al: Pulmonary circulation during adult respiratory distress syndrome, in Zapol WM, Falke KJ (eds): *Acute Respiratory Failure*. New York, Marcel Dekker, 1985, vol 24, pp. 241–73.
132. Wood LDH, Prewitt RM: Cardiovascular management in acute hypoxemic respiratory failure. *Am J Cardiol* 47:963, 1981.
133. Kramer GC, Herndon DM, Linares HA, Traber DL: Effects of inhalation injury on airway blood flow and edema formation. *J Burn Care Rehabil* 10:45, 1989.
134. Ghignone M, Girling L, Prewitt RM: Effects of vasodilators on canine cardiopulmonary function when a decrease in cardiac output complicates an increase in right ventricular afterload. *Am Rev Respir Dis* 131:527, 1985.
135. Bishop MJ, Huang T, Cheney FW: Effect of vasodilator treatment on the resolution of oleic acid injury in dogs. *Am Rev Respir Dis* 131:421, 1985.
136. Pruitt BA Jr, Mason AD, Moncrief JA: Hemodynamic changes in the early postburn patient: The influence of fluid administration and of a vasodilator (hydralazine). *J Trauma* 11:36, 1971.
137. Summer WR, Mizus I, Gurtner G: Effects of B-agonists and aminophylline on lung fluid balance. *Acute Lung Injury: Pathogenesis of Adult Respiratory Distress Syndrome*, 1986, pp. 219–32.
138. Demling RH: Burns. *N Engl J Med* 313:1389, 1985.
139. Demling RH, Kramer G, Harms B: Role of thermal injury-induced hypoproteinemia on fluid flux and protein permeability in burned and nonburned tissue. *Surgery* 95:136, 1984.
140. Mizus I, Summer WR, Gurtner GH: Isoproterenol or aminophylline attenuate pulmonary edema after acid lung injury. *Am Rev Respir Dis* 131:256, 259, 1985.
141. Berthiaume Y, Staub NC, Matthay MA: Beta-adrenergic agonists increase lung liquid clearance in anesthetized sheep. *J Clin Invest* 79:335, 1987.
142. Wright PW, Bernard GR: Increased airway resistance contributes to impaired lung mechanics in the adult respiratory distress syndrome. *Am Rev Respir Dis* 137(4):137, 1988.
143. Wright PW, Bernard GR: Effects of metaproterenol, atropine and ibuprofen on lung function during the late phase of endotoxemia in sheep. *Am Rev Respir Dis* 137(4):179, 1988.
144. Southorn PA, Powis G, Phil D: Free radicals in medicine: II. Involvement in human disease. *Mayo Clin Proc* 63:390, 1988.
145. Bernard GR, Lucht WD, Niedermeyer ML, et al: Effect of N-acetylcysteine on the pulmonary response to endotoxin in the awake sheep and upon in vitro granulocyte function. *J Clin Invest* 73(6):1772, 1984.
146. Lucht WD, English DK, Bernard GR, et al: Prevention of release of granulocyte aggregates into sheep lung lymph following endotoxemia by *n*-acetylcysteine. *Am J Med Sci* 294:161, 1987.
147. Bernard GR, Brigham KL: Pulmonary edema: Patho-

physiologic mechanisms and new approaches to therapy. *Chest* 89(4):594, 1986.
148. Lee CT, Fein AM, Lippmann M, et al: Elastolytic activity in pulmonary lavage fluid from patients with adult respiratory-distress syndrome. *N Engl J Med* 304(4):192, 1981.
149. Haagsman HP, van Golde LMG: Lung surfactant and pulmonary toxicology. *Lung* 163:275, 1985.
150. Avery ME, Taeusch HW, Floros J: Surfactant replacement. *N Engl J Med* 315(13):825, 1986.
151. Horbar JD, Soll RF, Sutherland JM, et al: A multicenter randomized, placebo-controlled trial of surfactant therapy for respiratory distress syndrome. *N Engl J Med* 320:959, 1989.
152. Melot C, Lejeune P, Leeman M, et al: Prostaglandin E_1 in the adult respiratory distress syndrome. *Am Rev Respir Dis* 139:106, 1989.
153. Holcroft JW, Vassar MJ, Weber CJ: Prostaglandin E_1 and survival in patients with the adult respiratory distress syndrome. *Ann Surg* 203:371, 1986.
154. Mandell GL: ARDS, neutrophils, and pentoxifylline. *Am Rev Respir Dis* 138:1103, 1988.
155. Welsh CH, Lien D, Worthen GS, Weil JV: Pentoxifylline decreases endotoxin-induced pulmonary neutrophil sequestration and extravascular protein accumulation in the dog. *Am Rev Respir Dis* 138:1106, 1988.
156. Andreadis N, Petty TL: Adult respiratory distress syndrome: Problems and progress. *Am Rev Respir Dis* 132:1344, 1985.
157. Baumann WR, Jung RC, Koss M, et al: Incidence and mortality of adult respiratory distress syndrome: A prospective analysis from a large metropolitan hospital. *Crit Care Med* 14:1, 1986.
158. Fowler AA, Hamman RF, Zerbe GO, et al: Adult respiratory distress syndrome. *Am Rev Respir Dis* 132:472, 1985.
159. Montgomery AB, Stager MA, Carrico J, Hudson LD: Causes of mortality in patients with the adult respiratory distress syndrome. *Am Rev Respir Dis* 132:485, 1985.
160. Johanson Jr WG: Prevention of respiratory tract infection. *Am J Med* 69, 1984.
161. Elliott CG, Rasmussen BY, Crapo RO: Upper airway destruction following adult respiratory distress syndrome: An analysis of 30 survivors. *Chest* 94:526, 1988.
162. Ghio AJ, Elliott G, Crapo RO, et al: Impairment after adult respiratory distress syndrome: An evaluation based on American Thoracic Society recommendations. *Am Rev Respir Dis* 139:1158, 1989.
163. Bell RC, Coalson JJ, Smith JD, Johanson WG: Multiple organ system failure and infection in adult respiratory distress syndrome. *Ann Intern Med* 99(3):293, 1983.
164. Campbell GD, Coalson JJ, Johanson WG: The effect of bacterial superinfection on lung function after diffuse alveolar damage. *Am Rev Respir Dis* 129:974, 1984.
165. Seidenfeld JJ, Pohl DF, Bell RC, et al: Incidence, site, and outcome of infections in patients with the adult respiratory distress syndrome. *Am Rev Respir Dis* 134:12, 1986.
166. van Uffelen R, van Saene HKF, Fidler V, Lowenberg A: Oropharyngeal flora as a source of bacteria colonizing the lower airways in patients on artificial ventilation. *Intensive Care Med* 10:233, 1984.
167. Stoutenbeek CP, van Saene HKF, Miranda DR, Zandstra DF: The effect of selective decontamination of the digestive tract on colonization and infection rate in multiple trauma patients. *Intensive Care Med* 10:185, 1984.
168. ARDS: A clinical view, editorial. *Lancet* 2:439, 1986.
169. Johanson Jr WG, Seidenfeld JJ, de Los Santos R, et al: Prevention of nosocomial pneumonia using topical and parenteral antimicrobial agents. *Am Rev Respir Dis* 137:265, 1988.
170. Nelson S, Chidiac C, Summer WR: New strategies for preventing nosocomial pneumonia. Which common interventions leave patients at increased risk? *J Crit Illness* 3(4):12, 1988.
171. Torres A, de La Bellacasa JP, Rodriguez-Roisin R, et al: Diagnostic value of telescoping plugged catheters in mechanically ventilated patients with bacterial pneumonia using the metras catheter. *Am Rev Respir Dis* 138:117, 1988.
172. Fagon JY, Chastre J, Hance AJ, et al: Detection of nosocomial lung infection in ventilated patients: Use of a protected specimen brush and quantitative culture techniques in 147 patients. *Am Rev Respir Dis* 138:110, 1988.
173. Johanson Jr WG, Seidenfeld JJ, Gomez P, et al: Bacteriologic diagnosis of nosocomial pneumonia following prolonged mechanical ventilation. *Am Rev Respir Dis* 137:259, 1988.
174. Klastersky J, Thys JP: Endotracheal administration of aminoglycosides. *Kidney Dis* 511, 1982.
175. Prewitt RM: Pathophysiology and treatment of pulmonary hypertension in acute respiratory failure. *J Crit Care* 2(3):206, 1987.
176. Spragg RG, Cochrane CG: Human neutrophil elastase and acute lung injury. *Lung Biol Health Dis* 24:379, 1985.
177. Zwillich CW, Pierson DJ, Creagh CE, et al: Complications of assisted ventilation—a prospective study of 354 consecutive episodes. *Am J Med* 57:161, 1974.
178. Powner DJ: Pulmonary barotrauma in the intensive care unit. *J Intensive Care Med* 3:224, 1988.
179. Suter PM, Fairley HB, Isenberg MD: Effect of tidal volume and positive end-expiratory pressure on compliance during mechanical ventilation. *Chest* 2:158, 1978.
180. Ralph DD, Robertson HT, Weaver LJ, et al: Distribution of ventilation and perfusion during positive end-expiratory pressure in the adult respiratory distress syndrome. *Am Rev Respir Dis* 131:54, 1985.
181. Qvist J, Pontoppidan H, Wilson RS, et al: Hemodynamic responses to mechanical ventilation with PEEP: The effect of hypervolemia. *Anesthesiology* 42:45, 1975.
182. Jones WG, Madden M, Finkelstein J, et al: Tracheostomies in burn patients. *Ann Surg* 209:471, 1989.
183. Colice GL, Munster AM, Haponik EF: Tracheal stenosis complicating cutaneous burns: An underestimated problem. *Am Rev Respir Dis* 134:1315, 1986.
184. Rinaldo JE, Rogers RM: Adult respiratory distress syn-

drome: Changing concepts of lung injury and repair. *N Engl J Med* 306:900, 1982.
185. Matuschak GM, Rinaldo JE, Pinsky MR, et al: Effect of end-stage liver failure on the incidence and resolution of the adult respiratory distress syndrome. *J Crit Care* 2(3):162, 1987.
186. Marshall WG, Dimick AR: The natural history of major burns with multiple subsystem failure. *J Trauma* 23:102, 1983.
187. DeCamp MM, Demling RH: Posttraumatic multisystem organ failure. *JAMA* 260:530, 1988.
188. Zuckerman L, Caprini JA, Lipp V, Vagher JP: Disseminated intravascular multiple system activation (DIMSA) following thermal injury. *J Trauma* 18:432, 1978.
189. Aikawa, Shinozawa Y, Ishibiki K, et al: Clinical analysis of multiple organ failure in burned patients. *Burns* 13:103, 1987.
190. Field BE, Rackow EC,Astiz ME, Weil MH: Original observations: Early systolic and diastolic dysfunction during sepsis in rats. *J Crit Care* 4(1):3, 1989.
191. Jardin F, Genevray B, Brun-Ney D, Bourdarias JP: Influence of lung and chest wall compliances on transmission of airway pressure to the pleural space in critically ill patients. *Chest* 88(5):653, 1985.
192. Eddy AC, Rice CL: The right ventricle: An emerging concern in the multiply injured patient, review. *J Crit Care* 4(1):58, 1989.
193. Raper R, Sibbald WJ, Driedger AA, Gerow K: Relative myocardial depression in normotensive sepsis. *J Crit Care* 4(1):9, 1989.
194. Parker MM, Suffredini AF, Natanson C, et al: Responses of left ventricular function in survivors and nonsurvivors of septic shock. *J Crit Care* 4(1):19, 1989.
195. Reilly JM, Cunnion RE, Burch-Whitmen C, et al: A circulating myocardial depressant substance is associated with cardiac dysfunction and peripheral hypoperfusion (lactic acidemia) in patients with septic shock. *Chest* 95:1072, 1989.
196. Cunnion RE, Parillo JE: Myocardial dysfunction in sepsis: Recent insights. *Chest* 95:941, 1989.
197. Martyn JAJ, Snider MT, Szyfelbein SK, et al: Right ventricular dysfunction in acute thermal injury. *Ann Surg* 191:330, 1980.
198. Wise RA, Robotham JL, Bromberger-Barnea B, Permutt S: Effect of PEEP on left ventricular function in right-heart-bypassed dogs. *J Appl Physiol* 51:541, 1981.
199. Dhainaut JF, Bricard C, Monsallier FJ, et al: Left ventricular contractility using isovolumic phase indices during PEEP in ARDS patients. *Crit Care Med* 10(10):631, 1982.
200. Robotham JL, Lixfeld W, Holland L, et al: The effects of PEEP on right and left ventricular performance. *Am Rev Respir Dis* 121:677, 1980.
201. Gill JB, Cairns JA: Prospective study of pulmonary artery balloon flotation catheter insertions. *J Intensive Care Med* 3:121, 1988.
202. Shuman RB, Schuster DP, Zuckerman GR: Prophylactic therapy for stress ulcer bleeding. A reappraisal. *Ann Intern Med* 106:562, 1987.
203. Craven DE, Kunches LM, Kilinsky V, et al: Risk factors for pneumonia and fatality in patients receiving continuous mechanical ventilation. *Am Rev Respir Dis* 133:792, 1986.
204. Driks MR, Craven DE, Celli BR, et al: Nosocomial pneumonia in intubated patients given sucralfate as compared with antacids or histamine type 2 blockers: The role of gastric colonization. *N Engl J Med* 317:1376, 1987.
205. Howard RL, Anderson RJ: Continuous arteriovenous hemofiltration and multiple organ failure, editorial. *J Crit Care* 3(3):161, 1988.
206. Burchiel KJ, Steege TD, Wyler AR: Intracranial pressure changes in brain-injured patients requiring positive end-expiratory pressure ventilation. *Neurosurgery* 8:443, 1981.

Chapter 6

Pulmonary Host Defenses in Burn Injury

Steve Nelson

Despite significant advances in the care of patients with burn injuries and the development of ever more powerful antibiotic therapies, infection continues to be the most frequent cause of morbidity and mortality in these patients.[1] In fact, pneumonia is the most frequent life-threatening infection encountered in burn patients.[2] The cause of this apparent increased susceptibility to infection is directly related to the underlying depression of both humoral and cellular host defenses following burn injury. Current therapeutic modalities, such as topical antibiotics and early excision and grafting of the burn wound, have decreased the mortality directly related to bacterial infections in thermally injured patients.[3] However, further progress in reducing burn mortality due to bacterial infection is dependent upon increasing our understanding of the basic mechanisms whereby burns depress host defenses against invading pathogens and developing new approaches to counteract these processes.

Infection is the clinical manifestation of multiple interactions involving immunologic defenses, metabolism, nutrition, and therapeutic interventions. In order to understand the sequence of pathophysiologic events that lead to the acquired immunodeficiency state of the burn-injured patient, it is first necessary to review how the lung maintains the sterility of the distal airways in the normal host. Bacterial challenges that enter the lower respiratory tract rarely cause pneumonia in healthy individuals. This is because the invading pathogens encounter a highly integrated system of defense mechanisms composed of both mechanical and immunologic components that are remarkably effective under normal circumstances.

NORMAL LUNG HOST DEFENSES

The lower respiratory tract is the largest epithelial surface exposed to the external environment. Inspired air contains not only oxygen but also particulates, noxious gases, and microorganisms. Additionally, the lungs are repeatedly inoculated with bacteria that are aspirated from the oropharynx. Essential components of the pulmonary host defense system are distributed throughout the respiratory tract from the point of air entry to the point of gas exchange (Table 6-1). There are five major defense mechanisms: aerodynamic filtration, airway reflexes that cause cough and bronchospasm, the mucociliary system, soluble factors in airway secretions, and phagocytic cells.[4,5]

The conducting airways of the lung extend from the nasopharynx to the respiratory bronchioles. The surfaces of conducting airways are lined with mucosa consisting of a specialized fluid layer, ciliated epithelial cells, a basement membrane, and a submucosa containing organized structures such as secretory glands and aggregates of plasma cells and lymphocytes. This ciliated epithelium is interspersed with goblet cells and orifices leading from the submucosal bronchial glands. Approximately 100 to 200 cilia per epithelial cell beat up to 1000 times each minute in a coordinated sequential, wavelike motion with a rapid action stroke directed toward the glottis and a slower oppositely directed recovery stroke. Mucus is produced by specialized cells in the respiratory epithelium and the submucosal glands. Mucus is composed of complex mucopolysaccharides that coalesce together and float on the aqueous fluid layer that bathes the ciliated epithelial cells. It has viscoelastic properties, stretching and contracting as it is moved up the airway surface by ciliary activity. The state of hydration of mucus and the ionic composition of respiratory secretions are important factors that govern the viscosity of mucus. Ciliary activity and the output of secretions by mucosal glands are under neurohumoral control. Because ciliated epithelium ends proximal to the terminal bronchioles, mucociliary clearance is of importance for particulates that are deposited in the airways but is responsible for little clearance of organisms from alveolar surfaces.[4] At the junction of the terminal and respiratory bronchioles, the mucosa abruptly changes to a delicate, single layer of flattened, nonciliated epithelial cells which line the gas exchange surfaces of the alveolar structures. This epithelial layer contains freely moving, detachable phagocytic cells and lymphocytes on the alveolar surface. Host defenses in the upper airways principally consist of mechanical barriers and the mucociliary clearance mechanism. Beyond the level of the respiratory bronchioles, phagocytes provide essential host defense capabilities.

Table 6-1 Lung Antibacterial Defense Mechanisms

Upper airway
Aerodynamic filtration
IgA
Lower respiratory tract
Aerodynamic filtration
Mucociliary escalator
Airways reflexes
IgG, IgA
Alveolar surface
Alveolar macrophages
IgG
Complement
Cytokines
Arachidonic acid metabolites
Surfactant
Alveolar lining fluid
Influx of neutrophils and phlogistic mediators
Initiation of immune responses

A majority of particles 10 μm or greater in diameter are either removed by filtration in the nose during inspiration or are deposited by inertial impaction on the surfaces of the upper airways. Those less than 10 but greater than 1.0 μm are deposited by sedimentation on the mucosal surfaces of the conducting airways. Inertial impaction occurs in large airways particularly at points of bifurcation, while sedimentation occurs in small conducting airways where air flow is low. Following their deposition on mucosal surfaces, particles are mechanically removed by cough or by their entrapment and cephalad transport via the mucociliary escalator. Vagally mediated airway reflexes that cause bronchoconstriction narrow airway caliber and limit the penetration of inhaled particles into the lung. Cough causes high shear forces along the airway epithelium, which forcefully ejects mucus from the lungs. In the sol layer of mucus, lysozymes and immunoglobulins bind, neutralize, and degrade particulates, preventing their penetration of the mucosa and thereby isolating them from the host.[6] Secretory antibodies, particularly immunoglobulin A (IgA), and glycoproteins present in the mucus layer provide essential host defenses in the larger airways. IgA is the predominant immunoglobulin in the nasopharynx and salivary secretions.[7] IgA is produced by plasma cells in the respiratory mucosa, then taken up by serous cells in mucosal glands, where it is linked to a protein that facilitates the transport of IgA and renders it less susceptible to proteolytic digestion by bacterial proteases. The primary function of IgA is to neutralize inhaled particles and toxins. It agglutinates large particle antigens, neutralizes bacterial toxins and some viruses, and reduces bacterial adherence to buccal and airway epithelial cells. This is an important effect because bacterial adherence to buccal and airway epithelial cells increases in critically ill patients, and this may be the first step in the pathogenesis of nosocomial pneumonia.[8] All of these nonspecific mechanisms of defense provide an effective physical barrier against inhaled particulates and serve to maintain the sterility of the respiratory tract. However, these physical barriers per se offer little resistance to invasion by virulent microorganisms deposited in the gas exchange regions of the lung. The cells lining the alveoli having been modified for efficient gas exchange and lack cilia. Particles or microbes of small dimensions (>0.5 μm and <1.0 μm in size) in inspired air elude the trapping mechanisms in the conducting airways and reach the alveolar surface.

Alveolar lining fluid contains a variety of substances with antimicrobial properties and plays an important role in host defense within alveolar air spaces.[9] These include surfactant and other glycoproteins (fibronectin), free fatty acids, lysozyme, transferrin, lactoferrin, and humoral immune factors. Surfactant and fragments of fibronectin can function as nonimmune opsonins. Complement, particularly C3b, can promote receptor-mediator attachment to a macrophage or, in the presence of antibody, augment receptor interaction and enhance bacterial binding. Transferrin interferes with bacterial cell growth. Lysozyme hydrolyzes bacterial cell wall mucopolysaccharides. Immunoglobulins with antibody specificity in alveolar lining material function as immune opsonins and serve to enhance phagocytosis. The concentrations of IgG increase distally in the conducting airways, so that IgG predominates in the gas exchange parenchyma.[5] IgG is abundant in alveolar fluid and can be produced locally within the lung by plasma cells as well as derived from the vascular space. IgG binds to alveolar macrophages and neutrophils to augment phagocytosis and also activates the complement cascade. Immunoglobulin G is the principal opsonic antibody in the alveolar fluid. Macrophages can ingest inanimate particles without prior opsonization, but they will not ingest many viable bacteria, particularly gram-negative species, without an opsonic coating. Clearly, a specific opsonin increases the effectiveness of phagocytosis significantly.

Alveolar macrophages (AM) are uniquely equipped for the efficient processing of particulates that reach the gas exchange units of the lung. The AM has classically been described as the primary defender of the lung against bacteria that reach the alveolar surface.[10] AM are the principal phagocyte on the air exchange surface of the lung. Bronchoalveolar lavage (BAL) in a normal nonsmoking subject yields approximately 10^7 cells of which 90 to 95 percent are AM. About 5 to 10 percent are lymphocytes, and less than 3 percent are neutrophils (PMN). It is important to realize that AM harvested by BAL may represent a subset of cells that is loosely adherent because of senescence or other local factors. To what extent the cells recovered by this technique are representative of the "actual" cell population within the alveoli is unclear. Studies looking at resident AM have demonstrated heterogeneity of morphological, cytochemical, and functional properties.

Traditionally, the macrophage has been viewed primarily as a phagocytic cell. However, macrophages are active secretory cells and can influence almost every aspect of the immune and inflammatory responses, from the first breach of the epithelium to its eventual repair.[11,12] Ingestion of inhaled microorganisms as well as inorganic particles by the AM clearly constitutes an important first line of host defense. This role has been confirmed in several in vivo animal investigations demonstrating that the resident AM population is capable of phagocytosing massive numbers of microorganisms and that other mechanisms of pulmonary defense, such as mucociliary clearance, are relatively less important.[10,13] In vitro studies utilizing human AM have demonstrated that these cells' phagocytic capacity following exposure to bacteria is greater than that of human neutrophils on a cell-for-cell basis.[14] Opsonization of microorganisms by immunoglobulin is the single most important factor in promoting their phagocytosis by AM.[10,13–15] During phagocytosis, the cell membrane of the AM invaginates to form a phagosome which fuses with intracellular lysosomes, creating a phagolysosome rich in acidic proteases, neutral proteases, and lysozyme that act to degrade the ingested particle. Phagocytosis by the AM is associated with a dramatic change in oxidative metabolism, usually referred to as the respiratory burst. Highly reactive oxygen radicals generated by the AM are utilized for intra- and extracellular killing of microbes.[16] While AM play a pivotal role in cleansing gas exchange surfaces of the lung parenchyma, the precise fate of these cells after having phagocytosed foreign materials is not absolutely clear. The majority of particle-laden phagocytes appear to be propelled by respiratory movements to the bronchoalveolar junction, where they gain access to the mucociliary escalator and are removed from the lung. Some AM may gain entry to the interstitial spaces, where they drain proximally via lymphatics to the lymph nodes.

The AM can also process and present antigen for the induction or augmentation of specific immune responses.[17] The soluble end products of B lymphocyte–mediated immunity are specific antibodies that serve to enhance phagocytosis, promote microbial killing, and neutralize toxins. Although opsonins will enhance phagocytic uptake by macrophages, additional factors are sometimes required to activate macrophages so that they can more effectively contain or kill microorganisms, particularly intracellular pathogens.[18] In their response to immunologic stimuli, macrophages and lymphocytes interact through a complex series of stimulatory and inhibitory signals. T-lymphocyte activation frequently requires the release of mediators by macrophages, and macrophage activation, as defined by bactericidal capacity, in turn depends on specific lymphokines. Lymphokines are polypeptide products of activated lymphocytes that participate in a variety of cellular responses, including the regulation of the immune system.[19] Following release from lymphocytes, these soluble mediators convert quiescent macrophages to efficient microbicidal phagocytes. Mediators from airway lymphocytes, such as interferon-γ, are important for this activation, which stimulates greater antimicrobial action and can also stimulate the macrophage to secrete a variety of other mediators, including cytokines, thus enhancing their immune effector power.

Inflammatory cytokines, including interleukin-1 (IL-1) and tumor necrosis factor-alpha (TNF), are produced by macrophages in response to numerous agents, including microorganisms, microbial products, lipopolysaccharide, complement, and lymphokines.[12,20,21] At the site of infection, the production of these inflammatory cytokines most likely benefits the host by promoting the microbicidal functions of both AM and PMN. These cytokines may also be produced within the vascular compartment in response to systemic stimuli, such as endotoxin, and exert profound effects ranging from phagocyte activation to tissue injury and shock. The excessive or unregulated production of cytokines, particularly TNF, likely contributes to the pathogenesis of septic shock.[22]

Macrophages are also a rich source of arachidonic acid metabolites known to be potent mediators of the inflammatory response.[23] These metabolites can be divided into two major groups: (1) products of the cyclooxygenase pathway, the prostaglandins, and (2) those of the lipoxygenase pathway, the leukotrienes and hydroxyeicosatetraenoic acids. The actions of these arachidonic acid products in the lung are extremely complex. Thromboxane, the predominant product of the cyclooxygenase pathway in human AM, has been proposed as a key mediator of microvascular injury in noncardiogenic pulmonary edema.[11] It can cause pulmonary vasoconstriction, neutrophil adherence, and platelet aggregation, all of which have been implicated in this syndrome. Leukotriene B_4, the major lipoxygenase pathway of human AM, is a chemotactic agent for neutrophils comparable in potency to the complement-derived peptide C5a.[24] As such it may play a major role in the recruitment of neutrophils to inflammatory foci in the lung in response to bacterial invasion.

The inflammatory response of the lung is an essential component of host defense that functions to remove microorganisms or particles that have reached the distal airways and alveolar surface. It augments the usual function of alveolar macrophages, immunoglobulins, and other defense mechanisms such as a mucociliary clearance. The mobilization of inflammatory cells and phlogistic factors from the intravascular compartment into the lung is critical for effective pulmonary host defense. Any factor which impairs PMN responsiveness will be predictably associated with infectious complications.

Once the macrophage has encountered a microbe and ingested it, the phagocyte may be able to kill it or contain it and the problem is resolved. Alternatively, conditions that favor proliferation of the microorganism, that is, large inoculum, virulence, or virgin exposure of the host, may require that the macrophage recruit additional phagocytic help. One mechanism for accomplishing this is the elaboration of chemotactic factors that attract PMN into the alveoli.[25] Expression of the antimicrobial function of the PMN is contingent upon the ability of these cells to leave the circulation and enter infected sites. PMN movement into the alveoli is an orderly reaction initiated from the alveolar side. Chemotactic factors from PMN may be released from either bacterial or host cells, or they may be generated enzymatically from components of plasma and bronchial secretions (Fig. 6-1). The net effect is a local increase in the alveolus of several factors that possess potent chemoattractant activity. Either maintenance of a large concentration gradient across the air-blood interface or diffusion of these factors into the vascular compartment could initiate an influx of inflammatory cells into the alveolus.

A small percentage of PMN is usually found among the respiratory cells retrieved by bronchoalveolar lavage from lungs of nonsmokers (about 1 percent). Because lavage may not recover all the PMN, the actual in situ number on the alveolar and peripheral airway surfaces is probably greater. Whereas few PMN are normally in the tissue of the lung or reside on the alveolar surfaces, a large number are located in the pulmonary vasculature as part of a transient and dynamic population that comprises the marginated pool. Approximately 20 percent of the body's marginated supply of PMN is within the lung vasculature ready to be mobilized into a potential inflammatory site.[26] A complex series of steps enables the PMN to bind to the endothelium and move through the alveolar-capillary membrane into the airways. PMN adherence, a vital prelude to immigration into the alveoli, is an active process and is modulated by complement products, arachidonic acid metabolites, cytokines, and endothelial factors.

Components of the complement system have been identified in bronchoalveolar lavage fluid obtained from humans and may be centrally involved in lung host defenses.[4,25] The presence of an intact alternative pathway is an extremely useful resident defense mechanism because this pathway can be activated by many bacteria and/or bacterial products in the absence of specific antibody. Therefore, this pathway plays a critical role in preventing infection with bacteria for which prior humoral immunity does not exist. Within the lung, complement components may act as opsonins or as chemotaxins. Complement activation products can promote phagocytosis of certain bacteria by the alveolar macrophage in the presence of low IgG levels. A major chemoattractant of host origin is C5a, a polypeptide derived from the enzymatic cleavage of C5. C5 is known to be present in bronchial secretions.

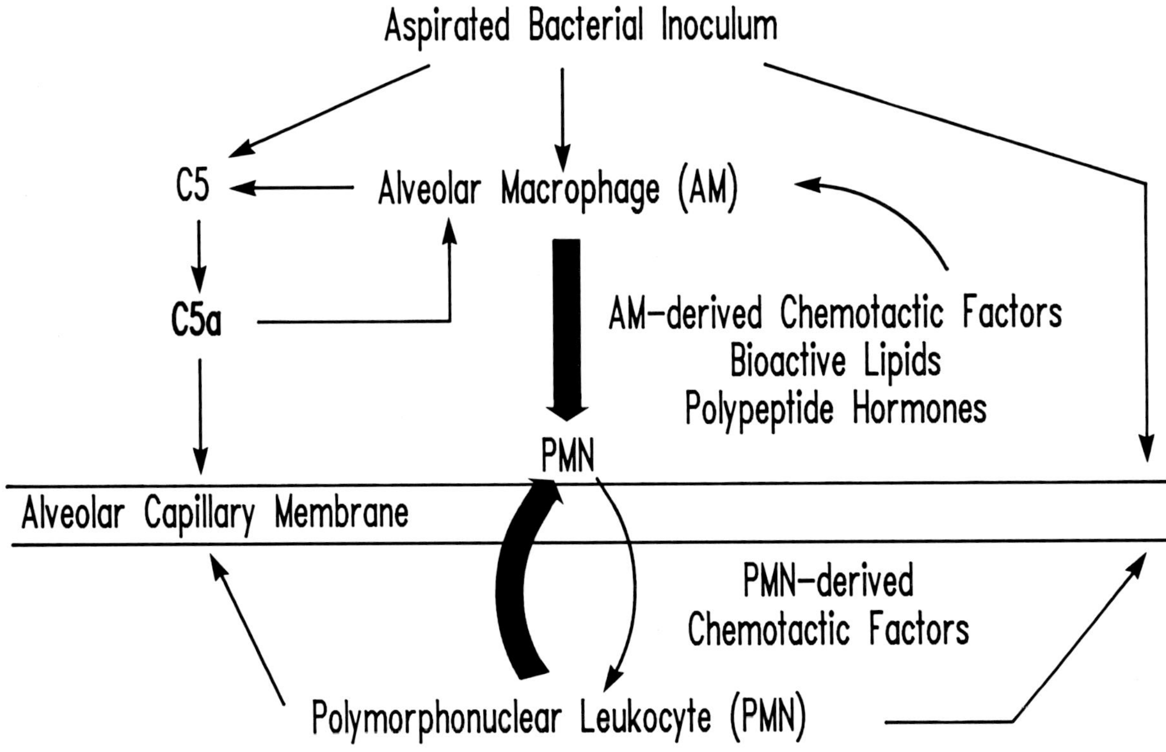

Figure 6-1 Potential pathways of initiating alveolar inflammation.

Among the substances secreted by the AM are a number of lysosomal enzymes able to activate C5 to generate C5a. Thus, the AM is an indirect source of the chemoattractant C5a.[25] Recent investigations also suggest that C5 may have a potential role in modulating the release of other inflammatory mediators by the AM including TNF and IL-1 in addition to its role as a primary chemoattractant.[27]

The AM-derived polypeptide hormones IL-1 and TNF are potent mediators of the inflammatory response.[20,21] IL-1 is a chemoattractant, and its release induced by TNF.[28] IL-1 is a highly inflammatory molecule and stimulates phagocyte functions.[21] TNF has also been demonstrated to have diverse effects on phagocyte functions. TNF activates PMN and enhances their phagocytic and bactericidal activities.[29] Recently, TNF has been demonstrated to directly stimulate PMN chemotaxis in vitro and in vivo.[30,31] These effects appear to be dose-dependent. Low concentrations markedly stimulate while higher levels inhibit chemotaxis.[32] This dual effect may be a potential mechanism for the initiation and subsequent localization of the inflammatory response. We have recently reported that TNF activity in BAL precedes the recruitment of PMN into the alveoli in response to an intrapulmonary challenge.[33] Furthermore, TNF activity following either intravenous or intratracheal lipopolysaccharide administration is confined to the challenged compartment and may be an essential factor in compartmentalizing and localizing the host's inflammatory response at a specific tissue site. Additionally, preliminary studies in our laboratory indicate that intrapulmonary instillation of TNF can augment the microbicidal activity of the lung against certain bacterial pathogens.

Chemotactic factors may also be derived from or secreted by PMN during the inflammatory response. PMN homogenates contain a heat-stable nondialyzable molecule that is chemotactic for PMN, and PMN releases chemotactic factors during phagocytosis.[4] Additionally, certain bacteria including *Streptococcus pneumoniae*, *Staphylococcus aureus*, and *Haemophilus influenzae* have all been shown to release chemotaxins during bacterial growth.[34]

Granulocytes and macrophages are secretory cells that are intimately involved in antibacterial defenses and the immune response. The resident phagocyte population of the uninfected lung is almost exclusively composed of alveolar macrophages. The stimulation of the AM by invading pathogens ignites a cascade of events that leads to the immigration of PMN from the vascular compartment into the alveoli to provide essential auxiliary phagocytic defenses. Clearly, this inflammatory response may be initiated by several different mechanisms. Different chemotaxins may be generated in sequence such that certain factors are involved in the initial response while others are essential only in the late phases. Certain mediators not only alter cellular components of the inflammatory reaction but also change membrane permeability, vascular responses, and bronchomotor tone. While the major components involved in the generation of the pulmonary inflammatory response to bacteria are beginning to be identified, little is known about how the secretion of these factors is controlled and coordinated. Furthermore, the means by which this response is regulated once it is activated in order to prevent inadvertent tissue injury are poorly understood. Clearly, excessive or chronic inflammation in the lung may create pathology leading to the adult respiratory distress syndrome and other inflammatory-mediated lung diseases.

In summary, removal of microorganisms that reach the mucosa of the naso-oropharynx and conducting airways is accomplished by mechanical mechanisms (mucociliary clearance, cough) and local secretion of IgA and other substances that contribute to the physical coating of the mucosa. At the level of the respiratory bronchioles where the airways change from serving as conduits for airflow to adapting for efficient air exchange, host defenses change. On the alveolar surface, the sterility of the lungs is maintained by the combined function of phagocytic cells which have significant immune effector activities and secretory functions. When pneumonia develops, some element of this normal defense apparatus has failed.

HOST DEFENSE ALTERATIONS IN BURN INJURY

Pneumonia results from aspiration of the oropharyngeal flora, inhalation of airborne pathogens, direct spread from a contiguous source, or hematogenous spread. In burn patients, prior to the utilization of topical chemotherapeutic agents and improved wound management techniques, the majority of pulmonary infections were secondary to hematogenous dissemination of the pathogen from the wound to the lungs.[3] At the present time, hematogenous pneumonia is relatively infrequent. This change in the predominant type of pneumonia reflects not only the decrease in burn wound infections but the improved early survival of patients with severe airway damage due to inhalational injury and the more frequent use of mechanical ventilatory support. Aspiration of the oropharyngeal flora in a susceptible patient is recognized as the predominant mechanism. Colonization of the oropharynx, followed by aspiration into the lungs of a burn patient whose normal antibacterial defenses have been impaired, represents the most common pattern in the development of pneumonia (Fig. 6-2).

Clearly, burn injury can alter pulmonary host defenses by at least four separate, specific mechanisms. Cutaneous thermal injury directly leads to a rapid depression of systemic host defenses. Second, systemic sepsis resulting from invasive infection of the burn wound can lead to pulmonary dysfunction and subsequent nosocomial pneumonia. This results from both alterations in components of the immune response induced by sepsis and the end-organ effects of sepsis on the lung. Third, in-

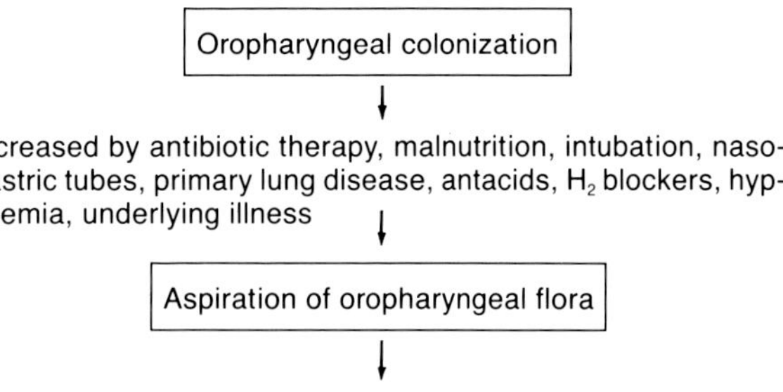

Increased with depressed consciousness, impaired gag or cough reflexes, nasogastric tubes, endotracheal tubes, hypnotics, narcotics, neuroleptics, tracheostomy

Pneumonia

Related to
1. Inoculum
2. Bacterial virulence factors
3. Impaired host defenses secondary to
   a. Cutaneous burn injury
   b. Inhalational injury
   c. Underlying illnesses
   d. Pharmacologic therapy and interventional procedures

Figure 6-2 Pattern in the development of pneumonia.

Table 6-2 Potential Pathways of Impairing Lung Host Defenses in Burn-Injured Patients

Depression of antibacterial defenses by remote cutaneous burns
Systemic sepsis-induced suppression of lung host defenses
Inhalational injury
Nonspecific risk factors in critically ill patients

halation injury can directly impair lung host defenses and result in serious pulmonary compromise and pneumonia. In any individual patient, all of these pathways may be involved and place the patient at an extreme risk for fatal pneumonia. Finally, burn patients are subject to the same nosocomial risks for pneumonia as other critically ill patients such as colonization, poor nutritional status, intubation, pharmacologic therapy, and other underlying medical illnesses (chronic obstructive pulmonary disease, diabetes, alcoholism) (Table 6-2).

Burn injury not only causes skin damage and tissue necrosis but also exerts deleterious effects on every organ system, including those involved in the response to and defense against microbial invasion. In addition to disrupting the mechanical barrier of the skin, an extensive burn injury affects the function of all other components of the immune system.[1] The susceptibility to infection increases in a sigmoid dose-dependent fashion as the extent of the burn increases.[35] The severity and duration of altered organ function are similarly related to burn size, and this induced dysfunction of the host defense system predisposes the burn patient to septic complications.[36]

The burn wound is frequently the site of initial bacterial colonization of the patient, which may progress to invasion with systemic dissemination.[37] Both local wound factors and microbial factors influence the rate of proliferation, and the balance between host defense capacity and the invasive capabilities of the bacterial population of the wound determines whether invasive infection will occur. The denatured protein of the burn eschar serves as an excellent culture medium to support the growth and proliferation of the colonizing microorganisms, and the avascularity of the burned tissue limits the delivery of both endogenous and exogenous antibacterial agents to the site of microbial proliferation.[38]

The microorganisms present within the wounds of these patients change with time. Gram-positive organisms are initially prevalent but are gradually superseded by the gram-negative opportunists that appear to have a greater propensity to invade.[35] These pathogens frequently possess certain virulence factors which promote the invasion of underlying viable tissue. These include lipopolysaccharide, exotoxin A, proteases, and elastases. If bacterial growth reaches a level of 10^5 organisms per gram of tissue, invasion with bloodstream dissemination is likely.[3] This syndrome is termed "burn wound sepsis." Topical antimicrobial agents do not sterilize the burn wound but maintain the microbial density below 10^5 organisms per gram of tissue, a level which even the immunocompromised burned host can reasonably defend.[39] The advent of topical antimicrobial therapy, the development of more effective topical and systemic antibiotics, and early excision and grafting of the burn wound have dramatically decreased the frequency of pneumonia in burn patients resulting from direct hematogenous dissemination from the wound to the lungs.[38] However, systemic infection continues to be frequently associated with the subsequent development of nosocomial pneumonia. Extrapulmonary sepsis induces several significant effects on pulmonary host defenses that may contribute to the development of subsequent bacterial pneumonias in susceptible patients. Studies by our laboratory have shown that sepsis impairs AM bactericidal capacity, causes neutrophil sequestration in the pulmonary vascular bed, and inhibits PMN recruitment into the lung in response to bacterial challenge.[40,41] Clearly, the inability of the host to initiate an effective intrapulmonary inflammatory response during systemic sepsis markedly suppresses the antibacterial defenses of the lung. These defects in essential host defense mechanisms provide a potential mechanism for the clinical association of burn injury, sepsis, and pneumonia.

Recently, it has been determined that the bacteria colonizing the gastrointestinal tract penetrate the epithelial mucosa of the bowel and spread to visceral organs following a moderate thermal injury.[42–44] This process is termed bacterial translocation. Therefore, not only may the burn wound serve as a focus of sepsis in these patients but the patient's own gastrointestinal tract microflora may be a reservoir for nosocomial infections and a primary source of sepsis following burn injury.

Further progress in reducing burn mortality due to the bacterial infection is dependent upon understanding the fundamental processes whereby burns depress host defense mechanisms against infection. Depressed immunity occurs in patients with severe traumatic injuries and in those who have sustained major surgical procedures.[45] In these patients, immunologic changes are dramatic and leave the host susceptible to life-threatening infections. The immunologic changes that occur secondary to thermal injuries share a common pathway with the immune consequences of other types of tissue injury. Evidence indicates that burn injuries often precipitate a profound multicentric depression of host defenses that predisposes these patients to systemic infection.[1] Impairment of immune function is almost certain in patients with greater than 40 percent total body surface area burns. Clearly, patients with significant underlying disease or those at the extremes of life are more susceptible than an otherwise normal host. These alterations in the immune system are listed in Table 6-3. This hyporesponsiveness of the immune system following an acute burn injury may, under most conditions, serve to protect the host. Clearly, it would not be advantageous to the host to either nonspecifically or continually activate the inflammatory cascade, as this may inadvertently injure the host. Furthermore, this mechanism may serve to localize the inflammatory response at a specific site or within a selective compartment. However, this adaptive mechanism may render the burn-injured patient vulnerable to subsequent infection at an adjacent or distant site, such as the lung or abdomen.

Table 6-3 Effects of Burn Injury on Host Defenses

Depression of cell-mediated immunity
Activation (and subsequent depletion) of the complement system
Suppression of phagocyte (macrophage, neutrophil) functions
Release of immunosuppressive mediators
Increased consumption of immunoglobulin
Depletion of fibronectin and serum opsonic activity
Increased T-suppressor cell activity

The complement system is essential for normal host defense.[4] A number of investigators have noted hypocomplementemia after burn injury both in animals and in humans.[1,46,47] There are two major pathways of complement activation. The classical complement pathway is activated by the interaction of antigen with IgG or IgM antibody and thus usually requires a specific immunologic response. The alternative complement pathway may be initiated by the polysaccharide moiety of bacterial endotoxin or by thermally damaged cells or serum proteins. Activation products of the complement system directly contribute to inflammatory responses and to host defenses against invasion by pathogenic organisms.

In an animal model utilizing a 25 percent body surface area, full-thickness scald wound, massive activation of the alternative complement pathway, but not the classic pathway, was seen.[48] The observed depletion of the alternative pathway was primarily due to activation and not simple protein loss. Furthermore, in human burn patients with 30 to 90 percent full-thickness burns, complement levels on admission demonstrated that alternative pathway hemolytic activity was significantly more depleted than classic pathway activity.[49] It is of interest that in all patients with depleted activity of the alternative pathway, bacteremia, pneumonia, or the adult respiratory distress syndrome developed.

These data suggest that burn injury results in massive complement activation, primarily by the alternative pathway. The resultant alternative pathway deficiency may contribute to impaired host defense against bacterial pathogens for which the patient has no preformed antibody. Furthermore, the fact that the classical pathway is largely intact suggests that passive or active immunization may be useful in burn patients by recruiting classic pathway opsonic, chemotactic, and bactericidal activities.

The massive, unregulated complement activation that follows burn injury most likely directly contributes to burn morbidity and mortality. In animal studies, complement depletion prior to burn injury reduces early mortality from 65 to 10 percent.[50] Massive activation of the complement system has been implicated as a contributing factor in septic shock and in the development of injury involving the lung and bowel.[51] The sequestration of neutrophils within the vasculature of affected organs together with activation of their microbicidal activities may very well be central to the pathogenesis of tissue injury and multiple organ failure in burn and septic patients.[52–54] Furthermore, the observed defects in phagocyte function following burn injury may be a consequence of their prior in vivo exposure to stimuli that are abnormal in magnitude, creating systemic rather than localized activation. Initial activation may render the phagocytes refractory to further stimulation, resulting in an impaired capacity to respond to a second, localized infected site, such as the lung (Fig. 6-3).

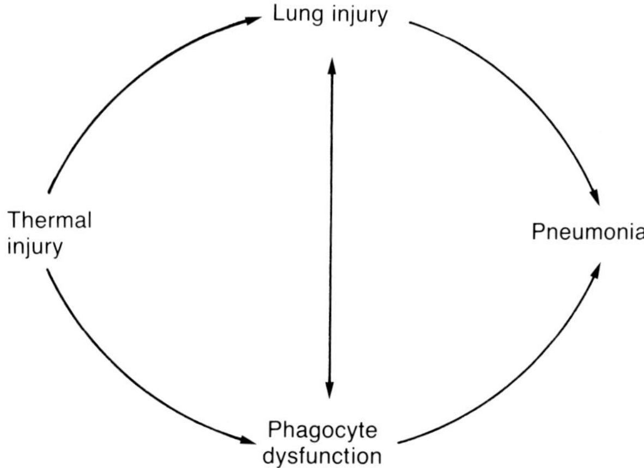

Figure 6-3 Schematic diagram illustrating the interactions of thermal injury, phagocyte dysfunction, and the development of lung injury and/or pneumonia.

The acute post burn period is marked by a suppression of macrophage and lymphocyte function and vigorous suppressor T-cell activity.[1,45] The prolonged survival of skin cell grafts used to cover major thermal injuries is secondary to these alterations in cellular immunity. Graft survival appears to be proportional to the size of the burn and correlates with the altered responsiveness of the lymphocytes.[55] A further indication of suppressed T-lymphocyte function is that patients with a burn size of 20 percent or greater typically fail to respond with delayed cutaneous hypersensitivity following skin testing with certain antigens.[56] In these burn patients the in vitro production of lymphokines by their peripheral blood lymphocytes is also significantly depressed.[52,57] These mediators are important activators of the host defense system. This decrease in lymphokine activity is strongly correlated with a depressed bactericidal activity of phagocytic cells in burned patients. The abnormal function of these lymphocytes from burn patients precedes clinical evidence of sepsis and indicates that depressed cell-mediated immunity significantly increases the threat of sepsis.[58,59] Suppressor T lymphocytes appear to play a major role in the depression of cell-mediated immunity following thermal injury. Although the number of circulating T cells is decreased in burn patients regardless of the extent of the burn, the absolute number of suppressor T cells is increased in patients with burns exceeding 25 percent of total body surface area.[60] Even normal T lymphocytes can become nonspecific suppressor T lymphocytes when they are incubated in the presence of serum from thermally injured patients.

There is increasing evidence to indicate that immunosuppressive substances are present in the sera of patients with burn injuries (Table 6-4).[1,45,61–63] The activity of these factors is directly related to the severity of burn injury and persist for extended periods of time. The identification of these suppressors is a major area of burn research.[64] Potential candidates include endotoxin, arachidonic acid metabolites, neuropeptides, cytokines, and endogenous glucocorticoids. Iatrogenic immune suppression may also result from topical agents, drugs, antibiotics, blood products, anesthesia, and fluid resuscitation. To the extent that any of these immunoregulatory factors, either singly or in combination, contribute to the immunologic depression observed in burn-injured patients, the hope remains that selective intervention may be a potential therapeutic approach.

As previously noted opsonins are factors that stimulate phagocytosis and render bacteria more susceptible to phagocytic uptake by neutrophils and macrophages. The most important opsonins are specific immunoglobulins, complement, and opsonic fibronectin. A transient depression in B-lymphocyte cell populations and immunoglobulin production has been described in thermally injured patients.[1] However, recent evidence indicates that an increase in the clearance or catabolism of serum antibody may be one mechanism for depressed serum levels and that, in fact, synthesis is normal or even elevated in postburn injury.[65] Kinetic studies of administered human IgG to burned patients have shown a decreased serum half-life. Serum from burn patients has been shown in vitro to be defective in its ability to promote the opsonization of bacteria. Opsonization is improved by adding exogenous IgG to the assay suggesting that the phagocytic depression is secondary to an acquired opsonic deficiency. However, while intravenous infusion of gamma globulin can restore circulating levels of IgG to normal in the postburn period, there are no convincing data to indicate that it reduces the subsequent occurrence of infection.[66]

The polymorphonuclear leukocyte is the major component of the body's defense against acute infections. In humans, the turnover time of the whole granulocyte system in the bone marrow, from the first precursor cell to the mature granulocyte that leaves the circulation, is approximately 10 days.[67] Average PMN production is 1.6×10^9 cells per kilogram body weight per day. In addition, the marrow reserve pool contains 8.8×10^9 cells per kilogram body weight which can be rapidly mobilized in response to an acute infection. After completion of maturation, the PMN enter the circulation. In the circulation, the PMN equilibrate with the marginated pool. The cells then migrate into tissue sites or are removed by the reticuloendothelial system. The migration of PMN into tissue sites is an end-stage activity, there is no return to the vascular compartment. The mature neutrophil is highly specialized to respond to microbial invasion by means of chemotaxis, phagocytosis, intracellular killing, digestion, and extracellular release of leukocytic products in-

Table 6-4 Potential Immunosuppressive Mediators following Thermal Injury

Bacterial endotoxin
Prostaglandins (PGE_2)
Endogenous glucocorticoids
Cytokines (tumor necrosis factor, interleukins, interferon)
Histamine
Immune complexes
Neuropeptides
Autoantibodies
Suppressor peptides
Iatrogenic factors

cluding lysosomal enzymes, oxygen free radicals, and potent mediators of inflammation.

Leukocytosis is a common initial finding occurring within a few hours after a burn is sustained.[68] The white blood cell count usually then falls on the fourth postburn day. This early leukocytosis occurs largely as a result of a shifting of the marginal granulocyte pool in the vessels to the free circulating pool and a release of granulocytes from the bone marrow to the blood circulation. The subsequent rapid fall in the blood white blood cell count reflects invasion of tissue sites by the PMN where they may play a major role in burn pathophysiology (such as adult respiratory distress syndrome — ARDS) as well as exhaustion of the granulocyte reserve. In experimental burns, indium-labeled PMN have been shown to localize in burn areas and other organs and become trapped in capillaries and venules, causing obstruction.[69] They cause poor perfusion and increase microvascular permeability. They release their enzyme content and oxygen free radicals into the local environment and clearly contribute to the autodestructive consequences of thermal injury.[70]

Suppression of granulocyte production in infected burns was first reported several decades ago. Later it was demonstrated that there is a strong depression of DNA synthesis in the bone marrow cells during the first few hours after an uncomplicated burn injury.[71] Since the turnover time in humans of the whole granulocyte system is 10 days, the massive outflow of mature granulocytes from the marrow with simultaneous inhibition in production leads to an exhaustion of the granulocyte system before the first week post injury, when the patient typically develops his or her initial septic episode. The mechanisms of postburn marrow failure are not clear. It is likely that the pathophysiology of postburn marrow failure is multifactorial in etiology and reflects the combined actions of numerous other physiologic and immunologic factors. In a model of *Pseudomonas* burn wound sepsis, administration of recombinant human granulocyte colony-stimulating factor (G-CSF), which stimulates the growth of granulocyte precursors and activates mature neutrophils, has been shown to augment the myelopoietic response and improve survival.[72] In our laboratory, administration of murine recombinant G-CSF markedly enhances pulmonary bactericidal activity and PMN recruitment in an animal model of *Pseudomonas aeruginosa* pneumonia. This agent may increase the immunological reserve of the burned patient and decrease septic morbidity and mortality.

The roles of granulocytes in burn pathology are multiple. An initial leukocytosis contributes to the autodestruction of tissues and subsequent inhibition in production causes exhaustion of the bone marrow and heightened susceptibility to overwhelming infection. In addition to the abnormalities in granulocyte kinetics in burn-injured patients, there are numerous reports demonstrating that PMN from severely burned patients exhibit reduced chemotactic responses, compromised phagocytosis, and decreased intracellular microbicidal capacity.

Decreases in chemotactic response of PMN from thermally injured patients have been repeatedly observed.[1] One of the vital host defense functions adversely affected by thermal injury is the ability of circulating leukocytic phagocytes to emigrate to extravascular sites of infection such as the lung. Leukocyte chemotactic dysfunction ex vivo is a consistent laboratory observation for patients with major degrees of burn injury and is associated with a high frequency of bacterial sepsis and death.[73]

Evidence for a generalized loss of PMN chemotactic function in burn patients has been demonstrated by the inability of their neutrophils to respond to multiple attractants including zymosan-activated serum, the *N*-formyl tripeptide FMLP, and casein. Recent investigations indicate that loss of chemotaxis in response to C5a is the result of down-regulation of receptors for the C5a and of reduced motility.[74] In contrast, the loss of chemotaxis to the tripeptide FMLP is the result of reduced motility alone. Specific deactivation results from selective loss of surface receptors for a chemoattractant, a phenomenon known as desensitization. Stimulated random motility (chemokinesis) is a component of any chemotactic response and a reduced motility alone would limit chemotactic responses nonspecifically to several factors. Nonspecific deactivation could be related to the initial excessive stimulation of the respiratory or secretory functions of the cell, or both. Stimulated respiration results in production of reactive products of oxygen metabolism which may chemically modify cellular components required for cell motility — a process termed "auto-oxidation."[75] Considering the evidence for activation of the complement cascade after thermal injury, complement components are likely candidates in effecting PMN down-regulation. Other agents with the potential to effect nonspecific deactivation include a number of cytokines and arachidonic acid metabolites, which are known to influence the function and responses of the neutrophil. These data suggest that the initial global activation of neutrophils occurring after burn injury may leave neutrophils refractory to a subsequent inflammatory stimulus, such as a localized site of infection, and thereby increase host susceptibility. Further investigations clarifying the factors involved in inducing this hyporesponsiveness of the host may offer new and innovative approaches to the therapy of the immunosuppressive state that characterizes the burn-injured patient.

Neutrophil adherence is a critical early component of bacterial host defense. Diminished neutrophil adhesiveness may contribute, in part, to the poor localization of infection and increased risk of sepsis after thermal injury in humans. Initially there is an up-regulation of receptors mediating adherence of the PMN in burn patients.[76] Mobilization of a large number of receptors or circulating neutrophils may render the cells hyperadherent and lead to sequestration and tissue injury. Furthermore, plasma from burn patients significantly increases the attachment of unstimulated PMN compared with plasma from normal controls. This hyperadhesive effect of plasma is transient and does not appear to last beyond the first day of injury.[77] The identity of the adhesive augmenting factor or factors in plasma from burn patients is unknown, but activated complement components and certain cytokines, such as TNF and IL-1, appear to be likely candidates.

This initial period of augmented PMN adhesiveness is followed by a period of hypoadherence of the neutrophil. Within 24 hours of injury, neutrophils from burn patients demonstrate a marked reduction in adherence, and this defect appears to last as long as 2 weeks after the burn injury is sustained.[77] This impairment of neutrophil adhesion is not stimulus specific. Several investigators have documented a decrease in the quantity of circulating plasma fibronectin soon after thermal injury and have noted that the onset of sepsis in burn patients is heralded by a precipitous decline in plasma fibronectin.[78,79] Fibronectin is a glycoprotein that has been implicated in the adhesive interactions of neutrophils with various substrates during inflammation. However, exogenous plasma fibronectin failed to improve the defect in adherence of neutrophils from burn patients.[77] These results may reflect an inability of exogenous plasma fibronectin to affect the intracellular or membrane concentrations. Cellular fibronectin possesses 100 times the agglutinating activity of plasma fibronectin and is more active in promoting adhesion. Recent data indicate that neutrophil fibronectin is significantly reduced within 24 hours of thermal injury.[77] Restoring cellular fibronectin concentrations may be a therapeutic approach to restoring neutrophil adherence after thermal injury.

Neutrophil phagocytosis of gram-negative and gram-positive bacteria has been demonstrated to be impaired in severely burned patients. Certain data suggest the presence of a direct inhibitor of phagocytosis in the sera of these patients.[1] Suppression of the bactericidal activity of neutrophils isolated from burn patients or experimental animals against *S. aureus* and *P. aeruginosa* has also been reported by several investigators.[1,80] Decreases in the oxidative metabolism of neutrophils have been demonstrated in thermally injured patients. This suppression of the bactericidal capacity of the PMN has been reported to occur as early as 24 hours post-burn injury and remain significantly reduced at least 9 days post-burn.[81] Recently it has been proposed that prostaglandins of the E series may be involved in the pathogenesis of the immunosuppressive effects of thermal injury. PGE_1 and PGE_2 have been shown to inhibit various functions of PMN, including aggregation, chemotaxis, superoxide production, and lysosomal enzyme release. These mediators are primary products of arachidonic acid metabolism via the cyclooxygenase pathway. In a recent investigation, therapy with nonsteroidal anti-inflammatory drugs to inhibit production of these compounds by the cyclooxygenase pathway initiated 3 hours postburn injury fully restored the bactericidal activity of neutrophils from thermally injured animals.[82] Other studies have demonstrated beneficial effects of these blockers on cell-mediated immune responses in thermally injured animals.[83,84] These data suggest that the use of these agents as adjuncts to standard therapy may be of therapeutic benefit in treating thermally injured humans.[88]

Perhaps the most common cause of postburn death is pneumonia secondary to an acquired immunodeficiency state induced by thermal injury. As the alveolar macrophage is the primary resident defender of the lung against microbial invasion, one would speculate that this phagocyte would be profoundly affected by burn injury. However, limited investigations to date have demonstrated that the in vitro microbicidal activity of the AM is not inhibited by a 30 percent total body surface area, full-thickness scald burn. In contrast, both phagocytosis and chemotaxis of AM were markedly impaired under these experimental conditions. These studies suggest that the altered pulmonary host resistance after thermal injury may not be due to an impaired macrophage microbicidal function but instead to a phagocytic defect.[85–87] Further in vivo studies in experimental models and in AM obtained by lavage from burn patients are needed to clarify the effects of thermal injury on alveolar macrophage function. It is important to note that systemic sepsis does in itself lead to a suppression of lung host defenses. Therefore, impairment of pulmonary antibacterial defense may be the sequelae of a septic event in a burn-injured patient rather than a direct result of the burn injury itself.

As noted thermal injury profoundly depresses the defense mechanisms of the body that under normal conditions protect the host against microbial infection. In addition, body surface burns can cause damage to lung vascular endothelium and/or alveolar epithelial lining cells, resulting in ARDS. The pathogenesis of lung injury subsequent to remote skin burns is the subject of another contributing author. However, it is important to note that ARDS is a major risk factor for the subsequent development of pneumonia. Pneumonia is one of the most common secondary infections in these patients and is associated with the poorest survival rate. The prognosis of infected patients with ARDS is poor, as compared with that of uninfected persons, with currently employed treatment modalities. In a recent report, the mortality of patients with ARDS and nosocomial infections was not affected by antibiotic administration, indicating that host defense and underlying disease factors may be critical determinants of susceptibility and survival in these patients.[88]

HOST DEFENSE ALTERATIONS IN INHALATIONAL INJURY

Inhalation injury was not well described prior to the Cocoanut Grove fire, in Boston in 1942. Presently, respiratory complications have emerged as the dominant killer of individuals with major thermal injury.[89] The presence or absence of inhalation injury may be a stronger determinant of mortality than the size of burn injury. With increasing burn size, there is a corresponding rise in the incidence of inhalation injury. In one recent study, inhalation injury affected mortality more prominently than the surface area of the burn.[90] The incidence of inhalation injury is approximately 33 percent of all thermally injured patients admitted to burn units. The presence of inhalation injury in a burn patient has been estimated to increase mortality by 30 to 40 percent.

The clinical course of patients with severe inhalation injury typically proceeds through three stages: acute pulmonary insufficiency, pulmonary edema, and finally bronchopneumonia in those patients who survive the initial injury.[91] Pulmonary infection is a leading cause of death in patients with smoke inhalation. Bronchopneumonia appears in 15 to 60 percent of these patients and has a reported mortality of 50 to 86 percent. In a recent report, 38 percent of patients diagnosed by bronchoscopy and/or ventilation perfusion lung scan with inhalation injury developed pneumonia. Among patients without evidence of inhalation injury in this study, only 8.8 percent developed pneumonia. In this investigation, inhalation injury alone increased mortality by 20 percent and pneumonia by 40 percent, with a maximum increase of approximately 60 percent when both were present. These data indicate that inhalation injury and pneumonia have significant, independent, additive effects on burn mortality.[92]

The most common type of inhalation injury from fires is chemical injury from toxic products of pyrolysis contained in smoke. Areas involved in inhalation injury may include the oropharynx, tracheobronchial tree, and/or parenchyma. Inhalation injury is primarily a chemical injury due to smoke poisoning and not a thermal injury. Inhalation of heated air usually results in burns that are confined to the face, oropharynx, and upper airway. Heat damage to the pulmonary parenchyma generally is prevented by laryngeal reflexes and efficiency of heat dissipation in the upper respiratory tract.[93]

Smoke is composed of gases and suspended particulate materials. These carbonaceous particles are not themselves damaging. However, they are often coated with aldehydes, ketones, and organic acids. Volatile gases, as well as those adsorbed on particles, may gain entry into the lower respiratory tract, and within minutes of exposure, cilia cease functioning, resulting in impaired mucus clearance. Bronchospasm frequently occurs, and the resultant airway obstruction combined with retained secretions further impairs effective pulmonary toilet, increasing susceptibility to pneumonia. Chemotactic substances and inflammatory mediators are released and neutrophils are recruited into the airways and parenchyma and most likely potentiate airway injury.[94] Bronchoscopic examination in the initial 24 hours shows edematous tracheobronchial mucosa and/or shedding of the mucosa with almost complete de-epithelialization. Smoke inhalation may produce a large spectrum of upper and lower airway injury, ranging from congestion and edema to a complete necrosis and shedding of the respiratory epithelium. This epithelium begins to regenerate within 24 hours of injury and is usually complete by 7 days. The damaged epithelium forms pseudomembranous casts, causing a complete or partial obstruction of the airway, resulting in patchy areas of atelectasis. Studies have demonstrated an immediate reduction in pulmonary surfactant after smoke inhalation.[95,96] This may also contribute to the early development of peripheral atelectasis in many fire victims. Chemical injury resulting from inhalation of toxic products of pyrolysis also may occur at the alveolar level, although it is less common than injury to the airways. Such injury involves damage to both the epithelial and endothelial membranes and can result in increased permeability and edema. It is clear that alveolar flooding may occur even when pulmonary capillary hydrostatic pressure is normal in these patients. With disruption of the alveolar capillary membrane, protein-rich plasma exudes into the tracheobronchial tree and may serve as a medium for bacterial growth. The high incidence of pneumonia in patients with inhalation injury most likely results from these pulmonary histopathologic changes combined with the global immunosuppression induced by the accompanying burn injury.

As previously noted, the alveolar macrophage is the principal phagocyte on the air-exchange surface of the lung. Efficient functioning of this cell is essential in the control of respiratory tract infection. Smoke inhalation has a depressive effect on pulmonary host defense mechanisms. Inhalation of complex mixtures of tobacco smoke and other gases (nitrogen dioxide, sulfur dioxide, and ozone) can enhance susceptibility to infection through functional alterations of pulmonary macrophages.[97–102] After exposure to these toxic substances, macrophages exhibit abnormalities of their surface membrane and develop reduced chemotaxis, decreased phagocytosis, and inhibition of their bactericidal activity. After smoke inhalation, impairments in the functional characteristics of mucociliary transport of the upper respiratory tract and of the alveolar macrophage impair

Table 6-5 Alterations Induced by Inhalation Injury on Lung Host Defense

Upper respiratory tract
Mucosal burns
Laryngeal obstruction
Lower respiratory tract
Tracheobronchitis
Paralysis of mucociliary escalator
Bronchorrhea
Mucosal sloughing
Bronchospasm
Airway edema
Atelectasis
Phagocyte dysfunction
Alveolitis
Decreased surfactant

lung defenses and increase susceptibility to infection (Table 6-5).

The antibacterial properties of pulmonary macrophages are adversely affected by exposure to wood pyrolysis.[103] The local response of the bronchoalveolar cell population after acute exposure to wood smoke has been recently reported in experimental animals. These macrophages have a diminished phagocytic potential, are less adherent, and have a marginal decrease in their bactericidal function when assessed by in vitro methods. Other investigations have demonstrated that exposure to both carbon particles and the toxic aldehyde of wood pyrolysis, acrolein, results in a PMN alveolitis that occurs several hours after exposure. Recent studies have demonstrated that smoke inhalation induces the release of chemotactic factors from alveolar macrophages, which in turn mediate an influx of neutrophils into the lung. The production and release of proteolytic enzymes and oxygen free radicals from these neutrophils may in all likelihood contribute to the severity of pulmonary complications following smoke inhalation.

As can be readily seen, the burn-injured patient is in all respects an immunocompromised host. The host defense system is markedly suppressed as a direct consequence of specific alterations induced by both the burn and inhalational injuries. Furthermore, the subsequent development of systemic sepsis further compromises the already precarious pulmonary antibacterial defense system. Finally, there are numerous other commonly employed therapeutic interventions and general risk factors that affect all critically ill patients that leave the burn-injured patient at increased risk for pneumonia.[104,105]

RISK FACTORS FOR NOSOCOMIAL PNEUMONIA

Although the lung is the third most frequent site of infection in hospitalized patients (15 percent of all cases), pneumonia is the most lethal infection and accounts for nearly 20 percent of all hospital deaths.[106,107] Colonization of the oropharynx, followed by aspiration into the lungs of a patient whose normal antibacterial defenses have been impaired, represents the most common pattern in the development of nosocomial pneumonia. Aspiration occurs in up to 70 percent of patients with depressed consciousness and is increased by a diminished or absent gag or cough reflex, and by the presence of endotracheal and nasogastric tubes.[108]

Available data show a predominant rate for gram-negative bacilli in nosocomial pneumonia.[109–112] The normal bacterial flora of the oropharynx of healthy individuals is stable, and gram-negative bacilli are rarely isolated. The prevalence of nasocarriage of these bacteria in normal subjects is approximately 2 percent, and it is experimentally difficult to induce colonization in healthy individuals.[113,114] It is now known that several factors may significantly alter the oropharyngeal flora in selected patients.[115] Risk factors for colonization include leukopenia, antibiotic therapy, hypoxemia, poor nutritional status, intubation, nasogastric tubes, and primary respiratory disease. Colonization remains relatively stable once established in an individual. As many as 90 percent of patients with gram-negative pneumonia have had previous oropharyngeal colonization by the same organism, and pneumonia develops five to eight times more frequently in these patients.[116] Approximately 50 percent of patients hospitalized in a critical care unit are eventually colonized with gram-negative bacteria, and a positive correlation exists between the duration of stay and subsequent colonization and pneumonia.

Many commonly used pharmacologic agents are capable of disrupting normal pulmonary host defenses.[117] They can impair the host at each step in the evolution of a pneumonia from colonization to aspiration and defensive response. Antibiotics are known to suppress the normal resident flora (and thus predispose the patient to colonization with more virulent bacteria) and to increase the ability of gram-negative bacteria to adhere to the oropharynx. Hypnotics, narcotics, and neuroleptics predispose the patient to aspiration by altering his or her level of consciousness and by depressing the gag and cough reflexes.

While the presence of significant underlying disease is usually the major factor in weakening pulmonary host defenses in thermally injured patients, certain medical interventions may make things even worse. Many commonly employed drugs including aspirin, aminophylline, and corticosteroids can impair the bactericidal capacity of the alveolar macrophage.[117–119] Similarly, a number of pharmacologic agents including certain antibiotics, nonsteroidal anti-inflammatory drugs, corticosteroids, aspirin, digoxin, and aminophylline have been shown in experimental models of pneumonia to impair the generation of the pulmonary inflammatory response to bacteria and thus to increase susceptibility to infection.[117,118,120,121] These deleterious effects of pharmacologic agents may be significant determinants of clinical outcome in certain situations, particularly in the case of patients with life-threatening disease or who are already immunocompromised by burn injury.

Many interventional procedures commonly employed in the management of critically ill patients also have adverse effects on the patient's antibacterial defenses. Early intubation for airway management and ventilatory support is frequently utilized in patients with inhalation injury. Endotracheal tubes disrupt the normal epiglottic function and impair the ciliary escalator and cough mechanism. Moreover, contaminated oral secretions frequently collect above the cuff of the endotracheal tube and the posterior pharynx. Deflation of the cuff or the use of low-pressure cuffs allow these secretions to enter the tracheobronchial tree. It has recently been determined that the endotracheal tube itself may serve as a reservoir for the persistent contamination of the tracheobronchial tree. The surface binding characteristics of polyvinyl chloride endotracheal tubes allow aggregates of pathogenic bacteria to adhere to the tube within 48 hours in virtually 100 percent of intubated patients.[122] Frequent endotracheal suctioning most likely dislodges these bacterial aggregates and instills them within the lung. Indeed, this may be one explanation for the extraordinarily high incidence of nosocomial pneumonia in intubated patients. Patients receiving mechanical ventilation have a 21-fold greater incidence of nosocomial pneumonia than nonventilated patients, and this risk increases with the duration of respiratory assistance.[123,124] After 5 days of mechanical ventilation, the rate of nosocomial pneumonia is 60 percent.

Antacids and H_2 blockers, which are often used as prophylaxis against stress-induced bleeding in critically ill patients, raise gastric pH and allow overgrowth of gram-negative bacteria in the stomach. This rise in gastric pH increases the risk of tracheal bacterial colonization as well. Retrograde movement of bacteria from the stomach to the oropharynx has been shown to occur, particularly in those patients who have nasogastric tubes. Nasogastric tubes are frequently required in burn patients for gastric decompression or enteral feeding. Cimetidine is also a significant risk factor for the development of nosocomial pneumonia in patients who require the assistance of mechanical ventilation. A recent study has reported that nosocomial pneumonia occurs twice as frequently among patients receiving antacids or H_2 blockers as among patients receiving sucralfate, which does not alter gastric pH.[125]

The stomach has also been shown to be colonized in critically ill patients with acute respiratory failure who were being supported by mechanical ventilation and who were receiving enteral feedings.[126] Tracheal colonization occurs in almost 90 percent of long-term intubated patients, and one-third of these bacteria originate from the stomach. Thus, early enteral nutrition (which has been recently emphasized) may lead to gastric flora colonizing the trachea and thus contribute to the development of nosocomial respiratory infection.

In summary, the predominant mechanism of acquiring nosocomial pneumonia is aspiration of the oropharyngeal flora in colonized patients with impaired lung defenses. Burn patients have an enormous risk because of the environmental flora; rapid colonization of the oropharynx and stomach; and use of endotracheal intubation, tracheostomy, and nasogastric intubation, which facilitate aspiration. Impairment of pulmonary antibacterial defenses induced by their primary disease and use of specific pharmacologic agents further reduces the patient's defenses, allowing aspirated bacteria to proliferate and cause invasive disease.

The care and management of the burn-injured patient represents a formidable challenge to the physician. As long as the basic underlying host defense defects in burn patients remain elusive, the clinician's approach will remain symptomatic and empirical. Further knowledge of the underlying pathophysiology of burn injury will undoubtedly provide innovative approaches to both the prevention and the early and effective treatment of their infectious complications. Clearly, the development of a multimodal approach, including components of immune restoration and immune modulation, is needed to improve the multiple defects in the host defense system induced by burn injury (Table 6-6).[127–129] However, it must be remembered that the normal host defense system operates in a delicate balance. Efforts to nonselectively stimulate the immune system may prove to be as deleterious to the burn-injured patient as the negative effects of immunosuppression.

Table 6-6 Potential Therapeutic Approaches to Enhance Host Defenses in Burn Patients

Modulation of the complement cascade
Restoration of serum deficiencies
Antagonists of proinflammatory mediators
Plasmaphoresis
Blockade of immunosuppressive mediators
Fibronectin replacement
Passive immunization (hyperimmune IgG)
Active immunization
Nonsteroidal anti-inflammatory drugs
Nutritional replacement
Neutrophil transfusions
Human recombinant granulocyte colony-stimulating factor
Immunopotentiators

REFERENCES

1. Till GO: Cellular and humoral defense systems and inflammatory mechanisms in thermal injury. *Clin Lab Med* 3:801, 1983.
2. Pruitt BA: The diagnosis and treatment of infection in the burn patient. *Burns Incl Therm Inj* 11:79, 1984.
3. Luterman A, Dacso CC, Curreri PW: Infections in burn patients. *Am J Med* 81(suppl 1A):45, 1986.
4. Toews GB: Determinants of bacterial clearance from the lower respiratory tract. *Semin Respir Infect* 1:68, 1986.
5. Reynolds HY: Host defense impairments that may lead to respiratory infections. *Clin Chest Med* 8:339, 1987.
6. Green GM, Jakab GJ, Low RB, Davis GS: Defense mechanisms of the respiratory membrane. *Am Rev Respir Dis* 115:479, 1977.
7. Kaltreider HB, Chan MKL: The class specific immunoglobulin composition of fluids obtained from various levels of the canine respiratory tract. *J Immunol* 116:428, 1976.
8. Johanson WG: Prevention of respiratory tract infection. *Am J Med* 76:69, 1984.
9. Coonrod JD: The role of extracellular bactericidal factors in pulmonary host defense. *Semin Respir Infect* 1:118, 1986.
10. Goldstein E, Lippert W, Warshauer D: Pulmonary alveolar macrophage: Defender against bacterial infection of the lung. *J Clin Invest* 54:519, 1974.
11. Fels AOS, Cohn ZA: The alveolar macrophage. *J Appl Physiol* 60:353, 1986.
12. Nathan CF: Secretory products of macrophages. *J Clin Invest* 79:319, 1987.
13. Green GM, Kass EH: The role of the alveolar macrophage in the clearance of bacteria from the lung. *J Exp Med* 119:167, 1964.
14. Hoidal JR, Schmeling D, Peterson PK: Phagocytosis, bacterial killing and metabolism by purified human lung phagocytes. *J Infect Dis* 144:61, 1981.

15. Davis-Scibienski C, Beaman BL: Interaction of alveolar macrophages with *Nocardia asteroides*: Immunological enhancement of phagocytosis, phagosome-lysosome fusion, and microbicidal activity. *Infect Immun* 30:578, 1980.
16. Shepherd VL: The role of the respiratory burst of phagocytes in host defense. *Semin Respir Infect* 1:99, 1986.
17. Kaltreider HB: Immune defenses of the lung, in Sande MA, Hudson LD, Root RK (eds): *Respiratory Infections*. New York, Churchill Livingstone, 1986, pp 47–90.
18. Murray HW: Interferon-gamma, the activated macrophage, and host defense against microbial challenge. *Ann Intern Med* 108:595, 1988.
19. Dinarello, CA, Mier JW: Lymphokines. *N Engl J Med* 317:940, 1987.
20. Beutler B, Cerami A: Cachectin: More than a tumor necrosis factor. *N Engl J Med* 316:379, 1987.
21. Dinarello CA: Biology of interleukin 1. *FASEB J* 2:108, 1988.
22. Tracey KJ, Fong Y, Hesse DG, et al: Anti-cachectin/TNF monoclonal antibodies prevent septic shock during lethal bacteraemia. *Nature* 330:662, 1987.
23. Martin TR: Arachidonic acid metabolism in lung phagocytes. *Semin Respir Infect* 1:89, 1986.
24. Ford-Hutchinson AW: Leukotrienes: Their formation and role as inflammatory mediators. *Fed Proc* 44:25, 1985.
25. Nelson RD, Herron MJ: Chemotaxis and motility of lung phagocytes. *Semin Respir Infect* 1:79, 1986.
26. Reynolds HY: Lung inflammation: Normal host defense or a complication of some diseases? *Annu Rev Med* 38:295, 1987.
27. Okusawa S, Yancey KB, vander Meer JWM, et al: C5a stimulates secretion of tumor necrosis factor from human mononuclear cells *in vitro*. *J Exp Med* 168:443, 1988.
28. Dinarello CA, Cannon JG, Wolff SM, et al: Tumor necrosis factor (Cachectin) is an endogenous pyrogen and induces production of interleukin 1. *J Exp Med* 163:1433, 1986.
29. Shalaby MR, Palladino MA, Hirabayashi SE, et al: Receptor binding and activation of polymorphonuclear neutrophils by tumor necrosis factor-alpha. *J Leukocyte Biol* 41:196, 1987.
30. Figari IS, Palladino MA: Stimulation of neutrophil chemotaxis by recombinant tumor necrosis factors alpha and beta. *Fed Proc* 46(A):562, 1987.
31. Averbook B, Ulich T, Jeffes E, et al: Human alpha lymphotoxin and TNF induce different types of inflammatory responses in normal tissue. *Fed Proc* 46(A):562, 1987.
32. Yonemaru M, Zheng H, Stephens KE, et al: Biphasic effect of tumor necrosis factor on polymorphonuclear leukocyte chemotaxis. *Am Rev Respir Dis* 137:42, 1988.
33. Nelson S, Bagby GJ, Bainton BG, et al: Compartmentalization of intraalveolar and systemic lipopolysaccharide-induced tumor necrosis factor and the pulmonary inflammatory response. *J Infect Dis* 159:189, 1989.
34. Ward PA, Lepow IH, Newman LJ: Bacterial factors chemotactic for polymorphonuclear leukocytes. *Am J Pathol* 52:725, 1968.
35. Pruitt BA, McManus AT: Opportunistic infections in severely burned patients. *Am J Med* 77:146, 1984.
36. Pruitt BA: The burn patient: I. Initial care. *Curr Probl Surg* 16:8, 1979.
37. Hansbrough JF: Burn wound sepsis. *J Intensive Care Med* 2:313, 1987.
38. Pruitt BA, Lindberg RB, McManus WF, Mason AD: Current approach to prevention and treatment of *Pseudomonas aeruginosa* infections in burned patients. *Rev Infect Dis* 5:S889, 1983.
39. Moncrief JA, Lindberg RB, Switzer WE, Pruitt BA: Use of topical antibacterial therapy in the treatment of the burn wound. *Arch Surg* 92:558, 1966.
40. White JC, Nelson S, Winkelstein JA, et al: Impairment of antibacterial defense mechanisms of the lung by extrapulmonary infection. *J Infect Dis* 153:202, 1986.
41. Harris SE, Nelson S, Astry CL, et al: Endotoxin-induced suppression of pulmonary antibacterial defenses against *Staphylococcus aureus*. *Am Rev Respir Dis* 138:1439, 1988.
42. Deitch EA, Maejima K, Berg R: Effect of oral antibiotics and bacterial overgrowth on the translocation of the GI tract microflora in burned rats. *J Trauma* 25:385, 1985.
43. Ziegler TR, Smith RJ, O'Dwyer ST, et al: Increased intestinal permeability associated with infection in burn patients. *Arch Surg* 123:1313, 1988.
44. Deitch EA, Berg R: Bacterial translocation from the gut: A mechanism of infection. *J Burn Care Rehabil* 8:475, 1987.
45. Ninnemann JL: Trauma, sepsis, and the immune response. *J Burn Care Rehabil* 8:462, 1987.
46. Dhennin C, Pinon G, Greco JM: Alterations of complement system following thermal injury: Use in estimation of vital prognosis. *J Trauma* 18:129, 1978.
47. Bjornson AB, Altemeier WA, Bjornson HS: Complement, opsonins, and the immune response to bacterial infection in burned patients. *Ann Surg* 191:323, 1980.
48. Gelfand JA, Donelan M, Hawiger A, Burke JF: Alternative complement pathway activation increases mortality in a model of burn injury in mice. *J Clin Invest* 70:1170, 1982.
49. Gelfand JA, Donelan M, Burke JF: Preferential activation and depletion of the alternative complement pathway by burn injury. *Ann Surg* 198:58, 1983.
50. Gelfand JA, Donelan MB, Hawiger A, Burke JF: Role of complement activation in early mortality from burns. *Surg Forum* 31:80, 1980.
51. Ward PA: Host-defense mechanisms responsible for lung injury. *J Allergy Clin Immunol* 78:373, 1986.
52. Demling RH: Burns. *N Engl J Med* 313:1389, 1985.
53. Aikawa N, Shinozawa Y, Ishibiki K, et al: Clinical analysis of multiple organ failure in burned patients. *Burns Incl Therm Inj* 13:103, 1987.
54. Demling RH: Wound inflammatory mediators and multisystem organ failure. *Prog Clin Biol Res* 236A: 525, 1987.
55. Ninnemann JL, Fisher JC, Frank HA: Prolonged survival of human skin allografts following thermal injury. *Transplantation* 25:69, 1978.
56. Rapaport FT, Milgorm F, Kano K, et al: Immunologic

sequelae of thermal injury. *Ann NY Acad Sci* 150:1004, 1968.
57. Baker CC, Yamada AH, Faist E, Kupper TS: Interleukin-1 and T cell function following injury. *J Burn Care Rehabil* 8:503, 1987.
58. Baker CC, Miller CL, Trunkey DD: Identity of mononuclear cells which compromise the resistance of trauma patients. *J Surg Res* 26:478, 1979.
59. Miller CL, Baker CC: Changes in lymphocyte activity after thermal injury: The role of suppressor cells. *J Clin Invest* 63:202, 1979.
60. Sukhtankar AY, Sengupta SR: Cellular immunity in burns. *Burns Incl Therm Inj* 8:168, 1981.
61. Ozkan AN, Hoyt DB, Ninnemann JL: Generation and activity of suppressor peptides following traumatic injury. *J Burn Care Rehabil* 8:527, 1987.
62. Green DR, Wang N, Zheng H: A suppressor-inducer factor produced by burn trauma-associated T cells. *J Burn Care Rehabil* 8:521, 1987.
63. Horgan PG, Rodrick ML, Ellwanger K, et al: *In vivo* effects of an immunosuppressive factor isolated from patients following thermal injury. *Surg Forum* 39:96, 1988.
64. Hoyt DB, Ozkan AN, Ninnemann JL: Immunologic monitoring of infection risk in trauma patients: Research questions and an approach to the problem. *J Burn Care Rehabil* 8:549, 1987.
65. Hansbrough JF, Field TO, Gadd MA, Soderberg C: Immune response modulation after burn injury: T-cells and antibodies. *J Burn Care Rehabil* 8:509, 1987.
66. Burleson DG, Mason AD, McManus AT, Pruitt BA: Lymphocyte phenotype and function changes in burn patients after intravenous IgG therapy. *Arch Surg* 123:1379, 1988.
67. Graddock CG: Production, distribution and fate of granulocytes, in Williams WJ, Beutler E, Erslev AJ, Rundles RW (eds): *Hematology*. New York, McGraw-Hill, 1972, pp 607–18.
68. Asko-Seljavaara S: Granulocyte kinetics in burns. *J Burn Care Rehabil* 8:492, 1987.
69. Dominioni L, Alexander JW, Ogle CK, et al: *In vivo* chemotaxis and body compartment distribution of indium-111 labelled polymorphonuclear leukocytes in burned guinea pigs. *J Trauma* 23:911, 1983.
70. Demling RH: The role of mediators in human ARDS. *J Crit Care* 3:56, 1988.
71. Asko-Seljavaara S: Granulocyte kinetics in burned mice: Inhibition in granulocyte growth studied *in vivo* and *in vitro*. *Scand J Plast Reconstr Surg Hand Surg* 8:185, 1974.
72. Mooney DP, Gamelli RL, O'Reilly M, Herbert JC: Recombinant human granulocyte colony-stimulating factor and *Pseudomonas* burn wound sepsis. *Arch Surg* 123:1353, 1988.
73. Warden GD, Mason AD, Pruitt BA: Evaluation of leukocyte chemotaxis *in vitro* in thermally injured patients. *J Clin Invest* 54:1001, 1974.
74. Nelson RD, Hasslen SR, Ahrenholz DH, Solem LD: Mechanisms of loss of human neutrophil chemotaxis following thermal injury. *J Burn Care Rehabil* 8:496, 1987.
75. Hinshaw DB, Sklar LA, Bohl B, et al: Cytoskeletal and morphologic impact of cellular oxidant injury. *Am J Pathol* 123:454, 1986.
76. Moore FD, Davis C, Rodrick M, et al: Neutrophil activation in thermal injury as assessed by increased expression of complement receptors. *N Engl J Med* 314:948, 1986.
77. Marino JA, Gerding RL, Fratianne RB, Spagnuolo PJ: Neutrophil adhesive dysfunction in thermal injury: The role of fibronectin. *J Infect Dis* 157:674, 1988.
78. Lanser ME, Saba TM, Scovill WA: Opsonic glycoprotein (plasma fibronectin) levels after burn injury: Relationship to extent of burn and development of sepsis. *Ann Surg* 192:776, 1980.
79. Saba TM, Blumenstock FA, Shah DM, et al: Reversal of opsonic deficiency in surgical, trauma, and burn patients by infusion of purified human plasma fibronectin. *Am J Med* 80:229, 1986.
80. Alexander JW, Ogle CK, Stinnett JD, MacMillan BG: A sequential, prospective analysis of immunologic abnormalities and infection following severe thermal injury. *Ann Surg* 188:809, 1978.
81. Bjornson AB, Bjornson HS, Knippenberg RW, Cardone JS: Temporal relationships among immunologic alterations in a guinea pig model of thermal injury. *J Infect Dis* 153:1098, 1986.
82. Bjornson AB, Knippenberg RW, Bjornson HS: Nonsteroidal anti-inflammatory drugs correct the bactericidal defect of polymorphonuclear leukocytes in a guinea pig model of thermal injury. *J Infect Dis* 157:959, 1988.
83. Hansbrough J, Peterson V, Zapata-Sirvent R, Claman HN: Postburn immunosuppression in an animal model: II. Restoration of cell-mediated immunity by immunomodulating drugs. *Surgery* 95:290, 1984.
84. Zapata-Sirvent RL, Hansbrough JF: Postburn immunosuppression in an animal model: III. Maintenance of normal splenic helper and suppressor lymphocyte subpopulations by immunomodulating drugs. *Surgery* 97:721, 1985.
85. Loose LD, Turinsky J: Macrophage dysfunction after burn injury. *Infect Immun* 26:157, 1979.
86. Loose LD, Turinsky J: Depression of the respiratory burst in alveolar and peritoneal macrophages after thermal injury. *Infect Immun* 30:718, 1980.
87. Loose LD, Megirian R, Turinsky J: Biochemical and functional alterations in macrophages after thermal injury. *Infect Immun* 44:554, 1984.
88. Seidenfeld JJ, Pohl DF, Bell RC, et al: Incidence, site, and outcome of infections in patients with the adult respiratory distress syndrome. *Am Rev Respir Dis* 134:12, 1986.
89. Herndon DN, Langner F, Thompson P, et al: Pulmonary injury in burned patients. *Surg Clin North Am* 67:31, 1987.
90. Herndon DN, Thompson PB, Traber DL: Pulmonary injury in burned patients. *Crit Care Clin* 1:79, 1985.
91. Pecha BS, Raffin TA: Smoke inhalation: Averting long-term damage. *J Respir Dis* 8:87, 1987.
92. Shirani KZ, Pruitt BA, Mason AD: The influence of inhalation injury and pneumonia on burn mortality. *Ann Surg* 205:82, 1987.

93. Wald PH, Balmes JR: Respiratory effects of short-term, high-intensity toxic inhalations: Smoke gases, and fumes. *J Intensive Care Med* 2:260, 1987.
94. Stein MD, Herndon DN, Stevens JM, et al: Production of chemotactic factors and lung cell changes following smoke inhalation in a sheep model. *J Burn Care Rehabil* 7:117, 1986.
95. Matsuura Y, Najib A, Lee WH: Pulmonary compliance and surfactant activity in thermal burns. *Surg Forum* 17:86, 1966.
96. Nieman GF, Clark WR, Wax SD, Webb SR: The effect of smoke inhalation on pulmonary surfactant. *Ann Surg* 191:171, 1980.
97. Demarest GB, Hudson LD, Altman LC: Impaired alveolar macrophage chemotaxis in patients with acute smoke inhalation. *Am Rev Respir Dis* 119:279, 1979.
98. Dressler DP, Skornik WA: Alveolar macrophage in the burned rat. *J Trauma* 14:1036, 1974.
99. Loke J, Paul E, Virgulto JA, Smith GJW: Rabbit lung after acute smoke inhalation. *Arch Surg* 119:956, 1984.
100. Pollok AJ, Gemmell CG, Clark CJ, et al: Functional status of pulmonary alveolar macrophages following exposure to toxic gases. *Br J Anaesth* 59:943P, 1987.
101. Gemmell CG, Pollok AJ, McMillan F, et al: Structural and functional changes in alveolar macrophages following exposure of fire victims to smoke. *Eur J Clin Invest* 17:A56, 1987.
102. Janoff A, Pryor WA, Bengali ZH: Effects of tobacco smoke components on cellular and biochemical processes in the lung. *Am Rev Respir Dis* 136:1058, 1987.
103. Fick RB, Paul ES, Merrill WW, et al: Alterations in the antibacterial properties of rabbit pulmonary macrophages exposed to wood smoke. *Am Rev Respir Dis* 129:76, 1984.
104. Nelson S, Chidiac C, Summer WR: New strategies for preventing nosocomial pneumonia. *J Crit Illness* 3:12, 1988.
105. Martin TR: Lung antibacterial defense mechanisms in critically ill patients. *Pulmon Crit Care Update* 3:(lesson 24), 1988.
106. Haley RW, Culver DH, White JW, et al: The nationwide nosocomial infection rate: A new need for vital statistics. *Am J Epidemiol* 121:159, 1985.
107. Gross PA, Neu HC, Aswapokee P, et al: Deaths from nosocomial infections: Experience in a university hospital and a community hospital. *Am J Med* 68:219, 1980.
108. Huxley EJ, Viroslav J, Gray WR, Pierce AK: Pharyngeal aspiration in normal adults and patients with depressed consciousness. *Am J Med* 64:564, 1978.
109. Stamm WE, Martin SM, Bennett JV: Epidemiology of nosocomial infections due to gram-negative bacilli: Aspects relevant to development and use of vaccines. *J Infect Dis* 136:S151, 1977.
110. Sanford JP, Pierce AK: Lower respiratory tract infections, in Bennett JV, Brachman PS (eds): *Hospital Infections*. Boston, Little Brown, 1979, pp 255–86.
111. Centers for Disease Control: *National Nosocomial Infections Study Report, Annual Summary, 1979*. Atlanta, Centers for Disease Control, 1982, pp 2–13.
112. Bartlett JG, O'Keefe P, Tally FP, et al: Bacteriology of hospital-acquired pneumonia. *Arch Intern Med* 146:868, 1986.
113. Johanson WG, Pierce AK, Sanford JP: Changing pharyngeal bacterial flora of hospitalized patients: Emergence of gram-negative bacilli. *N Engl J Med* 281:1137, 1969.
114. LaForce FM, Hopkins J, Trow R, Wang WLL: Human oral defenses against gram-negative rods. *Am Rev Respir Dis* 114:929, 1976.
115. Johanson WG: Prevention of respiratory tract infection. *Am J Med* 76:69, 1984.
116. Johanson WG, Pierce AK, Sanford JP, Thomas GD: Nosocomial respiratory infections with gram-negative bacilli: The significance of colonization of the respiratory tract. *Ann Intern Med* 77:701, 1972.
117. Esposito AL: The effect of common pharmacologic agents on pulmonary antibacterial defenses: Implications for the geriatric patient. *Clin Chest Med* 8:373, 1987.
118. Nelson S, Summer WR, Jakab GJ: Aminophylline-induced suppression of pulmonary antibacterial defenses. *Am Rev Respir Dis* 131:923, 1985.
119. White JC, Lanser ME, Nelson S, Jakab GJ: Methylprednisolone impairs the bactericidal activity of alveolar macrophages. *J Surg Res* 39:46, 1985.
120. Nelson S, Summer WR, Terry PB, et al: Erythromycin-induced suppression of pulmonary antibacterial defenses: A potential mechanism of superinfection in the lung. *Am Rev Respir Dis* 136:1207, 1987.
121. Esposito AL: Digoxin disrupts the inflammatory response in experimental pneumococcal pneumonia. *J Infect Dis* 152:14, 1985.
122. Sottile FD, Marrie TJ, Prough DS, et al: Nosocomial pulmonary infection: Possible etiologic significance of bacterial adhesion to endotracheal tubes. *Crit Care Med* 14:265, 1986.
123. Stoutenbeek CP, van Saene HKF, Miranda DR, et al: The effect of oropharyngeal decontamination using topical nonabsorbable antiobiotics on the incidence of nosocomial respiratory tract infections in multiple trauma patients. *J Trauma* 27:357, 1987.
124. Dixon RE: Nosocomial respiratory infections. *Infect Control* 4:376, 1983.
125. Driks MR, Craven DE, Celli BR, et al: Nosocomial pneumonia in intubated patients given sucralfate as compared with antacids or histamine type 2 blockers: The role of gastric colonization. *N Engl J Med* 317:1376, 1987.
126. Pingleton SK, Hinthorn DR, Liu C: Enteral nutrition in patients receiving mechanical ventilation: Multiple sources of tracheal colonization include the stomach. *Am J Med* 80:827, 1986.
127. Hansbrough JF, Zapata-Sirvent RL, Peterson VM: Immunomodulation following burn injury. *Surg Clin North Am* 67:69, 1987.
128. Waymack JP, Miskell P, Gonce SJ, Alexander JW: Immunomodulators in the treatment of peritonitis in burned and malnourished animals. *Surgery* 96:308, 1984.
129. Donati L, Lazzarin A, Signorini M, et al: Preliminary clinical experiences with the use of immunomodulators in burns. *J Trauma* 23:816, 1983.

Chapter 7

Clinical and Functional Assessment

Edward F. Haponik

The clinical diagnosis of inhalation injury is based upon knowledge of the spectrum and temporal development of respiratory problems; classic, historically useful bedside predictors of the presence of injury; and the results of objective diagnostic tests. The first two of these factors largely determine the pretest probability of inhalation injury and previously had represented the sole means of establishing the diagnosis. In the absence of any further information, these data still serve to identify individuals with increased risks and, consequently, help to direct early empiric therapy. In many instances, however, they provide insufficient information for precise, timely diagnosis; moreover, they are often inadequate for the important purposes of triage. The latter requires diagnostic information with a high negative predictive value (that is, a low false-negative rate) and a high diagnostic sensitivity. While patients with catastrophic early respiratory injuries are usually identified easily—recognition and treatment of their respiratory problems are incorporated in initial life-saving efforts—the insidious nature of inhalation injury makes diagnosis difficult in other circumstances.

Technologic progress has provided an array of diagnostic tests that permits rapid measurement of asphyxiants and both direct and indirect demonstration of airway injury; all are generally available in a timely manner. Carboxyhemoglobin measurements can be performed within minutes using modern co-oximetry, and progress in the rapid detection of cyanide assists identification of other individuals with asphyxia. Pharyngeal and tracheobronchial inflammatory changes can be seen endoscopically, documenting major airway injury directly and immediately. Inhomogeneity of radionuclide deposition, physiologic demonstration of airflow obstruction, and, less often, focal abnormalities of the chest roentgenogram provide other important, albeit indirect, evidence of airway injury. To a degree, the relationships of these findings to late-onset parenchymal injury assist planning in the absence of more precise early diagnostic and prognostic indicators. All of this diagnostic information is complementary, and the clinician must be aware of its optimum applications and practical limitations.

SPECTRUM AND TIME COURSE OF RESPIRATORY PROBLEMS

The diversity of respiratory complications of smoke inhalation has been addressed in previous chapters; primary injuries are classified as asphyxia, upper and lower airway damage, and parenchymal effects and may occur either alone or in various combinations, with or without cutaneous burns.[1–17] These anatomic and physiologic derangements due to injury have implications for diagnostic strategies.[18–28] Injuries to discrete levels of the respiratory tract vary in their clinical manifestations, severity, and amenability to detection by one test or another. In addition, the presence of cutaneous burn bears an important relationship to not only an increased likelihood that respiratory injury will be present but also influences the types of diagnostic tests necessary, their feasibility, and the settings in which they will be performed and interpreted.

Categorization of respiratory problems with respect to the time which has elapsed after injury is a clinically useful guide to the diagnostic evaluation (Chap. 2). Because carbon monoxide intoxication, upper airway obstruction, and tracheobronchial obstruction are early events, usually present during the initial hours after exposure, timely detection must focus upon these problems. Moreover, as Clark and Framm have noted, the diagnosis of inhalation injury becomes progressively easier during the patient's clinical course[17]: either manifestations of respiratory damage develop or they don't. Thus, the time elapsed after the initial injury has added implications for the need for diagnostic testing.

Although this chapter will emphasize the physician's initial clinical and functional assessment, principles and tests valuable in early diagnosis also serve useful roles as part of the serial reevaluation of the patient so integral to effective management and may assist evaluations of residual pulmonary injury during convalescence. For example, flow volume curves and endoscopic procedures contribute to assessment of patients with chronic upper airway obstruction, while spirometric demonstration of obstructive and/or restrictive ventilatory defects may clarify the nature of long-term respiratory symptoms or help select surgical candidates. Furthermore, some tests which have less value as initial diagnostic or screening procedures (e.g., the chest roentgenogram, arterial blood gas analysis) may have an enhanced usefulness in the detection and management of later-onset respiratory problems such as pulmonary edema, pneumonia, and pulmonary embolism. These diagnostic applications are considered in other chapters.

CLASSIC CLINICAL INDICATORS OF INHALATION INJURY

Early descriptions of inhalation injury relied nearly exclusively upon the historical characteristics of the exposure, the presence or absence of signs and symptoms related to the respiratory tract, burns involving the face or neck, and the expectoration of carbonaceous sputum. In a recent report of experience from the Brooke institute,[29] 373 of 487 (76.6 percent) patients with major risk factors for inhalation injury (facial burns, structural fires, closed-space setting, and mental or physical impairment at the scene of exposure) had inhalation injury confirmed at fiberoptic bronchoscopy and/or xenon scans. In comprehensive experiences from different parts of the world, Heimbach and Waeckerle and Clark et al. have also stressed the role of such clinical information in patients with cutaneous burns.[28–30] Thus, these familiar markers of increased risk are quite valuable, so long as their limitations are recognized. The predictive values of some of these clinical indicators are outlined in Table 7-1. Such clinical findings are often present in combinations, enhancing the bedside predictation of inhalation injury. In their recent review of a selected group referred to a burn center, Clark and coworkers noted

Table 7-1 Relative Predictive Values (PV) of Some "Classic" Markers of Inhalation Injury

	Positive PV* (%)	Negative PV† (%)
Enclosed space setting	47–62	80–93
Facial burns	25–69	50–96
Carbonaceous sputum	81–100	33–83

*Proportion of burn victims with the finding who prove to have inhalation injury.

†Proportion of burn victims without the finding who prove to not have inhalation injury.

that only 15 percent of patients with inhalation injury had only a single finding, while 56 percent of patients had 3 or more, and 32 percent had 4 or more such findings.[17a]

Historical Clues

Detailed information about the setting of injury is essential and should be sought from not only the patient but also other victims, witnesses, and members of evacuation and rescue teams. Exposures which have occurred in a closed space, particularly in association with entrapment (such as in an automobile or locked room) suggest that an intense exposure to high concentrations of toxic combustion products has occurred. Residential and other structural fires, automobile fires, and ship and airline disasters are examples of such circumstances. Prolonged exposures in these settings mandate particularly careful clinical monitoring even in the absence of either surface burn or of abnormalities of most initial objective tests. The positive predictive value of a closed-space setting has varied, however, from approximately 47 to 62 percent. Moreover, the absence of this historical clue does not ensure a low likelihood of inhalation injury: several authors have reported severe respiratory injury to occur following outdoor exposures.

Some situations connote direct respiratory injury. Facial exposures to either direct flame or to irritant gases of high water solubility are especially hazardous. Transient, high-intensity "flash exposures" (e.g., as with explosions during priming of automobile carburetors or lighting of household appliances (e.g., lighting gas burners) present increased risks of upper airway obstruction despite the limited extent of cutaneous burn. Aspiration of hot liquids presents similar obvious risks.[31–33] As noted in Chap. 3, exposures to live steam, fires in hyperoxic environments, and those related to explosive gases (e.g., propane, ether) or liquid aspirations may be associated with a true thermal injury to the lower respiratory tract.

Unconsciousness and altered sensorium are additional major predispositions for severe injury.[34] Alcohol intoxication is a well-recognized offender in residential fire scenarios.[35] Neurologic impairment can also be a manifestation of asphyxia, shock, trauma sustained in fight or flight from the burn scene, or combinations of these factors. Moreover, this finding helps to identify an individual who is especially likely to have experienced an intense exposure.

On some occasions (e.g., following industrial accidents), the precise nature of the toxic gases generated at the burn scene might suggest particular respiratory hazards.[36] For example, recognized exposures to low water solubility gases like oxides of nitrogen or phosgene increase the likelihood of delayed onset pulmonary edema (even in the absence of early abnormalities). Alternatively, appreciation of a predominant fuel and, by inference, the combustion products most likely to have been generated might yield similar diagnostic information (Chap. 3). In addition, predispositions for inhalation injury might be expected to be modified with societal practices; thus physicians must appreciate emergence of potentially new risk factors. Severe upper airway injury has been associated with the ignition of widely used petrolatum-based hair greases.[37] Recently, severe thermal injury to both upper and lower conducting airways has followed the practice of free-basing of cocaine.[38] Chemical injury induced by smoke and/or the intratracheal ignition of the highly flammable ether vehicle has caused severe reactive airways disease and tracheal stenosis requiring reconstructive surgery.

In the clinical appraisal of the likelihood of smoke inhalation injury in fire fighters, several unique occupational clues to the severity of exposure should be sought.[23] These include the duration of work in "danger areas" with especially high concentrations of smoke, the number of air tanks used during the fire, and whether or not any "pastings" or "shellackings" (i.e., episodes of being overcome by smoke) had occurred. Work habits during the "mop up" or "overhaul" phase of the fire should be investigated in detail: the continued smoldering (i.e., pyrolysis) which is encountered typically generates high concentrations of often unrecognized toxic products and is a particularly deceptive, hazardous environment.[39] In addition, the fire fighters' pattern of use of self-contained breathing apparatus (i.e., whether it is worn continuously or intermittently) and the mode with which it is used—low flow versus demand—are important.[23] The former mode reduces exposure to smoke by effectively pressurizing the mask and "flushing" air around its sides but also more rapidly depletes the compressed air supply. This contributes to the fire fighters' tendency to either use masks intermittently or else conserve the compressed air supply through use of the demand mode. It has been noted that intermittent mask use is as effective as no mask at all, providing virtually no protection against carbon monoxide intoxication.[40]

Details about the patient's behavior at the fire scene are often quite informative and may vary considerably depending upon whether the exposure occurs in familiar surroundings (e.g., residential fires) or an unfamiliar environment (public place). Unusual behaviors in which patients inexplicably remain at the scene of exposure, rather than flee from obvious danger, have been observed in the former setting,[41] predisposing to more severe inhalation injury. If remembered, the victim's degree of activity; pattern, frequency, and depth of breathing; perceptions about the density of smoke and duration of exposure; and whether or not specific efforts were made to minimize inhalation of toxic gases (e.g., by covering the mouth with a handkerchief or wet towel) should all be noted as possible indices of the dosages of toxic inhalants. Finally, general characteristics of each patient's previous health status are key determinants of how well even a minor inhalation injury might be tolerated and thus have an important influence on management. Increased age or the presence of underlying cardiopulmonary or cerebrovascular disease or other chronic illnesses may lessen the patient's physiologic reserve considerably. Unfortunately, too little is known at present about the effects of varying susceptibility among individuals to the pulmonary and systemic effects of inhaled toxic products.

General Appearance of the Patient

The critical nature of many patients' injuries is usually obvious from their initial general appearance. Simple inspection may be definitive: a tachypneic, dyspneic patient who is either covered with soot or whose clothing has the characteristic acrid odor of smoke must be suspected to have inhalation injury until proven otherwise. It has been noted that fire victims prefer the semi-Fowler's position and that individuals who favor upright postures are more likely to have inhalation injury.[12] Cyanosis is recognized uncommonly and may be difficult to detect in the hypotensive, soot-covered victim. Even profound hypoxemia is not associated with cyanosis in the presence of severe anemia. The cherry-red color classically sought as a sign of carbon monoxide intoxication is present uncommonly. Obvious abnormalities of neurologic status, including mental confusion, hallucinations, dizziness, headache, seizure activity, and altered consciousness, should be noted as important clues to asphyxiants. Apparent abdominal pain, nausea, or vomiting may reflect not only inhaled toxins but also trauma. The evaluation for manifestations of inhalation injury must be coupled with a careful survey of the total patient for other injuries which may be obscured by predominant signs of respiratory distress.

Respiratory Symptoms and Signs

The relative frequencies of respiratory symptoms or signs in representative, large published series are summarized in Table 7-2 but should be expected to vary considerably. While these findings do not always document the presence of inhalation injury with certainty, their presence may be particularly useful and complements other information. Dyspnea, cough, and hoarseness are commonly reported among fire victims but are often transient, self-limited findings which clear spontaneously during the patient's evacuation from the scene of exposure to smoke. Thus, although dyspnea might suggest early parenchymal injury, wheezing might represent an indicator of early chemical bronchitis, and hoarseness more strongly suggests oropharyngeal injury, these symptoms do not always establish whether major damage at these sites has occurred. Chest pain has been reported in up to one-third of exposed individuals. Worsened angina pectoris or acute myocardial infarction, especially in the presence of carbon monoxide or cyanide intoxication and/or hypoxemia; pneumothorax related to vascular access procedures, chest trauma, or artificial airway placement; as well as primary inhalation injury must be considered in the differential diagnosis. Hemoptysis may accompany particularly severe mucosal injury or lung contusion (if coexisting chest trauma is present) or may follow traumatic, emergency airway placement; later in the course, it might suggest pulmonary embolism with infarction or necrotizing pneumonia.

Table 7-2 Presenting Symptoms and Signs of Inhalation Injury

	Relative frequency (%)
Dyspnea	3–71
Hoarseness	19–61
Throat pain	10–13
Chest pain	32–41
Cough	9–76
Hemoptysis	6–18
Carbonaceous sputum	9–80
Cyanosis	6–15
Tachypnea	25–80
Stridor	5–33
Wheezing	13–47
Rhonchi	23–52
Crackles	23–35

Tachypnea should always suggest inhalation injury and is a sensitive indicator but may also be due to anxiety with hyperventilation in the stressful fire setting. Tachypneic fire victims usually breathe with low tidal volumes; the presence of hyperpnea should suggest concomitant metabolic acidosis. Recruitment of accessory respiratory muscles (e.g., the presence of sternocleidomastoid, supraclavicular, infraclavicular, and/or intercostal retractions, flaring of the alae nasi) is an even more important bedside sign of respiratory distress. Paradoxical thoracoabdominal excursions, the movement of chest and abdomen in opposite directions, might suggest either upper airway obstruction (inward thoracic and outward abdominal displacement durng inspiration), increased diaphragmatic loads, or muscle instability (outward thoracic, inward abdominal displacement during inspiration). Pulsus paradoxus exceeding 10 mmHg is a sphygnanometric sign of accentuated swings of pleural pressure and can accompany upper or lower airway obstruction or worsening thoracic compliance. Clearly, an unstable pattern of breathing or apnea is a poor prognostic sign requiring prompt supportive therapy. Asymmetric movement of a hemithorax should suggest not only major atelectasis, pneumothorax, pleural effusion, mainstem bronchial intubation, or splinting due to chest wall burn but also occult subdiaphragmatic injury.

Auscultatory Findings

Despite more recent de-emphasis of chest auscultation in favor of imaging procedures, valuable information with direct implications for management is derived from carefully performed examinations. Auscultation is often difficult in patients who have limited mobility because of their burn distribution, in individuals with chest wall burns, or in those requiring mechanical ventilation. Nevertheless, even partial examinations with particular attention to the presence or absence of symmetry of breath sound intensity may be quite informative. Development of gross, unilateral reduction of breath sounds, for example, requires exclusion of atelectasis, pneumothorax, effusion, or pneumonia. Phillips et al. have observed that the presence of adventitious breath sounds ("rattles or rhonchi") at the time of presentation of patients with large burns is associated with a poor outcome.[34]

Stridor is, fortunately, uncommon among "all-comers" exposed to smoke but must always be sought. When present, this characteristic inspiratory sign demands immediate response because of the catastrophic, rapidly progressive nature of upper airway obstruction in this setting. Altered voice quality, dysphagia, and/or odynophagia are often associated with stridor and frequently precede it. Stridor has been associated with an adult upper airway less than 5 mm in diameter. Auscultation over the neck during both inspiration and expiration should be performed routinely. This maneuver while the patient pants may help to elicit subclinical upper airway obstruction which is not apparent from the examination during quiet breathing. Coarse, high-frequency breath sounds transmitted from the upper airway should be appreciated and often precede evolution to obvious stridor.

It has been said that nearly half of patients with inhalation injury have demonstrated wheezing at some time during their courses. These continuous, musical adventitious sounds cannot be distinguished from those occurring in asthma or other chronic obstructive airways diseases. Although there is considerable variability from patient to patient, DiVincenti et al. have reported that inspiratory and expiratory wheezes and crackles were usually appreciated by the second postburn day in patients with inhalation injury[9]. That audible wheezing usually develops after the physiologic demonstration of airflow obstruction has occurred, and clears before physiologic abnormalities resolve, is similar to observations in asthmatics and suggests that the abnormal physical examination detects a higher grade of inhalation injury of conducting airways. Focal wheezes might reflect local airway obstruction by impacted mucus in these patients, but wheezing is generally diffuse in this situation. Smoke inhalation can also induce exacerbations of bronchospasm in individuals with preexisting asthma or chronic obstructive pulmonary disease, functioning as a nonspecific airway irritant. Left ventricular failure (e.g., due to carbon monoxide intoxication or overhydration) may present as "cardiac asthma," while the new onset of wheezing late in the course should suggest pulmonary embolism. Rhonchi are lower-pitched continuous sounds which are commonly present. Early on, rhonchi reflect the bronchorrhea which often develops after smoke inhalation; later, they suggest secretions due to purulent bronchitis or pneumonia.

Crackles may be present in up to a third of patients with inhalation injury and presumably occur in all with severe parenchymal damage. Caused by the abrupt, explosive opening of closed lung units, these discontinuous sounds should suggest focal atelectasis and secretions as well as alveolar flooding by pulmonary edema or pus. Their characterization as "wet or dry" has no accurate relationship to the patient's intravascular volume status and may be misleading in this regard. Their timing as early (bronchitis) or late (pulmonary edema, fibrosis) during inspiration can be helpful. Crackles may accompany either permeability, low pressure (noncardiogenic) edema or hydrostatic (cardiogenic) edema, pneumonia, or partial atelectasis. Pleural friction rubs, usually heard later in the course, are uncommonly appreciated but might suggest either pleural-based pneumonia or pulmonary infarction.

Perhaps because of disproportionate overreliance on diagnostic tests, there has been surprisingly little recent discussion of the relationship of changes in the chest examination to alterations of the physiologic status of the patient. Phillips et al., however, warned of the importance of a "silent chest" as an ominous prognostic indicator in Cocoanut Grove victims.[34] This transition retains such significance: as in the acutely ill asthmatic, the clearing of wheezes with decreased intensity of breath sounds often represents marked deterioration, rather than clinical resolution. Airflow may be insufficient to generate a wheeze, and generalized closure of lung units may be too severe to allow opening crackles.

Facial Burns

The presence of facial burns has assumed particular historical importance in the clinical diagnosis of inhalation injury (Fig. 7-1).[42–45] Because of the frequency of facial burns, present in over half of patients with thermal injury,[46] however, this distribution of cutaneous burn has had only a variable relationship to respiratory damage. When the latter is diagnosed with objective tests, rather than clinical criteria, the positive predictive value of the presence of facial burns (i.e., the proportion of individuals with facial burns who prove to have inhalation injury) has ranged from 41 to 69 percent.[46] Moreover, the negative predictive value of this finding (i.e., the proportion of individuals at risk without facial burns who do not have inhalation injury) is only about 50 percent.[46] In some studies in which upper airway obstruction was documented endoscopically, neither the presence of facial burns nor the existence of pharyngeal inflammation at physical examination accurately differentiated those patients with upper airway obstruction. Singed nasal vibrissae or singed or lost eyebrows or beard also suggest, but do not establish, that an inhalation injury has occurred. Thus, the criterion of facial burns alone does not provide the level of certainty that is necessary for either diagnosing or excluding the presence of inhalation injury reliably.

Nevertheless, among varying series, the presence of facial burns has correlated with the development of objectively diagnosed inhalation injury, late onset pulmonary edema, and pneumonia. This apparent paradox can be reconciled if one recognizes the importance of burns of the "respiratory area," those second- and third-degree burns involving the area between the nose and lips (including full-thickness burns of the lips) and often extending to the neck. Such involvement connotes an inability to escape direct flame and/or entrapment and has been associated with the presence of large body surface area burns (which, themselves, portend an increased

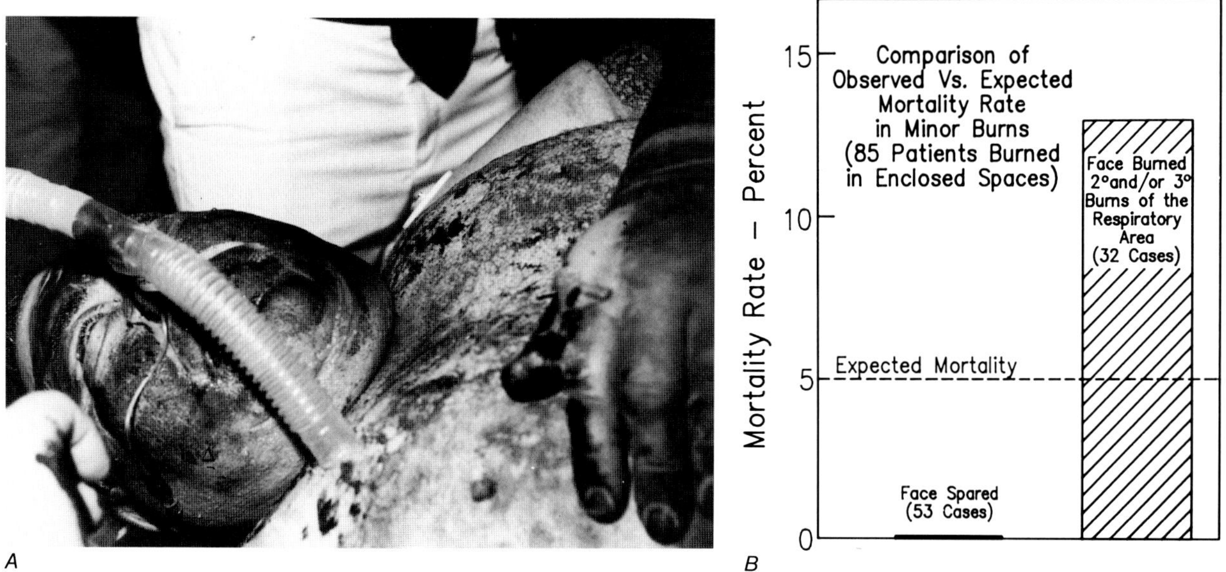

Figure 7-1 Although facial burns (*A*) are inexact predictors of inhalation injury, the presence of involvement of the "respiratory area" suggests a major risk (*B*). The high likelihood of rapid progression of edema requires early, elective endotracheal intubation. (*Reprinted with permission from Refs. 26 and 42.*)

risk of inhalation injury).[47–50] Burns with this distribution are more likely to be associated with upper airway edema and suggest a major airway emergency. Thus, when this more restricted criterion is used, facial burns retain their historically important diagnostic and therapeutic implications.

Pharyngeal Examination

Nasal and oropharyngeal inflammation identified by an experienced observer also suggests strongly that major pharyngeal edema is present and that the patient has an increased risk for upper airway obstruction. However, because of the limitations of subjective assessment of pharyngeal inflammation by physical examination alone, one must be cautious in interpreting such findings. We and others have found that in many patients the physical examination alone represents an inaccurate estimate of the presence or absence of upper airway edema and does not substitute for careful, direct visualization of airway patency with endoscopic procedures. These issues are addressed in more detail later in this chapter.

Carbonaceous Secretions

Carbonaceous sputum is often expectorated following smoke inhalation (Fig. 7-2). This finding is most accurately interpreted as a marker of exposure rather than as one synonymous with inhalation injury. Sooty secretions may be produced immediately after intense exposure or else have a more delayed appearance several days following injury, as airways are cleared spontaneously by the mucociliary escalator. This material may be produced for 2

Figure 7-2 Carbonaceous secretions, while "classic" predictors of inhalation injury are a nonspecific marker of exposure. (*Reprinted with permission from Ref. 26.*)

to 3 weeks following smoke inhalation and, apart from potential direct airway injuries due to inhalation of hot cinders, mechanical airway obstruction, and theoretically important prolongation of the residence time of adsorbed gaseous products, is of uncertain clinical significance.

Efforts to enhance diagnosis of inhalation injury through the examination of sputum for cytopathologic evidence of cellular deterioration and carbonaceous material ingested by alveolar macrophages has been performed[51–53] but is impractical for most settings. We have found that individuals with such abnormal cytologic changes in endotracheal aspirates already have otherwise obvious manifestations of respiratory disease, and the laboratory finding does not contribute substantially to management. Although grossly purulent sputum might herald superinfection, to date, the careful study of either expectorated sputum or aspirated tracheobronchial secretions has been unreliable in the early detection of parenchymal injury or pneumonia in this setting.

PREDICTION OF RESPIRATORY DAMAGE

A variety of clinical scoring systems has been developed in efforts to enhance diagnostic criteria for inhalation injury, to improve prognosticating ability, and to establish more consistent classifications of patients for clinical investigations. Typically, point values and relative weights are assigned for the presence of historical findings, pertinent signs or symptoms, and abnormal test results to estimate the likelihood and severity of inhalation injury. The advanced preparation with simple questionnaires and checklists may ensure the complete recording of such epidemiologic information and findings of initial examination and contribute to the application of such scores. Some of these classification schemes are summarized in Table 7-3.[3,30,54] In the initial evaluation of Cocoanut Grove victims, it was noted that such a clinical grade of respiratory involvement often correlated with the severity of roentgenographic abnormalities.[3] However, symptomatic severity exceeded that suggested by radiographic signs in approximately one-third of individuals. Subsequent reports have also documented variable relationships of these classifications to results of objective diagnostic tests and outcome.[44–49] Nevertheless, these approaches are informative for their systematic consideration of clinical observations and have been helpful in designing research protocols. Although some of these systems are clinically valuable at individual (originating) institutions, none are yet applied universally. Furthermore, there has been no validation of any scoring system through prospective study, nor have the advantages of their use been documented.

More promising has been the formal incorporation of clinical parameters into prediction equations which estimate the likelihood of inhalation injury. Such equations have been derived from the retrospective analyses of large populations at burn centers. While their value in prospectively assessing an individual patient is also presently unclear, they provide important insights about the interactions and relative impact of easily identified clinical factors upon prognosis. With the assistance of microcomputer software, complex analyses of an individual patient's risks can now be achieved at the bedside. In a comprehensive analysis by Shirani et al.,[29] the probability (p) of inhalation injury was determined from a stepwise logistic regression algorithm:

$$p = \frac{e^y}{1 + e^y}$$

where

$$y = 4.4165 + 1.61(\text{CLSP}) + 1.77(\text{FB}) + 0.0237(\text{TBS}) + 0.0268(\text{age})$$

This relationship takes into account the historically recognized significance of the presence (1 point) or

Table 7-3 Some Clinical Grading Systems of Smoke Inhalation Injury

Cocoanut Grove Victims[3]

Grade
0 No signs or symptoms referable to the respiratory tract.
1 Signs and symptoms limited to the upper respiratory passages, including mild laryngitis.
2 Evidence of involvement of the trachea and bronchi or abnormal signs in the lungs other than those of frank consolidation.
3 Dyspnea, cyanosis, wheezing or transient stridor, or frank signs of consolidation.
4 Evidence of extensive pulmonary involvement or of obstruction to the airways necessitating tracheotomy or resulting in severe asphyxia.

Recent Clinical Investigations — *Assigned Point Values*

Finding	Lund et al.[110]	Venus et al.[54]	Whitener et al.[77]	Clark et al.[30]
History	0–0.5			
Closed space	0.2	2	1	1
Flame/fume	0.05		1	
Choking/coughing	0.1			
Dyspnea		1		1
Altered consciousness	0.15			1
Hoarseness		1	1	1
Physical examination	0–0.5			
Facial burns	0.05	1	1	1
Singed nasal vibrissae	0.1	1		
Nasal/oropharyngeal		1	1	
Mucosal inflammation	0.15			
Carbonaceous sputum	0.2	1	1	1
Stridor		1		
Wheezing/auscultatory changes		1		1
Elevated carboxyhemoglobin			1	
Bronchoscopic evidence of injury	0–2		4	
Larynx	0.5			
Trachea-carina	0.5–1.5			
Bronchial involvement	1.5–2.0			
Xenon scan	0–1			
Slight-moderate, unilateral	0.5			
Bilateral involvement or severe unilateral	0.5–1.0			
Maximum total score	4.0	10	11	7
Score at which inhalation injury presumed	≥1	not stated	≥4	>2

absence (0 points) of closed-space setting (CLSP), facial burns (FB), burn size (TBS), and patient age.

Clark and coworkers have recently described a clinical score of the likelihood of smoke inhalation that subsequently was incorporated in a regression equation to predict the probability of death.[30] In this system, one point was assigned for the presence of each of the following characteristics: (1) enclosed space, entrapment in a residential or industrial fire; (2) carbonaceous sputum; (3) perioral (nose, lips, mouth, throat) facial burns; (4) confusion or other altered level of consciousness; (5) symptoms of respiratory distress ("sense of suffocation, choking, breathlessness, wheezing") or discomfort affecting the eyes or throat; (6) signs of respiratory distress (including tachypnea, labored breathing, and/or auscultatory abnormalities); (7) hoarseness or voice loss. Using this scale, scores ranged from 0 to 7 points; patients whose scores exceeded 2 points were considered to have "unequivocal smoke inhalation." Interestingly, the clinical score derived in this manner correlated with the estimated COHb concentration at the time of exposure (Figs. 7-3, 7-4). The latter was determined from the direct measurement of COHb at the time of presentation and, using a previously validated nomogram (Fig. 7-5), back-calculation to the COHb level at the time of exposure. When the sympton score of Clark et al. was coupled with other clinical characteristics of 128 carefully described patients, stepwise linear logistic regression analysis showed the following equation to best predict the probability of death:

$$p = \frac{e^z}{1 + e^z}$$

where

$$z = -7.9 + 0.78(\text{symptom score}) + 0.094(\text{BSA}) + 0.034(\text{age})$$

Using similar multivariate analytical methods, Heimbach and coworkers have reported that the combination of COHb levels exceeding 10 percent, carbonaceous sputum, and enclosed-space setting have a 96-percent correlation with bronchoscopically diagnosed inhalation injury.[55–57] When fewer clinical criteria were found, in their referral population the accuracy of clinical prediction worsened (70 percent for the presence of two positive criteria, 36 percent for one only).

As can be seen from these experiences which confirm intuitive impressions, the presence of multiple clinical risk factors increases the likelihood of inhalation injury and amplifies the power of the bedside evaluation considerably. More complete determination of the usefulness of these and other

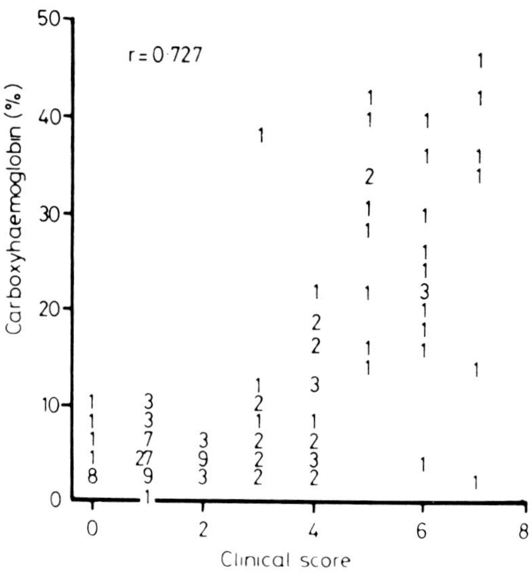

Figure 7-3 The clinical score of the likelihood of smoke inhalation correlates with the carboxyhemoglobin concentration (estimated) at the time of exposure. Numbers denote numbers of patients; score ranges from 0 to 7. (See text for details.) (*Reprinted with permission from Ref. 30.*)

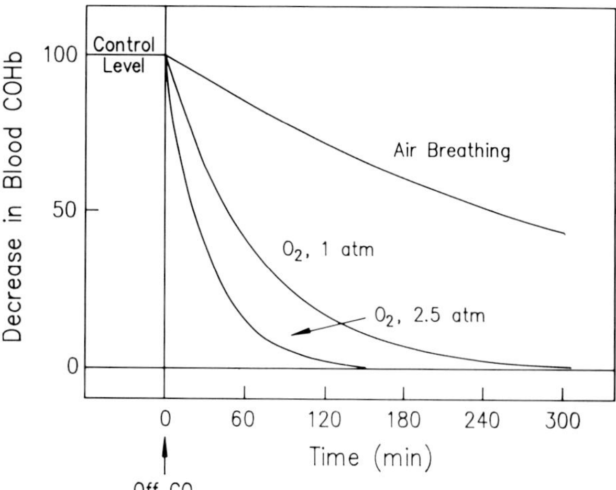

Figure 7-4 Changes in arterial carboxyhemoglobin measurements vary as a function of time, during breathing of air or oxygen. Slopes of such curves might assist either estimates of the severity of initial exposures or predictions of the expected times by which carboxyhemoglobin should be cleared with appropriate oxygen therapy. (*Adapted with permission from Ref. 62*)

predictors which might be applied to individual patients still requires prospective study. It seems likely that the early computer-assisted estimation of the likelihood of inhalation injury employing such epidemiologic data and, when known, other details of the fire scenario (Chap. 19) will further improve clinical assessments. Such determinations might contribute to the early and accurate triage of injured patients into groups with low, intermediate, and high risks for respiratory injury and influence allocations of critical care resources.[30]

INHALATION INJURY: COMMON DIAGNOSTIC TESTS

At one major burn center where diagnosis was based upon objective criteria, approximately one-fourth of patients with "classic" risk factors for inhalation injury, carefully documented on a regular basis by experienced personnel, did not prove to have it.[29] When evaluation is performed episodically by less experienced individuals, the accuracy of clinical assessment alone might be expected to be considerably lower. At a major consensus conference regarding inhalation injury a decade ago, the diagnosis of inhalation injury on the basis of clinical criteria alone was equated to a coin toss.

Although clinical assessments of risk factors permit specific diagnoses in some patients and lead to worthwhile modifications of therapy in many others, accurate detection of inhalation injury and identification of exposed individuals who have not sustained significant respiratory damage have been advanced further by the widespread availability of several objective tests. Useful in both community hospitals and tertiary referral centers, these studies permit prompt, on-the-scene diagnoses and, in many instances, also present immediate guides to early management. Moreover, such objective tests may be particularly useful in the serial reevaluation of patients with cutaneous burns, inhalation injury, and their combinations.

Co-oximetry and arterial blood gas analysis are provided by most pathology laboratories, while standard chest roentgenography is also available routinely. Fiberoptic bronchoscopy and experienced individuals skilled in its use are also generally available to most practitioners via pulmonary, otolaryngology, or surgery associates. More dependent upon supportive resources and generally requiring the activation of additional personnel, radionuclide scanning and pulmonary function studies are other objective procedures of proven value in the early assessment of patients with possible inhalation injury.

Measurement of Asphyxiants

Although the clinical history and details of exposure might strongly suggest intoxication due to tissue asphyxiants, measurement of carbon monoxide and, more recently, of cyanide, are essential components of acute evaluations of patients at risk.

Carbon Monoxide Because of the priority of carbon monoxide (CO) intoxication as the primary cause of early deaths from smoke inhalation, COHb levels must be measured by co-oximetry in all smoke inhalation victims.[58] To this end, portable breath analyzers which can detect carbon monoxide have been useful in both the field and emergency room screening of exposed individuals.[59] Co-oximetry is performed more universally. Although there are general relationships between the presence of particular signs and symptoms and arterial COHb levels (Chap. 9), these can vary considerably; in any individual patient, this measurement cannot be predicted reliably on the basis of clinical findings alone.[58–65] In the recent analysis of a 5-year experience encompassing 247 patients, it has been suggested that psychometric testing is a more accurate measure of the severity of CO intoxication.[65] It has been well established that a normal or elevated Pa_{O_2} does not exclude severe CO intoxication. Moreover, the hemoglobin oxygen saturation reported with arterial blood gas results is usually determined by nomogram and infrequently represents direct measurement. This information does not take into consideration COHb, methemoglobin, or sulfhemoglobin levels, all of which may be elevated after smoke inhalation (depending upon the fuels burned). Thus, unless it has been measured directly, a normal Sa_{O_2} might be reported erroneously in the presence of carbon monoxide intoxication.

Several factors influence the COHb level, detracting somewhat from its potential usefulness in early diagnosis. The measurement is altered by the time elapsed after exposure and the predictable, rapid falls with CO displacement by the oxygen therapy which, ideally, is initiated empirically immediately at the scene of exposure (Fig. 7-4). This dynamic aspect makes the designation of a single COHb measurement as a diagnostic value difficult (and inherently unreliable); approaches to this dilemma vary among institutions. Nomograms are available which permit estimation of the CO concentration encountered at the fire and extrapolation of the time necessary to clear current CO levels with oxygen therapy (Fig. 7-5). This information is helpful and may enhance appraisals of either prognosis or predictions of other respiratory injury. Clark et al. have found that COHb concentration at exposure might, in the absence of other clinical information, assist prediction of mortality[30]: this estimated concentration derived from nomogram has been shown to be a better predictor of outcome than the COHb measurement at the time of hospital presentation.[30] The presumptive diagnosis of smoke inhalation has been based arbitrarily upon COHb concentrations exceeding 10 percent at the time of exposure.[30]

Just as COHb levels must be measured in all exposed individuals, it is desirable to monitor serial measurements confirming appropriate falls of COHb with treatment. The presence of elevations document one important, treatable manifestation of inhalation injury and thus, by definition, has a high positive predictive value. Although among individual series such measurements have correlated to varying degrees with the presence of nasopharyngoscopically identified upper airway edema[66] and pulmonary edema and have suggested that the length of hospital stay will be prolonged, even high CO levels have had an inexact relationship to the

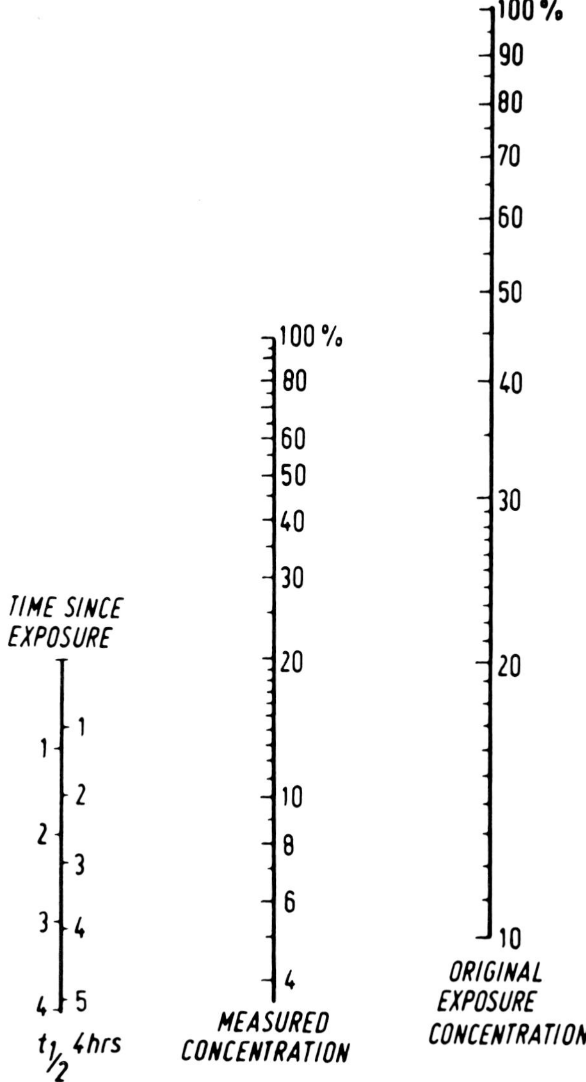

Figure 7-5 Knowledge of the COHb concentration at the time of presentation and the time interval from smoke exposure may allow estimation of the initial severity of CO exposure. (Left-hand time scale used if oxygen has been administered.)

development of other respiratory complications. Importantly, the presence of a low or normal COHb measurement is unhelpful in ruling out inhalation injury. In one series, fewer than 10 percent of individuals with objectively proven inhalation injury had elevated COHb measurements at the time of hospitalization, reflecting the effects of transportation time and prompt reductions of COHb levels with supplemental oxygen therapy. COHb levels may also be increased in cigar and cigarette smokers and city dwellers, but these elevations are usually mild (<10 percent) and should pose little diagnostic problem.

Cyanide Recently, Clark and others have also demonstrated a potentially useful relationship between COHb level and that of another less readily (and, historically, less often) measured toxic products, cyanide.[67] Others have not substantiated this relationship.[68] The presence of an elevated COHb level and persistent acidemia or obtundation that seems inappropriate for the level of CO might suggest concomitant cyanide intoxication and imply that empiric treatment for cyanide toxicity be considered. Rapid detection of cyanide by means of newly available assays assists this evaluation considerably and should be performed on a more regular basis in smoke inhalation victims.

Using the Conway diffusion technique,[69] Symington and colleagues measured cyanide (CN), thiocyanate, and COHb levels in 144 patients with clinically suspected smoke inhalation injury or smoke exposure.[70] Twenty-two percent of their patients had elevated CN levels, including 12 with "lethal" levels (greater than 1.0 mg/L) in the presence of sublethal COHb measurements. Eight of these latter individuals died. CN levels did not correlate with burn size (mean BSA 33 percent). In addition, 90 percent of 43 other burn victims who were dead on arrival had "abnormal" CN levels, and two-thirds of them had "lethal" levels. These observations are consistent with previous epidemiologic studies of the role of cyanide poisoning in burn deaths and support routine measurements of this asphyxiant in all patients at risk.

Arterial Blood Gas Analysis

Arterial blood gas analysis is another fundamental diagnostic study which must be performed in all patients clinically suspected of smoke inhalation injury. In addition, serial measurements are essential to objectively assess the course of respiratory involvement and to guide its management. A simple but clinically useful classification of acute respiratory failure as "hypoxemic failure," "hypoventilatory failure," or a mixed (combined) pattern can be performed on the basis of blood gas measurements and can facilitate early recognition of respiratory problems as they develop. Hypoxemic failure, characterized by a large physiologic shunt, is associated typically with the adult respiratory distress syndrome. Acute hypoventilatory failure, defined by presence of an elevated Pa_{CO_2} with respiratory acidosis, most often suggests upper and/or lower airway obstruction. Combinations of these patterns early in the course suggest severe respiratory injury with ominous prognosis.

Oxygenation Arterial hypoxemia, an increased alveolar-arterial oxygen gradient [(A-a) D_{O_2}], and reduced hemoglobin oxygen saturation (Sa_{O_2}) have been shown to accompany smoke inhalation, cutaneous burn injury, and their combinations.[71–81] Transient hypoxemia (mean Pa_{O_2}, 71 mmHg) has been documented following the exposure of 21 fire fighters to dense smoke.[71] Nineteen of these individuals were asymptomatic, and Pa_{O_2} normalized (to 91 mmHg) within 20 hours. Richards has been credited with the initial report of reduced arterial hemoglobin oxygen saturation in burn victims.[72] Twelve of 19 patients had reduced Sa_{O_2} (range, 81 to 88 percent) that persisted from 3 to 7 days after injury, often in the absence of apparent pneumonia or pathologic changes. Baxter reported that Pa_{O_2} and Sa_{O_2} were reduced following increasingly large surface burns and failed to improve to the degree expected during the administration of 100% oxygen, observing that "moderate arterial desaturation will often be present until resuscitation is begun."[73] Luce et al. confirmed that the (A-a) D_{O_2} was increased (>15 torr) during the first day after inhalation injury and worsened progressively.[74] Epstein et al. reported that the 17 hypoxemic individuals among 28 previously well young adults had larger cutaneous burns, more severe facial involvement, abnormal chest roentgenograms, and higher mortality.[75] Oxygenation failed to improve with administration of 95% oxygen in 10 of these patients, documenting the presence of severe shunt. Petroff et al. confirmed that admission Pa_{O_2} was lower and (A-a) D_{O_2} higher in patients with inhalation injury compared with those with burns alone.[76] More recently, Whitener and coworkers noted reduced Pa_{O_2} (room air breathing, 9 and 58 hours after injury) in patients who had large burns or burns with inhalation injury compared with those with small burns.[77] Shunt fraction increased during the initial 58 hours in patients with combined cutaneous and respiratory injury, with subsequent worsening of oxygenation paralleling deteriorations of pulmonary function measurements.

Thus, the presence of hypoxemia presents simultaneously an indicator of injury and a guide for supplemental oxygen therapy. Although hypoxemia may occur in acutely traumatized individuals without inhalation injury, this finding should be regarded as a sign of respiratory damage in burn victims until proven otherwise. Arterial oxygen tension is often normal during early evaluations of patients who have sustained significant inhalation injury.[78] Because the delayed onset of hypoxemia is a common problem, initial measurements of Pa_{O_2} represent insensitive indicators. In addition, although nonsurvivors often have worsened oxygenation early in the course,[79] such measurements do not predict outcome accurately. The patients of Whitener et al. who had smoke inhalation alone could not be differentiated by their initial Pa_{O_2} measurements 9 hours after exposure.[77] Although the patients of Moylan et al. with objectively documented respiratory injury had lower admission Pa_{O_2} measurements, these were all $\geqslant$74 mmHg,[46] a level which is deceptively high and which might be overlooked in a busy triage setting. Even more disturbingly, Hudson found that the onset of hypoxemia could be delayed for as much as 48 hours after admission and occurred despite the absence of either clinical or roentgenographic evidence of pulmonary edema.[80]

As with COHb determinations, arterial oxygen measurements must be interpreted not only absolutely but also with regard to their appropriateness for the inspired oxygen concentration (FI_{O_2}). The latter can be estimated from application of the alveolar gas equation or its simple, bedside form [$PA_{O_2} = (7)(FI_{O_2})(100) - Pa_{CO_2}$], from the use of nomograms, or from the Pa_{O_2}/FI_{O_2} index. The latter has recently been incorporated as an estimate of severity in a revised clinical classification of the adult respiratory distress syndrome.[83] With such estimates the severity and physiologic mechanism of hypoxemia can be assessed readily. Severe hypoxemia unimproved by supplemental oxygen suggests shunt due to pulmonary edema or major atelectasis, while milder hypoxemia (improved with oxygen administration) implies less severe ventilation/perfusion mismatch ($\dot{V}/\dot{Q}$), most often due to airways obstruction.[82] Heimbach and Waeckerle have reported that a reduced Pa_{O_2}/FI_{O_2} index is an early indicator of respiratory injury, with a ratio less than 300 suggesting "impending pulmonary problems," and one less than 250 representing an indication for "vigorous pulmonary therapy."[28] Serial changes of this index in carefully evaluated patients with smoke inhalation, cutaneous burns, and their combination are shown in Fig. 7-6.[84] Some investigators have suggested that the Pa_{O_2}/FI_{O_2} index might help to predict outcome, but this has generally been unreliable in individual patients with catastrophic respiratory failure. Nishimura and Hiranuma reported this ratio was normal at admission in survivors, declined rapidly to a nadir by the fourth day, and then improved; whereas nonsurvivors had worsened oxygenation throughout the course.[79]

Although hemoglobin oxygen saturation can be monitored noninvasively by means of pulse oximetry, there are practical limitations in this setting: currently available units do not permit the distinction between oxyhemoglobin and COHb, resulting in overestimates of the Sa_{O_2}.[85] In addition, potential problems with reduced local perfusion or edema

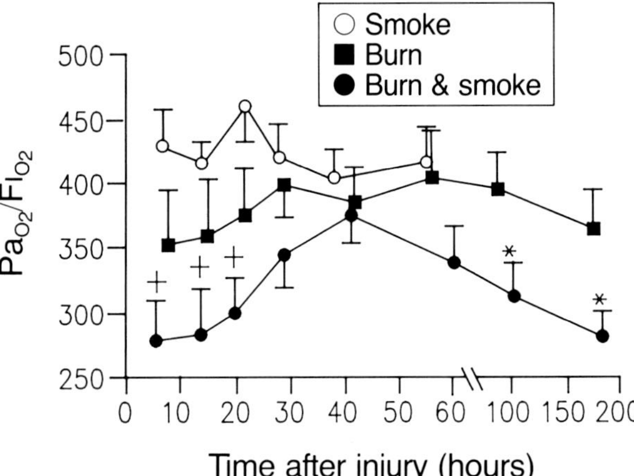

Figure 7-6 Serial managements of Pa_{O_2}/FI_{O_2} ratios in patients with smoke inhalation only, burns only (67% BSA), and both burns (55% BSA) and inhalation injury. (*Adapted with permission from Ref. 84.*)

which might hinder the proper fixation of the oximeter probe can lessen its usefulness even after COHb levels have fallen.

Alveolar Ventilation In most patients, the Pa_{CO_2} should be normal or reduced at the time of presentation. Alveolar hyperventilation will often accompany acute exposure and influences interpretation of the Pa_{O_2}, since an otherwise normal Pa_{O_2} might be inappropriately low if it occurs in the presence of marked hypocarbia. When documented, initial Pa_{CO_2} measurements have usually been similar in burn victims with and without inhalation injury. Serial measurements in one report have revealed progressive rises of Pa_{CO_2} after the sixth hospital day, with hypercapnia occurring after 8 days (despite therapy) in patients with fatal injuries.[79] A normal Pa_{CO_2} in a tachypneic, hyperpneic patient has the same ominous connotations which might be identified in an asthmatic during an acute exacerbation of airways disease: this finding is inappropriate for the clinical situation and identifies a fatiguing patient with little reserve and incipient respiratory failure. Similarly, even mild alveolar hypoventilation, defined by an elevated Pa_{CO_2}, must be regarded as a potential major risk; this finding might require intubation and prompt initiation of mechanical ventilation because of the additive dangers posed by combined respiratory and burn-related metabolic acidosis.

Alveolar hypoventilation in burn victims is often multifactorial, with components of upper airway obstruction, respiratory muscle weakness, splinting from pain, diminished effort, and/or concomitant administration of sedative/hypnotic agents and narcotic analgesics, as well as severe pulmonary injury. The related respiratory acidosis is particularly hazardous because of its potential superimposition upon the metabolic acidosis of burn shock. Acute alveolar hypoventilation might also indicate pneumothorax, cardiogenic edema, exacerbated chronic obstructive pulmonary disease (COPD), or the preterminal stages of adult respiratory distress syndrome (ARDS). When hypoxemia and/or acute hypoventilation occurs in patients already treated with mechanical ventilation, an array of problems must be considered immediately.[86a] Alveolar hyperventilation can also accompany the mild hyperchloremic metabolic acidosis induced with topical mafenide administration or, later in the clinical course, suggests sepsis, pneumonia, or pulmonary embolism. Respiratory alkalosis is commonly induced iatrogenically in patients treated with ventilators. Thus, careful interpretation of measurements from arterial blood gases within the context of the other physiologic events occurring in the patient is essential.

Comprehensive experience with transcutaneous measurements of Pa_{CO_2} has not been reported in this setting. Capnography, continuous monitoring of expired CO_2, can provide added insights about dead space[86] and alveolar ventilation, but its role in burn victims has not been elucidated.

Chest Roentgenograms

A spectrum of focal and diffuse roentgenographic abnormalities has been described in burn victims with inhalation injury.[87–95] These radiologic patterns are reviewed in detail in Chap. 8. Although some authors have reported the presence of relatively subtle roentgen signs of disease, most series have underscored that the chest roentgenogram is an insensitive early indicator of the presence of pulmonary injury. This discrepancy probably reflects differences in patient populations (e.g., smoke inhalation only versus smoke inhalation with burn) and the timing of studies after exposure, as well as institutional differences in the thresholds used to call abnormalities. Admission chest roentgenograms are generally normal in this setting, and early pulmonary edema is an especially uncommon finding, usually limited to patients who are trapped in environments with very high concentrations of noxious gaseous products. In our review of 191 patients admitted to the Baltimore Regional Burn Center with risk factors for inhalation injury, only 5 had abnormal initial chest roentgenograms.[94] In three of them, pneumothoraces had complicated intravenous access procedures or placement of artificial airways, while a fourth patient had a pleural effusion. Only one of these individuals had pulmonary edema at the time of presentation. A similar experience was reported following the Las Vegas Hotel fires, when minor roentgenographic abnormalities were found in only 2 to 7 percent of patients, and none had abnormalities at the time of presentation to the hospital.[93] This paucity of early roentgenographic abnormalities has led some authors to suggest that chest roentgenograms be reserved only for hospitalized patients.[86] When either more severely injured patients are surveyed or more subtle roentgenographic abnormalities are sought, it is possible that the predictive value of the admission chest roentgenogram might be improved. Lee and O'Connell have noted that 33 of 44 (73 percent) patients hospitalized after a major fire disaster had abnormal studies, with bronchial wall thickening (87 percent) and subglottic edema (39 percent), the most commonly identified abnormalities.[95a] Recently, in an elegant study, Peitzman and coworkers developed a grading system for radiographic abnormalities and documented abnormal findings in 84 percent of their severely ill burned patients (two-thirds of whom had fatal injuries), within 48 hours of smoke inhalation.[95b] The radiographic grade of severity correlated with increases of extravascular lung water and decreases of static pulmonary compliance. When any roentgenographic abnormality was observed, nearly all (92 percent) patients had other abnormal objective evidence of pulmonary dysfunction. The predictive value of these findings in patients with less severe burns requires further evaluation.

Because it might help to exclude otherwise unsuspected thoracic injuries sustained at the burn scene and provides an important baseline for subsequent evaluations of patients (in whom there are relatively few other objective means of monitoring), the chest roentgenogram remains a useful early diagnostic procedure. If abnormalities are demonstrated on the admission chest roentgenogram, the clinician should assume that respiratory injury has occurred and that these abnormalities are likely to progress, particularly if accompanied by large cutaneous burns and large resuscitative fluid requirements. From the outset, such abnormalities might present earlier indications for hemodynamic monitoring and the rigorous exclusion of concomitant cardiac injury and other acute complications.

We have found that serial measurements from the chest roentgenogram can yield valuable early monitoring information which might lessen the need for invasive tests (Table 7-4).[94] The width of the vascular pedicle (VP), the mediastinal silhouette of the great vessels, has been shown to correlate with circulating blood volume and assists in the radiographic categorization of patterns of pulmonary edema.[96] We identified 42 burn victims in whom reproducible technique of serial chest roentgenograms permitted reliable comparisons of the VP (Table 7-4) on their serial films. In 24 patients who did not develop pulmonary edema during their courses, the VP measured on the second hospital day was similar to that on admission. However, in 18 others who developed pulmonary edema during the first three hospital days, coinciding with the period of mobilization of burn edema fluid, the VP had widened significantly during the initial 24 hours. Importantly, none of the patients had pulmonary edema at the time pedicle enlargement had been

Table 7-4 Roentgenographic Prediction of Pulmonary Edema

	Pulmonary edema* (n = 18)	No pulmonary edema (n = 34)	p
Age (year)	44.2 ± 1.57	28.9 ± 18.1	<0.025
Body surface area burn	43.1 ± 19.9	31.6 ± 17.7	NS
Resuscitative volume, initial 24 h (L)	16.0 ± 9.7	8.9 ± 4.7	<0.005
Vascular pedicle width (cm) during initial 24 h			
Baseline	5.9 ± 0.9†	6.0 ± 1.0	NS
Follow-up	6.9 ± 1.2†	5.8 ± 0.7	<0.001

*Onset during initial 24–72 hours of injury.
†$p < 0.001$.

demonstrated, and 12 of the 13 patients in whom VP width changed greater than 1 cm during the first day subsequently developed pulmonary edema. These findings strongly implicated excessive fluid resuscitation in the genesis of this early form of pulmonary edema and permit the noninvasive identification of individuals at risk for this problem. Interestingly, such net fluid retention during the initial 48 hours of crystalloid resuscitation recently has been shown to be an accurate predictor of burn mortality, with 230 cm^3/kg lean body mass discriminating survivors from nonsurvivors.[97] Since this observation, such objective analysis of the chest roentgenogram has been incorporated in decision making regarding adjustments of fluid administration in patients at the Baltimore Regional Burn Center.

As in other critical care settings, many authors have also documented the importance of serial chest roentgenograms in detection of not only late onset respiratory injuries but also of iatrogenic problems related to intravenous access procedures, invasive diagnostic studies, endotracheal tube malposition, and mechanical ventilatory support. These applications are considered in further detail in Chap. 8 and 16.

Endoscopic Procedures

Because of the early, primary onset of tracheobronchial abnormalities in the pathogenesis of inhalation injury, bronchoscopic findings antedate abnormalities of chest roentgenograms and arterial blood gases and can be particularly useful diagnostically. In addition, because of the priority of objective assessment of the upper airway in this setting (and the potential need for prompt endotracheal intubation), endoscopy yields direct information of immediate therapeutic relevance. Laryngoscopy was performed in Cocoanut Grove victims[2]: in those with fatal injuries, patchy adherent debris; edema; and reddening of the hypopharynx, larynx, and epiglottis were found. Two patients had swelling of the tongue, while in "several" others, the larynx could not be visualized because of the severity of edema. Bedside laryngoscopic examination remains a useful, universally available tool for the emergency evaluation of patients at risk for inhalation injury. However, because of the potential risks of worsening pharyngeal obstruction by traumatizing the airway with the instrument, such examinations must be performed by skilled personnel. At training institutions in particular, this most critical aspect of examination is too often performed by the least experienced individuals. The advent of the fiberoptic era has improved capability for safe assessment of the airway. An extensive endoscopic experience in persons with smoke inhalation injury has established the value of this procedure.[46,56,66,98–108]

Fiberoptic Bronchoscopy Fiberoptic bronchoscopy permits the immediate, direct visualization of airway injury and has become a definitive, final arbiter of the presence of inhalation injury at many centers. This widely available test may demonstrate a spectrum of mucosal and extramucosal abnormalities (Table 7-5, Fig. 7-7). The frequency of these findings vary with the reporting institution, its referral populations, and the degree of detail described by individual endoscopists. There are variable classification schemes for description of the severity of pharyngeal and endobronchial changes,

Table 7-5 Endoscopic Findings Associated with Acute Inhalation Injury

I. Categorization of involvement
   A. Mucosal: erythema, edema, ulceration, hemorrhage
   B. Submucosal: hemorrhage
   C. Extramucosal: carbonaceous material (soot, cinders) secretions, casts, blood
II. Anatomic level of injury
   A. Supraglottic
      1. Nasopharyngeal
      2. Oropharyngeal
      3. Hypopharyngeal, epiglottic
   B. Glottic
   C. Subglottic
      1. Tracheal
      2. Bronchial
III. Grading severity of injury
   A. Arbitrary scales: mild, moderate, severe
   B. Degree of airway obstruction

and at some centers the addition of Polaroid photography or motion pictures obtained with compact video cameras has further enhanced diagnostic as well as investigational uses of these procedures. In patients with severe injuries, global damage to the upper and lower airways may be present. Hunt et al. have described obliteration of recognizable anatomic landmarks (e.g., pyriform sinuses) and massive swelling of the epiglottis and arytenoepiglottic and ventricular folds.[99] In one-fourth of his patients, visualization of the glottis was difficult because of the severity of this edema. Subglottic changes have included soot deposition and inflammation ranging from the trachea to subsegmental bronchi. Some authors have associated the presence of these objective signs of airway injury with prolonged entrapment, violent explosion, or recognized noxious fume release at the scene of exposure but have also recorded that such "classic" clinical predictors do not identify all individuals with bronchoscopically documented respiratory injury.[92,96,99,103] True thermal injury of the proximal airways seems to correlate best with the history of an explosion, flash, or steam burns and with clinically obvious head and neck involvement. Some endoscopists have associated mucosal discoloration and focal hemorrhage with a history of blasts and explosion-related injuries. Mucosal pallor has been observed following blasts or during systemic hypotension and might lead to an underestimation of the severity of airway involvement.[92,96]

Complications of endoscopy are unusual when it is performed in the appropriately monitored circumstances by experienced personnel. Topical anesthesia with lidocaine or, in the presence of significant nasopharyngeal edema, cocaine is achieved easily in most patients. Rigorous technical expertise and meticulous attention to detail are essential to ensure safe examinations in this setting. Despite the absence of major procedure-related complications in large published series, unpublished fatalities have occurred with injudiciously attempted endoscopy. Clinicians must recognize the importance of not attempting to bypass an obviously obstructed proximal airway because of the risks of exacerbating airway edema by mechanical trauma with the bronchoscope. Rather, if lower airway examination is contemplated, an endotracheal tube must first be placed in order to ensure a patent upper airway. Concurrent with examination, the bronchoscope may be used to achieve otherwise unfeasible intubations by functioning as a stylette.[99,101,102,105–107] With this approach, the bronchoscope is passed through the edematous supraglottic and glottic apertures and the endotracheal tube is passed over this instrument. As with other objective diagnostic tests, serial bronchoscopy has proved quite useful in this setting. Fiberoptic bronchoscopy has been performed safely in children with inhalation injury but is potentially more hazardous because of the size of the pediatric airway. The availability of smaller instruments has been helpful in this regard, but in general, endoscopy has a more limited role in children.

Fiberoptic Nasopharyngoscopy We have had particular interest in the use of the fiberoptic nasopharyngoscope.[66,104,108] The small size (4 mm in diameter) of this instrument makes it quite suitable for examining narrowed, edematous airways without compromising the patient's respiratory status. Dur-

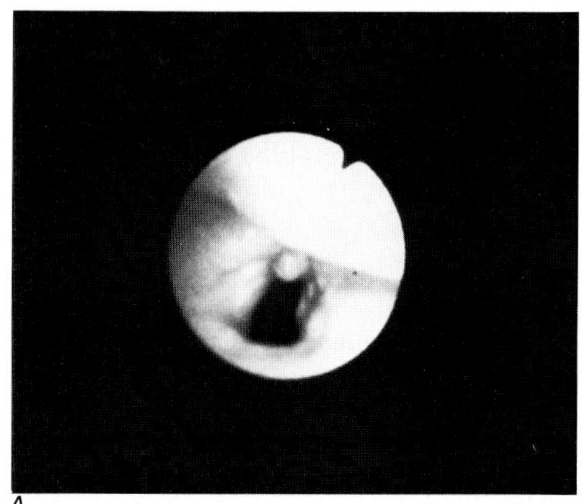

A

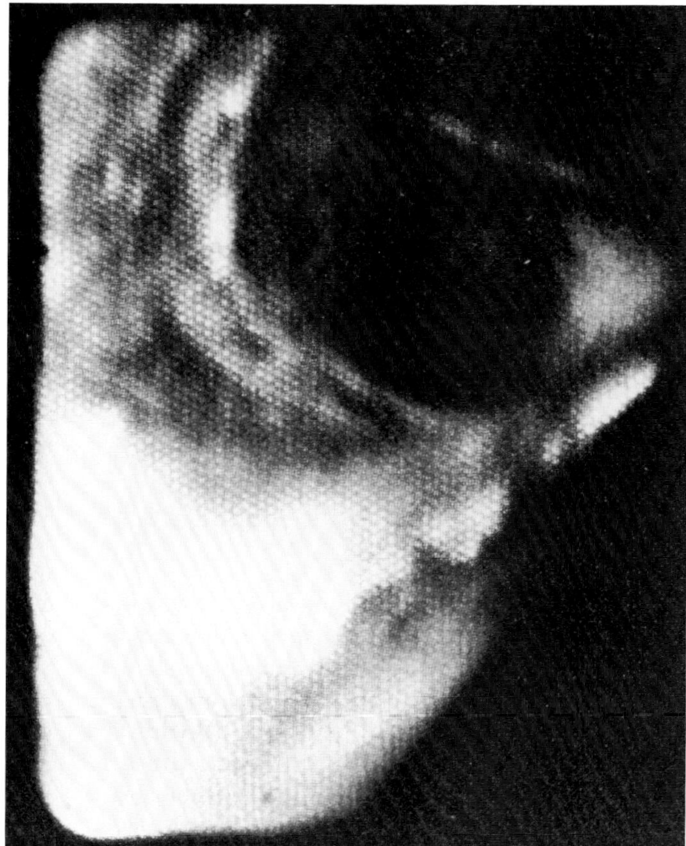

B

Figure 7-7 Diagnostic bronchoscopic demonstration of upper airway edema (*A*) and tracheobronchial smoke inhalation injury (*B*). (*B is reprinted with permission from Ref. 99.*)

ing a 4-year period, we performed 235 fiberoptic nasopharyngoscopies at the time of patients' initial emergency room or burn unit presentations.[108] There were no complications of these procedures, and they provided sufficient information to guide management in all patients. During this period, only one individual required fiberoptic bronchoscopy; life-threatening upper airway obstruction necessitated bronchoscopic intubation after other attempts had failed.

This experience has shown a consistent spectrum of upper airway responses to acute injury (Table 7-6). The severity of these upper airway inflammatory changes has correlated with the presence of facial burns and with admission measurements of elevated COHb concentrations.[66] Although edema of the true vocal folds is present occasionally, in most instances the predominant anatomic changes occur in the immediate supraglottic area: in general, edematous, boggy, mucosa prolapses during inspiration to occlude the airway. Epiglottic edema may sometimes be severe and, when this finding is present, assumes a diagnostic and therapeutic importance similar to that of acute infectious epiglottitis. More often, obscuration of the arytenoid eminences is seen as an early development and is frequently associated with edema of the interarytenoid area. The propensity for involvement of this location may have particular functional significance, because this site immediately overlies the posterior arytenoid

Table 7-6 Fiberoptic Nasopharyngoscopy in Acute Smoke Inhalation Injury

	Mild (n = 29)	Moderate–severe (n = 13)	Total
Clinical characteristics			
Percent BSA burn	17.9 ± 15.7	23.0 ± 15.5	
Facial burns, n(%)	19 (65.5%)	9 (69.2%)	
Pharyngeal inflammation, n(%)	4 (13.8%)	3 (23.1%)	
Nasopharyngoscopy results			
No inflammatory changes	5	0	5
Mucosal inflammation present			
Pharynx	5†	8†	13
Epiglottis	15	4 (3)*	19
Arytenoids	17 (2)*‡	11 (4)*	28
True vocal cords	4	3	7
Extramucosal carbon present	3	3	6

*Numbers in parentheses are the number of patients who required endotracheal intubation.

†$p < 0.01$.

‡Follow-up nasopharyngoscopy in two patients in Group A demonstrated progression from mild to severe supraglottic edema (Group B), which required intubation.

muscles, which are responsible for abduction of the vocal cords. Thus, focal injury to this area might interfere with normal motion at the cricoarytenoid joint, leading to physiologic upper airway obstruction even in the absence of massive upper airway swelling. These changes are generally accompanied by varying degrees of mucosal hyperemia, and deposition of upper airway carbonaceous material is often present as well. Occasionally, large accumulations of soot might mechanically obstruct the glottis, but this event is unusual.

Serial nasopharyngoscopic examinations are usually very well tolerated and provide useful information.[104] Not surprisingly, progressive edema of the upper airway is associated with an increased body surface area of burn and an increased rate of resuscitative fluid administration (Fig. 7-8).[104] Patients who have anatomically stable upper airways generally have experienced smaller burns and, consequently, have received less fluid. Interestingly, the introduction (and immediate availability) of such objective means of direct airway monitoring with endoscopy not only ensures prompt, accurate identification of burn victims with life-threatening pharyngeal obstruction but also lessens the need for empiric intubation of those who do not. In this way, late-onset problems due to mechanical airway trauma or synergistic damage caused by combined effects of tube trauma and inhalation injury of the trachea might be avoided.[109]

Later during the course endoscopy can contribute substantially to decisions about the timing of the removal of endotracheal tubes in patients with inhalation injury. We have performed fiberoptic nasopharyngoscopy immediately before and after extubation and have deferred extubation when examination reveals continued prolapse of edematous supraglottic mucosa around the tube. On the other hand, a well-visualized "glottic chink," demonstrating a patent supraglottic and glottic lumen adjacent to the tube, suggests (but does not always guarantee) that extubation will be successful. Following removal of the tube, the patient is reexamined to confirm a patent airway and assess the severity of residual supraglottic and laryngeal abnormalities. Patterns of injury due to smoke inhalation are, in our experience, quite distinctive from airway trauma due to endotracheal tubes. Nasopharyngoscopic examinations following endotracheal intubation in burn victims significantly more often demonstrate glottic abnormalities, often with "kissing ulcerations" of the true vocal cords, bilat-

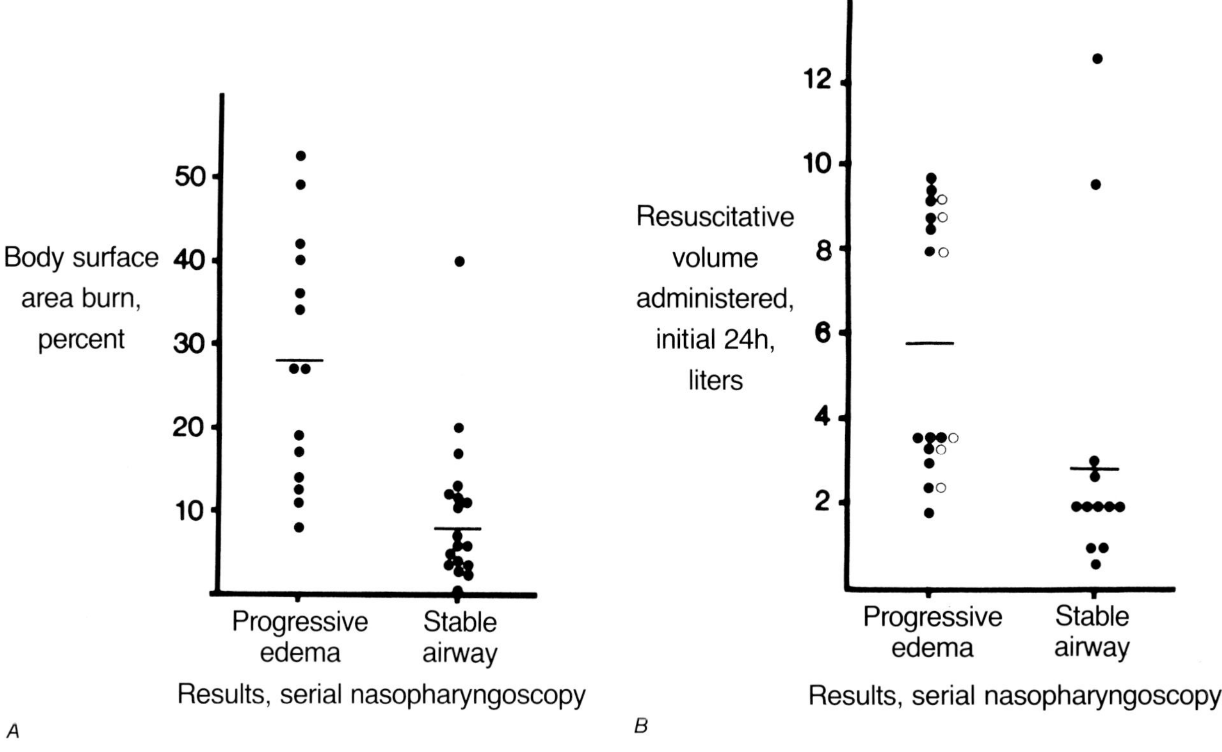

Figure 7-8 The severity and progression of upper airway inflammatory changes seen at fiberoptic nasopharyngoscopy correlate with the extent of cutaneous burn (*A*) and with the need for rapid administration of large volumes of resuscitative fluid (*B*). (*Reprinted with permission from Ref. 104.*)

eral arytenoid ulcerations, and, occasionally, anterior commissural injury.[108] Lund et al. have recommended evaluation of the anatomic status of the upper airway in all burn victims intubated for longer than 3 weeks, with bronchoscopy the preferred mode of examination.[110]

General Observations Experience at multiple centers has confirmed that supraglottic airway injury is generally more severe than that sustained by the tracheobronchial tree. These findings support the important protective role of the glottis during acute exposure and are consistent with reflex laryngospasm demonstrated in animal models. Furthermore, this typical distribution of inflammatory changes has practical implications for the extent of airway examination that should be performed routinely. For example, when careful endoscopic inspection of the pharynx has shown either no injury or only very minor abnormalities, continuation of the procedure to complete a tracheobronchial survey may not be necessary because its yield is likely to be exceedingly low. If the most important information needed for acute management decisions is gleaned from upper endoscopy alone (with demonstration, for example, of severe edema which documents the need for endotracheal intubation), the benefits of completing a lower airway examination for diagnostic purposes are questionable, particularly in view of the nonspecificity of management of the latter. The tracheobronchial survey of already-intubated patients who have acceptable oxygenation is usually rapidly and safely performed. Although diagnostic of inhalation injury, however, the finding of tracheobronchial inflammation is itself nonspecific and has variable relationships to the development of late onset parenchymal injury and to overall outcome. In his evaluation of 189 procedures performed in 104 patients (mean BSA, 45.8 percent; mortality, 47.8 percent), Head observed that bronchoscopy results did not always predict either the degree of parenchymal injury or prognosis.[100] Diffuse subglottic injury (seen in 55 percent), "distal airways" abnormalities (19 percent), and proximal subglottic injury (26 percent) resolved during the 2 weeks after exposure. The degree of mucosal damage, however, demonstrated "only fair" correlation with the development of fatal respiratory failure. In their recent prospective study of 27 patients who underwent early bronchoscopy with numerical grading of endobronchial findings, Bingham and coworkers found that bronchoscopic indices did not correlate with survival, the duration of endotracheal intubation, or the level of PEEP required to maintain acceptable oxygenation.[110a] Thus, the precise impact on management (and, consequently, the purposes served by such study) is unclear and requires further investigation. These uncertainties have led to diametrically opposed attitudes regarding bronchoscopy: while some authorities regard it as essential and advocate repeated procedures for diagnosis, monitoring the patient's course, and as an aid to tracheobronchial toilet, others are more conservative in the use of this procedure. Despite claims that early and repeated bronchoscopy leads to "improved" survival,[111] complete bronchoscopy is generally not prerequisite to the appropriate management of most patients and is not performed routinely at a number of leading centers.[54,112]

By contrast, careful, direct examination of the *upper* airway is an essential part of the initial evaluation that must not be deleted in patients at risk for inhalation injury. Clinical studies in which the status of the upper airway has been predicted on the basis of bedside examinations by experienced clinicians (often including even rigid laryngoscopy) have confirmed that objective assessment is necessary. Oropharyngeal inflammation with severe edema, erythema, and blistering of the tongue and palate in patients with respiratory area burns indicates direct thermal injury to the upper airway. However, unless such obviously severe changes are evident from simple inspection or laryngoscopic examination, interpretations of less marked pharyngeal abnormalities are often inaccurate. Bartlett et al. have noted that the empiric intubation of every patient with facial burns, singed nasal vibrissae, or oropharyngeal soot would "result in unnecessary intubation of the vast majority of patients."[43] Although 85 percent of Head's patients with bronchoscopically confirmed inhalation injury had abnormal oropharyngeal examinations, simple inspection was correct in only 38 percent of those with negative bronchoscopy.[100] We have found that in most instances, clinical predictions based on simple inspection have tended to underestimate the degree of injury found at nasopharyngoscopy. Nine of 13 patients with moderate to severe upper airway inflammation had been believed to have suffered only minimal airway damage, and 5 of these 9 eventually required endotracheal intubation for severe upper airway obstruction.[66] Moylan et al. have reported a similar experience.[46] Thus, unless obvious pharyngeal obstruction is present, clinical predictors are unacceptably unreliable in their assessment of the presence or absence of upper airway injury. Because of the dynamic changes of upper airway anatomy and function that occur in the early postburn period, the capability of performing serial examinations, preferably by the same endoscopist to appropriately assess changes, must be available. Alternatively, if this cannot be ensured and there is any doubt about whether significant edema is present, risk-benefit considerations favor early, empiric, elective endotracheal intubation.

Other Applications In addition to its diagnostic functions, bronchoscopy retains important therapeutic and investigative applications. As an aid to intubation, bronchoscopy may help to avert tracheostomy. In addition, the copious secretions encountered in patients with inhalation injury may require repeated therapeutic bronchoscopic procedures when more conservative approaches are unsuccessful or unfeasible. In general, it has been our practice to avoid bronchoscopy in the management of atelectasis unless either the problem is unresponsive to standard chest physiotherapy or the severity of resulting gas exchange abnormalities does not allow time for this therapeutic approach. Because practical limitations by chest wall burns are often imposed upon respiratory therapists, therapeutic bronchoscopy for purposes of pulmonary toilet truly may be indicated more often in burn victims than in other critical care settings.

As with acute pulmonary injury incurred in other situations, analysis of bronchoalveolar lavage (BAL) fluid obtained at the time of diagnostic bronchoscopy might prove useful, particularly through the identification of either cell populations or mediators associated with delayed-onset permeability edema. Measurement of alveolar fluid protein concentrations might assist clinical differentiation of hydrostatic pulmonary edema (BAL/serum concentration ratio < 0.6) from ARDS (BAL/serum > 0.6).[113] Head has used detection of systemically administered indocyanine green in bronchial fluid to document increased lung permeability accompanying cutaneous burns.[100] Although currently BAL is a helpful probe for the investigation of inhalation injury in animal models, it is premature to advocate this as a routine, clinically useful diagnostic technique in burn victims. Perhaps more promising will be the role for BAL with quantitative bacterial cultures in the assessment of possible nosocomial pneumonia. While colonization is the rule in patients hospitalized in the ICU/burn center environment, even when the best of bedside preventative measures are observed, the early definition of the presence of bacterial pneumonia remains difficult in this setting in which chest roentgenograms are often either of suboptimal quality or are already abnormal. Quantitative bacterial cultures of BAL fluid or the use of specialized, protected bronchoscopic brushes and catheters for retrieval of uncontaminated specimens may assist in this long-standing clinical dilemma[114,115] and requires critical evaluation in burn victims.

Radionuclide Scanning

While endoscopic techniques provide direct visualization of airway injury, the presence of tracheobronchial obstruction can be inferred from demonstration of inhomogeneous ventilation and delayed clearance of radionuclide tracers from the lung (Fig. 7-9)[116–120] Introduced by Moylan and coworkers and validated in a series of investigations at Brooke Institute, abnormalities of such scans may antedate roentgenographic changes, have correlated with mortality from inhalation injury in some studies, and complement other objective diagnostic tests. The favored approach has been the intravenous administration of xenon 133. Following appearance of the tracer within the lung, the documentation of patchy uptake (implying inhomogeneous ventilation), segmental retention, and/or delayed clearance

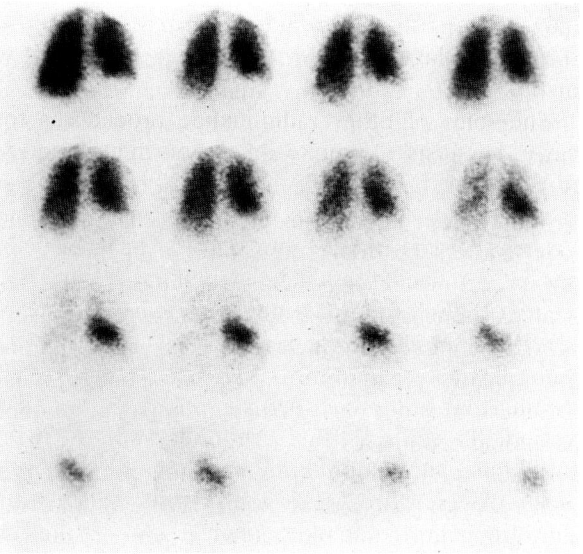

Figure 7-9 Xenon 133 scans diagnostic of smoke inhalation injury. Note the inhomogeneous, segmental distribution of isotope and its prolonged retention, both suggesting tracheobronchial obstruction.

(greater than 90 seconds in most studies) suggests that airflow obstruction and, hence, tracheobronchial injury, has occurred. The accuracy of the tests may be increased by requiring a longer period of "hang-up" of tracer (greater than 150 seconds) for a diagnostic result.[120] Intravenous methods of administering the radionuclide have been preferred because they minimize the need for patient cooperation and are performed more readily in anxious, hyperventilating or poorly compliant patients than are standard ventilation scanning techniques.

False positive examinations are most often due to the presence of chronic obstructive pulmonary disease but may also be caused by early alveolar edema (unrelated to inhalation injury), pneumonia, or aspiration of blood and secretions. False negatives may also occur, but these have, for the most part, been attributed to delays in performing the scans. Because xenon scanning has seemed to add little useful diagnostic or prognostic information in patients with abnormal fiberoptic bronchoscopy, it has been suggested recently that such lung scans should be reserved for individuals who have normal bronchoscopy.[29] Nevertheless, radionuclide scanning remains an important noninvasive option in the early diagnosis of inhalation injury at many institutions.

The roles of other radionuclide procedures for early diagnosis of smoke inhalation injury require further evaluation.[121] A dose-responsive increase of the pulmonary clearance of aerosolized ^{99m}Tc diethylenetriamine pentacetate (DTPA) has been observed in a canine model of smoke inhalation, suggesting that an early permeability injury had been identified.[122] However, seven burn victims with smoke exposure had normal DTPA clearance, suggesting that this procedure may not be a practical option. By contrast, increased clearance of tracer from lung into blood has been documented in a group of seven fire fighters, prompting speculation that their chronic smoke exposure had resulted in subclinical increases in alveolar capillary membrane permeability.[123] It is premature to assign a clinical role to this test in the evaluation of smoke inhalation victims.

Pulmonary Function Tests

Just as radionuclide testing allows graphic demonstration of the presence of airflow obstruction, the bedside performance of physiologic studies permits direct quantitation of these abnormalities. It was noted in Cocoanut Grove fire victims that a reduced "expiratory push" could be sensed by the examiner's palm placed before the patient's open mouth.[2] Formal physiologic testing with spirometry and flow volume curves allows more precise measurement of the same phenomenon and is complemented by other objective functional measurements. Aub et al. have observed that "the vital capacity test represents our best quantitative index of the severity of lung burns, even though it obviously cannot be used in the first few days after an accident."[2] With minor modifications of procedures for this acutely ill population, and with recognition of some practical limitations of these studies, physiologic testing can be a valuable bedside procedure in the early detection and quantitation of inhalation injury.[64,76,77,104,124–134]

Spirometry During spirometry, forced expiration is assessed by measurement of exhaled volume as a function of time (Fig. 7-10). Obstructive ventilatory defects, characterized by a reduction of the forced expiratory volume in 1 second (FEV_1) as a percentage of the total volume exhaled with the maneuver (the forced vital capacity, FVC), and a reduced $FEV_1/FVC\%$, occur early after inhalation injury. These findings, seen typically during the initial 4 to 6 hours after exposure, usually precede roentgenographic abnormalities and changes of arterial blood gases and are sensitive indicators of injury due to smoke. In addition, the severity of injury is suggested by the degree of physiologic abnormality. Interpretation of the significance of spirometric changes usually requires reference to the normal values predicted for a patient's sex, age, and height. These standards are incorporated in the software of widely available portable, computerized systems for pulmonary function measurements. In the absence of such information, however, an FEV_1 less

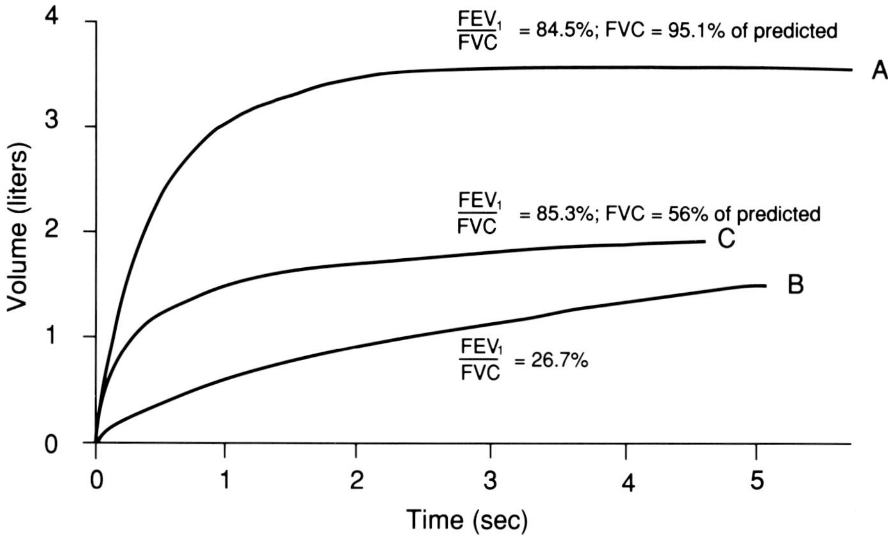

Figure 7-10 Representative spirometric patterns seen in burn and smoke inhalation victims: (*A*) normal tracing; (*B*) obstructive pattern (decreased FEV_1/FVC%); (*C*) restrictive ventilatory defect (normal FEV_1/FVC%, decreased FVC.)

than 1 L (such as <10 cm^3/kg) in patients with airflow obstruction should be regarded as a severe defect, and an FVC below 15 cm^3/kg in the absence of obstruction suggests a severe restrictive defect in most adults. Such objective measurements have correlated with injuries diagnosed by bronchoscopy and xenon scans and, in other acute settings, with an increased likelihood that mechanical ventilation will be necessary.

Later in the course, spirometry often suggests restrictive ventilatory defects that are characterized by a reduction of the FVC with preservation of the FEV_1/FVC%. At some institutions, these findings have been confirmed with more precise measurements of lung volumes, revealing reduced total lung capacity and functional residual capacity. Not surprisingly, the presence of such restrictive abnormalities has been associated with increased body surface area burn, chest wall and abdominal distribution of burns, the development of fluid retention, and decreased colloid osmotic pressure.[77,133] These observations suggest that the primary restrictive defects seen in patients with the combination of burns and inhalation injury are truly multifactorial, likely reflecting effects of airway inflammation, chest wall and muscular abnormalities, and increased lung water. Although it has been suggested that serial measurements of the severity of restriction might present a noninvasive guide for adjustments of fluid resuscitation, the multiplicity of factors which might cause restriction suggest that this would be difficult. There is no prospective documentation of the use of this approach. Quinby has incorporated documentation of restrictive ventilatory defects as a criterion for surgical release procedures in patients with burn scar contractures.[125] Serial pulmonary function studies might also contribute to the use of bronchodilator therapy in patients with tracheobronchial obstruction, but neither the bronchodilator responsiveness of this smoke-induced lesion nor the benefits of such physiologic testing has been demonstrated conclusively.

The extent of reductions of all spirometric measurements has been shown to be worse in the presence of combined smoke inhalation injury and cutaneous burns,[77] and their resolution parallels and may even precede obvious clinical improvement. In the most comprehensive documentation of these serial physiologic measurements in burn victims, Whitener and coworkers found that vital capacity fell 12 hours after inhalation injury, with "significant impairment" developing by 72 hours in all except two patients with the smallest burns.[77] In the remaining 26 patients, combined surface burns and smoke inhalation caused the most marked deterioration of pulmonary function; however, either problem alone was associated with physiologic evidence of respiratory dysfunction. It should also be appreciated that these physiologic changes are not specific for inhalation injury. For example, obstruction might indicate an exacerbation of underlying obstructive airways disease, and restrictive and obstructive defects may also occur with cardiogenic edema or pneumonia.

Flow Volume Curves Complementary physiologic information may be presented in another way by means of flow volume curves recorded simultaneously with spirometry. These studies graphically demonstrate flow rates as a function of the lung volume at which they are measured. Petroff et al. placed particular emphasis upon the usefulness of expiratory flow rates in burn victims and found them to be low in patients with inhalation injury.[76] Reduced expiratory flow rates at low lung volumes are seen typically with variable intrathoracic obstruction and are similar to findings in patients with chronic obstructive lung disease. Complete flow volume curves which include inspiratory, as well as expiratory, flow rate measurements provide still more insights (Fig. 7-11).[66] Because variable extra-

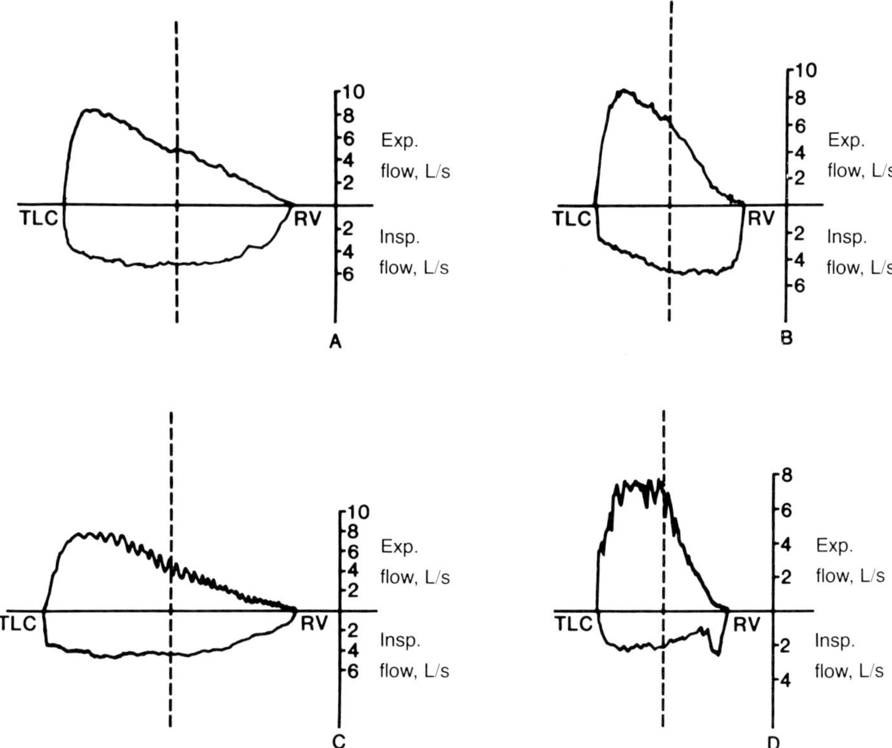

Figure 7-11 Flow volume curve patterns seen in smoke inhalation victims: *A*, normal; *B, C,* and *D*, variable extrathoracic airway obstruction; *C* and *D*, sawtoothing (*reprinted with permission from Ref. 64*).

thoracic obstruction is predominantly an inspiratory limitation, the documentation of such complete flow volume curves allows more complete analysis of upper airway, as well as lower airway, events. Several characteristic patterns of the flow volume curve may be seen (Figs. 7-11 and 7-12)[66]: variable extrathoracic obstruction is associated with preferential reduction of inspiratory flow rates (and relative preservation of expiratory flows), while fixed extrathoracic obstruction is characterized by marked reductions of both expiratory and inspiratory flow rates and suggests a more severe degree of injury. In addition, irregular, remarkably reproducible oscillations of flow rates, "sawtoothing" of flow volume curves, provide other graphic evidence of upper airway dysfunction. Comparisons of flow volume curves performed during breathing of air and helium-oxygen mixtures have been employed in the detection of small airways disease in burn victims,[130] but the complexity of this test limits its usefulness.

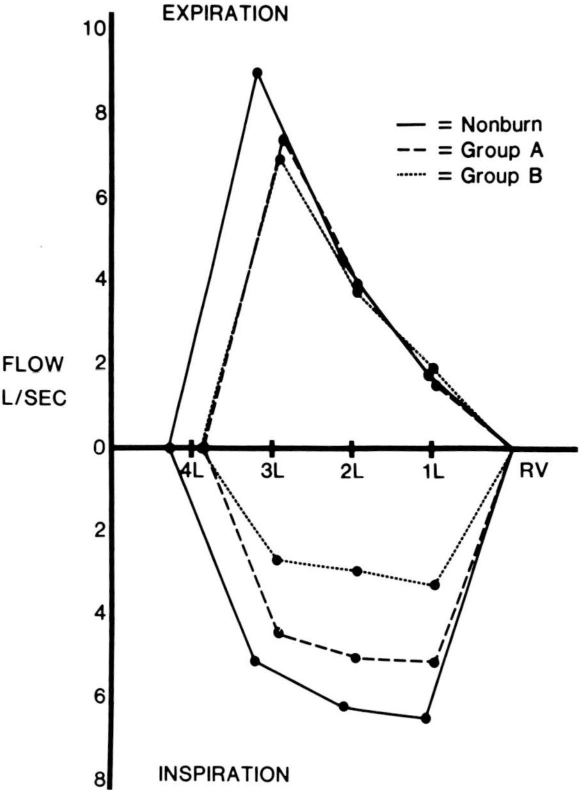

Figure 7-12 Flow volume curve patterns derived from mean inspiratory and expiratory flow rates and forced vital capacity measurements in nonburn controls, Group A (17.9 ± 15.7% BSA, mild upper airway injury at nasopharyngoscopy) and Group B (23.0 ± 15.5% BSA, moderate-to-severe upper airway inflammatory changes visualized) burn patients. Curves are plotted from residual volume (RV). (*Reprinted with permission from Ref. 64.*)

We have found that abnormal flow volume curves and/or spirometry often occur in patients with clinical risks for inhalation injury, underscoring the diagnostic sensitivity of physiologic testing shown by previous investigators.[66,104] Such changes develop early (within hours) after exposure to smoke, often preceding visible endoscopic abnormalities. This observation is similar to the demonstrations of the high sensitivity of physiologic measurements in other acute and chronic respiratory diseases. The degree of compromise of flow rates suggesting upper airway obstruction has correlated with the severity of pharyngeal edema and with subsequent needs for endotracheal intubation (Table 7-7).[66,134] In 221 patients with clinical risk factors for inhalation injury, 161 (72.8 percent) had abnormal flow volume curves and/or spirometry at the time of their hospitalizations within hours of injury.[134] Seventeen of these individuals (10.5 percent) required endotracheal intubation because of objective upper airway compromise. Anatomic airway obstruction visualized at nasopharyngoscopy was used as the primary, independent criterion for their intubation. Among the 60 patients who had normal acute measurements of their pulmonary function, only 1 was intubated; in this individual with massive cutaneous burns, the resuscitative fluid requirement influenced the decision to intubate despite a patent-appearing upper airway. The negative predictive value of normal pulmonary function studies was 98.3 percent in this study of patients with small body surface area burns. Serial physiologic studies have also paralleled nasopharyngoscopic changes.[104] Stable measurements are associated with anatomic stability, whereas reductions of flow rates connote

Table 7-7 Relationship of Pulmonary Function Tests (PFT) to Acute Endotracheal (ET) Intubation,* Baltimore Regional Burn Center†

	Normal PFT	Abnormal PFT	Total
ET tube	1	17	18
No tube	59	144	203
Total	60	161	221

*Intubation performed for endoscopically confirmed upper airway edema.

†$p < 0.01$.

worsening pharyngeal obstruction. Not surprisingly, progression of both anatomic upper airway edema and physiologic dysfunction has correlated with the presence of facial burns, the extent of surface burn, and rapid fluid resuscitation (Fig. 7-10), supporting long-standing clinical impressions that these factors influence upper airway structure and function.

These observations are consistent with other suggestions that physiologic measurements obtained during the acute phase of the illness are useful prognostically. Petroff and coworkers found that patients who had expiratory flow rates at 50 percent of the vital capacity ($\dot{V}_{50}$) which were below 50 percent of predicted values more often developed severe hypoxemia, abnormal radionuclide scans, and subsequent pneumonia or atelectasis.[76] Patients with well-maintained admission flow rates (exceeding 70 percent of predicted) had these findings rarely. Whitener et al. have observed that acute respiratory failure with noncardiogenic pulmonary edema developed in patients who had the lowest FVC and FEV_1 measurements.[77] Moreover, all patients who had an FVC below 60 percent of predicted died, in contrast to only one death among patients exceeding this level.

Surprisingly, there have been no published reports of the role of perhaps the easiest and most economical means of measuring airway function. Simple peak flow meters have long been effective in both the emergency room evaluation of acutely ill asthmatics and in the home self-monitoring of these patients' pharmacologic therapy, but their usefulness in burn victims is unknown. The high predictive values of flow rate measurements obtained with flow volume curves suggest that bedside use of peak flow meters could be an even more cost-effective option, obviating the need for either a technician or sophisticated equipment. In this way, more complex procedures might be reserved (if used at all) for individuals in whom initial, screening measurements obtained by peak flow meter showed reduced flow rates.

Complementary Respiratory Studies Rapid progress in the technologic resources available to monitor critically ill patients has occurred,[135,136] but the precise roles of these resources in burn victims require clarification. Several diagnostic studies of respiratory mechanics have been applied in both experimental models and clinical investigations of inhalation injury. These might assist evaluation of carefully selected patients, but the studies' present roles are more restricted, often because of the increased technologic requirements or costs of the tests or because either their clinical utility or superiority over more readily available studies has not been established.

For example, demonstration of increased closing volumes and closing capacities, as well as increased airway resistance and abnormal helium/air flow volume curves, might suggest the presence of small airway disease. Airway inhalation challenge procedures have occasionally demonstrated nonspecific bronchial hyperreactivity as a residual effect of inhalation injury, and reductions of static and dynamic compliance can be used to confirm chronic parenchymal and airway disease, respectively. Complete pressure volume curves, in which the relationships between changes in lung volume and changes in pleural pressure (determined by means of an esophageal balloon) are measured, permit detection of interstitial edema or fibrosis by demonstrating increasing stiffness (i.e., reduced compliance) of the lung. Approximations of thoracic compliance are more frequently obtained indirectly in acutely ill individuals who are already intubated and treated with mechanical ventilation. In this latter circumstance, the compliance, $\Delta V/\Delta P$, can be estimated serially from the plateau pressures (minus any positive end-expiratory pressure applied to the system) associated with the delivery of a known tidal volume. Such bedside determinations may be useful in differentiating acute problems which primarily worsen compliance (e.g., pneumothorax, pulmonary edema, pneumonia) from those predominantly worsening resistance (e.g., mucous plug, bronchospasm).

Documentation of increased work of breathing might not only assist the recognition of respiratory injury but also affect assessments of patients' caloric needs. Measurement of maximum inspiratory and expiratory airway pressures can help to gauge respiratory muscle strength; the former has proved valuable as one of the several mechanical criteria used for assessing whether patients are ready for weaning from mechanical ventilation. Maximum negative inspiratory pressures greater than -20 to -30 cmH_2O have, by convention, suggested that respiratory muscle strength is sufficient to make spontaneous ventilation feasible. It should be recognized that many other integrated factors such as neurologic function, patient effort, pain, and superimposed medication influence this measurement, and it does not reflect respiratory status alone. Expired gas analysis allows the calculation of physiologic dead space (V_D/V_T) and because V_D/V_T is an important determinant of alveolar ventilation, assists the evaluation of patients' ventilatory reserve.[86] While normal V_D/V_T is approximately 33 percent, patients with measurements exceeding 60 to 70 percent ordinarily cannot maintain alveolar ventilation. Recently, dead space measurements have contributed to the evaluation of burn victims. Expired gas analysis also allows indirect calorimetry for purposes of evaluating patients' nutritional needs[86,137] and the effects of various substrates upon oxygen consumption and CO_2 production. Such measurements have been used to assist both ventilator care and nutritional therapy in critically ill patients with and without cutaneous burns. Although some authorities feel strongly that such technologic input has enhanced patient care, support for this assertion is not yet so convincing as to recommend routine use of all these monitoring procedures.

Other Physiologic Measurements

Refinements in still other bedside tools recently applied to the management of critically ill patients may contribute to the diagnosis and management of burn victims with inhalation injury.

Hemodynamic Monitoring Just as the clinical role of hemodynamic monitoring with the Swan-Ganz catheter is being reevaluated in other critically ill populations,[138] its optimum use in burn victims has not been defined. Although the hazards of overhydration in patients with inhalation injury are well appreciated, most management protocols are not adjusted routinely for the dynamic responses of the pulmonary microcirculation that occur during different phases of burn injury and recovery. Fluid restriction to lower hydrostatic driving pressure might minimize pulmonary edema in patients with ARDS due to smoke, but major limitations of resuscitative fluid administration based on measurements of pulmonary capillary wedge pressure might conceivably worsen outcome. These issues are addressed in detail in Chap. 10.

Despite the widespread availability of Swan-Ganz catheters to guide such difficult decisions, there are surprisingly few published data regarding their use in burn victims. Noe and Constable initially reported this application of right heart catheterization,[139] and German et al. monitored pulmonary arterial pressure for 2 to 5 days in 10 patients (60% BSA; 9 with fatal injuries).[140] In extrapolations made from the use of Swan-Ganz catheters in other settings, such hemodynamic monitoring has been recommended for burn victims whose fluid management is complicated by cardiac, pulmonary, or renal disease; smoke inhalation; or associated major injuries, or for individuals with burns exceeding 50% BSA.[140,141] Although these indicants seem reasonable, improved outcome as a result of such monitoring has not been documented, and better criteria for the application of Swan-Ganz catheters are needed.

In contrast to noninvasive diagnostic and monitoring studies, significant hazards associated with pulmonary arterial catheterization are of particular concern in burn victims. In addition to the usual complications of cardiac arrhythmias and pneumothoraces associated with line insertions, burn victims are predisposed to central line-related infections and have an increased propensity for central venous thrombosis.[142,143] In one report, 8 Swan-Ganz catheter–related complications were described in 39 patients (61% mean BSA).[141] Problems included balloon ruptures (4), tricuspid and pulmonic valvular vegetations (2), subacute bacterial endocarditis (1), and persistent ventricular irritability (1). Moreover, one-third of catheter tip cultures were positive. As in other critically ill populations, positive cultures and line-related infections were associated with prolonged use (exceeding 3 days in duration). Thus, a careful risk-benefit assessment is central to the decision about whether pulmonary artery catheterization should be performed.

Clinical Lung Water Measurements In efforts to improve the early detection of increased permeability of the alveolar capillary membrane, techniques for estimating extravascular lung water (EVLW) have evolved. One of the more popular of these approaches has been the thermal green-dye double-indicator dilution method, in which the changes of diffusible (heat) and nondiffusible indicators are compared to estimate increases of lung water.[144] This technique has been applied to small numbers of burn victims; such estimates have varied considerably with the timing and techniques of measurement, mode of fluid resuscitation, presence and severity of inhalation injury, and, in particular, the clinical onset of sepsis. Because of the dependence of this method upon the homogeneity of lung perfusion, and the well-documented inhomogeneity of lung perfusion that accompanies smoke inhalation, it is not surprising that measurements of EVLW have varied considerably among studies.

Following an initial report of reductions of EVLW in 7 patients,[145] Tranbaugh et al. reported measurements in 14 patients (37% BSA) with clinically severe inhalation injury.[146] EVLW was normal at the time of hospitalization in 13 of them and subsequently increased in 5, 4 of whom had sepsis. In nine patients, Morgan et al. reported EVLW to increase during the period of maximum weight gain.[147] In their study of 26 patients (50% BSA), Pietzman and coworkers found that EVLW rose within hours of smoke exposure in their hypoxemic patients but did not correlate with the clinical severity of respiratory damage in the 18 patients with inhalation injury.[148] EVLW increased further following the onset of sepsis. Most recently, Herndon and coworkers have compared EVLW measurements in patients with smoke inhalation only, massive burns without smoke inhalation, and burns with inhalation injury.[84] Patients had been resuscitated to similar urine outputs and plasma colloid oncotic pressures and had similar central venous pressure (CVP) and cardiac index measurements during the early postburn period. These investigators found that EVLW rose in both groups with smoke injury during the first 24 hours after exposure, confirming clinical suspicions that pulmonary edema results from toxic effects of smoke. EVLW remained normal throughout the period of study in patients with cutaneous injuries alone. Despite these preliminary investigations, there is no firm support for the routine measurement of EVLW or criteria for its use in guiding management decisions.

DO TESTS REFLECT GRADATIONS OF INHALATION INJURY?

Differences in the sensitivity of diagnostic tests appear to reflect gradations in the severity of respiratory injury, as well as variations among the tests themselves in their amenability to this application. This concept is presented schematically in Fig. 7-13 and not only has implications for selection of one test over another but also reinforces the notion that manifestations of inhalation injury represent a continuum in many patients. This gradation in severity

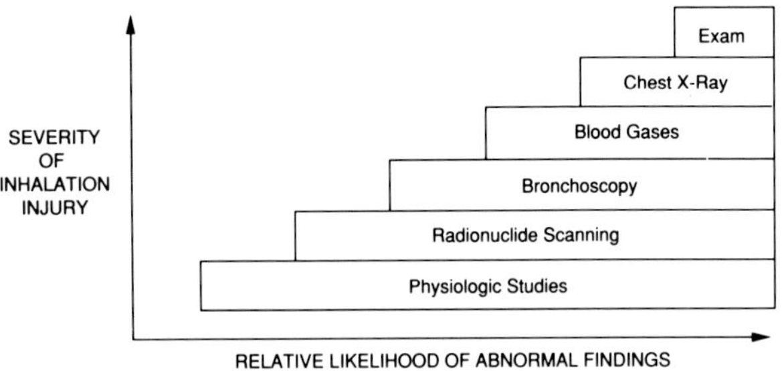

Figure 7-13 Postulated relationship between diagnostic test results and clinical gradation of inhalation injury. While diverse combinations of test results may be seen, data from numerous clinical investigations suggest that abnormalities of physiologic tests and radionuclide scans more sensitively detect subtle injury. Abnormalities of chest roentgenograms and clinical examination demonstrate more severe, established respiratory change.

of injury, together with local differences in patient populations and the thresholds used for defining abnormal results, also helps to account for institutional variations in the yields of various diagnostic tests. The usefulness (and need for) tests will vary according to whether one is evaluating patients with large surface burns at a referral burn center or individuals with smoke inhalation and minor cutaneous injuries seen in the emergency room setting. In the former circumstance, decisions about diagnosis, hospitalization, and early management are relatively straightforward, as clinical criteria reveal the gravity of the situation. In the latter, these initial decisions may be more difficult.

Physiologic tests and radionuclide scans appear to detect the earliest, functional effects of clinically important respiratory injury. These primary airway effects are consistent with the early anatomic and physiologic changes demonstrated in laboratory models following acute exposures to smoke in animals: acute physiologic airway obstruction may precede recognizable mucosal inflammation. With more severe injury, however, such endobronchial damage is seen readily at bronchoscopy. That such visible abnormalities in patients represent more severe injury is supported by the more consistent relationships shown between the presence of abnormal bronchoscopy and mortality. While these primary airway effects of injury may cause mismatching of ventilation and perfusion sufficient to alter oxygenation, it has been found in many investigations that they antedate gross abnormalities of arterial blood gases. A widened alveolar-arterial oxygen gradient and arterial hypoxemia are usually manifest before either roentgenographic evidence of more severe airway (atelectasis or focal emphysema) or parenchymal (interstitial and alveolar edema) injury are detectable. Finally, after severe exposures, damage to the alveolar capillary membrane will be clinically manifest, usually in combination with signs of injury to both proximal airways and lung parenchyma evident at physical examination.

Thus, patients who have abnormal arterial blood gas measurements and/or chest roentgenograms at the time of presentation are not likely to benefit substantially from indiscriminate use of all tests for inhalation injury. Their diagnosis is already apparent, and the information fundamental to management decisions has already been obtained. The results of more sensitive tests are unlikely to influence management, unless other conditions (e.g., congestive heart failure, chronic obstructive pulmonary disease) which might cause hypoxemia or radiographic abnormalities in the absence of inhalation injury are present. By contrast, individuals who have normal arterial blood gases and chest roentgenograms despite clinical risk factors for inhalation injury usually require further testing.

PRACTICAL APPLICATIONS OF DIAGNOSTIC TESTING

The integrated use of objective diagnostic tests in the evaluation of patients with suspected inhalation injury provides the physician with considerable latitude, allowing for diagnostic strategies which can be adapted to differing clinical circumstances. Agee and others have shown that these studies are complementary: the diagnostic accuracies of radionuclide scanning (87 percent), fiberoptic bronchoscopy (86 percent), and expiratory flow volume curves (91 percent) were uniformly high, and combinations of these tests (scanning plus bronchoscopy—93 percent; scanning, bronchoscopy, and flow volume curves—96 percent) have afforded even more accuracy.[16,119] This complementarity should not be surprising, since these various tests together with clinical findings assess differing sites of respiratory injury (Table 7-8).

Although all of these tests are available and are performed regularly in investigative settings, not all are clinically indicated. Neither are they necessary in all patients suspected of inhalation injury. Several basic factors influence the approach to testing that any one individual clinician will select. Some of these include the timely availability of the test, an awareness of practical limitations for each test (in each patient), the clinician's pretest suspicions and pretest probabilities of the likelihood of inhalation injury, the diagnostic performance characteristics of the test, and the utility of the information generated (its pragmatic impact on patient management).

Advantages and Disadvantages of Specific Tests

It has been well-established that bronchoscopy, radionuclide scanning, and pulmonary function testing can be performed easily at the bedside. We have performed endoscopic and physiologic studies in settings ranging from the emergency room and tub room to the intensive care unit; they can be coordinated easily with initial acute assessment and debridement of patients with surface burns. The combination of the light source, nasopharyngoscope, medications needed for local anesthesia, and a spirometer and oscilloscope used for physiologic testing on a compact portable cart makes all equipment necessary for evaluation available on a moment's notice for these studies. This equipment is transported readily by the pulmonary laboratory

Table 7-8 Acute Inhalation Injury: General Relationships between Pathophysiologic Events, Clinical Findings, and Diagnostic Tests

Event	Common clinical finding	Diagnostic test results
Asphyxia	Altered sensorium, coma, nausea, vomiting	Increased COHb, CN
Upper airway obstruction (UAO)	Stridor, hoarseness, dyspnea, sore throat, painful swallow, respiratory area burns, flash exposure, pharyngeal edema/erythema	COHb often increased; N, increased Pa_{CO_2} (when severe); CXR usually N (occasionally subglottic edema, pulmonary edema); laryngoscopy, nasopharyngoscopy abnormal; flow volume curves: UAO patterns, decreased flow rates (especially inspiratory)
Lower airway obstruction	Dyspnea, tachypnea, wheezing, rhonchi, carbonaceous sputum	COHb often increased; decreased Pa_{O_2} (mild); decreased, N, increased Pa_{CO_2} (when severe); CXR usually N, occasional focal atelectasis or hyperinflation; spirometry: obstructive defect (decreased FEV_1, decreased FVC, decreased FEV_1/FVC%); flow volume curves: decreased $\dot{V}_{Exp}$; bronchoscopy: tracheobronchial inflammation ± soot; radionuclide scans: inhomogenous uptake, retention
Parenchymal injury	Dyspnea, tachypnea, crackles	COHb often increased; Pa_{O_2}: N (early), decreased late; Pa_{CO_2}: decreased, N, increased; CXR: N early, pulmonary edema late; spirometry: restrictive defect; flow volume curves: reduced flow rates; bronchoscopy, radionuclide scans usually abnormal

N = normal, CXR = chest x-ray.

technician to the burn unit or emergency room for evaluation of any new admission at risk for inhalation injury or, alternatively, may be maintained on site in the unit for its ongoing use in the serial monitoring of the status of each patient. Appropriate operational relationships have also permitted similar prompt access to radionuclide scanning at many centers.

Practical limitations include those related to equipment and personnel needs and the suitability and adaptability of the tests for an acutely ill patient population. Portable radionuclide scans are available, but there are additional requirements which must allow for the venting of exhaust gas from the unit. The need for radionuclide tracers (dictated by the half life of the radiopharmaceutical) and for specialized personnel and equipment usually makes bronchoscopy and physiologic testing more accessible than radionuclide scanning at most institutions. Not only is the timely performance of the test essential, but even more importantly, its interpretation must be available at a time that allows it to influence management decisions optimally. Bronchoscopy, with its direct anatomic demonstration of the airway, would seem to have an advantage over the interpretations of either flow volume curve patterns or ventilation scans; the latter procedures would be more likely to require input from the specialist. However, even with relatively little experience, gross abnormalities of physiologic studies and radionuclide tests can be recognized easily and provide valuable information. Furthermore, measurements of flow rates can be performed reproducibly with simple peak flow meters, obviating the technical needs posed by spirometry or flow volume curves.

Endoscopic procedures have added advantages in that they might be performed readily with less patient cooperation. The effort-dependence of many of the physiologic measurements (e.g., forced vital capacity, peak expiratory and inspiratory flow rates) limits their usefulness and demands that the quality of physiologic studies be monitored closely. Pulmonary function studies must be reproducible in order to avoid misinterpretations due to patients' weakness, splinting from pain, or the suppressive effects of already-administered narcotics. In these settings effort-dependent measurements would be underestimated, leading to an erroneous diagnosis of airway injury. If the forced expiratory maneuver is too brief (<7 seconds), the $FEV_1/FVC\%$ might be overestimated, with resulting failure to diagnose airways obstruction. We and others have found that from 10 to 15 percent of acutely injured burn victims are unable to provide pulmonary function studies of reproducible quality. Nevertheless, for the remaining 85 to 90 percent of individuals, these tests retain substantial value.

The financial costs of diagnostic procedures are also important considerations, particularly since many of them will be performed serially through the patient's course. In addition, the frequent need to expeditiously (and economically) evaluate large numbers of patients nearly simultaneously injured often occurs following mass exposures (e.g., after a hotel fire or industrial accident). While complete fiberoptic bronchoscopy ($300 to $400) and radionuclide scanning ($300 to $500) are relatively costly, nasopharyngoscopy ($150) and spirometry ($50) are comparatively inexpensive. By this criterion, the low relative costs of spirometry and flow volume curves, together with their diagnostic sensitivity, appears to make them preferable screening procedures. The expense of more technologically oriented tests detracts from their value for this indication.

The selection of tests will also be influenced by the clinical setting, characteristics of the patient population evaluated and the circumstances of their evaluation, and the results of previous tests. The clinical likelihood of inhalation injury may be so overwhelmingly high that nonspecific, symptomatic therapy is indicated in the absence of confirmatory information. In many patients the obvious severity of overall injury (e.g., clinical presentations with moribund status, large burns, shock with respiratory distress) obviates the needs for detailed tests. In other individuals with apparently minor injuries and/or respiratory complaints, or in those without obvious respiratory injury, more comprehensive studies may be necessary. It is the patient in whom the diagnosis is most in question that testing has the greatest impact on management decisions. This concept is outlined in Table 7-9. In patients with already apparent respiratory dysfunction, objective tests may provide very important guidance for resuscitative, supportive care, but their diagnostic role is somewhat limited. When it is less clear whether the patient has sustained significant respiratory injury (e.g., following a transient exposure to smoke with minimal symptoms), such tests assume added importance because of their greater impact upon early triage decisions. Perspectives about the usefulness of testing would be expected to vary according to locales at which patients are seen (e.g., general emergency room populations versus regional burn center referrals).

The diagnostic performance characteristics of the tests used to confirm or exclude inhalation injury are another important consideration. While their utility in published series can be both helpful and instructive, the predictive values of tests as they are performed at one's own institution are of foremost importance. Clearly, local resources will determine not only what is available but what is truly reliable for the clinician's own routine bedside evaluations. Because the presence of abnormalities of co-oximetry, arterial blood gas analyses, chest roentgenograms, radionuclide scans, endoscopy, and physiologic tests are generally incorporated in the definitions of inhalation injury at most institutions, the positive predictive values when abnormalities of these tests are found are uniformly high. Of particular importance, especially to the physician in a triage position, are the negative predictive values of these tests. To what extent does a normal result exclude the presence of inhalation injury? The negative predictive values of these studies in large clinical investigations, the proportion of individuals with normal test results who do not have inhalation injury, are summarized in Table 7-10. As can be seen, the negative predictive values of chest roentgenograms and arterial blood gas analyses are low: normal test results do not exclude inhalation injury. By contrast, radionuclide scans, fiberoptic bronchoscopy, and physiologic studies (spirometry, flow volume curves) have considerably higher negative predictive values, a finding documented consistently in published series. These relationships must influence strategies used for diagnosis of inhalation injury. In patients with clinical risk factors for smoke inhalation injury, completely normal spirometry and flow volume curves appear to effectively

Table 7-9 Relationship of Diagnostic Testing to Clinical Presentations and Management Priorities

Clinical presentation	Management priority	Relative importance and roles of diagnostic tests*	
Asphyxiant death at burn scene	—	—	—
Cardiopulmonary arrest; successful CPR (grade V)†	Resuscitative	(+)	Monitoring
Clinically obvious established respiratory dysfunction (grades II to IV)†	Supportive	(++)	Confirmatory, monitoring
Exposure history; possible delayed-onset respiratory dysfunction (grade I)†	Accurate triage	(+++)	Exclusion of significant injury

*Grade 0 to 3+ in ascending levels of importance.

†Severity of anatomic/physiologic injury as described in Chap. 2, Table 2-13.

Table 7-10 Smoke Inhalation: Negative Predictive Values of Common Diagnostic Tests

	%
Chest roentgenogram	38–59
Arterial blood gases	40–74
Radionuclide scan	85–97
Fiberoptic bronchoscopy	88–100
Spirometry, flow volume curves	94–100

exclude significant respiratory injury. Increasing experience suggests that such individuals might be discharged safely from the emergency room if no other related problem (e.g., carbon monoxide intoxication, significant cutaneous burn) requires hospitalization.

Potential Diagnostic Algorithms

While several appropriate algorithms for the initial evaluation of patients have been designed,[149–150] diagnostic tests might be regarded in the following manner (Fig. 7-14): a first echelon or tier of testing would include studies that are uniformly, readily available and should be performed in virtually all patients at risk for inhalation injury. These essential studies include measurement of asphyxiants, arterial blood gas analysis, and the chest roentgenogram. Although the negative predictive values of these tests are low, the presence of abnormalities would identify individuals with early-onset, already established respiratory problems. Another essential study should include the direct visualization of the upper airway by the most reliable means available. This is regarded as necessary because of the unreliability of clinical predictors of upper airway obstruction and the disastrous consequences of overlooked and untreated pharyngeal edema. This "first tier" of tests, coupled with the complete appraisal of clinical risk factors and carefully performed

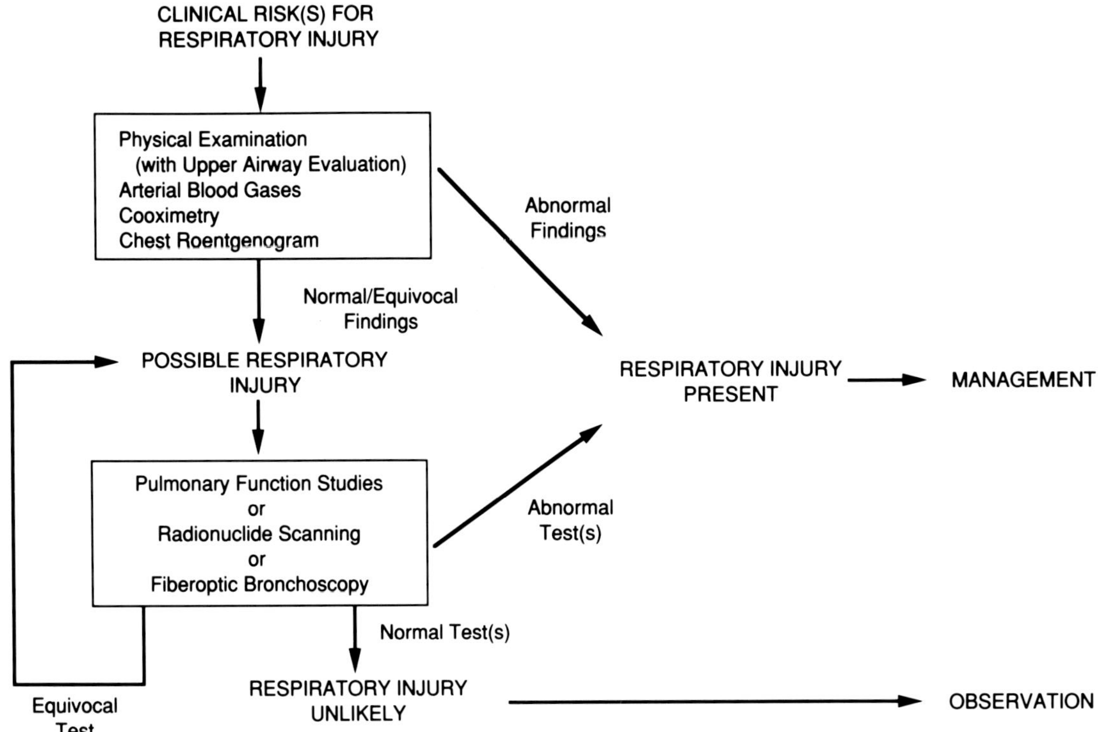

Figure 7-14 Algorithm for potential use of common diagnostic tests. In general, the more severe the patient's obvious degree of injury, the fewer the diagnostic studies which will be required. The major role of tests is in the screening of large numbers of exposed individuals and in excluding those who have not sustained inhalation injury. These applications require sensitive tests with high negative predictive values (see text for details).

physical examination, may be all that is necessary to identify most individuals with moderate or severe respiratory injury.

When the combination of these results with the clinical history and findings at physical examination identifies injuries requiring hospitalization and treatment, no further diagnostic testing is needed. If however, this initial database fails to establish whether inhalation injury has occurred, a second echelon of testing (radionuclide scan, lower endoscopy, spirometry/flow volume curves) should be performed, with the particular study to be determined by institutional factors. Generally, a normal test result, in combination with the negativity of first echelon clinical information, would exclude inhalation injury for practical purposes, since normal findings substantially lessen its likelihood. In the absence of other indications for hospitalization or treatment, such individuals might be observed as outpatients and are likely to do well. If doubt remains, or if clinical factors have identified a high-risk patient (e.g., elderly, preexisting systemic disease, limited return access to care), an additional second echelon test might be necessary for confirmation. This approach offers considerable flexibility to the clinician.

After extensive experience with the integrated use of fiberoptic nasopharyngoscopy and bedside physiologic testing, the following diagnostic approach was adopted in patients admitted to the Baltimore Regional Burn Center with clinical risks for inhalation injury but without stridor or already established hypoxemic or hypoventilatory respiratory failure. Simultaneous flow volume curves and spirometry are performed initially, either in the emergency room or at the time of the patient's arrival to the unit. If physiologic studies are completely normal, then the patient is monitored carefully through the combination of careful bedside observations of nursing staff and physicians and with follow-up flow volume curves. If either initial or follow-up physiologic studies are abnormal, of suboptimal quality, or unobtainable, then nasopharyngoscopy is performed. When upper airway injury is demonstrated, management focuses upon its severity, within the context of the patient's overall status, burn size, age, etc. Immediate nasotracheal intubation is performed in all patients with anatomic upper airway obstruction. The approach to less severe degrees of pharyngeal inflammatory changes is modified according to burn size and distribution, resuscitative requirements, mental status, estimated pulmonary reserve and related factors, and the overall status of the patient. When mild or moderate inflammation is seen in individuals with large burns or otherwise compromised status, prophylactic intubation is performed electively because of the increased likelihood of progressive airway compromise. When these findings are present in patients with small burns and no other risk factors, intubation is deferred and the patient is monitored carefully. Physiologic studies and/or nasopharyngoscopy are repeated if symptoms or signs suggest progressive upper airway inflammation (e.g., altered voice quality, worsening hoarseness, painful swallowing).

The latter algorithm, feasible only because of the continuous availability of the diagnostic tests and, even more importantly, of experienced physicians, nursing staff, and other paramedical personnel, has allowed prompt identification and treatment of all patients with upper airway obstruction. Moreover, it has reduced the frequency with which empiric intubation is performed. Importantly, with the use of this selective strategy based upon objective, rather than subjective, criteria, no patient has developed undiagnosed (and untreated) upper airway obstruction, many individuals with clinically unsuspected airway injury have been diagnosed, and unnecessary intubation has been avoided in others who were erroneously thought to have upper airway obstruction on clinical grounds alone. If this supportive environment cannot be ensured, safety demands early intubation based upon "classic" indicators (i.e., when in doubt, intubate). Although such an approach will result in the overdiagnosis and overtreatment of some individuals, those with inhalation injury will be managed appropriately. Thus, the setting in which the diagnostic evaluation (and treatment based upon it) is performed has an important, sometimes overlooked impact. Factors such as the overall work load and appropriateness of staffing in a burn unit or emergency room facility, for example, will also influence whether time-consuming diagnostic testing or empiric treatment would be safest and in the patient's best interests. Whatever approach is adopted, advance formulation of a plan integrating diagnosis with acute management is essential for each institution. Such preparations must accommodate the needs of each patient and, at designated centers, those of large numbers of individuals injured in community disasters.

UNRESOLVED DIAGNOSTIC ISSUES

Despite major progress in the diagnosis of inhalation injury, several problems remain to be resolved. First, the optimum testing strategy must be determined. There have been no prospective comparisons of one diagnostic approach with another, from which it might be determined whether one or another of the second echelon tests would have priority. It seems likely that all would be diagnostically equivalent when performed by suitable laboratories and that cost considerations would favor physiologic testing as the initial procedure of choice. Lower endoscopy would be the next option either for individuals with nondefinitive physiological tests or for patients who are unable to perform them. The end point of such comparative studies should not be limited to determining which test is most accurate. Rather, it must be determined whether any one diagnostic strategy results in more favorable outcomes for patients. In this regard, prospective use of computer-assisted prediction equations based on clinical observations requires further evaluation. Clarification of the best approaches to diagnostic testing requires not only more definitive diagnosis of inhalation injury but also more accurate identification of those low-risk individuals who are not likely to develop problems. Consequently, this latter group might be spared the low but finite risks of unnecessary empiric therapy.

Perhaps the greatest unresolved diagnostic problem relates to the needs for earlier identification of patients likely to develop delayed-onset parenchymal changes. The major diagnostic tests currently in use are directed appropriately at asphyxiants and the primary airway sites of early injury but provide only indirect inference of increased risks for parenchymal disease. The earlier detection of increased lung water might be facilitated by measurements of thermal space and have been performed in some clinical investigations, but definition of the best, reproducible, clinically applicable method (and, for that matter, the true meaning of this study) requires further investigation. Whether computed chest tomography or other imaging techniques will fill the current void in early detection of parenchymal injury remains to be seen. Whether detection of cells or cell products, or demonstration of mediators documenting activated humoral cascades in either lung fluids or serum will enhance detection of early pulmonary injury is unclear at present. Development of practical, clinically applicable diagnostic tools requires not only technologic progress but also further delineation of the pathogenesis of inhalation injury. Such anticipated advances can be expected to enhance but not substitute for clinical judgment.

REFERENCES

1. Cope O: Management of the Cocoanut Grove burns at the Massachusetts General Hospital. *Ann Surg* 117:801, 1943.
2. Aub JC, Pittman H, Brues AM: The pulmonary complications: A clinical description. *Ann Surg* 117:834, 1943.
3. Finland M, Davidson CS, Levenson SM: Clinical and therapeutic aspects of the conflagration injuries to the respiratory tract sustained by victims of the Cocoanut Grove disaster. *Medicine* 25:215,1946.
4. Stone HH, Reame DW, Corbitt JD, et al: Respiratory burns: A correlation of clinical and laboratory results. *Ann Surg* 165:157,1967.

5. Stone HH, Martin JD: Pulmonary injury associated with thermal burns. *Surg Gynecol Obstet* 129:1242, 1969.
6. Pruitt BA, Flemma RJ, DiVincenti FC, et al: Pulmonary complications in burn patients. *J Thorac Cardiovasc Surg* 59:7, 1970.
7. Pruitt BA, DiVincenti FC, Mason AD, et al: The occurrence and significance of pneumonia and other pulmonary complications in burned patients: Comparison of conventional and topical treatments. *J Trauma* 10:519, 1970.
8. Achauer BM, Allyn PA, Furnas DW, Bartlett RH: Pulmonary complications of burns: The major threat to the burn patient. *Ann Surg* 177:311, 1972.
9. DiVincenti FC, Pruitt BA, Reckler JM: Inhalation injuries. *J Trauma* 11:109, 1971.
10. Pruitt, BA, Erickson DR, Morris A: Progressive pulmonary insufficiency and other pulmonary complications of thermal injury. *J Trauma* 15:369, 1975.
11. Moylan JA, Chan CK: Inhalation injury—an increasing problem. *Ann Surg* 188:34, 1977.
12. Haponik EF, Summer W: Respiratory complications in burned patients: Pathogenesis and spectrum of inhalation injury. *J Crit Care* 2:49, 1987.
13. Loke J, Matthay RA, Smith GJW: The toxic environment and its medical implications with special emphasis on smoke inhalation, in Loke J (ed): *Pathophysiology and Treatment of Inhalation Injuries*. New York, Marcel Dekker, 1988, pp 453–504.
14. Haponik E, Crapo RO, Traber DL, et al: Smoke inhalation. *Am Rev Respir Dis* 138:1060, 1988.
15. Kinsella J: Smoke inhalation. *Burns* 14:269, 1988.
16. Artz CP, Moncrief JA, Pruitt BA (eds): Pulmonary disease in the patient, in *Burns: A Team Approach*. Philadelphia, W.B. Saunders, 1979, pp 97–105.
17. Clark WR, Framm BS: Burn mortality: Experience at a regional burn unit. Literature Review. *Acta Chir Scand* 537(suppl):1, 1987.
17a. Clark WR, Bonaventurea M, Myers W: Smoke inhalation and airway management at a regional burn unit. 1974-1983. Part I: Diagnosis and consequences of smoke inhalation. *JBCR* 10:52, 1989.
18. Trunkey DD: Inhalation injury. *Surg Clin North Am* 58:1133, 1978.
19. Bartlett RH: Types of respiratory injury. *J Trauma* 19:918, 1979.
20. Powers SR: Consensus summary on smoke inhalation. *J Trauma* 19:921, 1979.
21. Fein A, Leff A, Hopewell PC: Pathophysiology and management of the complications resulting from fire and the inhaled products of combustion: Review of the literature. *Crit Care Med* 8:94, 1980.
22. Crapo RO: Smoke inhalation injuries. *JAMA* 246:1694, 1981.
23. Crapo RO, Ellis N (ed): *Management of Smoke Inhalation Injuries*. Salt Lake City, Intermountain Thoracic Society, 1980.
24. Cahalane M, Demling RH: Early respiratory abnormalities from smoke inhalation. *JAMA* 251:771, 1984.
25. Herndon DN, Thompson PB, Traber DL: Pulmonary injury in burned patients. *Crit Care Clin* 1:79, 1985.
26. Haponik EF, Summer W: Respiratory complications in burned patients: Diagnosis and management of inhalation injury. *J Crit Care* 2:121, 1987.
27. Shirani KZ, Moylan JA, Pruitt BA: Diagnosis and treatment of inhalation injury in burn victims, in Loke J (ed): *Pathophysiology and Treatment of Inhalation Injuries*. New York, Marcel Dekker, 1988.
28. Heimbach DM, Waeckerle JF: Inhalation injuries. *Ann Emerg Med* 17:1316, 1988.
29. Shirani KZ, Pruitt BA, Mason AD: The influence of inhalation injury and pneumonia on burn mortality. *Ann Surg* 205:82, 1987.
30. Clark WR, Reid WH, Gilmour WH, Campbell D: Mortality probability in victims of fire trauma: Revised equation to include inhalation injury. *Br Med J* 292:1303, 1986.
31. Jung RC, Gottlieb LS: Respiratory tract burns after aspiration of hot coffee. *Chest* 72:125, 1977.
32. Garland JS, Rice TB, Kelly KJ: Airway burns in an infant following aspiration of microwave-heated tea. *Chest* 90:621, 1986.
33. Desai MN, Nichols MM, Herndon DN: Scald injury of the respiratory tract: An unusual occurrence. *J Burn Care Rehabil* 8:210, 1987.
34. Phillips AW, Tanner JW, Cope O: Burn Therapy: IV. Respiratory tract damage (an account of the clinical, x-ray and postmortem findings) and the meaning of restlessness. *Ann Surg* 158:799, 1963.
35. Birky MM, Clarke FB: Inhalation of toxic products from fires. *Bull NY Acad Med* 57:997, 1981.
36. Summer W, Haponik E: Inhalation of irritant gases. *Clin Chest Med* 2:273, 1981.
37. Bascom R, Haponik EF, Munster AM: Inhalation injury related to use of petrolatum-based hair grease. *J Burn Care Rehabil* 5:327, 1984.
38. Taylor RF, Bernard GR: Airway complications from free-basing cocaine. *Chest* 95:476, 1989.
39. Dyer RF, Esch VH: Polyvinyl chloride toxicity in fires. *JAMA* 235:393, 1976.
40. Levine MS: Respirator use and protection from exposure to carbon monoxide. *Am Ind Hyg Assoc J* 40:832, 1979.
41. Mawson AR: Is the concept of panic useful for scientific purposes? In Levin BM, Paulson RL (eds.), *International Seminar on Human Behavior in Fire Emergencies*. U.S. Dept. of Commerce; National Bureau of Standards Special Publication, Washington, DC, pp. 208–211, 1980.
42. Phillips AW, Cope O: Burn therapy: III. Beware the facial burn. *Ann Surg* 156:759, 1962.
43. Bartlett RH, Niccole M, Tavis MJ, et al: Acute management of the upper airway in facial burns and smoke inhalation. *Arch Surg* 111:744, 1976.
44. Wroblewski DA, Bower GC: The significance of facial burns in acute smoke inhalation. *Crit Care Med* 7:335, 1979.
45. Waymack JP, Law E, Park R, et al: Acute upper airway obstruction in the postburn period. *Arch Surg* 120:1042, 1985.
46. Moylan JA, Adib K, Birnbaum M: Fiberoptic bronchoscopy following thermal injury. *Surg Gynecol Obstet* 140:541, 1975.

47. Sochor FM, Mallory GK: Lung lesions in patients dying of burns. *Arch Pathol* 75:303, 1963.
48. Feller I, Hendrix RC: Clinical pathologic study of sixty fatally burned patients. *Surg Gynecol Obstet* 119:1, 1964.
49. Foley FD, Moncrief JA, Mason AD: Pathology of the lung in fatally burned patients. *Ann Surg* 167:251, 1968.
50. Foley FD: The burn autopsy: Fatal complications of burns. *Am J Clin Pathol* 52:1, 1969.
51. Cooney W, Dzuira B, Harper R, Nash G: The cytology of sputum from thermally injured patients. *Acta Cytol* 16:433, 1972.
52. Ambiavagar M, Chalon J, Zargham I: Tracheobronchial cytologic changes following lower airway thermal injury: A preliminary report. *J Trauma* 14:280, 1974.
53. Faling LJ, Medici TC, Chodosh S: Sputum cell population measurements in bronchial injury: Observations in acute smoke inhalation—closed space. *Chest* 66(suppl):565, 1974.
54. Venus B, Matsuda T, Copiozo J, Mathru M: Prophylactic intubation and continuous positive airway pressure in the management of inhalation injury in burn victims. *Crit Care Med* 9:519, 1981.
55. Heimbach DM: Burns, in Condon RE, DeCosse JJ (eds): *Surgical Care*. Philadelphia, Lea & Febiger, 1985, pp 323–50.
56. Sharer SR, Hudson LD: Pulmonary injury from burns and smoke inhalation. *Pulmonary Crit Care Update* 4(8):1, 1988.
57. Robinson MB, Myers GC, Demarest GB, et al: The diagnosis of early airway complications following thermal injury. *Chest* 80:382A, 1981.
58. Zikria BA, Weston GC, Chodoff AM, et al: Smoke and carbon monoxide poisoning in fire victims. *J Trauma* 12:641, 1972.
59. Stewart RD, Scot R, Stamm W, Seelen RP: Rapid estimation of carboxyhemoglobin level in firefighters. *JAMA* 235:390, 1976.
60. Jackson DL, Menges H: Accidental carbon monoxide poisoning. *JAMA* 243:772, 1980.
61. Strohl KP, Feldman NT, Saunders NA, O'Connor N: Carbon monoxide poisoning in fire victims: A reappraisal of prognosis. *J Trauma* 20:78, 1980.
62. Winter PM, Miller JN: Carbon monoxide poisoning. *JAMA* 236:132, 1976.
63. Coburn RF: Mechanisms of carbon monoxide toxicity. *Prev Med* 8:310, 1979.
64. Radford EP, Levine MS: Occupational exposures to carbon monoxide in Baltimore firefighters. *J Occup Med* 18:628, 1976.
65. Myers RAM, Britten JS: Are arterial blood gases of value in treatment decisions for carbon monoxide poisoning? *Crit Care Med* 17:139, 1989.
66. Haponik EF, Munster AM, Wise RA, et al: Upper airway function in burn patients: Correlation of flow volume curves and nasopharyngoscopy. *Am Rev Respir Dis* 129:251, 1984.
67. Clark CJ, Campbell D, Rein WH: Blood carboxyhaemoglobin and cyanide levels in fire survivors. *Lancet* 1:1332, 1981.
68. Barillo DJ, Goode R, Rush BF, et al: Lack of correlation between carboxyhaemoglobin and cyanide in smoke inhalation injury. *Curr Surg* 43:421, 1986.
69. Feldstein M, Klendshaj MJ: The determination of cyanide in biologic fluids by microdiffusion analysis. *J Lab Clin Med* 44:116, 1954.
70. Symington IS, Anderson RA, Oliver JS, et al: Cyanide exposure in fires. *Lancet* 2:91, 1978.
71. Genovesi MG, Tashkin DP, Chopra S, et al: Transient hypoxemia in firemen following inhalation of smoke. *Chest* 71:441, 1977.
72. Richards DW: The circulation in traumatic shock in man: The Harvey Lectures. Springfield, Science Press Printing Co., 1943–44.
73. Baxter CR: Fluid volume and electrolyte changes of the early postburn period. *Clin Plast Surg* 1:693, 1974.
74. Luce EA, Su CT, Hoopes JE: Alveolar-arterial oxygen gradient in the burn patient. *J Trauma* 16:212, 1976.
75. Epstein BS, Hardy DL, Harrison HN, et al: Hypoxemia in the burned patient: A clinical-pathologic study. *Ann Surg* 158:924, 1963.
76. Petroff PA, Hander EW, Clayton WH, Pruitt BA: Pulmonary function studies after smoke inhalation. *Am J Surg* 132:346, 1976.
77. Whitener DR, Whitener LM, Robertson J, et al: Pulmonary function measurement in patients with thermal injury and smoke inhalation. *Am Rev Respir Dis* 122:731, 1980.
78. Tripathi FM, Pandey K, Paul PS, et al: Blood gas studies in thermal burns. *Burns* 10:13, 1983.
79. Nishimura N, Hiranuma N: Respiratory changes after major burn injury. *Crit Care Med* 10:25, 1982.
80. Hudson L: Delayed hypoxemia in smoke inhalation. *Clin Res* 19:191, 1971.
81. Robinson TJ, Bubna-Kasteliz B, Stranc MF: Alterations in pulmonary ventilation and blood gases in acute burns. *Br J Plast Surg* 25:250, 1972.
82. Robinson NB, Hudson LD, Robertson HT, et al: Ventilation and perfusion alterations after smoke inhalation injury. *Surgery* 90:352, 1981.
83. Murray JF, Matthay MA, Luce JM, Flick MR: An expanded definition of the adult respiratory distress syndrome. *Am Rev Respir Dis* 138:720, 1988.
84. Herndon DN, Barrow RE, Traber DL, et al: Extravascular lung water changes following smoke inhalation and massive burn injury. *Surgery* 102:341, 1987.
85. Parker SJ, Tremper KK, Hufstedler S, et al: The effects of carbon monoxide on non-invasive oxygen monitoring. *Anesth Analg* 65:S12, 1986.
86. Stollery DE, Jones RL, King EG: Deadspace ventilation: A significant factor in respiratory failure after thermal inhalation. *Crit Care Med* 15:260, 1987.
86a. Glauser FL, Polatty RC, Sessler CN: Worsening oxygenation in the mechanically ventilated patient: Causes, mechanisms, and early detection. *Am Rev Respir Dis* 138:458, 1988.
87. Schatzki R: Roentgenologic report of the pulmonary lesions. *Ann Surg* 117:841, 1943.
88. Finland M, Ritvo M, Davidson CS, Levenson SM: Roentgenologic findings in the lungs of victims of the Cocoanut Grove disaster. *Am J Roentgenol* 55:1, 1946.

89. Putman CE, Loke J, Matthay RA, Ravin CE: Radiographic manifestations of acute smoke inhalation. *Am J Roentgenol* 129:865, 1977.
90. Kangarloo H, Beachley MC, Ghahremani GG: The radiographic spectrum of pulmonary complications in burn victims. *Am J Roentgenol* 128:441, 1977.
91. Teixidor HS, Rubin E, Novick GS, Alonso DR: Smoke inhalation: Radiologic manifestations. *Radiology* 149:383, 1983.
92. Teixidor HS, Novick G, Rubin E: Pulmonary complications in burn patients. *J L Assoc Can Radiol* 34:264, 1983.
93. Miller EJ: Management of patients with smoke inhalation: The Las Vegas experience, in O'Donohue WJ (ed): *Current Advances in Respiratory Care*. Park Ridge, Ill., American College of Chest Physicians, 1984.
94. Haponik EF, Adelman M, Munster A, Bleecker ER: Vascular pedicle widening preceding burn-related pulmonary edema. *Chest* 90:649, 1986.
95. Lee MJ, O'Connell DJ: The plain chest radiograph after acute smoke inhalation. *Clin Radiol* 39:33, 1988.
95a. Peitzman AB, Shires GT, Teixidor HS, Currier PW, Shires GT: Smoke inhalation injury: Evaluation of radiographic manifestations and pulmonary dysfunction. *J Trauma* 29:1232, 1989.
96. Milne ENC, Pistolesi M, Miniati M, Guintinin C: The radiologic distinction of cardiogenic and noncardiogenic edema. *Am J Roentgenol* 144:879, 1985.
97. Carlson RG, Finley RK, Miller SF, et al: Fluid retention during the first 48 hours as an indicator of burn survival. *J Trauma* 26:840, 1986.
98. Wanner A, Cutchavaree A: Early recognition of upper airway obstruction following smoke inhalation. *Am Rev Respir Dis* 108:1421, 1973.
99. Hunt JL, Agee RN, Pruitt BA: Fiberoptic bronchoscopy in acute inhalation injury. *J Trauma* 15:641, 1975.
100. Head JM: Inhalation injury in burns. *Am J Surg* 139:508, 1980.
101. Moylan JA: Inhalation injury. *J Trauma* 21:720, 1981.
102. Moylan JA, Alexander LG: Diagnosis and treatment of inhalation injury. *World J Surg* 2:185, 1978.
103. Grozel JM, Marichy J, Nombret T, Banssillon V: Fibroscopie et brulures pulmonaires: Etude préliminaire, à propos de 44 observations. *Ann Fr Anesth Reanim* 1:407, 1982.
104. Haponik EF, Meyers DA, Munster AM, et al: Acute upper airway injury in burn patients: Serial changes of flow-volume curves and nasopharyngoscopy. *Am Rev Respir Dis* 135:360, 1987.
105. Clark CJ, Reid WH, Telfer ABM, Campbell D: Respiratory injury in the burned patient: The role of flexible bronchoscopy. *Anesthesiology* 38:35, 1983.
106. Lee KC, Weedman D, Peters WJ: Use of the fiberoptic bronchoscope to change endotracheal tubes in patients with burned airways: Case report. *JBCR* 7:348, 1986.
107. Schneider W, Berger A, Maihnder P, Tempka: Diagnostic and therapeutic possibilities for fiberoptic bronchoscopy in inhalation injury. *Burns* 14:53, 1988.
108. Haponik EF, Munster AM, Britt EJ, Bleecker ER: Fiberoptic nasopharyngoscopy in the acute assessment of burn victims: Experience in 235 procedures. (Unpublished data.)
109. Colice GL, Munster AM, Haponik EF: Tracheal stenosis complicating cutaneous burns: An underestimated problem. *Am Rev Respir Dis* 134:1315, 1986.
110. Lund T, Goodwin CW, McManus WF, et al: Upper airway sequelae in burn patients requiring endotracheal intubation or tracheostomy. *Ann Surg* 201:374, 1985.
110a. Bingham HG, Gallagher TJ, Powell MD: Early bronchoscopy as a predictor of ventilatory support for burned patients. *J Trauma* 27:1286, 1987.
111. Weill RB, Capozzi A, Falces E., et al: Smoke inhalation study. *Ann Plast Surg* 4:121, 1980.
112. Herndon DN, Thompson PB, Brown M, Traber DL: Diagnosis pathophysiology, and treatment of inhalation injury, in Boswick JA (ed): *The Art and Science of Burn Care*. Rockville, Md, Aspen Publishers, 1987.
113. Fein A, Grossman R, Jones JG, et al: The value of edema fluid protein measurements in patients with pulmonary edema. *Am J Med* 67:32, 1979.
114. Johanson WG, Seidenfeld JJ, Gomez P, et al: Bacteriologic diagnosis of nosocomial pneumonia following prolonged mechanical ventilation. *Am Rev Respir Dis* 137:259, 1988.
115. Fagon JY, Chastre J, Hance AJ, et al: Detection of nosocomial lung infection in ventilated patients: Use of a protected specimen brush and quantitative culture techniques in 147 patients. *Am Rev Respir Dis* 138:110, 1988.
116. Moylan JA, Wilmore DW, Mouton DE, Pruitt BA: Early diagnosis of inhalation injury using ^{133}xenon lung scan. *Ann Surg* 176:477, 1972.
117. Milstein D, Nusynowitz ML, Lull RJ: Radionuclide diagnosis in chest disease resulting from trauma. *Semin Nucl Med* 4:339, 1974.
118. Lull RJ, Agee RN, Long JL, et al: Radionuclide evaluation of inhalation injury in patients with thermal injury. *J Nucl Med* 16:A547, 1976.
119. Agee RN, Long JM, Hunt JL, et al: Use of ^{133}xenon in early diagnosis of inhalation injury. *J Trauma* 16:218, 1976.
120. Schall GL, McDonald HD, Carr LB, Capozzi A: Xenon ventilation-perfusion lung scans: The early diagnosis of inhalation injury. *JAMA* 240:2441, 1978.
121. Witten ML, Quan SF, Sobonya RE, Lemen RJ: New developments in the pathogenesis of smoke inhalation induced pulmonary edema. *West J Med* 148:33, 1988.
122. Clark WR, Grossman ZD, Ritter-Hincirik C, Warner F: Clearance of aerosolized ^{99m}Tc-Diethylenetriamine pentacetate before and after smoke inhalation. *Chest* 94:22, 1988.
123. Minty BD, Royston D, Jones JG, et al: Changes in permeability of the alveolar-capillary barrier in firefighters. *Br J Ind Med* 42:631, 1985.
124. Garzon AA, Seltzer B, Song IC, et al: Respiratory mechanics in patients with inhalation burns. *J Trauma* 10:57, 1970.
125. Quinby WC: Restrictive effect of thoracic burns in children. *J Trauma* 12:646, 1972.
126. Landa J, Avery WG, Sackner MA: Some physiologic observations in smoke inhalation. *Chest* 61:62, 1972.

127. Morris AH, Spitzer KW: Lung function in convalescent burn patients. *Am Rev Respir Dis* 108:989, 1973.
128. Horovitz JH: Abnormalities caused by smoke inhalation. *J Trauma* 19:915, 1979.
129. Prashad J, Young RC, Laster HC, et al: Respiratory effects of a single moderately acute smoke inhalation episode. *J Natl Med Assoc* 71:251, 1979.
130. Horovitz JH: Diagnostic tools for use in smoke inhalation. *J Trauma* 21:717, 1981.
131. Elwood RK, Johnson AJ, Abboud RT, et al: Pulmonary function and bronchial reactivity in survivors of smoke inhalation. *Am Rev Respir Dis* 123:77A, 1981 (suppl).
132. Tripathi FM, Pardey K, Paul PS, et al: Respiratory functions in thermal burns. *Burns* 9:401, 1983.
133. Demling RH, Crawford G, Lind L, Read T: Restrictive pulmonary dysfunction caused by the grafted chest and abdominal burn. *Crit Care Med* 16:743, 1988.
134. Haponik EF, Munster AM, Wise RA, Bleecker ER: Pulmonary function following acute smoke inhalation injury: The predictive value of normal studies. (Unpublished data.)
135. Tobin MJ: Respiratory monitoring in the intensive care unit. *Am Rev Respir Dis* 138:1625, 1988.
136. Vender JS (ed): Intensive care monitoring. *Crit Care Clin* 4:411, 1988.
137. Saffle JR, Medina E, Raymond J, et al: Use of indirect calorimetry in the nutritional management of burned patients. *J Trauma* 25:32, 1985.
138. Matthay MA, Chatterjee K: Bedside catheterization of the pulmonary artery: Risks compared with benefits. *Ann Intern Med* 109:826, 1988.
139. Noe JM, Constable JD: A new approach to pulmonary burns: A preliminary report. *J Trauma* 13:1015, 1973.
140. German JC, Allyn PA, Bartlett RH: Pulmonary artery pressure monitoring in acute burn management. *Arch Surg* 106:788, 1973.
141. Alikawa N, Martyn JAJ, Burke JF: Pulmonary artery catheterization and thermodilution cardiac output determination in the management of burned patients. *J Trauma* 25:32, 1985.
142. Warden GD, Wilmore DW, Pruitt BA: Central venous thrombosis: A hazard of medical progress. *J Trauma* 13:620, 1973.
143. Moncrief JA: Femoral catheters. *Ann Surg* 147:166, 1958.
144. Cutillo AG: The clinical assessment of lung water. *Chest* 92:319, 1987.
145. Tranbaugh RF, Lewis FR, Christensen JM, Elings VB: Lung water changes after thermal injury: The effects of crystalloid resuscitation and sepsis. *Ann Surg* 192:479, 1980.
146. Tranbaugh RF, Elings VB, Christensen JM, Lewis FR: Effect of inhalation injury on lung water accumulation. *J Trauma* 23:597, 1983.
147. Morgan A, Knight D, O'Connor N: Lung water changes after thermal burns: An observational study. *Ann Surg* 187:288, 1978.
148. Peitzman AB, Shires T, Crobett WA, et al: Measurement of lung water in inhalation injury. *Surgery* 90:305, 1981.
149. Boutros AR, Hoyt JL, Boyd WC, et al.: Algorithm for management of pulmonary complications in burn patients. *Crit Care Med* 5:89, 1977.
150. Jelenko C III, McKinley JC: Postburn respiratory injury. *J Am Coll Emerg Physician* 5:455, 1976.

Chapter 8

Radiologic Evaluation

Craig L. Coblentz
Caroline Chiles
Charles E. Putman

Patients brought to the emergency room from the site of a fire or an industrial accident can be placed into one of three categories: those with surface burns, those with recognized pulmonary injury, and those with injury to both skin and lungs. The hospital course of these three groups of patients will vary. The prognosis of patients with surface burns is largely dependent upon the percentage of body surface area involved, with mortality increasing as the extent of involved skin surface increases. The burn patient may have escaped pulmonary injury for two reasons: (1) inspired air is rapidly cooled by the tracheal mucosa, so that thermal injury is rarely present below the level of the vocal cords, and (2) laryngospasm may prevent inhalation of the toxic products of combustion present in smoke.[1] The major pulmonary complication in burn patients is due to sepsis, with resulting capillary leak.

The second group of patients has sustained pulmonary injury alone, usually due to either smoke inhalation or exposure to a chemical spill.[2,3] In this patient population, the extent of pulmonary injury, and therefore clinical outcome, is difficult to predict. Oxygenation may prove to be difficult in this patient, requiring increased oxygen delivery. This carries with it a risk of barotrauma and oxygen toxicity, again resulting in noncardiogenic pulmonary edema.

The patient with both dermal and pulmonary injury has an even poorer prognosis, with clinical management complicated by large fluid requirements in the face of a decreased arterial oxygen saturation.[4-8]

These three groups of patients do have in common complications frequently encountered in the intensive care unit population. These include aspiration, pneumonia, cardiogenic or noncardiogenic pulmonary edema, drug toxicity, barotrauma, and complications related to catheter placement. Days or weeks into the hospital course, the chest radiographs of all three patient groups are likely to reveal unchanging bilateral airspace opacities characteristic of adult respiratory distress syndrome (ARDS). On a chronic basis, these patients have an increased incidence of pulmonary fibrosis, cicatricial emphysema, and bronchiolitis obliterans.

In this chapter, we will review the radiographic appearance of patients with suspected pulmonary injury. Confirmation of injury to the major airways is possible with fiberoptic bronchoscopy.[9] However, the diagnosis of parenchymal injury is more difficult to establish; abnormalities of blood gas levels may be delayed giving equivocal results, and the administration of oxygen may normalize the burn victim's carboxyhemoglobin level.[10] A variety of imaging modalities have been used in the evaluation of burn victims, including radionuclide studies, pulmonary angiography, bronchography, computed tomography (CT), magnetic resonance imaging (MRI), and chest radiographs. Because burn patients are often clinically unstable, chest radiographs obtained at bedside with a portable unit are the most frequently used imaging modality. Nuclear imaging is also frequently used.

CHEST RADIOGRAPH

In ours and others' experience, the conventional chest radiograph is generally an insensitive means of determining pulmonary injury by smoke inhalation. [2,11,12] Despite its limitations, a chest radiograph should be performed on all burn patients at the time of admission to hospital. Although frequently normal, an abnormal chest radiograph at admission suggests a poor prognosis. The admission chest radiograph serves as a baseline for subsequent radiographs. Abnormalities seen on a chest radiograph can be divided into three categories, based on time of development: acute, subacute, and chronic phases.[8] Chest radiographs may also allow detection of iatrogenic complications.

Acute Phase

The acute phase can be defined as the first 24 hours following the injury. Damage to the major airways, while best assessed by fiberoptic bronchoscopy, is occasionally recognized radiographically by (1) thickening of the tracheal wall and (2) indistinctness and irregularity of the luminal surface.[12] On chest radiographs, patchy pulmonary opacities, either focal or diffuse, may be present (Fig. 8-1). If the acute phase is not complicated by ARDS, also called progressive pulmonary insufficiency, these opacities typically clear within 3 days[8] (Figs. 8-1 and 8-2). Such rapid clearing suggests the opacities are due to atelectasis.

Evidence that these opacities are in part atelectatic in nature has been provided by animal models; gross atelectasis can be seen within seconds of the onset of smoke exposure and is invariably present at the end of a 5-minute period of smoke inhalation.[13] Further, cinephotomicroscopy suggests that the alveolar walls become unstable, and measurement of minimum surface tension increases. This can be explained by a decrease in available surfactant and/or inactivation of the surfactant present resulting in adhesive atelectasis. Obstructive atelectasis also occurs and may result from (1) reflex bronchoconstriction and (2) inspissation of secretions secondary to mucociliary dysfunction.[2,11]

Bilateral diffuse airspace disease can also be seen acutely and most often indicates noncardiogenic pulmonary edema (Figs. 8-3 and 8-4). Its presence in the first 24 hours is often ominous. Noncardiogenic edema can also be focal (Fig. 8-5). Capillary permeability edema is one form of noncardiogenic edema; this results from alveolar epithelial and capillary endothelial damage which, by increasing the permeability of the alveolar-capillary membrane, allows fluid to escape into the alveolar spaces. Edema from any cause may produce bilateral diffuse airspace opacities, but noncardiogenic edema may be distinguished from cardiogenic edema by the absence of (1) cardiomegaly, (2) septal lines, (3) a widened vascular pedicle, and (4) pleural fluid (Fig. 8-4).[14] Other features helpful in differentiating cardiogenic from permeability pulmonary edema are listed in Table 8-1.

Cardiogenic edema can also occur. One of the products of combustion is carbon monoxide, which by raising the patient's carboxyhemoglobin level, shifts the oxygen dissociation curve to the left. This

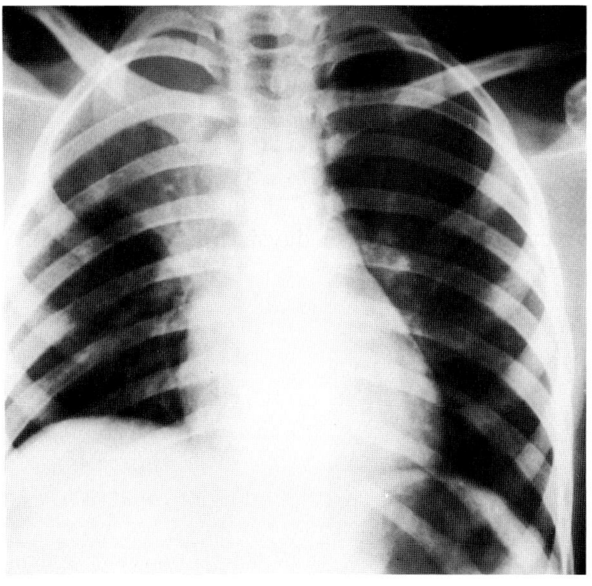

Figure 8-1 Atelectasis of the right upper lobe in a 10-year-old boy developed within 4 hours of smoke inhalation. The chest radiograph returned to normal 24 hours later. (*Reprinted with permission from AJR 129:865, 1977.*)

may give rise to myocardial ischemia and left ventricular dysfunction, especially in patients with underlying coronary artery disease. Congestive heart failure and myocardial infarction may result in cardiogenic pulmonary edema.

Pleural fluid collections are sometimes seen in the acute phase, particularly in patients with extensive cutaneous burns. These appear to be unrelated to inhalation injury and may result from vigorous intravenous fluid administration, especially in patients who may have hypoproteinemia from extensive cutaneous burns.[10]

Subacute Phase

Days 2 to 5 comprise the subacute phase. During this period the radiologist's goal is to identify secondary pulmonary complications such as infection, fluid overload, and ARDS.

ARDS may be incited by a diverse group of conditions including inhaled toxins, aspiration, and in-

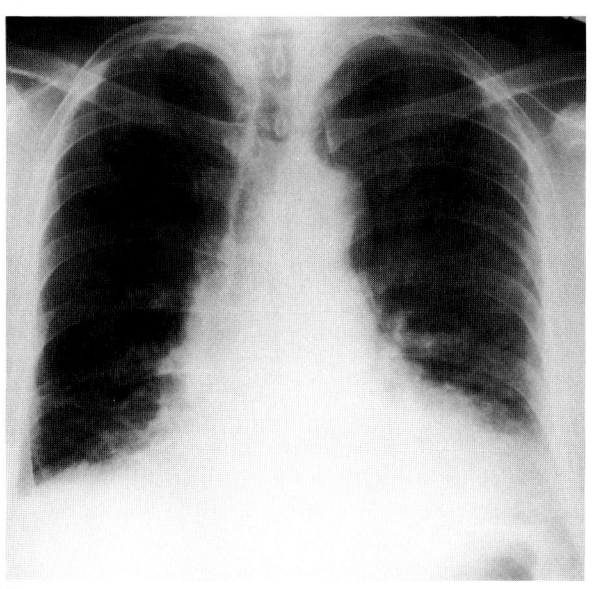

A

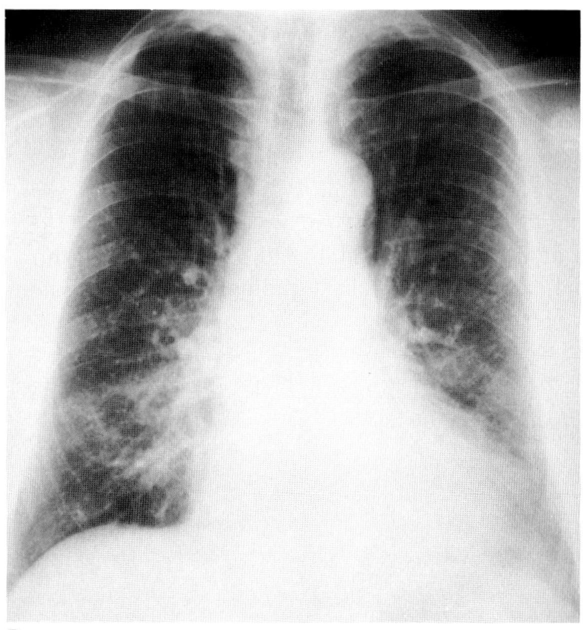

B

Figure 8-2 *A.* Bibasilar atelectasis demonstrated on a baseline radiograph of a 74-year-old man obtained within 24 hours of smoke inhalation. *B.* Atelectasis cleared in 3 days.

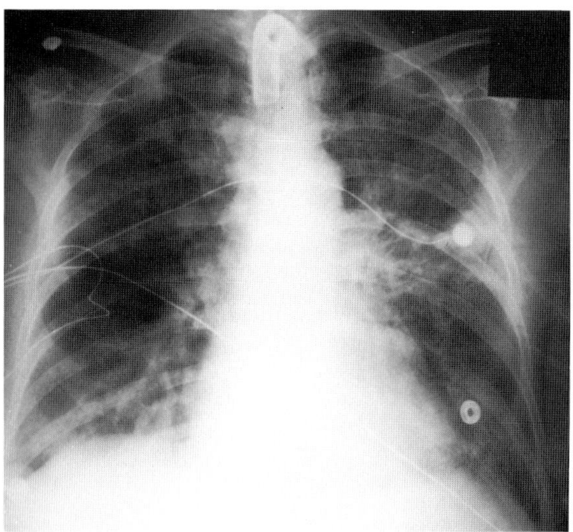

Figure 8-3 Noncardiogenic pulmonary edema in a 53-year-old woman developed within 24 hours of smoke inhalation. The lung changes are in part caused by capillary injury. The tracheostomy was required because of upper airway injury and severe hypoxemia. The patient subsequently did well.

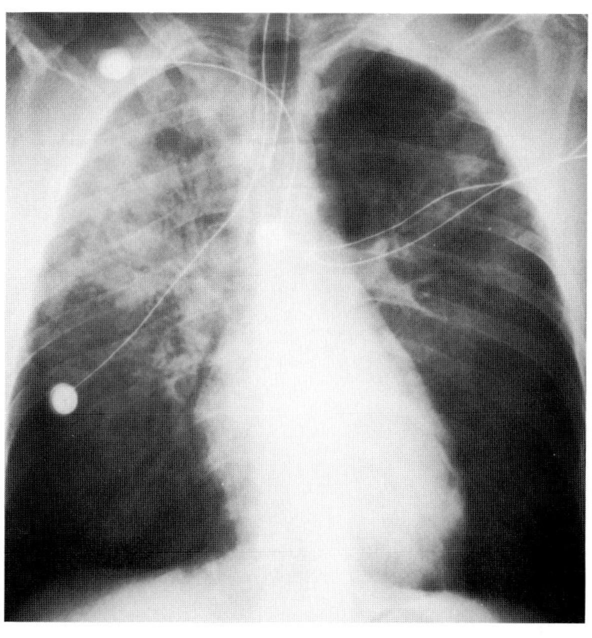

Figure 8-4 Noncardiogenic edema in a 35-year-old man following smoke inhalation. Note normal size heart and vascular pedicle and absence of septal lines distinguishing noncardiogenic edema from cardiogenic edema.

Table 8-1 Radiographic Features of Pulmonary Edema

	Overhydration	Permeability	Cardiac
Heart size	Enlarged	Nonenlarged	Enlarged
Vascular pedicle	Enlarged	Normal or reduced	Normal or enlarged
Pulmonary blood flow distribution	Balanced	Normal or balanced	Inverted
Pulmonary blood volume	Increased	Normal	Normal or increased
Septal lines	Not common	Absent	Not common
Peribronchial cuffs	Very common	Not common	Very common
Air bronchogram	Not common	Very common	Not common
Lung edema, regional distribution (horizontal axis)	Central	Peripheral	Even
Pleural effusions	Very common	Not common	Very common

SOURCE: Modified from Ref 14.

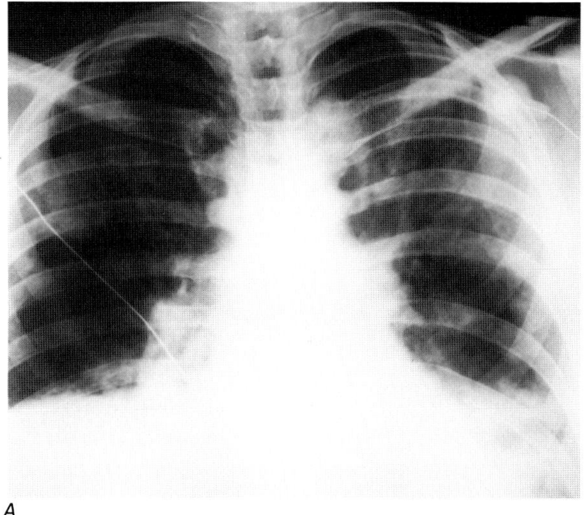

A

Figure 8-5 *A.* Chest radiograph 6 hours after smoke inhalation in a 28-year-old fireman shows bibasilar and predominantly left upper lobe airspace disease. These findings probably represent a combination of atelectasis and noncardiogenic edema. *B.* Bronchography of the right lung was performed 10 months later despite a normal chest radiograph because of bronchorrhea and repeated respiratory infections. This shows cylindrical and saccular bronchiectasis. *C.* ^{133}Xe ventilation scanning also performed 10 months later shows unequal ventilation with air trapping predominantly in the right lower lung. (*Reprinted with permission from AJR 129:867, 1977.*)

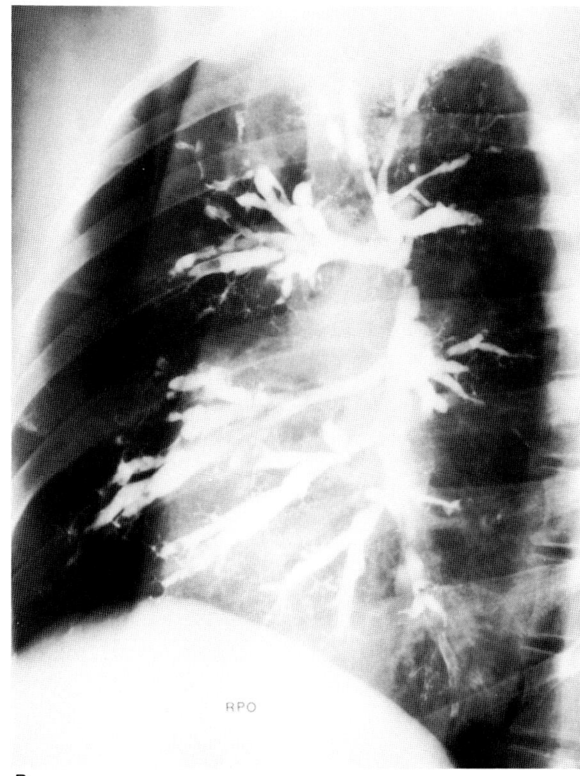

B

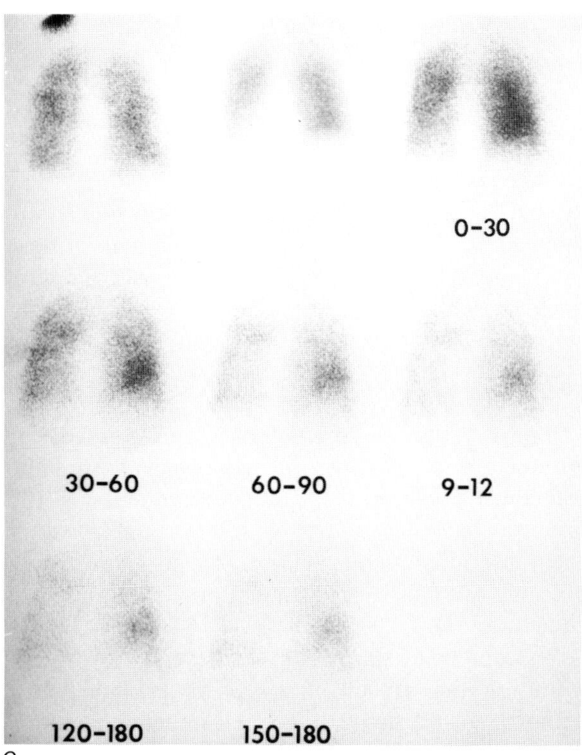

C

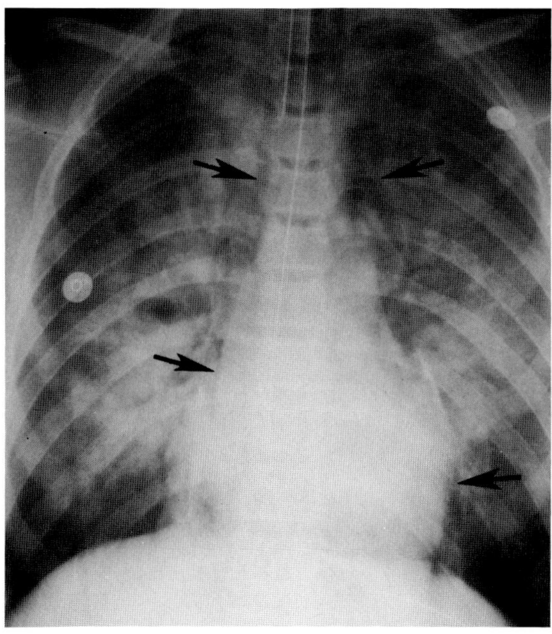

Figure 8-6 Diffuse bilateral airspace disease of ARDS in an 11-year-old girl. Note pneumomediastinum (arrows) resulting from high ventilatory pressure.

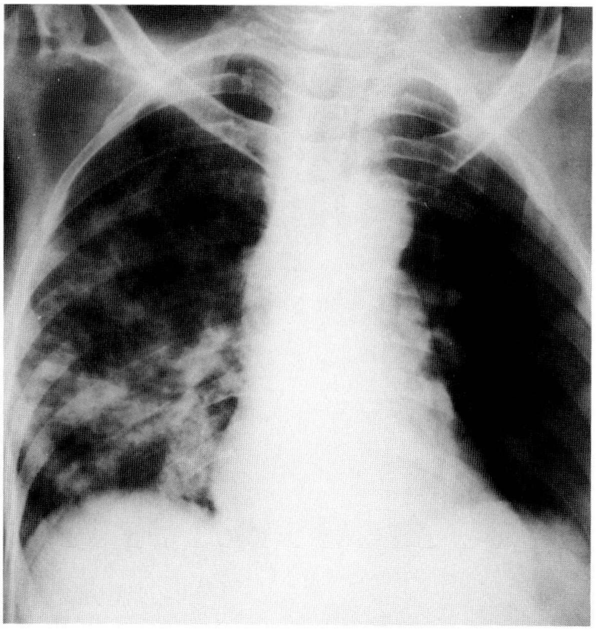

Figure 8-7 Aspiration pneumonia; 3 hours following inhalation injury, the patient was noted to aspirate gastric contents resulting in patchy airspace disease. This cleared in 3 days.

fection and can be considered as the final pathway in acute lung injury.[15] Because the syndrome is recognized not just on clinical and functional criteria but also by radiographic abnormalities, the radiologist plays a key role.[16]

Typically, radiographic abnormalities are not seen for 24 hours following the onset of the clinical signs of respiratory distress. After 24 hours, bilateral patchy, ill-defined pulmonary opacities appear. Although focal areas of lung may be spared initially, frequently these, too, will become involved as the process becomes more widespread (Fig. 8-6). Pleural fluid is characteristically absent and, when present, should suggest infection or cardiogenic edema.

Widespread airspace disease does not always represent ARDS. It can also be seen in pulmonary hemorrhage, cardiogenic edema, infection, and aspiration.[17] Because exposure to smoke and noxious gases can result in asphyxia and loss of consciousness, patients may aspirate oropharyngeal secretions and gastric contents (Fig. 8-7). The sequelae of aspiration depend on the material aspirated and the status of the pulmonary defense mechanisms. The defenses of the lung are multiple and complex. Reflex mechanisms of the upper airways prevent aspiration, and specialized cells of the airways and alveoli remove and neutralize aspirated material. When aspiration of oropharyngeal secretions does occur, it may result in a primary pneumonia. The pathogens may be anaerobic or aerobic; patients who aspirate outside the hospital usually demonstrate anaerobic organisms on culture, while hospitalized patients frequently have both aerobic and anaerobic organisms. Among the most frequently recovered anaerobic organisms are *Bacteroides* species, *Fusobacterium nucleatum, Peptostreptococcus,* and microaerophilic streptococci.

Radiographically, these pneumonias produce seg-

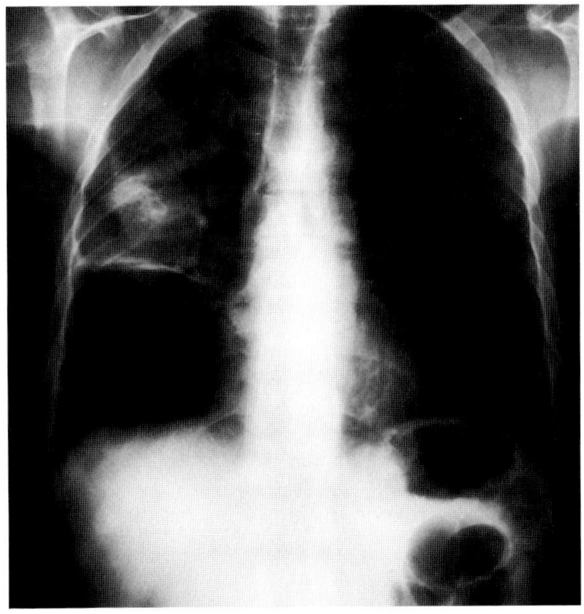

Figure 8-8 Air bronchograms within right upper lobe pneumonia.

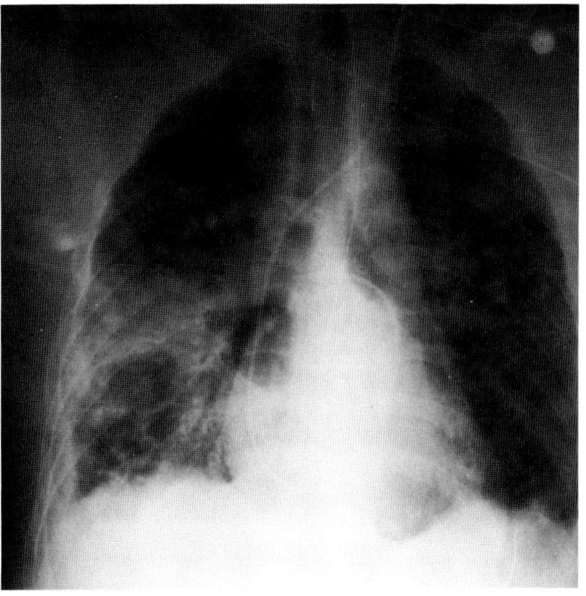

Figure 8-9 Aspiration pneumonia predominantly in superior segment of right lower lobe.

mental or lobar consolidation with preservation of lung volume (Fig. 8-8). Air bronchograms may be absent, and the opacity may appear masslike. Cavitation with or without an air-fluid level may occur. The predilection of aspiration pneumonia for the posterior segment of the right upper lobe and the superior segment of the right lower lobe is due to the influences of gravity in the supine patient and the branching pattern of the tracheobronchial tree (Figs. 8-9 and 8-10). The middle lobe and lingula are uncommonly involved because these segmental bronchi branch anteriorly from the bronchial tree. Ipsilateral hilar adenopathy may accompany aspiration pneumonia.

Pleural fluid in association with a documented anaerobic pneumonia is invariably an exudate. When pleural fluid collections are large, they must be drained. These fluid collections are frequently loculated; in this circumstance, placement of a chest tube is facilitated by computed tomography (CT) or ultrasound. Both cavitary pneumonia and empyema with a bronchopleural fistula may contain an air-fluid level, and differentiation may be difficult by chest radiograph alone (Fig. 8-10). Development of an air-fluid level at the site of a previously seen pleural fluid collection usually indicates a bronchopleural fistula. The fluid level in an empyema extends to the chest wall, and because an empyema is usually lenticular in shape, the dimensions of the fluid level are different on the frontal and lateral radiographs. A lung abscess is more likely to be round, and the length of the air-fluid level in a lung abscess is similar in both frontal and lateral projections.

CT is more accurate in differentiating abscess from empyema.[18] The most reliable CT features for differentiating abscess from empyema are wall characteristics, pleural separation, and lung compression. Empyemas typically have a thin, smooth, and uniform wall, in contrast to the wall of an abscess which is usually thick and irregular. The actual separation of uniformly thickened visceral from pari-

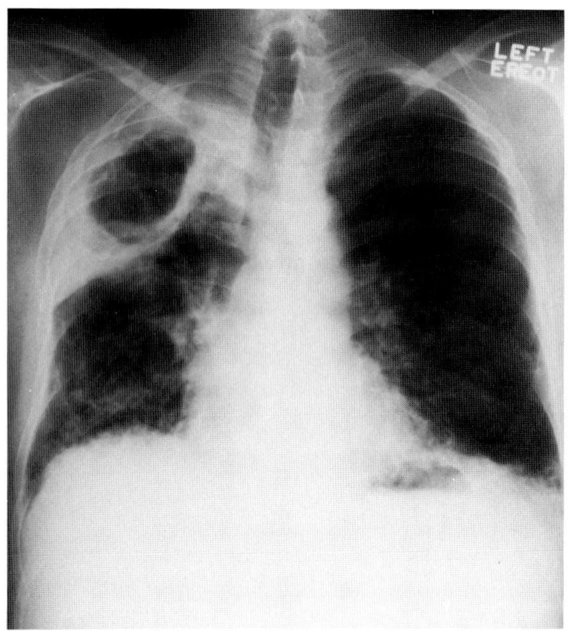

Figure 8-10 Cavitary right upper lobe pneumonia. Culture yielded *Klebsiella.*

etal pleura by empyema can often be seen. This has been called the "split pleura" sign and is best seen on CT when intravenous contrast material is administered. An empyema, particularly when large, causes compression of adjacent lung, with distortion and bowing of bronchovascular structures around the periphery of the lesion. This feature is typically absent in lung abscess.

Aspiration of nontoxic materials has fewer complications, particularly as it rarely has sufficient bacterial inoculum to cause infection. Radiographic abnormalities are usually absent or nonspecific. The most common abnormality is bilateral basilar, subsegmental atelectasis which resolves over several days.

Aspiration of toxic substances results in Mendelson's syndrome. This most commonly results from aspiration of gastric acid, but inhaled substances such as highly soluble gases (for example, ammonia, chlorine, sulfuric acid, nitrous oxide, and phosgene) also cause bronchial and alveolar toxicity. Aspiration of such toxic agents rapidly induces hypoxia from reflex bronchoconstriction. Hemorrhage and exudation of fluid into the alveoli and interstitium then occurs from loss of alveolar capillary integrity. Alveolar capillary damage causes a decrease in surfactant and, therefore, atelectasis. The end result of these events is decreased lung compliance and increased pulmonary vascular resistance.

The radiographic appearances of Mendelson's syndrome are those of permeability pulmonary edema (Table 8-1). The radiographic abnormalities may be unilateral or bilateral. An interesting appearance is the development of bilateral disease resembling congestive heart failure when unilateral disease was present initially. One explanation for this is a pulmonary vascular reflex phenomenon, secondary to either hypoxia or released biochemical mediators. In the absence of superimposed infection, the chest radiograph returns to normal 3 to 7 days after gastric aspiration.

In addition to pneumonia from aspiration, victims with inhalation injury are very susceptible to airborne infection due to hypoventilation, damaged mucosa, and mucociliary dysfunction. Radiographic features which suggest pulmonary infection include cavitation, increased focal opacity, bulging fissures, and pleural fluid[12,19] One of the most common bacterial infections acquired in tertiary care hospitals is caused by *Pseudomonas aeruginosa*. Organisms may infect the lung by hematogenous spread or inhalation. Inhalation usually occurs secondary to contaminated suction or tracheostomy devices. Although there is a predilection for the lower lobes, airspace disease may spread rapidly to involve the lung diffusely. Atelectasis and pleural fluid are uncommon. Cavitation and empyema may develop.

When the patient's burn involves a large percentage of body area, fluid losses from the skin surface are great and the patient may require support with large volumes of intravenous fluid. This and other reasons for intravenous fluid administration may result in inadvertent fluid overload. The radiographic features of overhydration pulmonary edema are those of cardiogenic edema, including (1) central perihilar airspace opacity, (2) prominent pulmonary vessels, (3) cardiomegaly, and (4) pleural fluid. In addition, the width of the vascular pedicle may be increased (Table 8-1).

The vascular pedicle is seen on the frontal chest radiograph as the midline structures extending from the thoracic inlet to the heart. Its right-hand border is formed by the right brachiocephalic vein above, and by the superior vena cava below. The left-hand border is formed by the left subclavian artery above the aorta.[20] The normal vascular pedicle width on an erect posteroanterior radiograph obtained at 6 feet in full inspiration is 43 to 53 mm. Because of the tremendous range of normal, measurement of the vascular pedicle on a single radiograph is of less use than detecting a change on subsequent radiographs. When examinations comparable in patient positioning and tube-to-film distance are obtained, an increase of 5 mm in the width of the vascular pedicle is equivalent to an increase of 1.0 L in total blood volume.[21] The usefulness of the vascular pedicle in burn patients has been evaluated.[22] Forty-two patients with cutaneous burns at risk for inhalation injury had chest radiographs performed on admission and 24 hours later. No patient had pulmonary edema on admission. The vascular pedicle increased in width from 6.0 $\pm$ 1.0 cm to 6.9 $\pm$ 1.2 cm in patients who subsequently developed pulmonary edema, while the vascular pedicle width remained the same in patients who did not develop pulmonary edema. The edema did not occur on average until 3.3 days after admission. From these results the authors concluded that enlargement of the vascular pedicle might provide a clinically useful predictor of this complication in burn patients.

In contrast to overhydration pulmonary edema, pulmonary edema due to increased capillary permeability has a more peripheral and patchy distribution of airspace opacity, and the pulmonary vessel caliber, heart size, and vascular pedicle width are normal (Table 8-1). Because of similarities in the radiographic appearance between ARDS, infection and pulmonary edema and also because mixed patterns are common, radiographic differentiation between these processes is often impossible.

Chronic Phase

After day 5, infection, ARDS, and/or pulmonary thromboembolism usually account for any radiographic abnormality. The chest radiograph is neither sensitive nor specific in the diagnosis of acute pulmonary thromboembolism. Ventilation-perfusion scans with a radiopharmaceutical are more sensitive; however, because patients with burns and inhalation injury frequently have coexisting pulmonary disease, the results may be indeterminate, requiring pulmonary angiography for definitive diagnosis.

In the months to years following injury, patients may continue to exhibit upper airway and pulmonary dysfunction. Residual structural damage to the trachea and bronchi may result in tracheal stenosis, bronchiectasis, and bronchiolitis obliterans.[11,23]

Tracheal stenosis can result from mucosal injury secondary to inhalation of noxious gases and less commonly, thermal injury. Tracheal stenosis is best evaluated by linear tomography, positive contrast tracheography, or bronchoscopy. The trachea can also be examined by CT; however, CT tends to overestimate the severity of stenosis and does not provide additional information in the detection or characterization of tracheal stenosis beyond that obtained from conventional studies.[24]

Bronchiectasis, like tracheal stenosis, usually results from inhalation rather than thermal injury. The primary imaging modality for the evaluation of bronchiectasis is bronchography[25]; it is accurate, easy, and safe to perform. Using oily propyliodine (Dionosil) as a contrast material, cylindrical and saccular bronchiectasis of segmental and subsegmental bronchi can be demonstrated (Fig. 8-5). Cylindrical bronchiectasis is manifested by fairly uniform dilation of the bronchi and represents mild disease. More severe disease is indicated by saccular (or cystic) bronchiectasis, which is seen as markedly dilated bronchi with a ballooned outline. Cystic spaces up to 2 cm in diameter, occasionally containing fluid levels, may be seen. In addition to dilated bronchi, fewer bronchi than usual are visualized in bronchiectasis, since small branches are destroyed and obliterated by fibrosis.

Acute infection may be accompanied by reversible tubular dilatation of bronchi. Because true bronchiectasis is irreversible, the optimal time for performing bronchography is 4 to 6 months following acute pneumonia, to allow time for bronchi to return to normal.

Recently, high resolution CT has been advocated as a less invasive procedure to establish the diagnosis and extent of bronchiectasis.[26] However, because both false positives and negatives occur, its exact role remains to be clarified.[25,27]

Bronchiolitis obliterans results when injury to the terminal airways, such as from inhalation of toxic fumes, is repaired by proliferation of granulation tissue. This granulation tissue along with organized purulent secretions may obliterate the lumina of bronchioles and alveolar ducts. This may be accompanied by (1) emphysema and pulmonary fibrosis that further engulfs vessels and terminal airways and/or (2) organizing pneumonia which is manifested by variable degrees of interstitial infiltration by mononuclear cells.[28] The radiographic features of bronchiolitis obliterans are variable[29] and are probably related to the varying degrees of organizing pneumonia present.[30] In its absence the radiograph may be normal or demonstrate a reticular-nodular pattern. When organizing pneumonia is present, patchy areas of airspace disease having a "ground glass" appearance are seen.[28,31] Hyperinflation, unilateral disease, cavitation, and pleural fluid are uncommon.

Iatrogenic Complications

A variety of therapeutic interventions such as endotracheal intubation and intravenous catheterization may be required in this patient population. The placement and optimal positioning of these tubes and lines are easily monitored on chest radiographs. The chest radiograph is also useful in detecting any complications resulting from these procedures.

The rapid accumulation of mediastinal or pleural fluid after venous line placement may indicate hemorrhage from vascular injury or infusion of fluid from aberrant line placement (Fig. 8-11). Endotracheal intubation of a mainstem bronchus can result in collapse of the opposite lung, a potentially life-threatening complication in a patient whose respiratory status may already be compromised by preexisting lung injury (Fig. 8-12). High ventilatory pressures may result in barotrauma including interstitial emphysema, subcutaneous emphysema, pneumomediastinum, pneumothorax, and, rarely, pneumopericardium.

Although most commonly seen in children, the earliest manifestation of extraalveolar air is interstitial emphysema. This results from high airway pressure causing alveolar rupture and dissection of alveolar air into the interstitial space.[32] The risk of interstitial emphysema is increased as the ventilatory pressures increase and if there is underlying disease of the alveoli (e.g. bullae as may occur with obstructive lung disease). Radiographic features of pulmonary interstitial emphysema include lucent lines coursing toward the hilum, perivascular and peribronchial halos, pneumatocele formation, and subpleural emphysema. The subpleural emphysema may appear as a cyst or as a radiolucent line. These vesicular or bubbly lucencies of interstitial emphysema should not be mistaken for air bronchograms in an area of parenchymal consolidation.

Subpleural air cysts may appear abruptly. They are usually peripherally located, particularly at the lung bases, either medially or along the diaphragm. The subpleural air cyst portends the development of pneumothorax.[33] By identifying the air cyst it may be possible to prevent a pneumothorax which may be life threatening; up to 90 percent of pneumothoraces in mechanically ventilated patients are under tension.

While the chest radiograph is very useful for its detection, should a pneumothorax develop, the findings may be subtle. In one study of critically ill

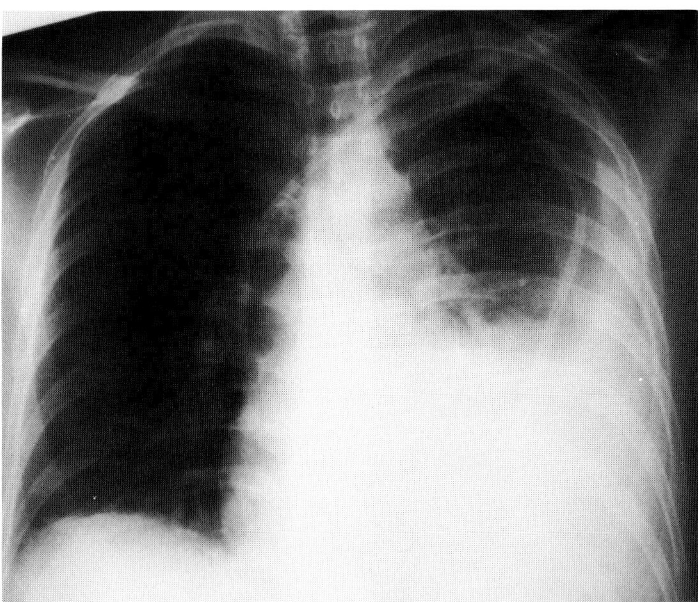

Figure 8-11 Left tension hemothorax resulting from traumatic central line placement.

patients with pneumothorax, 30 percent were missed initially.[34] This is because in the supine patient air may not appear in the classic location over the lung apices and lateral to the lungs. Instead, because air accumulates in the highest portion of the thorax, in the supine patient pneumothoraces will most often be seen in the anteromedial and subpulmonic recesses (Fig. 8-13).

Tracheostomy and prolonged tracheal intubation may result in tracheal stenosis and tracheomalacia (Fig. 8-14). The stenosis usually occurs at the level of the stoma or at the inflatable cuff. Rarely, it occurs at the tip of the tube. Although the stenosis may be seen on a chest radiograph, it is best demonstrated by bronchoscopy or linear tomography. Tracheomalacia results from either excess removal of cartilage at the time of tracheostomy and/or from destruction of cartilage by pressure necrosis or infection.[35] Without cartilaginous support, the compliance of the trachea is increased allowing it to change caliber with respiration. This may be observed fluoroscopically or by cine CT.[36]

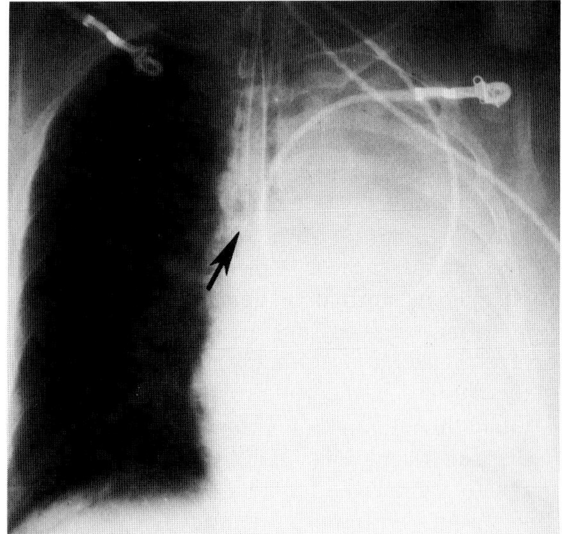

Figure 8-12 Left lung collapse from malpositioning of distal tip of endotracheal tube (arrow) down right main stem bronchus.

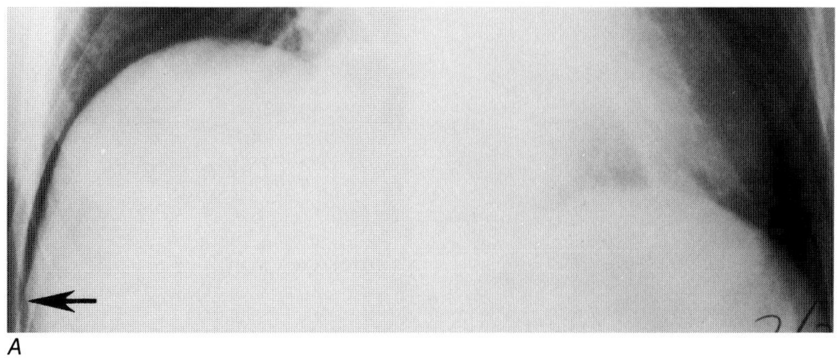

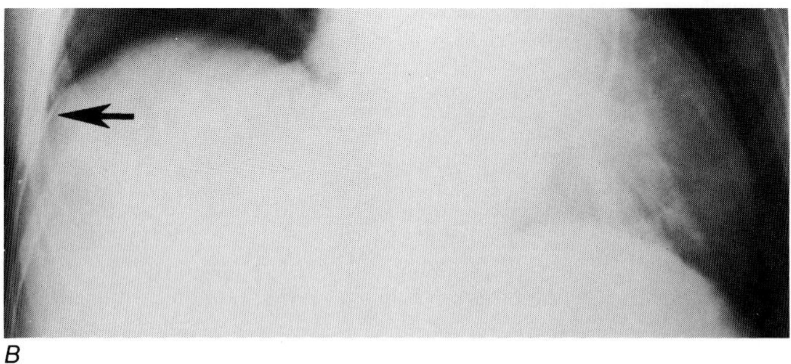

Figure 8-13 *A.* Deep sulcus sign (arrow) of pneumothorax in a supine patient following attempt at central line placement. *B.* A baseline radiograph shows normal right sulcus (arrow).

The administration of oxygen can directly damage the lung, especially if prolonged and in high concentrations as is often required in the intensive care population.[37] This results pathologically in edema, hemorrhage, hyaline membranes, and fibrosis. Patchy opacities typically develop 3 to 5 days following initiation of therapy, but there are no characteristic radiographic features of this complication.

Although not really a complication, physicians should be aware of the radiographic changes that can occur with positive end-expiratory pressure (PEEP) so as not to misinterpret these as either improving or worsening disease. Radiographs obtained at tidal volume appear "worse," while those with PEEP appear "better." Changes that occur with PEEP include lowered hemidiaphragms, decreased size and increased sharpness of pulmonary vessels, decreased heart size and mediastinal width, and disappearance of the silhouette sign.[38] The apparent improvement seen with mechanical ventilation is probably related to the improved lung volumes which occur on PEEP. The physician should note the parameters of ventilation prior to interpreting the radiograph so as not to ascribe radiographic improvement to clinical improvement when, in fact, increasing levels of PEEP required for worsening respiratory failure are responsible.

NUCLEAR IMAGING

Although the chest radiograph has many uses in the management of burn victims, it is an insensitive

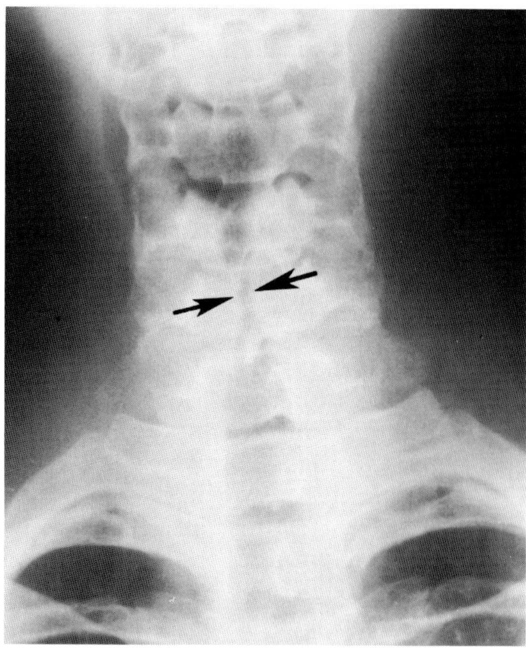

Figure 8-14 Tracheal stenosis (arrows) resulting from tracheostomy.

means for the early diagnosis of inhalation injury. A more sensitive method of detecting lung injury before the chest radiograph becomes abnormal is nuclear imaging with the gas xenon 133 (^{133}Xe).[39-41]

In this technique, 10 to 20 μCi of ^{133}Xe are dissolved in saline and injected intravenously. Imaging of the lung is then obtained with a gamma camera every 6 seconds for the first 30 seconds to monitor bolus arrival, followed by serial images every 30 seconds to evaluate regional washout. Following injection, virtually all the xenon enters the alveolar airspace during its first pass through the lung. From there the xenon can then be cleared, which in a normal person is complete by 150 seconds after injection. Any delay in the clearance of ^{133}Xe indicates inhalation injury. The cause of the delayed clearance is postulated to be trapping of the xenon gas behind obstructed small airways. The obstruction results from bronchiolar epithelial inflammation and edema, which are characteristic of the early stages of inhalation injury.[41,43] If the inflammation results in fibrosis, the ventilatory defects may persist (Fig. 8-5).

In a review by Lull et al. of several series totaling 193 patients, the overall accuracy of the ^{133}Xe washout study was 92 percent with an 87 percent positive predictive value and a 96 percent negative predictive value.[42] False positives may occur in patients with (1) acute pulmonary disease such as pneumonia and (2) in chronic lung diseases such as emphysema, asthma, chronic bronchitis, and bronchiectasis.

In addition to the ^{133}Xe study, some investigators obtain a comparison perfusion image with technetium 99m macroaggregated albumin (MAA); however, because perfusion abnormalities are uncommon, this step is not essential. If a perfusion study is performed, it can be used as a baseline should pulmonary embolism be suspected at a later date.[43]

Another radiopharmaceutical for lung imaging is ^{99m}Tc diethylenetriamine pentacetate (DTPA). This radionuclide is dissolved in saline and delivered as an aerosol which the patient inhales. Serial images of the lungs are obtained with a gamma camera at 30 second intervals. Regions of interest within the lungs are then selected, and the clearance of DTPA from these areas is calculated. The rate of clearance represents absorption of DTPA through the alveolar surface into the pulmonary capillary and then into the systemic circulation, with values ranging from 0.5 to 2 percent per minute.[44]

The rate of clearance is increased in conditions that increase epithelial permeability to solutes, for example, ARDS. Because (1) inhalation injury is thought to represent a toxic or chemical injury at the pulmonary parenchymal level,[12] and (2) because cigarette smoke has been shown to increase the clearance of DTPA in humans,[45] it has been proposed that this test should be useful in the early diagnosis of smoke inhalation. Indeed, in an animal model, DTPA clearance after smoke inhalation was increased and was found to be more sensitive in detecting lung injury than either a chest radiograph or ^{133}Xe scanning.[46] Unfortunately, in a follow-up pilot clinical trial of patients with smoke exposure (seven patients), DTPA clearance was normal and was not helpful in establishing the degree of inhalation injury.[46] The clearance of DTPA is useful in differentiating cardiogenic edema from increased permeability edema of ARDS, but its role in diagnosing injury from acute smoke inhalation will require additional study.

In a setting of diffuse lung disease, it is often impossible to determine the presence of pulmonary infection based on clinical information and a chest radiograph alone. In this circumstance, pulmonary infection can sometimes be documented by indium 111–labeled white blood cell scanning.

EXPERIMENTAL METHODS

The chest radiograph is incapable of detecting small increases in lung density that may reflect pulmonary edema due to lung injury. CT is able to detect small changes in lung density because of its excellent contrast resolution. This has proved helpful in animal models in defining some of the early radiographic changes that result from lung injury.[47,48] Magnetic resonance imaging (MRI) has also been used to investigate lung injury.[49] CT and MRI are more sensitive than the chest radiograph for parenchymal injury and can detect focal disease before the patient develops blood gas abnormalities.

Both CT and MRI have demonstrated differences in the distribution of pulmonary edema depending on whether it is hydrostatic, embolic-hemorrhagic, or due to increased capillary permeability. For example, in dogs, after 2 hours of elevated left atrial pressure (>28 mmHg), CT demonstrated increased density in central and dependent areas of the axial lung image.[50] In contrast, embolic-hemorrhagic injury from vascular infusion of oleic acid in dogs and sheep resulted in a patchy peripheral pattern of increased lung density.[47,51] Alloxan infusion in dogs, resulting in capillary leak, causes a more uniform increase in lung density.[52] The difference in the distribution of pulmonary edema reflects, in part, differences in dispersal of toxic agents in the pulmonary vasculature[53,54] and the response of the lungs to elevated vascular pressure.[50]

CT and MRI have also demonstrated regional changes in the lungs following inhalation injury. CT of dogs exposed to phosgene gas demonstrated diffusely increased lung density centrally and around vascular and bronchial structures.[47] Spin-echo MRI of baboons exposed to 98 percent oxygen for 4 days showed diffusely increased signal intensity in the lung parenchyma and also in the peribronchial, perivascular, and subpleural areas consistent with interstitial edema. These findings were confirmed at autopsy.

These and other radiologic studies have increased our understanding of lung injury. Hopefully this new knowledge will allow for the development of better methods for early detection and for following the course and treatment of lung injury.

REFERENCES

1. Moritz ZR, Henriques FC, McLean R: Effects of inhaled heat on air passages and lungs: An experimental investigation. *Am J Pathol* 21:311, 1945.
2. Trunkey DD: Inhalation injury. *Surg Clin North Am* 58:1133, 1978.
3. Zikria BA, Ferrer JM, Floch HF: The chemical factors contributing to pulmonary damage in smoke poisoning. *Surgery* 71:704, 1972.
4. Pruitt BA, Flemma RJ, DiVincenti FC, et al: Pulmonary complications in burn patients: A comparative study of 697 patients. *J. Thorac Cardiovasc Surg* 59:7, 1970.
5. Shook CD, MacMillan BC, Altemeier WA: Pulmonary complications of the burn patient. *Arch Surg* 97:215, 1968.
6. Achauer BM, Allyn PA, Furnas DW, Bartlett RH: Pulmonary complications of burns: The major threat to the burn patient. *Ann Surg* 177:311, 1973.
7. Stone HH, Martin JD: Pulmonary injury associated with thermal burns. *Surg Gynecol Obstet* 129:1242, 1969.

8. Kangarloo H, Beachley MC, Ghahremani GG: The radiographic spectrum of pulmonary complications in burn victims. *AJR* 128:441, 1977.
9. Hunt JL, Agee RN, Pruitt BA: Fiberoptic bronchoscopy in acute inhalation injury. *J Trauma* 15:641, 1975.
10. Teixidor HS, Rubin E, Novick GS, Alonso DR: Smoke inhalation: Radiologic manifestations. *Radiology* 149:383, 1983.
11. Putman CE, Loke J, Matthay RA, Ravin CE: Radiographic manifestations of acute smoke inhalation. *AJR* 129:865, 1977.
12. Teixidor HS, Novick G, Rubin E: Pulmonary complications in burn patients. *J Can Assoc Radiol* 34: 264, 1983.
13. Nieman GF, Clark WR, Wax SD, Webb WR: The effect of smoke inhalation on pulmonary surfactant. *Ann Surg* 191:171, 1980.
14. Milne ENC, Pistolesi M, Miniati M, Giuntini C: The radiologic distinction of cardiogenic and noncardiogenic edema. *AJR* 144:879, 1985.
15. Greene R, Jantsch H, Boggis C, et al: Respiratory distress syndrome with new considerations. *Radiol Clin North Am* 21:699, 1983.
16. Greene R: Adult respiratory distress syndrome: Acute alveolar damage. *Radiology* 163:57, 1987.
17. Putman CE: Infectious pneumonias—Including aspiration states, in Putman CE, Ravin CE (eds): *Textbook of Diagnostic Imaging*. Philadelphia, Saunders, 1988, chap 45.
18. Stark DD, Federle MP, Goodman PC, et al: Differentiating lung abscess and empyema: Radiography and computed tomography. *AJR* 141:163, 1983.
19. Chiles C, Hedlund LW, Putman CE: Diagnostic imaging in inhalation lung injury, in Loke J (ed): *Pathophysiology and Treatment of Inhalation Injuries*. New York, Dekker, 1988, chap 5.
20. Milne ENC, Pistolesi M, Miniati M, Giuntini C: The vascular pedicle of the heart and the vena azygos. Part I: The normal subject. *Radiology* 152:1, 1984.
21. Pistolesi M, Milne ENC, Miniati M, Giuntini C: The vascular pedicle of the heart and the vena azygos. Part II: Acquired heart disease. *Radiology* 152:9, 1984.
22. Haponik EF, Adelman M, Munster AM, Bleecker ER: Increased vascular pedicle width preceding burn-related pulmonary edema. *Chest* 90:649, 1986.
23. Perez-Guerra F, Walsh RE, Sagel SS: Bronchiolitis obliterans and tracheal stenosis: Late complications of inhalation burn. *JAMA* 218:1568, 1971.
24. Gamsu G, Webb WR: Computed tomography of the trachea: Normal and abnormal. *AJR* 139:321, 1982.
25. Mueller NL, Bergin CJ, Ostrow DN, Nichols DM: Role of computed tomography in the recognition of bronchiectasis. *AJR* 143:971, 1984.
26. Grenier P, Maurice F, Musset D, et al: Bronchiectasis: Assessment by thin-section CT. *Radiology* 161:95, 1986.
27. Silverman PM, Godwin JD: CT/Bronchographic correlations in bronchiectasis. *J. Comput Assist Tomogr* 11:52, 1987.
28. Epler GR, Colby TV, McLoud TC, et al: Bronchiolitis obliterans organizing pneumonia. *N Engl J Med* 312:152, 1985.
29. Gosink BB, Friedman PJ, Liebow AA: Bronchiolitis obliterans: Roentgenologic-pathologic correlation. *AJR* 117:816, 1973.
30. Mueller NL, Guerry-Force ML, Staples CA, et al: Differential diagnosis of bronchiolitis obliterans with organizing pneumonia and usual interstitial pneumonia: Clinical, functional, and radiologic findings. *Radiology* 162:151, 1987.
31. McLoud TC, Epler GR, Colby TV, et al: Bronchiolitis obliterans. *Radiology* 159:1, 1986.
32. Macklin CC: Transport of air along sheaths of pulmonic blood vessels from alveoli to mediastinum: Clinical implications. *Arch Intern Med* 64:913, 1939.
33. Rohlfing BM, Webb WR, Schlobohm RM: Ventilator-related extra-alveolar air in adults. *Radiology* 121:25, 1976.
34. Tocino IM, Miller MH, Fairfax WR: Distribution of pneumothorax in the supine and semirecumbent critically ill adult. *AJR* 144:901, 1985.
35. Harley HRS: Laryngotracheal obstruction complicating tracheostomy or endotracheal intubation with assisted respiration: A critical review. *Thorax* 26:493, 1971.
36. Ell SR, Jolles H, Galvin JR: Cine CT demonstration of nonfixed upper airway obstruction. *AJR* 146:669, 1986.
37. Joffe N, Simon M: Pulmonary oxygen toxicity in the adult. *Radiology* 93:460, 1969.
38. Curtis AMcB: Adult respiratory distress syndrome, in Putman CE, Ravin CE (eds): *Textbook of Diagnostic Imaging*. Philadelphia, Saunders, 1988, chap 51.
39. Moylan JA, Wilmore DW, Mouton DE, Pruitt BA: Early diagnosis of inhalation injury using ^{133}Xenon lung scan. *Ann Surg* 176:477, 1972.
40. Agee RN, Long JM, Hunt JL, et al: Use of ^{133}Xenon in early diagnosis of inhalation injury. *J Trauma* 15:218, 1976.
41. Schall GL, McDonald HD, Carr LB, Capozzi A: Xenon ventilation-perfusion lung scans: The early diagnosis of inhalation injury. *JAMA* 240:2441, 1978.
42. Lull RJ, Tatum JL, Sugerman JH, et al: Radionuclide evaluation of lung trauma. *Semin Nucl Med* 13:223, 1983.
43. Lull RJ, Anderson JH, Telepak RJ, et al: Radionuclide imaging in the assessment of lung injury. *Semin Nucl Med* 10:302, 1980.
44. O'Brodovich H, Coates G: Pulmonary clearance of ^{99m}Tc-DTPA: A noninvasive assessment of epithelial integrity. *Lung* 165:1, 1987.
45. Jones JG, Lawler P, Crawley JCW, et al: Increased alveolar epithelial permeability in cigarette smokers. *Lancet* 1:66, 1980.
46. Clark WR, Grossman ZD, Ritter-Hrncirik C, Warner F: Clearance of aerosolized ^{99m}Tc-diethylenetriaminepentacetate before and after smoke inhalation. *Chest* 94:23, 1988.
47. Hedlund LW, Putman CE: Methods for detecting pulmonary edema. *Toxicol Ind Health* 1:59, 1985.
48. Hedlund LW, Vock P, Effmann EL: Computed tomography of the lung: Densitometric studies. *Radiol Clin North Am* 21:775, 1983.
49. Hedlund LW, Deitz J, Herfkens R, et al: Magnetic reso-

nance imaging of pulmonary edema following oleic acid injury. *Am Rev Respir Dis* 133:A403, 1986.

50. Hedlund LW, Vock P, Effmann EL, et al: Hydrostatic pulmonary edema: An analysis of lung density changes by computed tomography. *Invest Radiol* 19:254, 1984.
51. Hedlund LW, Effmann EL, Bates WM, et al: Pulmonary edema: A CT study of regional changes in lung density following oleic acid injury. *J Comput Assist Tomogr* 6:939, 1982.
52. Putman CE, Hedlund LW, Tsai J, Effmann EL: Pulmonary edema: A comparison of regional differences in the lung in three animal models, abstracted. *Chest* 86:338, 1984.
53. Chiles C, Hedlund LW, Kubek RJ, et al: Distribution of 15- and 137-μ diameter microspheres in the dog lung in the axial plane. *Invest Radiol* 21:618, 1986.
54. Tarver RD, Tsai J, Hedlund LW, et al: Regional pulmonary distribution of iodine-125-labeled oleic acid: Its relationship to the pattern of oleic acid edema and pulmonary blood flow. *Invest Radiol* 21:102, 1986.

Chapter 9

Management of Inhalation Injury in Patients with and without Burns

Sam R. Sharar
David M. Heimbach
Leonard D. Hudson

Inhalation injury presents in a variety of clinical scenarios and occurs in all age groups; thus the discussion of its multiple forms and therapies is often fragmented and complex. In this chapter we will consider only two groups of patients with inhalation injury — patients with isolated smoke inhalation and those with smoke inhalation and concomitant burn injury. This knowledge can be extrapolated to the many subgroups of patients seen in clinical practice. The purpose of this chapter is to outline the clinical assessment and treatment of each patient group based on a chronology of events that follow the inhalation of smoke. Thus, an initial discussion of field management will be followed by strategies of acute hospital management and conclude with the management of delayed sequelae. In this way a format for the overall management of inhalation injury will be presented that can be applied to all potential victims and modified according to the clinical situation.

The discussion of patients with isolated smoke inhalation emphasizes airway control and oxygenation, both of which must be established urgently and maintained aggressively throughout all phases of treatment. These are treatment priorities, since isolated inhalation injury is generally a self-limited process involving upper airway and bronchial inflammation and not significant parenchymal lung injury. This clinical scenario is supported by evidence from the 1982 Las Vegas hotel fires. Eighty-four victims died at the scene, primarily of carbon monoxide intoxication. However, of over 400 victims of these fires who were transported to hospitals, the mortality was less than 1 percent, and the incidence of myocardial infarction, ventilatory insufficiency, and pneumonia was each only 1 percent.[1]

Associated injuries and concurrent medical problems must also be considered. For example, the elderly, diabetic widow confined to her apartment by peripheral and coronary vascular disease can sustain a life-threatening injury when her cigarette ignites a mattress, causing it to smolder. Because of her underlying pathophysiology, mild inhalation injury without any concomitant burn becomes a serious problem.

Finally, an understanding of the management of isolated inhalation injury is requisite for our discussion of the patients with combined inhalation and burn injuries. In such a patient, the principal concern is the management of two *different* injuries. An understanding of each injury alone is necessary before this patient can be successfully managed because some treatment priorities coincide (e.g., the establishment of airway, breathing, and circulation—ABCs—during initial resuscitation) and some do not (e.g., limited fluid resuscitation after isolated smoke inhalation but aggressive resuscitation in burn patients). A discussion of the management of cutaneous burns is beyond the scope of this presentation, but a comprehensive review can be found elsewhere.[2] In the second section of this chapter the interaction of concurrent smoke and burn injuries will be discussed. Such patients constitute approximately 10 to 20 percent of all hospitalized burn patients and have an overall mortality of 48 to 77 percent.[3] Mortality is significantly greater among these patients compared to those with burns of similar size alone. A study of over 1000 consecutive admissions to the Shriners Burn Institute in Galveston, Texas, reported the mortality of patients with 40 to 80 percent body surface area burns to be 20 percent, while similar patients with associated inhalation injury experienced a 58 percent mortality.[4] It has been estimated that inhalation injury and subsequent pneumonia increase mortality in burn patients by 60 percent.[5]

Finally, management of these patients makes tremendous technical, personnel, financial, and emotional demands on a medical facility. Transfer to a tertiary care or burn center is requisite when both burn and inhalation injuries are present and may be necessary for many patients with only one injury. The third section of this chapter reviews protocols for transport of patients with smoke or burn injuries or both. These recommendations are designed to ensure patient safety and proper continuity of care.

INHALATION INJURY MANAGEMENT IN PATIENTS WITHOUT BURNS

Field Management

The basic tenets of field management of inhalation injury do not differ initially from those guiding the care of any traumatic injury. Airway patency, breathing, and circulation should be rapidly evaluated and established. Standard protocols are outlined in the manuals of both the Advanced Trauma Life Support (ATLS) and Advanced Burn Life Support (ABLS) courses. In fact, beyond these ABCs little specialized diagnosis and treatment of inhalation injury can be performed at the accident scene. The presence of other concurrent injuries must be noted and, if necessary, treated in the field. Although isolated inhalation injury most often presents without other concomitant injuries (e.g., carbon monoxide [CO] poisoning in a parked automobile with idling motor), emergency personnel must be aware of the possibility of other injuries such as closed head trauma, musculoskeletal trauma, or cardiac dysrhythmias that may require urgent treatment.

The focus of field management of isolated inhalation injury is respiratory stabilization — airway maintenance and ventilation. When upper airway obstruction occurs at the scene, it is most likely due to associated neurologic injury (severe CO poisoning and coma) or acute supraglottic and glottic edema secondary to smoke-induced or occasionally heat-induced mucosal injury. Endotracheal intubation is the treatment of choice in these cases and is of course dependent on the skill and knowledge of the paramedical staff. If this option is not available, manual airway assistance with either an oral or nasal airway is the preferable second choice. Once an airway is established, either spontaneous or assisted ventilation with 100 percent oxygen is begun. This can rapidly improve tissue oxygenation since ambient oxygen fractions may be as low as 2 percent at the fire scene.[6] In addition, oxygen reduces the blood half-life of CO in a dose-dependent fashion as discussed below. Prehospital mortality is primarily due to CO intoxication — 66 percent of all house fire deaths in 1980.[7] Thus, rapid field oxygen therapy is essential to survival. As soon as the patient's ABCs are stabilized, rapid transport with continuous oxygen therapy to the nearest appropriate medical center is undertaken.

Acute Hospital Management

Upon arrival in the emergency room, the ABCs are quickly reviewed and a pertinent history rapidly taken. Certain elements of the inhalation history are crucial in determining the presence and severity of respiratory injury. Emphasis should be placed on the following key points:

1. Circumstances of the inhalation — e.g., history of a suicide attempt warrants careful patient observation and suggests early involvement of psychiatric personnel.
2. The accident scene — Inhalation injuries sustained in "closed spaces" (e.g., buildings, automobiles) result in more severe respiratory abnormalities with much greater frequency than those sustained in "open spaces."
3. Duration of exposure — An estimation of the severity of inhalation injury can be made with this information, as shown in animal studies.[8]
4. Type of smoke involved (i.e., type of substrate burned) — Very severe parenchymal lung injuries have been reported after polyvinylchloride (plastics, plumbing, electrical insulation) and polyurethane foam (furniture padding) smoke exposures, [9,10] thus raising the index of suspicion for lower respiratory tract injury.
5. Time between initial resuscitation and hospital arrival — This, together with a knowledge of CO elimination half-life (largely based on estimates of the inspired O_2 fraction) and measured blood carboxyhemoglobin (COHb) level, allows an estimate of peak COHb level as discussed below. COHb level has been shown to correlate with inhalation injury.[8,11]
6. Pertinent past medical history — The presence of underlying bronchospastic lung disease, for example, may alter subsequent therapy.

A screening physical exam is also performed emphasizing the face, oropharyngeal airway, breath sounds, level of consciousness, and the presence of specific neurologic deficits.

Airway

Following isolated inhalation injury, the primary goal is maintenance of a patent upper airway, since lower airway injury (tracheobronchitis) is usually remediable, and life-threatening parenchymal lung injury is infrequently seen. Although inhalation injury can involve any or all of these pulmonary components, the indications for endotracheal intubation are almost always dependent on the clinical status of the patient's upper airway and not on the mere presence or absence of inhalation injury. Of key importance is the distinction between the diagnosis of lower airway or parenchymal lung injury and that of upper airway injury. The diagnosis of lower airway or parenchymal lung injury depends on the variety of examination techniques and laboratory tests available,[3,12] while clinically important upper airway injury can be determined by history and physical exam alone. To illustrate this point, we offer a brief review of the diagnostic aids available in the hospital setting. Chapter 7 more completely details these points.

The early physiologic changes of lower airway injury may be nonspecific and frequently are not detectable by standard clinical and laboratory evaluation. Chest roentgenograms, in the majority of cases, reveal few abnormalities.[13] Abnormal gas exchange, including clinically apparent hypoxemia, may be delayed as long as 72 hours.[14] Since symptoms of upper airway obstruction may be confused with those from the lower airway, a number of specialized studies have been suggested to identify the latter. These include xenon 133 nuclear scans[12,15] and technetium 99m diethylenetriamine pentacetate (DTPA) scans,[16] while many authors now consider fiberoptic bronchoscopy to be the "gold standard."[17–19] These studies may offer more specific evidence of pulmonary injury but also require special equipment and personnel, involving additional time and expense.

To help answer this diagnostic dilemma we used bronchoscopy on 100 consecutive patients admitted to our unit with any of the usual clinical warnings of smoke inhalation (closed space injury, facial burn, singed nasal vibrissae, perioral burn, pharyngeal edema, hoarseness, carbonaceous sputum, bronchorrhea, or wheezing). Carboxyhemoglobin levels were also measured. A 96-percent correlation was found between positive bronchoscopic findings (soot, erythema, or mucosal ulceration) and the clinical triad of closed space fire, COHb levels of >10 percent, and carbonaceous sputum. If only two of the clinical triad were present the correlation dropped to 70 percent, and if only one was present the correlation dropped to less than 30 percent. Multivariate analysis could not discern any other positive correlations. For these reasons we favor the use of history, clinical exam, and laboratory studies in the diagnosis of inhalation injury and reserve the use of fiberoptic bronchoscopy for exceptional cases (e.g., expansion of lobar atelectasis or removal of obstructing intrabronchial plugs). Furthermore, we advocate that management of these patients (e.g., endotracheal intubation and mechanical ventilation) also be based on clinical criteria, together with upper airway endoscopy or laryngoscopy in selected patients at high risk for laryngeal injury.

Upper airway injury is usually diagnosed by history (closed space fire) and physical exam. Of the techniques discussed above, only fiberoptic bronchoscopy can assist in the evaluation but is unnecessary in the majority of cases. We feel that if hoarseness or pharyngeal edema are present acutely after smoke inhalation, then endotracheal intubation for airway control should be performed. This should be done early rather than adopting a "wait-and-see" attitude, since the pathophysiology of inflammation dictates increasing edema with decreasing airway caliber in the first 24 to 36 hours after injury. This is particularly true in children, who already have an underlying degree of airway compromise due to anatomically small airway caliber. Observation of these patients only affords the possibility of unwitnessed airway compromise. For those patients with milder signs of upper airway injury (facial burn, singed nasal vibrissae, or perioral burn) without obvious hoarseness or pharyngeal edema, observation without endotracheal intubation may be undertaken. Such observation should take place in a high visibility unit (e.g., intensive care), with nursing staff alerted to a high index of suspicion for airway compromise. Laryngoscopy, either directly or via a flexible fiberoptic laryngoscope may also be warranted in these patients. Bedside equipment for endotracheal intubation and cricothyrotomy should be available, as well as appropriately skilled staff. These guidelines are summarized in Table 9-1.

Table 9-1 Guidelines for Acute Upper Airway Management following Isolated Injury

Findings on history/exam	Clinical response
History of closed space fire, or carbonaceous sputum	Raised index of suspicion for upper (and lower) airway injury
Facial burn, singed nasal vibrissae, or perioral burn	Possible upper airway injury — observe patient in high visibility unit with immediate availability of staff and equipment for securing the upper airway
Hoarseness, stridor, or pharyngeal edema	Probable upper airway injury — secure the upper airway (endotracheal intubation) as rapidly as possible

Endotracheal intubation may be performed by either oral or nasal route. Nasal endotracheal tubes are better tolerated and easier to care for in cases of long-term intubation. However, the upper airway swelling and edema of smoke injury usually resolve within 3 to 5 days so that oral tubes are not disadvantageous and in many hands are more easily placed. The usual contraindications to nasal intubation (apnea, coagulopathy, associated midface fractures, and frank hypoxemia) should be noted. In cases of failed endotracheal intubation, either emergency needle cricothyrotomy or surgical cricothyrotomy are preferred to the more complicated and time-consuming tracheostomy. Extubation can usually be performed after 3 to 5 days as airway edema resolves. Prior to extubation, airway patency can be assessed either by deflating the tube cuff and listening for ventilation around the tube or by visual inspection of the periglottic structures by laryngoscopy. Such assessment is difficult in children due to their anatomy and the use of uncuffed endotracheal tubes. Extubation should therefore take place in the presence of personnel skilled and equipped to re-secure the airway.

The administration of steroids acutely after smoke inhalation is not recommended, except in special circumstances. Their anti-inflammatory effects will not prevent acute upper airway compromise, although they may reduce the peak inflammatory response. Animal studies are conflicting, with decreased mortality reported in smoke-exposed rats[20] and rabbits[21] treated with steroids, yet no changes in lung histopathology,[21] surfactant dysfunction, or increased lung water.[22] After isolated inhalation injury in humans, however, steroids have been shown to be of no benefit,[1,23] and in cases of combined inhalation and burn injuries their use is associated with higher mortality and infection rates.[24] Therefore, we strongly recommend endotracheal intubation for control of the upper airway and do not rely on steroids. However, with isolated smoke inhalation in patients who are dependent on exogenous steroids or in those with severe bronchospasm (discussed later in this section) at initial presentation, steroids (methylprednisolone 2 to 5 mg/kg/day) may be advantageous for the first 24 hours.

Carbon Monoxide Poisoning

Carbon monoxide and carbon dioxide are the two most common gases liberated during fires, the former being produced most rapidly during pyrolysis or smoldering. Carbon monoxide is colorless and tasteless and has an affinity for hemoglobin 200 times that of oxygen. Its primary pathophysiology involves the reversible displacement of oxygen on the hemoglobin molecule (forming carboxyhemoglobin, COHb). It also interacts with the myoglobin of cardiac muscle,[25] as well as the mitochondrial cytochrome-oxidase a_3 complex[26] with additional effects on cellular oxygen metabolism and organ function.[27] Carboxyhemoglobin results in impaired oxygen delivery to tissues and decreased mixed venous oxygen content. These effects, and thus the clinical symptoms of CO poisoning, are dependent on the amount of COHb present (Table 9-2). Angina and syncope are particularly dangerous consequences of tissue hypoxia in those with underlying coronary or cerebral vascular disease. Despite obvious difficulties with human studies, COHb levels of 60 percent are considered lethal.[28] Carbon monoxide elimination is dependent on the inspired oxygen concentration (hence, alveolar oxygen partial pressure) and the law of mass action, as oxygen is

Table 9-2 Signs and Symptoms of Carbon Monoxide Intoxication

Carboxyhemoglobin level (percent)	Clinical manifestation
5–10	Mild headache, confusion
11–20	Throbbing headache, blurred vision, flushing of the skin
21–30	Disorientation, nausea, impaired manual dexterity
31–40	Irritability, dizziness, vomiting, syncope
41–50	Tachypnea, tachycardia
50 and above	Coma, seizures, respiratory failure, death

exchanged for CO on the hemoglobin molecule. Because of mass action CO elimination is minimally affected by changes in alveolar ventilation. Elimination occurs in two phases — a rapid redistribution phase to other tissues, followed by a slower excretion phase. The elimination half-life of CO breathing room air is 250 minutes,[29] 40 to 60 minutes in 100 percent oxygen,[30] and 30 minutes at 2 atmospheres hyperbaric oxygen. In fact, at 2.5 atmospheres oxygen the dissolved oxygen content of plasma alone (greater than 5 mL/100 mL) is sufficient to meet basal body oxygen requirements.[31]

All patients with suspected inhalation injury, loss of consciousness, or fire-related burns should have supplemental oxygen begun immediately after rescue and maintained throughout hospital evaluation. The diagnosis of CO poisoning is made by measurement of COHb level. Cherry red discoloration of the lips and skin is reported to be the classic physical finding of this disorder but is rarely seen. Carboxyhemoglobin levels should be drawn as soon as possible, remembering that transport time may allow the COHb level to fall considerably prior to measurement. It is often helpful to back-calculate the peak COHb (at the scene) using the hospital COHb measurement, along with knowledge of transport time and oxygen therapy (i.e., CO elimination half-life). This calculated COHb can offer insight regarding the hidden severity of inhalation injury that may appear mild at hospital presentation. Arterial blood gas analysis will confirm the decrease in oxyhemoglobin (with a normal Pa_{O_2}) and may suggest the presence of other parenchymal lung injury (abnormal Pa_{O_2}). However, this is only true if oxygen saturation of hemoglobin is measured directly (e.g., by co-oximeter) and not calculated from Pa_{O_2} and hematocrit. Pulse oximetry should not be relied upon in cases of CO poisoning, since COHb is not sensed by the device. Only oxy- and deoxyhemoglobin are measured, yielding a falsely high oxygen saturation reading in the presence of COHb.[32] Oxygen saturation can be accurately measured, however, on arterial blood samples using a co-oximeter (Fig. 9-1). Serial COHb determinations to ensure adequate therapy should be made in cases of COHb greater than 30 percent at hospital arrival. Regardless of peak COHb level, proper treatment with high normobaric oxygen concentrations should result in CO elimination to levels less than 10 percent within the first 1 to 3 hours after injury.

Of concern is the debate over the incidence and treatment of acute and delayed neuropsychiatric sequelae of CO poisoning. Features including Parkinsonism, cortical blindness, temporospatial disorientation, deafness, memory changes, mental retardation, and frank psychosis have been reported with an incidence of 0.2 to 11 percent.[33–35] Neither incidence nor severity correlate with COHb level or ultimate prognosis.[36–38] In general, victims either die or recover from their neuropsychiatric symptoms, but few develop permanent impairment.

The mechanism of central nervous system injury is not understood, and recommendations for treatment or prophylaxis are in debate. Some investigators recommend hyperbaric oxygen administration for the treatment of CO poisoning to prevent the development of neurologic sequelae.[39–42] Since these studies were nonrandomized and not controlled for previous psychiatric and neurologic conditions, this recommendation should be tempered. Hyperbaric oxygen therapy is not without risk, potentially complicated by middle ear and sinus occlusion, oxygen seizures, and air embolus during too rapid a recompression.[43] Furthermore, patient care personnel must also be exposed to these risks. Some patients, because of preexisting illness or concomitant burn injury, are too unstable to leave the personnel and resources of the intensive care unit for transport to and placement into a hyperbaric chamber with limited personnel and facilities. This is particularly true for patients (Table 9-3) with acute concomitant burn and inhalation injury, as shown in a recent report where 7 of 10 such patients undergoing hyperbaric therapy developed major complications of seizures, aspiration, hypoxemia, dysrhythmia, or cardiac arrest.[44]

Until the neurologic injury of CO poisoning is better understood and a controlled multicenter ran-

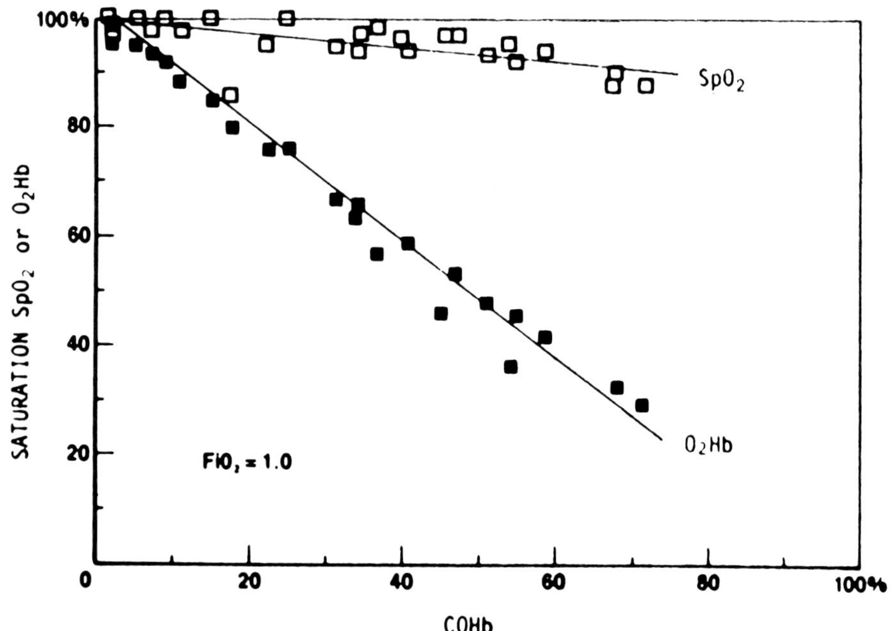

Figure 9-1 Oxyhemoglobin saturation as measured by pulse oximetry (Sp_{O_2}) and by co-oximeter (O_2Hb) in the presence of carboxyhemoglobin (COHb) in dogs ventilated with oxygen FI_{O_2} = 1.0 and varied concentrations of carbon monoxide. Sp_{O_2} consistently overestimates the true oxyhemoglobin saturation. Note that at FI_{O_2} = 1.0 the overestimation of O_2Hb is approximately 1 percent oxyhemoglobin for every 1 percent carboxyhemoglobin. (*Adapted from Barker SJ, Tremper KK: The effect of carbon monoxide inhalation on pulse oximetry and transcutaneous* P_{O_2}. *Anesthesiology 66:677, 1987.*)

Table 9-3 Complications Associated with Hyperbaric Oxygen Therapy in 10 Consecutive Patients Admitted to Harborview Medical Center/University of Washington Burn Center with Concomitant Burn Injury and Inhalation Injury*

	Case no.									
Complication	**1**	**2**	**3**	**4**	**5**	**6**	**7**	**8**	**9**	**10**
Barotrauma to ears		•	•							
Aspiration		•		•						
Seizure						•				
Hypocalcemia					•		•			
Decreased urine	•				•				•	
Metabolic acidosis						•		•	•	
Respiratory acidosis						•	•	•	•	
Decreased O_2						•	•			
Dysrhythmia	•							•	•	
Cardiac arrest								•	•	
Survival	•	•		•	•	•	•	•		

*Mean burn size, 18.5 ± 18% body surface area; carboxyhemoglobin levels, 32.0 ± 4.4%. The incidence of major complications (seizure, aspiration, hypoxemia, dysrhythmia, or cardiac arrest) during hyperbaric treatment was 70%, with an overall mortality of 70%.

SOURCE: Adapted from Grube BJ, Marvin JA, Heimbach DM: Therapeutic hyperbaric oxygen: Help or hindrance in burn patients with carbon monoxide poisoning? *J Burn Care Rehabil* 9:249, 1988.

domized clinical trial of hyperbaric oxygen therapy is performed, we recommend the following guidelines:

1. Patients with mild to moderate exposure (COHb < 30 percent, no coma, no neurologic findings) are probably treated adequately with 100 percent oxygen.
2. A patient who is comatose on admission, has a COHb level of greater than 30 percent, or has an existing neurologic deficit is at risk for permanent damage and, if a hyperbaric chamber is readily available, may benefit from a dive.
3. The patient with associated problems (burns greater than 40 percent of body surface area, other injuries, or airway compromise) should be considered for hyperbaric treatment only if there is no risk to life engendered by the delay in treatment of the other problems.

The hyperbaric oxygen treatment protocol at our institution consists of treatment for 5 hours starting at a pressure of 3 atmospheres and decreasing throughout. All patients who remain comatose after arrival in the emergency room, even if they have associated major burns, are treated with hyperbaric oxygen. Unfortunately, our results in this second group have been disappointing; recovery of neurologic function has been rare.

Cyanide Poisoning

The incidence of cyanide (CN) poisoning with inhalation injury is underappreciated. With the expanding use of synthetic polymers, particularly polyurethane, in the construction and furniture industries the incidence is increasing.[45] Cyanide inhibits the final step of oxidative phosphorylation by binding the cytochrome aa_3 complex and halting aerobic metabolism. The result is lactic acidosis and cellular asphyxia, despite normal blood oxygen content. Symptoms of intoxication consist of altered level of consciousness, dizziness, headache, tachycardia, and tachypnea. These symptoms are easily confused with those of either CO poisoning, hypoxemia, or anxiety. Diagnosis is made by history (closed space fire involving plastics or furniture), presence of unexplained metabolic acidosis, elevated venous oxygen content, and a high index of suspicion.

Blood CN levels may be determined with the Conway diffusion assay,[46] which, in our institution, currently takes 4 hours to perform. The lethal level is unresolved, but 1.0 to 3.0 mg/L is generally accepted.[45] Of greater concern is that CO and CN synergistically decrease oxygen consumption[47] so that sublethal levels of each may, in combination, be particularly deadly.

Treatment is indicated for any patient meeting the described clinical criteria or with CN levels greater than 0.20 mg/L. Cyanide is detoxified primarily by hepatic rhodanase and requires sulfate as a substrate. The resulting thiocynanate is inactive and excreted in the urine. Unfortunately, this reaction is slow and often limited by the availability of sulfate. Therefore, treatment involves the shunting of CN into other minor metabolic pathways while supplemental sulfate (thiosulfate) is given to accelerate the detoxification reaction. The Eli Lilly three-step cyanide antidote package is commonly available. Amyl nitrite is first administered by inhalation (15 to 30 seconds each minute) while sodium nitrite solution is prepared. This solution is injected (300 mg in 10 mL in an adult) over 2 to 4 minutes with careful blood pressure monitoring. These two steps produce methemoglobin, which combines with cytochrome-bound CN to yield nontoxic cyanomethemoglobin. The amount of sodium nitrite injected is limited to keep methemoglobin levels near 40 percent, a level above which toxic effects from hypoxia begin to appear.[48] Finally, sodium thiosulfate (12.5 g in 50 mL 5% dextrose) is injected over a 10-minute period. As a further supplement, hydroxycobalamin (vitamin B_{12}) may be given up to 400 μg/kg intravenously to produce the inactive cyanocobalamin[49]. Cyanide shunted to these minor pathways must eventually be detoxified by rhodanase, therefore careful observation of these patients is warranted (blood gases and CN levels) for 24 to 48 hours.

Bronchospasm

Inhalation injury to the lower airways results in a chemical tracheobronchitis that can produce wheezing. The decreased airway caliber, however, is often due to increased bronchial blood flow and airway edema, as opposed to bronchospasm. Thus, bronchodilators are variably effective, and no controlled clinical trials have compared their efficacy. Still, the smoke inhalation patient who develops wheezing deserves a trial of therapy. This is especially true for the victim who suffers from preexisting obstructive or reactive airway disease. The fastest route of administration is inhalation of standard nebulized $beta_2$ agonists (albuterol, metaproterenol, terbutaline, or isoetharine). Racemic epinephrine can also be helpful in cases where upper airway stridor is present. Terbutaline may also be given subcutaneously (0.25 to 0.5 mg every 4 to 6 hours). Aminophylline is the intravenous agent of choice (initial bolus of 5.6 mg/kg over 20 minutes, followed by 0.5 to 0.9 mg/kg/h continuous infusion) with careful monitoring of blood levels to maintain the therapeutic range (10 to 20 μg/mL). As previously mentioned, steroids are only indicated in the initial 24 hours after isolated inhalation injury (methylprednisolone 2 to 5 mg/kg/day) for those patients with severe bronchospasm despite treatment with standard bronchodilators, or those with preexisting dependence on exogenous steroids.

Bronchospasm occurs in response to airway irritation after smoke inhalation. There is chemical irritation of the airways, in addition to the irritation initiated by retained secretions due to poor mucociliary clearance. Therefore, the use of chest physiotherapy may be quite helpful. Parasympatholytic agents (atropine or glycopyrolate) may have some theoretical advantage as well, but their use is limited by their cardiac side effects and short duration of action. A new anticholinergic agent, ipratroprium bromide, is available in an inhaled preparation for maintenance therapy of bronchospasm. The inhaled route reduces the risk of cardiac side effects and drying. However, its efficacy in the setting of inhalation injury has not been studied.

Impaired Oxygenation

Injury to the lung parenchyma after isolated smoke inhalation is rare, seen particularly after inhalation of smoke generated from plastics (e.g., polyurethane, polyvinylchloride).[9,10] Parenchymal lung injury is also more common in those with combined smoke inhalation and burn injury.[11] Patients with underlying pulmonary disease, smokers, and the elderly are certainly at higher risk for parenchymal injury and abnormal oxygenation. Arterial blood gas analysis is the monitor of choice for assessing oxygenation since commonly used pulse oximeters only begin to show significant desaturation (oxyhemoglobin < 95 percent) at a Pa_{O_2} less than 80 mmHg (unusual since most patients receive supplemental oxygen) and are inaccurate in the presence of COHb.[32] Serial chest roentgenograms may also be helpful in diagnosis.

Needless to say, poor airway control and bronchospasm can contribute to the development of hypoxemia. Proper management of these two problems is essential. Another general recommendation that limits the development of both airway and alveolar edema is the restriction of volume intake to daily maintenance requirements in patients with isolated inhalation injury.[49,50] Such restriction is not the case when concomitant burn injury is present due to these patients' enormous fluid requirements.

Once rescued from the hypoxic fire environment and given supplemental oxygen via a patent airway, hypoxemia can result from either hypoventilation, the mismatch of ventilation and perfusion (V/Q), intrapulmonary shunt, or some combination of the three. The diagnosis and treatment of hypoventilation is usually uncomplicated. Differentiating V/Q mismatch and intrapulmonary shunt can be difficult, although the therapy for each is similar.

Hypoventilation is most commonly central in origin, secondary to CO or CN poisoning, or associated head injury. It is diagnosed by observation of slow or shallow respiratory pattern, a decreased level of consciousness, and the presence of CO_2 retention and hypoxemia on arterial blood gas analysis. Therapy is directed at the underlying problem, in conjunction with assisting ventilation, usually after endotracheal intubation.

The presence of V/Q mismatch after smoke inhalation can be predicted by the clinical observation of regional airway edema, bronchospasm, and retained secretions. The presence of V/Q mismatch has been demonstrated in such human victims, as well as animals, using multiple inert gas analysis.[51] Fluid restriction and bronchodilator therapy, as previously described, can limit the effects of airway edema and bronchospasm. Retained secretions are problematic after inhalation injury due to the sloughing of necrotic airway mucosa, reactive bronchorrhea, and dysfunction of the mucociliary clearance system. Therapy involves humidified oxygen, vigorous chest physiotherapy, and occasionally the use of fiberoptic bronchoscopy for removal of mucocellular casts. Supplemental oxygen is indicated in the hypoxemic patient. Endotracheal intubation and mechanical ventilation may be necessary in extreme cases, as described below in the management of intrapulmonary shunt.

Intrapulmonary shunt after isolated inhalation injury usually results from massive atelectasis but can occasionally be due to pulmonary edema or the adult respiratory distress syndrome (ARDS). Atelectasis may be due to small airway obstruction with distal alveolar collapse or a consequence of smoke-induced surfactant damage.[49,52] Isolated cases of pulmonary edema after polyvinylchloride smoke,[10] carbon monoxide,[53] and cyanide[54] have been reported clinically and described in some animal models.[55,56] Occult aspiration pneumonia, especially in patients with an altered level of consciousness, can also affect oxygenation through production of intrapulmonary shunt. The diagnosis of intrapulmonary shunt is made by arterial blood gas analysis. Whereas hypoxemia due to V/Q mismatch will correct when an $F_{I_{O_2}}$ of 1.0 is provided, the patient with shunt will remain hypoxemic when breathing such a mixture. Shunt tends to be a less reversible abnormality than V/Q mismatch and more often results in the use of high supplemental oxygen concentrations, mechanical ventilation, and possibly positive end-expiratory pressure (PEEP).

We have found that repeated blood gas measurements have been a sensitive indicator of the need to progress with pulmonary support. For each measurement the $Pa_{O_2}/F_{I_{O_2}}$ ratio is calculated, the normal value being in excess of 400. The P/F ratio is an approximation of, and well correlated ($r = 0.9$) with, measured shunt fraction (Q_s/Q_t).[57] An advantage of the P/F ratio is that its determination does not require invasive sampling of mixed venous blood via pulmonary artery catheter nor the tedious calculations of Q_s/Q_t. A P/F ratio between 200 and 400 indicates mild to moderate injury. Supplemental oxygen without mechanical ventilation is usually sufficient therapy at this level. However, a P/F ratio falling below 200 is evidence of potentially serious trouble, and respiratory support should progress.[58] Patients with increasing dyspnea, difficulty in handling secretions, or associated medical problems may require ventilatory assistance at P/F ratios greater than 200.

Ventilators are set with a tidal volume near the top of the compliance/tidal volume curve (10 to 15 mL/kg), and changes in compliance are carefully monitored. In our experience, the cause of early death following smoke inhalation has been rapidly progressive lung stiffness and difficulty with ventilation rather than with oxygenation. Steadily increasing pressure requirements to provide adequate tidal volumes may well represent decreasing lung compliance only, but the clinician must be alert to other mechanical causes, such as restriction of chest-wall motion by full-thickness burns, pneumothorax, mucous plugs, and mechanical difficulties with the endotracheal tube or ventilator.

To avoid both absorption atelectasis and pulmonary oxygen toxicity[59] we attempt to keep the $F_{I_{O_2}}$ at or below 0.5 and maintain a Pa_{O_2} of at least

70 mmHg. If these conditions cannot be met, the use of PEEP is indicated. If the primary problem is bronchiolitis, PEEP may increase the amount of air trapping and worsen hypoxemia. If, however, there is a predominance of atelectasis, interstitial and alveolar edema, and alveolar epithelial damage, PEEP may improve oxygenation, as has been documented in animal models of inhalation injury.[60] PEEP has been shown to be effective in the treatment of other forms of ARDS[61,62] in humans as well. If oxygenation is impaired (P/F ratio less than 200) we initiate PEEP and increase it in increments of 5 cmH_2O until there is improvement in the P/F ratio or until evidence of decreased cardiac output is apparent. Since PEEP may interfere with cardiac performance due to increased intrathoracic pressure and decreased venous return, a pulmonary artery catheter is indicated for all patients requiring greater than 10 cmH_2O PEEP. Determination of a "PEEP curve" may be helpful in these patients. By comparing Pa_{O_2} and cardiac output at increasing levels of PEEP, an "optimum PEEP" may be identified. Beyond this level, further increases can result in either a fall in cardiac output or minimal improvements in oxygenation. Lower PEEP levels are also desirable to avoid complication of barotrauma (e.g., pneumothorax, pneumomediastinum).

Continuous positive airway pressure (CPAP) was first developed to treat infant respiratory distress[63] and can be used in either intubated or nonintubated patients to improve oxygenation. CPAP is most effective in cases of pulmonary dysfunction characterized by decreased pulmonary compliance, decreased lung volume, increased work of breathing, and increased intrapulmonary shunt.[64] It has been shown to be effective in improving pulmonary function in an animal model of inhalation injury,[65] but its clinical utility in humans remains unclear. The best indication for the use of CPAP currently is in the unintubated patient with failing oxygenation, despite high Fi_{O_2}. CPAP by mask may stabilize oxygenation enough to avoid or delay endotracheal intubation and mechanical ventilation in appropriate patients where immediate intubation is not possible.

The prevention of parenchymal lung injury after smoke inhalation is being addressed in animal models but has not been studied clinically. Therapy is directed at circulating factors (e.g., thromboxane, antiproteases) that may be responsible for the lung injury. The prostaglandin-synthesis inhibitor ibuprofen,[66] the antiprotease gabexate mesylate,[67] the oxygen radical scavenger dimethylsulfoxide (DMSO)/heparin,[68] and the histamine type 2 receptor blocker cimetidine[50] have been shown useful in such a role in the laboratory but have yet to be studied clinically.

Fortunately, with careful fluid management and vigorous pulmonary therapy, reversal of severely impaired oxygenation begins 5 to 7 days after isolated inhalation injury. This course may be prolonged in the rare occurrence of ARDS or more likely in patients with concomitant burn and inhalation injury. In a stepwise fashion, PEEP is lowered when the patient can maintain an adequate P/F ratio. Using standard weaning parameters these patients can then be safely extubated to mask oxygen.

Antibiotics

Prophylactic antibiotics in the acute hospital treatment of inhalation injury are not indicated. Their use has not been shown to protect against subsequent pulmonary infection.[23] However, specific antibiotics are indicated for clinically apparent pneumonia that may subsequently develop.

Management of Delayed Sequelae

To reiterate, the vast majority of patients with isolated inhalation injury experience resolution of clinical airway and parenchymal lung abnormalities within 3 to 7 days. In contrast to patients with combined smoke and burn injuries, delayed pulmonary complications in the isolated inhalation injury group are rare. Histologic studies in animal models[9,69] and humans[17] show resolution of microscopic airway mucosal injury in 2 to 3 weeks. Pulmonary function tests are usually normal months after inhalation injury, although we occasionally see evidence of mild restrictive defects.

INHALATION INJURY MANAGEMENT IN PATIENTS WITH BURNS

Cutaneous burns act indirectly to perturb pulmonary function through the release of circulating factors (e.g., thromboxane, prostacyclin) and the development of intravascular hypoproteinemia. The latter occurs due to protein loss into the burn wound, and also into unburned tissues in patients with burns greater than 30 percent body surface area. The resultant pulmonary hypertension and decreased oncotic pressure, coupled with aggressive fluid resuscitation, result in a transient hydrostatic pulmonary edema.[70–72] Recent work in our laboratory confirms the absence of a pulmonary vascular protein permeability change after isolated burn injury, finding rather that the increased pulmonary lymph flow is dependent on burn size and the degree of hypoproteinemia. Clinically, patients with significant burns may show a mild decrease in oxygenation 24 to 48 hours after injury but with effective burn care (i.e., excision and grafting) experience little further pulmonary dysfunction. Those patients with combined burn and smoke injuries, however, can develop significant respiratory problems as discussed below.

Field Management

The field management of inhalation injury, when present with cutaneous burn, is no different than previously described. This includes identification of other associated musculoskeletal injuries that burned skin may disguise. The burns require additional treatment, however. Treatment begins with stopping the burning process. Since victims are often removed from fires with smoldering clothing still attached, it must be quickly removed. The burns should be temporarily dressed, covered with sterile bandages or towels. Although sterile saline- or water-soaked dressings may lessen discomfort from small burns, they will augment body heat loss in large burns with resultant hypothermia. Therefore, dry dressings are recommended for large burns. Finally, intravenous access is preferable for the early initiation of volume resuscitation but should not delay prompt transport to the hospital.

Acute Hospital Management

Concomitant burns most significantly complicate management of the airway, CO poisoning, and oxygenation in the acute postburn period of the smoke-exposed patient. Respiratory management, however, is still based on the principles outlined in the previous section on isolated inhalation injury.

Airway

Upper airway integrity may be directly affected by burn injury; however, the term "respiratory burn" is a misnomer. True thermal damage to the lower airway and lung parenchyma is extremely rare unless live steam or explosive gases are inhaled, or scalding liquid is aspirated.[73] The air temperature near the ceiling of a burning room may reach 1000°F or more, but air has such poor thermal capacity that most of the heat is dissipated in the nasopharynx and upper airway. As the heat is dissipated, however, burns of the pharynx and larynx may occur.

The presence of facial or pharyngeal burns should raise the index of suspicion of upper airway injury, as well as lower airway injury. Early endotracheal intubation, as indicated, is extremely important in patients with burns of the face and neck since postburn edema can rapidly develop in these tissues as fluid resuscitation progresses. Local anatomy and cervical range of motion may become disturbed to the point where intubation under direct laryngoscopy is not possible several hours after injury. Likewise, emergent tracheostomy is more difficult under these conditions and is associated with an increased incidence of pulmonary sepsis.[74] In addition, as the neck swells over the next few days, the danger of tracheostomy tube displacement and loss of airway is increased. Tracheostomy in cases of prolonged intubation is also associated with airway complications in burn patients but may be necessary to avoid permanent upper airway or vocal cord damage.[75] The decision to perform a tracheostomy is best individualized rather than based on an arbitrary number of days of intubation.

Muscle relaxants commonly used to achieve safe conditions for endotracheal intubation must be used carefully in patients with burns. Succinylcholine, a depolarizing muscle relaxant, can cause acute hyperkalemia and precipitate cardiac dysrhythmias.[76,77] This effect is not seen in acute burn victims but rather in those more than 24 hours beyond the time of the injury, and it lasts until burns are healed. Nondepolarizing muscle relaxants are therefore indicated for these patients, although larger than usual doses of atracurium,[78] *d*-tubocurarine,[79] and metocurine[80] may be necessary to achieve adequate conditions for intubation compared to nonburned patients.

Endotracheal tube stabilization can be difficult in patients with facial, scalp, and neck burns. Topical antibiotic cream makes common taping methods impractical. We prefer the weaving of a simple head sling using cotton tracheostomy tape (Fig. 9-2). Many such techniques have been suggested,[81] as has the use of intraoral wire stabilization of the tube.[82]

Carbon Monoxide Poisoning

As outlined in the previous section, prophylactic antibiotics and steroids are not indicated except in specific cases. Burn patients also pose a special challenge in the use of hyperbaric oxygen for the treatment of CO poisoning. As described previously, significant burns complicate the medical and nursing care of these patients and may contraindicate a tedious journey to the hyperbaric chamber.

Impaired Oxygenation

Oxygenation can become more severely impaired after combined injuries. The reasons for this observation in the immediate postburn period are unclear but may involve the development of interstitial pulmonary edema. Increased extravascular lung water (EVLW) has been documented in combined injury patients immediately after injury compared to those with burns alone.[83] A possible explanation is the greater amount of resuscitation fluid that these patients receive in order to meet standard endpoints of satisfactory resuscitation (e.g., adequate urine output). Scheulen and Munster found that combined injury patients received 37 percent more resuscitation volume than predicted by the Parkland formula compared to 6 percent more for those with equivalent burns alone.[84] Unpublished data from our laboratory confirm these clinical findings and suggest that EVLW is not elevated in goats with combined injuries that are restricted to only the resuscitation volume prescribed by the Parkland formula. The clinical utility of this strategy is, however, suspect since adequate organ perfusion is a vital priority after burn injury, and fluid restriction may be harmful. In an effort to reduce resuscitation volumes, the use of hypertonic crystalloid has been advocated, especially in the elderly.[85] However, hypernatremia is not an infrequent complication. Therefore, it is recommended that this technique only be used at a burn center and be guided by serial electrolyte determinations. In a more recent and unproven effort to improve the response to resuscitation, early plasma exchange has been suggested to remove rampant inflammatory mediators from the circulation.[86]

The presence of circumferential full-thickness thorax burns can also produce oxygenation and ventilation difficulties shortly after injury. Treatment of this restrictive lung defect involves chest wall escharotomies (Fig. 9-3). Escharotomies are made in the anterior axillary line bilaterally, extending from the clavicle to the costal margin. If the abdomen is involved with the burn, the inferior margins of the escharotomy may be connected transversely.

Management of Delayed Sequelae

Pneumonia and Burn Sepsis The most common cause of delayed morbidity and mortality in combined injury patients is sepsis, usually pulmonary or burn wound in origin. A recent study found that 9

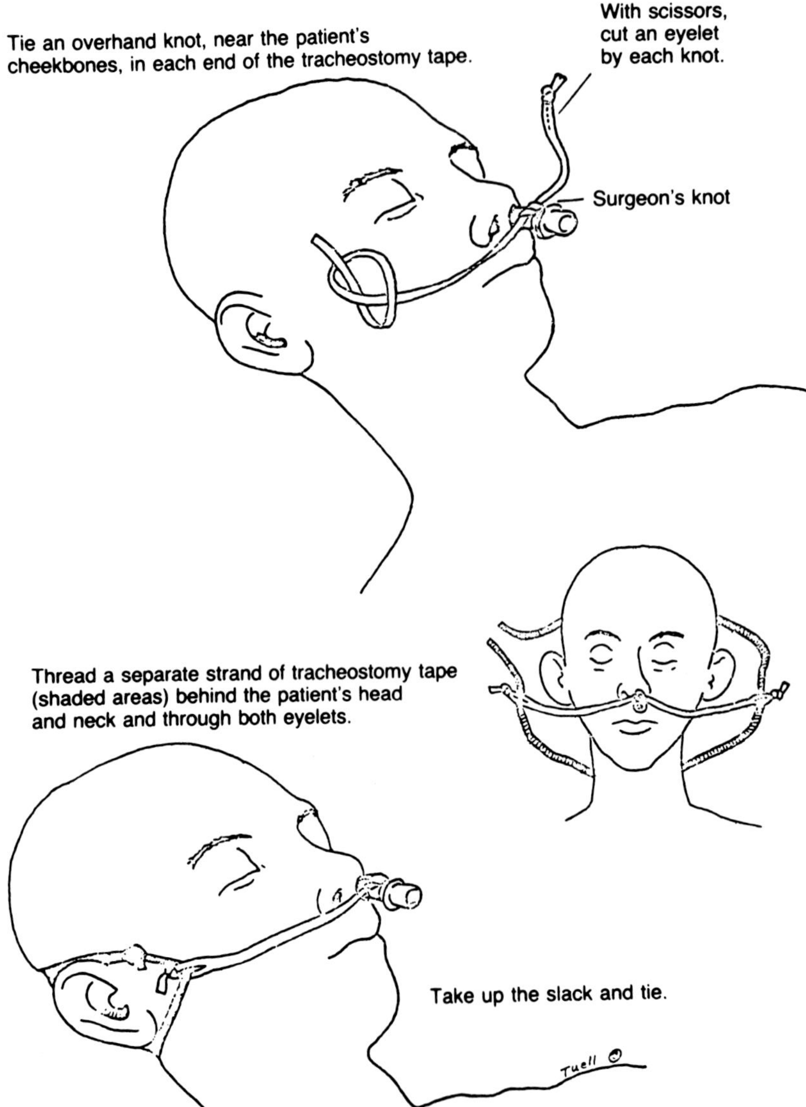

Figure 9-2 Illustration of one suggested method of securing an endotracheal tube in a patient with facial burns. The use of tape is avoided, yet head and neck movement are still possible. (*Adapted from Gordon MD (ed): Anchoring endotracheal tubes on patients with facial burns. J Burn Care Rehabil 8:233, 1987.*)

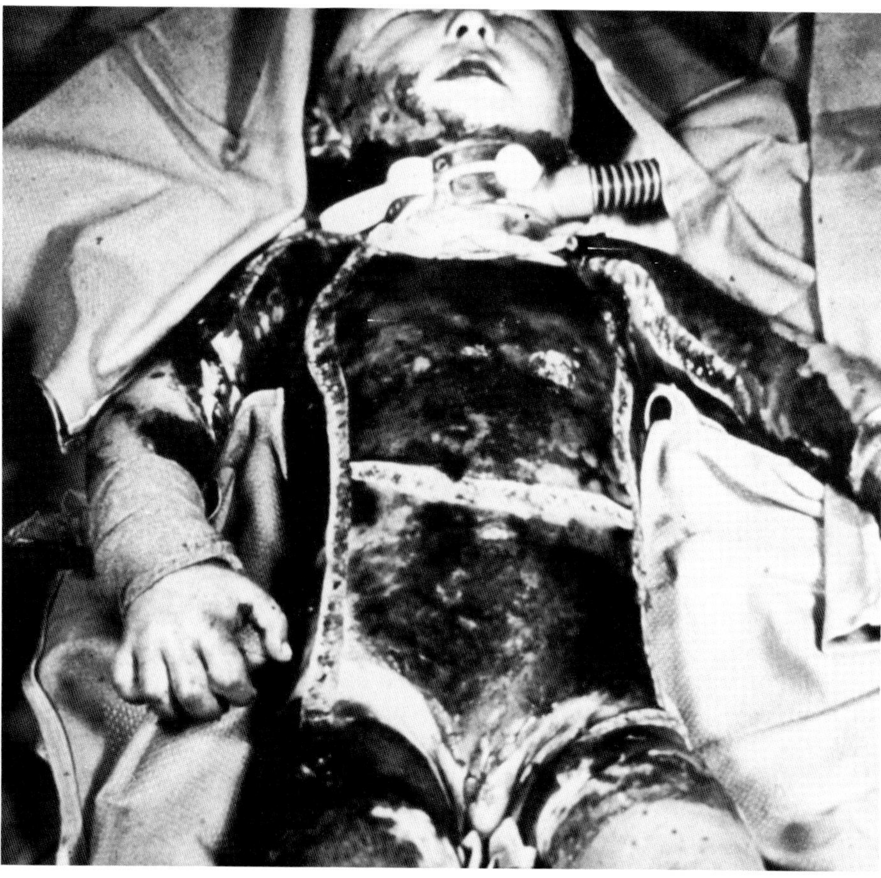

Figure 9-3 Escharotomy of the anterior chest and abdomen in a child with circumferential full-thickness burns of the torso that initially produced a restrictive defect to mechanical ventilation. Note the "H" shape of the incisions, as well as the absence of bleeding that is characteristic of escharotomy through a full-thickness burn.

percent of patients with isolated inhalation injury developed secondary pneumonia, whereas 46 percent of those with concomitant burns were affected.[5] This increased incidence is felt to be secondary to the combination of inhalation injury (structural epithelial damage, surfactant inactivation, and impaired mucociliary transport) and burn (global immunosuppression) resulting in a greater susceptibility to respiratory tract infection. In addition, EVLW increases dramatically in these patients with the onset of sepsis.[87,88] Thus, alveolar and interstitial edema combine with regional V/Q abnormalities and intrapulmonary shunt due to pneumonia. The result is poor oxygenation and potential ARDS.

Treatment begins with prevention — meticulous nursing care with respect to cleanliness and wound care, pulmonary toilet, early removal of central lines, and early extubation to avoid nosocomial infection. In susceptible individuals (greater than 20 percent body surface area burn plus inhalation injury) we monitor white blood cell count, sputum Gram stain, and chest x-ray daily, and obtain sputum cultures every 3 days. Second, the major source of bacteremia — the burn — must be removed. The burn serves as an unlimited source of recurrent bacteremia, allowing a daily "bolus" with every routine wound cleansing. In addition, the burn wound serves as a source of endotoxin. Burn wound endotoxin has been shown to cause distant lung dysfunction through the production of inflammatory mediators.[89] Excision and grafting of these wounds removes the source of trouble and should be pursued as soon after resuscitation as possible. Few burn patients are "too sick to operate on" given current intensive operating room monitoring, an understanding of the physiology and nutritional requirements of these extraordinarily ill patients, experience from excision and grafting of small burns, and skilled intensive care in the perioperative period. This aggressive posture has decreased not only the number of both infectious complications and days on potentially hazardous antibiotics[90] but also the length of hospital stay and hospital costs.[91] It is more difficult to prove that early excision improves mortality in patients with extensive burns (greater than 60 percent body surface area) and in the elderly. There are several reasons for this. The causes of death in patients with extensive burns are multiple. Although a decrease in burn wound–related sepsis has been reported, the incidence of pneumonia following smoke inhalation and the complications of treatment — intravascular sepsis related to central lines and aspiration of tube feedings — still remain significant. An interesting laboratory technique, not yet applied clinically, utilizes ibuprofen applied to burn wounds.[92] The therapy is associated with decreased burn wound prostanoid production, thus limiting lung dysfunction. However, the effects of the therapy on burn wound healing and infection are not known.

The most likely time for development of a resistant necrotizing bacterial pneumonia is during the second week after burn. Diagnosis is made by finding leukocytes in the sputum associated with the presence of a culturable pathogen. Chest x-ray usually shows a specific infiltrate, and the patient has evidence of clinical deterioration with a picture of sepsis. Treatment includes pulmonary toilet and possibly ventilatory support, as outlined in the previous section, and culture-specific antibiotics. Aspiration of gastric contents or tube feeding, and hematogenous pneumonia resulting from metastatic spread of infection from other sites can present with an identical picture. Once sepsis occurs, these patients are at 43-percent risk for developing ARDS[93] and also susceptible to multisystem organ failure.[94] The latter is frequently a terminal event in the lives of patients with extensive burns. Supportive treatment is the same as with other patients with ARDS, but only the most vigorous attempts to identify and treat the original source of infection will lead to a reversal of the process.

Other Respiratory Disorders Mafenide acetate (Sulfamylon), a common antimicrobial agent used against burns, is a potent carbonic anhydrase inhibitor. Metabolic acidosis is a potential side effect of its use, particularly in burns greater than 40 percent body surface area. Diagnosis is made by blood gas and serum bicarbonate determinations. This effect can be temporized by increasing minute ventilation mechanically but is best treated by changing to another topical agent.

The risk of pulmonary emboli in burn patients, reported to be as high as 4 to 7 percent,[95] is probably not greater than that found in other surgical or trauma populations. A recent review of 2106 burn victims found an incidence of only 0.4 percent.[96] Therefore, prophylactic anticoagulant therapy is not recommended. Rather, prevention should continue to be directed at patients with classic risk factors for pulmonary emboli: obesity, burns of the lower extremity, or prior history of thromboembolic disease.

TRANSPORT AND TRANSFER PROTOCOLS

Once an airway is established and resuscitation underway, burned patients are eminently suitable for transport. Resuscitation can continue en route and, for the most part, the patient will remain stable for several days. This was well proven during the Vietnam war, where burn victims were first transported from Vietnam to Japan and then from Japan to the military burn center in San Antonio, Texas. The decision of which patients require transfer to a burn center is based not only on the local surgical expertise but also on the technical and personnel resources available at the local hospital. The latter is particularly important due to the demanding care that these patients can require 24 hours a day. The American Burn Association has identified the following types of burn injuries that should be considered for referral to a burn center:

1. Patients with burns that involve more than 25 percent body surface area (20 percent in children under 10 years of age and adults over 40 years).
2. Full-thickness or third-degree burns involving more than 10 percent of the total body surface.
3. Partial-thickness or second-degree burns exceeding 20 percent of the body surface.
4. All burns involving the face, eyes, ears, hands, feet, or perineum.
5. Burns associated with significant fractures or other major injury.
6. High-voltage electrical burns (significant volumes of tissue beneath the surface may be injured and result in acute renal failure and other complications).
7. Inhalation injury.
8. Lesser burns in patients with significant preexisting disease.

Hospitals without specialized burn care facilities should decide where they will refer patients and work out transfer agreements and treatment protocols with the chosen burn center well in advance of need. If this is done, definitive care can begin at the initial hospital and continue without interruption during transport and at the burn center. In general, transfer should be from physician to physician, and contact should be established between them as soon as the patient arrives in the emergency room of the initial hospital. The mode of transport and arrangements for procuring it should be well known to all involved.

The mode of transport depends on vehicle availability, local terrain, weather, and the distances involved. For distances of less than 50 miles ground ambulance is usually quite satisfactory. Between 50 and 150 miles many people prefer helicopter transport. It should be noted that monitoring, airway management, and any changes in therapy can be difficult to achieve in a helicopter. However, safe transport of these critically ill burn patients has been documented.[97] All patients transported by air should have a nasogastric tube inserted and placed on dependent drainage, as nausea and vomiting are ever-present risks during the flight. Two large-bore IVs should be functional in case one stops working. For distances over 150 miles fixed-wing aircraft are usually most satisfactory. Modern air ambulances are completely equipped flying intensive care units, and the personnel are usually well trained for both critical care and the peculiarities of patient care during flight.[98]

All pertinent information should be forwarded from the initial hospital with the patient. This includes nursing flow sheets, laboratory test results, records of vital signs and urine output, and fluid administered. Any other information deemed important by the referring or receiving physician is also sent with the patient, thus avoiding duplication of therapy and ensuring continuity of care.

REFERENCES

1. Robinson NB, Hudson LD, Riem M, et al: Steroid therapy following isolated smoke inhalation injury. *J Trauma* 22:876, 1982.
2. Heimbach DM: Burns, in Condon RE, DeCosse JJ (eds): *Surgical Care*. Philadelphia, Lea & Febiger, 1985.
3. Herndon DN, Thompson PB, Linares HA, et al: Postgrad-

uate course: Respiratory injury Part I: Incidence, mortality, pathogenesis and treatment of pulmonary injury. *J Burn Care Rehabil* 7:184, 1986.

4. Thompson PB, Herndon DN, Traber DL, et al: Effect on mortality of inhalation injury. *J Trauma* 26:163, 1986.
5. Shirani KZ, Pruitt BA, Mason AD: The influence of inhalation injury and pneumonia on burn mortality. *Ann Surg* 205:82, 1987.
6. Davies JWL: Toxic chemical versus lung tissue — An aspect of inhalation injury revisited. *J Burn Care Rehabil* 7:213, 1986.
7. Baker SP: *The Injury Fact Book*, Lexington, Heath, 1984.
8. Shimazu T, Yukioka T, Hubbard GB, et al: A dose-responsive model of smoke inhalation injury. *Ann Surg* 205:89, 1988.
9. Alexeeff GV, Lee YC, Thorning D, et al: Pulmonary tissue reactions in response to smoke. *J Fire Sci* 4:427, 1987.
10. Dyer RF, Esch VH: Polyvinyl chloride toxicity in fires. *JAMA* 235:393, 1976.
11. Zawacki, BE, Jung, RC, Joyce J, et al: Smoke, burns and the natural history of inhalation injury in fire victims: A correlation of experimental and clinical data. *Ann Surg* 185:100, 1977.
12. Agee RN, Long JM, Hunt JL, et al: Use of ^{133}xenon in early diagnosis of inhalation injury. *J Trauma* 16:218, 1976.
13. Putnam CE, Loke J, Mathay RA, et al: Radiographic manifestations of acute smoke inhalation. *Am J Roentgenol* 129:865, 1977.
14. Hudson LD: Delayed hypoxemia in smoke inhalation. *Clin Res* 19:191, 1971.
15. Moylan JA, Wilmore DW, Morton DE, et al: Early diagnosis of inhalation injury using ^{133}xenon lung scan. *Ann Surg* 176:477, 1972.
16. Clark WR, Grossman ZD, Ritter-Hrncirik C, et al: Clearance of aerosolized ^{99m}Tc-diethylenetriaminepentacetate before and after smoke inhalation. *Chest* 94:22, 1988.
17. Hunt JL, Agee RN, Pruitt BA: Fiberoptic bronchoscopy in acute inhalation injury. *J Trauma* 15:641, 1975.
18. Moylan JA, Adib K, Birnbaum M: Fiberoptic bronchoscopy following thermal injury. *Surg Gynecol Obstet* 140:541, 1975.
19. Wanner A, Cutchavree A: Early recognition of upper airway obstruction following smoke inhalation. *Am Rev Respir Dis* 180:1421, 1973.
20. Dressler DP, Skornik WA, Cuppersmith S: Corticosteroid treatment of experimental smoke inhalation. *Ann Surg* 183:46, 1978.
21. Beeley JM, Crow J, Jones JG, et al: Mortality and lung histopathology after inhalation lung injury: The effect of corticosteroids. *Am Rev Respir Dis* 133:191, 1986.
22. Clark WR, Goyette DA, Nieman GF: The effects of methyl prednisolone on acute wood smoke inhalation. *Am Rev Respir Dis* 133:A284, 1986.
23. Levine BA, Petroff PA, Slade CL, et al: Prospective trials of dexamethasone and aerosolized gentamicin in the treatment of inhalation injury in the burned patient. *J Trauma* 18:188, 1978.
24. Moylan JA, Chan CK: Inhalation injury — An increasing problem. *Ann Surg* 183:34, 1978.
25. Haldane JBS: Carbon monoxide as a tissue poison. *Biochem J* 21:1068, 1927.
26. Estabrook RW, Franklin MR, Hildebrandt AG: Factors influencing the inhibitory effect of carbon monoxide on cytochrome P-450-catalyzed mixed function oxidation reactions. *Ann NY Acad Sci* 174:219, 1970.
27. Goldbaum LR, Orello T, Degal E: Mechanisms of the toxic reaction of carbon monoxide. *Ann Clin Lab Sci* 6:372, 1976.
28. Birch CA: *Emergencies in Medical Practice*. London, Churchill Livingstone, 1971.
29. Forbes WH, Sargent F, Roughton FJW: The rate of carbon monoxide uptake by normal men. *Am J Physiol* 143:594, 1945.
30. Mellins RB, Park S: Respiratory complications of smoke inhalation in victims of fires. *J Pediatr* 87:1, 1975.
31. Winter PM, Miller JN: Carbon monoxide poisoning. *JAMA* 236:1502, 1976.
32. Barker SJ, Tremper KK: The effect of carbon monoxide inhalation on pulse oximetry and transcutaneous P_{O_2}. *Anesthesiology* 66:677, 1987.
33. Choi IS: Delayed neurologic sequelae in carbon monoxide intoxication. *Arch Neurol* 40:433, 1983.
34. Shillito FH, Drinker CK, Shaughnessy TJ: The problem of nervous and mental sequelae in carbon monoxide poisoning. *JAMA* 106:665, 1936.
35. Smith JS, Brandon S: Morbidity from acute carbon monoxide poisoning at three-year follow-up. *Br Med J* 1:318, 1973.
36. Garland H, Pearce J: Neurological complications of carbon monoxide poisoning. *Q J Med* New Series XXXVI 144:445, 1967.
37. Ginsberg R, Romano J: Carbon monoxide encephalopathy: Need for appropriate treatment. *Am J Psychiatry* 133:317, 1976.
38. Sawa GM, Watson, CPN, Terbrugge K, et al: Delayed encephalopathy following carbon monoxide intoxication. *J Can Sci Neurol* 8:77, 1981.
39. Kindwall EP: Carbon monoxide poisoning treated with hyperbaric oxygen. *Respir Ther* 2:29, 1975.
40. Mathieu D, Nolf M, Durocher A, et al: Acute carbon monoxide poisoning risk of late sequelae and treatment by hyperbaric oxygen. *Clin Toxicol* 23:315, 1985.
41. Myers RA, Snyder SK, Emhoff, TA: Subacute sequelae of carbon monoxide poisoning. *Ann Emerg Med* 14:1163, 1985.
42. Norkool DM, Kirkpatrick JN: Treatment of acute carbon monoxide poisoning with hyperbaric oxygen: A review of 115 cases. *Ann Emerg Med* 14:1168, 1985.
43. Wiseman DH, Grossman AR: Hyperbaric oxygen in the treatment of burns. *Crit Care Clin* 1:129, 1985.
44. Grube BJ, Marvin JA, Heimbach DM: Therapeutic hyperbaric oxygen: Help or hindrance in burn patients with carbon monoxide poisoning? *J Burn Care Rehabil* 9:249, 1988.
45. Silverman SH, Purdue GF, Hunt JL, et al: Cyanide toxicity in burned patients. *J Trauma* 28:171, 1988.
46. Feldstein M, Klendshoj NJ: The determination of cyanide in biologic fluids by microdiffusion analysis. *J Lab Clin Med* 44:166, 1954.

47. Norris JC, Moore SJ, Hume AS: Synergistic lethality induced by the combination of carbon monoxide and cyanide. *Toxicology* 40:121, 1986.
48. Vogel SN, Sultan TR: Cyanide poisoning. *Clin Toxicol* 18:367, 1981.
49. Clark WR, Nieman GF, Goyette D, et al: Effects of crystalloid on lung fluid balance after smoke inhalation. *Ann Surg* 208:56, 1988.
50. Stewart RJ, Yamaguchi KT, Santibanez AS, et al: Effect of high-dose cimetidine on pulmonary extravascular water after acute smoke inhalation injury. *J Burn Care Rehabil* 7:484, 1986.
51. Robinson NB, Hudson LD, Robertson HT, et al: Ventilation and perfusion alterations after smoke inhalation injury. *Surgery* 90:352, 1981.
52. Nieman GF, Clark WR, Wax SD, et al: The effect of smoke inhalation on pulmonary surfactant. *Ann Surg* 191:171, 1980.
53. Fein A, Grossman RF, Jones JG, et al: Carbon monoxide effect on alveolar epithelial permeability. *Chest* 78:726, 1980.
54. Graham DL, Laman D, Theodore J, et al: Acute cyanide poisoning complicated by lactic acidosis and pulmonary edema. *Arch Intern Med* 137:1051, 1977.
55. Herndon DN, Traber DL, Neihaus GD, et al: The pathophysiology of smoke inhalation injury in a sheep model. *J Trauma* 24:1044, 1984.
56. Traber DL, Herndon DN, Stein MD, et al: The pulmonary lesion of smoke inhalation in an ovine model. *Circ Shock* 18:311, 1986.
57. Shirani KZ, Moylan JA, Pruitt BA: Diagnosis and treatment of inhalation injury in burn patients, in Loke J (ed): *Pathophysiology and Treatment of Inhalation Injuries*. New York, Marcel Dekker, 1988, pp 239–80.
58. Covelli HD, Nessan VJ, Tuttle WK III: Oxygen derived variables in acute respiratory failure. *Crit Care Med* 1:646, 1983.
59. Davis WB, Rennard SI, Bitterman PB, et al: Pulmonary oxygen toxicity: Early reversible changes in human alveolar structures induced by hyperoxia. *N Engl J Med* 309:878, 1983.
60. Nieman GF, Clark, WR, Goyette DA: Positive end expiratory pressure (PEEP) efficacy following wood smoke inhalation. *Am Rev Respir Dis* 133:A347, 1986.
61. Kumar A, Falke KJ, Geffin B, et al: Continuous positive pressure ventilation in acute respiratory failure: Effects on hemodynamics and lung function. *N Engl J Med* 283:1430, 1970.
62. Sugarman JH, Olofsson KB, Pollock TW, et al: Continuous positive end-expiratory pressure ventilation (PEEP) for the treatment of diffuse interstitial pulmonary edema. *J Trauma* 12:263, 1972.
63. Gregory GA, Kitterman JA, Phibbs RH, et al: Treatment of the idiopathic respiratory distress syndrome with continuous positive airway pressure. *N Engl J Med* 284:1333, 1971.
64. Downs JB, Seleny FL: Respiratory failure. *Curr Probl Anesth Crit Care Med* 10:1, 1978.
65. Davies LK, Poulton TJ, Modell JH: Continuous positive airway pressure is beneficial in treatment of smoke inhalation. *Crit Care Med* 11:726, 1983.
66. Shinozawa Y, Hales C, Jung W, et al: Ibuprofen prevents synthetic smoke-induced pulmonary edema. *Am Rev Respir Dis* 134:1145, 1986.
67. Kimura R, Lubbesmeyer H, Traber L, et al: Antiprotease inhibition of smoke induced lung lymph flow elevations. *Fed Proc* 46:1100, 1987.
68. Brown M, Desai M, Traber LD, et al: Dimethylsulfoxide with heparin in the treatment of smoke inhalation injury. *J Burn Care Rehabil* 9:22, 1988.
69. Walker HL, McLeod CG, McManus WF: Experimental inhalation injury in the goat. *J Trauma* 21:962, 1981.
70. Demling RH, Niehaus G, Perea A, et al: Effect of burn-induced hypoproteinemia on pulmonary transvascular fluid filtration rate. *Surgery* 85:339, 1979.
71. Demling RH, Will JA, Belzer FO: Effect of major thermal injury on the pulmonary microcirculation. *Surgery* 83:746, 1978.
72. Harms BA, Bodai BI, Kramer GC, et al: Microvascular fluid and protein flux in pulmonary and systemic circulations after thermal injury. *Microvasc Res* 23:77, 1982.
73. Desai MH, Nichols MM, Herndon DN: Scald injury of the respiratory tract: An unusual occurrence. *J Burn Care Rehabil* 8:210, 1987.
74. Eckhauser FE, Billote J, Burke JF, et al: Tracheostomy complicating massive burn injury: A plea for conservatism. *Am J Surg* 127:418, 1974.
75. Hunt JL, Purdue GF, Gunning T: Is tracheostomy warranted in the burn patient? Indications and complications. *J Burn Care Rehabil* 7:492, 1986.
76. Shaner PJ, Brown RL, Kirksey T, et al: Succinylcholine induced hyperkalemia in burned patients — 1. *Anesth Analg* 48:764, 1969.
77. Tolmie JD, Joyce TH, Mitchell GD: Succinylcholine changes in the burned patient. *Anesthesiology* 28:467, 1967.
78. Dwersteg JF, Pavlin EG, Heimbach DM: Patients with burns are resistant to atracurium. *Anesthesiology* 65:517, 1986.
79. Martyn JA, Matteo RS: Pharmacokinetics of *d*-tubocurarine in patients with thermal injury. *Anesth Analg* 61:241, 1983.
80. Martyn JA, Goudsouzian RS: Metocurine requirements and plasma concentration in burned paediatric patients. *Br J Anaesth* 55:263, 1983.
81. Gordon MD (ed): Burn care protocols anchoring endotracheal tubes on patients with facial burns. *J Burn Care Rehabil* 8:233, 1987.
82. Morgan RF, Persing, JA, Friedman RF, et al: Intraoral wire stabilization of the endotracheal tube in facial burns. *J Burn Care Rehabil* 5:446, 1984.
83. Peitzman AB, Shires GT III, Corbett WA, et al: Measurement of lung water in inhalation injury. *Surgery* 90:305, 1981.
84. Scheulen JJ, Munster AM: The Parkland formula in patients with burns and inhalation injury. J Trauma 22:869, 1982.
85. Bowser-Wallace BH, Cone JB, Caldwell FT: Hypertonic lactated Ringer's saline resuscitation of severely burned patients over 60 years of age. *J Trauma* 25:22, 1985.

86. Schnarrs RH, Cline CW, Goldfarb IW, et al: Plasma exchange for failure of early resuscitation in thermal injuries. *J Burn Care Rehabil* 7:230, 1986.
87. Tranbaugh RF, Elings VB, Christensen JM, et al: Effect of inhalation injury on lung water accumulation. *J Trauma* 23:597, 1983.
88. Tranbaugh RF, Lewis FR, Christensen JM, et al: Lung water changes after thermal injury: The effects of crystalloid resuscitation and sepsis. *Ann Surg* 192:479, 1980.
89. Demling RH, Wenger H, Lalonde CC, et al: Endotoxin-induced prostanoid production by the burn wound can cause distant lung dysfunction. *Surgery* 99:421, 1986.
90. Gray DT, et al: Early excision vs. conventional therapy in patients with 20–40% burns. *Am J Surg* 144:76, 1982.
91. Engrav LH, Heimbach DM, Reus JL, et al: Early excision and grafting vs. nonoperative treatment of burns of indeterminant depth: A randomized prospective study. *J Trauma* 23:1001, 1983.
92. Katz A, Ryan P, Lalonde C, et al: Topical ibuprofen decreases thromboxane release from the endotoxin-stimulated burn wound. *J Trauma* 26:157, 1986.
93. Maunder RJ, Hudson LD: The adult respiratory distress syndrome, in Simmons DH (ed): *Current Pulmonology.* Chicago, Yearbook Medical Publishers, 1986, vol. 7, pp 97–116.
94. DeCamp MM, Demling RH: Posttraumatic multisystem organ failure. *JAMA* 260:530, 1988.
95. Coon WW: Risk factors in pulmonary embolism. *Surg Gynecol* Obstet 143:385, 1976.
96. Purdue GF, Hunt JL: Pulmonary emboli in burned patients. *J Trauma* 28:218, 1988.
97. Treat RL, Sirinek KR, Levine BA, et al: Air evacuation of thermally injured patients: Principles of treatment and results. *J Trauma* 20:275, 1980.
98. Sharar SR, Luna GK, Rice CL, et al: Air transport following surgical stabilization: An extension of regionalized trauma care. *J Trauma* 28:794, 1988.

Chapter 10

Resuscitation of the Patient with Inhalation Injury

William G. Cioffi
Basil A. Pruitt, Jr.

The progressive loss of intravascular volume as edema forms in the area of thermally injured tissue necessitates intravascular fluid replacement. Failure to do so in patients with extensive burns will permit the hypovolemia to become of physiologic significance and burn shock to develop. Prompt administration of a balanced salt solution in an amount to replace the isotonic fluid shifts into the extravascular space, and the associated loss of plasma proteins, predominantly albumin, into the inju.ed tissue will correct the intravascular deficit and prevent burn shock. Appropriately administered and monitored fluid treatment can be considered the cornerstone of therapy for the prevention of burn shock. The presence of associated inhalation injury alters the fluid requirements and complicates the fluid resuscitation of such patients.

Many formulas exist for estimating the fluid needs of burn patients in the first 24 to 48 hours following injury, although none specifically address the patient with concomitant thermal and inhalation injury (Table 10-1). All formulas are based upon the size of the patient and the extent of the body surface burned. Even though the formulas vary greatly in the amount and composition of fluid recommended, each has been used successfully to resuscitate large numbers of burn patients. Examination of the volume and salt doses, calculated by each formula as being necessary for the first 24 hours following injury for a 70-kg patient with an 80 percent burn, reveals that the volumes vary by more than a factor of 2, as do the salt doses. It is the physiologic reserve of the average burn patient that allows this latitude in the early resuscitation. Regardless of

The opinions or assertions contained herein are the private views of the authors and are not to be construed as official or as reflecting the views of the Department of the Army or the Department of Defense.

Table 10-1 Formulas Commonly Used to Estimate Resuscitation Fluid Needs of Adult Burn Patients

Formula	First 24 hours			Second 24 hours		
	Electrolyte-containing solution	Colloid-containing fluid equivalent to plasma	Glucose in water	Electrolyte-containing solution	Colloid-containing fluid equivalent to plasma	Glucose in water
Burn budget of F. D. Moore	Lactated Ringer's 1000–4000 mL 0.5 normal saline 1200 mL	7.5% of body weight	1500–5000 mL	Lactated Ringer's 1000–4000 mL 0.5 normal saline 1200 mL	2.5% of body weight	1500–5000 mL
Evans	Normal saline 1.0 mL/kg/% burn	1.0 mL/kg/% burn	2000 mL	One-half of first 24-hour requirement	One-half of first 24-hour requirement	2000 mL
Brooke	Lactated Ringer's 1.5 mL/kg/% burn	0.5 mL/kg/% burn	2000 mL	One-half to ¾ of first 24-hour requirement	One-half to ¾ of first 24-hour requirement	2000 mL
Parkland	Lactated Ringer's 4.0% mL/kg/% burn	—	—	—	20 to 60% of calculated plasma volume	As necessary to maintain urinary output
Hypertonic sodium solution	Volume of fluid containing 250 meq of sodium per liter to maintain hourly urinary output of 30 mL	—	—	One-third isotonic salt solution orally up to 3500 mL limit	—	—
Modified Brooke	Lactated Ringer's 2.0 mL/kg/% burn	—	—	—	0.3 to 0.5 mL/kg/% burn	As necessary to maintain urinary output

what formula is adhered to, the goal of resuscitation should be the maintenance of vital organ function.

VASCULAR PERMEABILITY CHANGES

Exposure of tissue to temperatures of 43°C or greater and the vascular effects of materials, such as histamines, serotonin, prostaglandins, leukotrienes, the activation products of the coagulation and complement systems, and the products of activated neutrophils liberated from burn tissue increase vascular permeability in the area of injury that results in edema formation and a corresponding decrease in plasma volume.[1–6] Studies of the effects of burn injury on vascular permeability in tissues remote from the site of injury have produced conflicting data. Montero et al. in an ovine model have demonstrated a fourfold increase in lymph flow and a twofold increase in the lymph/plasma protein ratio from an unburned extremity following thermal injury, which suggests an alteration in vascular permeability.[7] The addition of smoke inhalation to this model resulted in a further doubling of the lymph flow from the unburned limb with maintenance of the elevated lymph/plasma protein ratio, suggesting an additive increase in systemic microvascular permeability in unburned tissue over that caused by burn injury alone. Data from this Institute have suggested that burn injury alone does not cause a generalized systemic increase in vascular permeability.[8] Carvajal et al. in a scald burn model demonstrated maximal burn wound edema at 3 hours following injury but documented neither albumin extravasation or water accumulation in unburned tissue.[9] Capillary permeability in the injured tissue returns to normal during the latter half of the first day, and functional capillary integrity is eventually restored during the second 24 hours following injury.[10] All resuscitation formulas recognize the time-related change in transcapillary fluid movement and recommend infusion of lesser volumes of fluid during the second day.

FLUID RESUSCITATION

Type of Fluid

Because of the persistent capillary leak which occurs in the first 24 hours following injury, most investigators feel that only isotonic crystalloid solutions should be infused during this time. Proponents of the use of colloid claim that infusion of colloid-containing fluid restores cardiac output to normal levels sooner by reducing the plasma volume deficit earlier. However, in the average burn patient, by 24 to 48 hours following injury, no clinically significant difference in cardiac output or plasma volume is noted between patients resuscitated with colloid-containing solution and those given only crystalloid fluids in the first 24 hours. In addition, no clinical study has shown a difference in survival attributable to either crystalloid- or colloid-containing solutions. The use of colloid in the first 24 hours may actually be detrimental. This study by Goodwin et al.[11] showed in a randomized series of patients that the long-term pulmonary complications and overall mortality were greater in those patients treated with colloid-containing solutions than those given only crystalloid fluids in the first 24 hours. This increase in morbidity was attributed to a significant increase in extravascular lung water which developed over the first week in those patients receiving colloid-containing solutions as compared to those receiving only crystalloid fluids during the first twenty-four hours following injury (Table 10-2). Those patients receiving colloid also exhibited a delayed mobilization of the administered fluid.

Although the predominant or even exclusive use of crystalloid solutions has been incriminated as cause of pulmonary edema following thermal injury, studies by Goodwin et al.,[12] Herndon et al.,[13] and Tranbaugh et al.[14] have indicated that lung water is little changed during the first 24 hours after injury even when the patient is resuscitated with large volumes of crystalloid-containing solutions alone. Goodwin used a soluble gas rebreathing technique, while Herndon and Tranbaugh used a thermal green-dye double-indicator dilution technique. Both techniques have been documented to underestimate the actual amount of extravascular lung water, especially in the presence of lung perfusion abnormalities.[15,16] In contrast, Sharar et al.,[17] using a goat model, found that a 30 percent total body surface burn injury produced a 30 percent increase in gravimetrically measured extravascular lung water with a threefold increase in lung lymph flow. The animals were resuscitated with 4.1 mL/kg/% body surface burn, which resulted in a urinary output response of 3 mL/kg/h. Although no adverse effect on oxygenation was noted, this excessive fluid resuscitation resulting in a prodigious urine output may partially explain the elevation seen in extravascular lung water. Clinically evident pulmonary edema is infrequent in the first 48 hours following injury even when the amounts of resuscitation fluid are far in excess of those estimated by the formulas. It is thought that the immediate elevation of pulmonary

Table 10-2 Postburn Changes in Lung Water and Cardiac Output as Related to Composition of Resuscitation Fluids

	Lung water, mL/mL of alveolar volume		Cardiac output, L/min	
Postburn day	Crystalloid resuscitation	Colloid resuscitation	Crystalloid resuscitation	Colloid resuscitation
0.5	0.13	0.13	4.07	4.30
1.0	0.122	0.125	4.55	5.28
1.5	0.124	0.120	4.29	4.51
2.0	0.137	0.123	4.89	4.65
2.5	0.138	0.141	5.45	5.30
3.0	0.139	0.144	6.83	6.74
5.0	0.149	0.167	8.28	7.70
7.0	0.137	0.173	9.19	10.20

vascular resistance after injury protects the lung from pulmonary edema during the resuscitation phase.[18] The consequences of administration of excessive amounts of resuscitation fluid may become evident only when pulmonary vascular resistance returns to normal and the edema in burned tissue is resorbed thus expanding the intravascular volume. In the study of Goodwin et al.,[11] delayed onset of pulmonary edema occurred in 20 percent of patients resuscitated with colloid-containing solutions compared to 5 percent of those resuscitated with crystalloid only. Further protection may be afforded by pulmonary lymphatic capacity sufficient to clear accumulated fluid and thus prevent significant lung edema.

The use of hypertonic saline for resuscitation has been suggested as a means to limit the amount of fluid administered. However, large series comparing standard resuscitation using isotonic salt solutions to that using hypertonic saline have shown that by 48 hours following injury most patients have received the same amount of free water and salt regardless of the initial fluid regimen.[19] Physiologic limits of the use of hypertonic saline in the resuscitation of burn patients appear to be cellular dehydration in excess of 15 percent or an increase in serum sodium concentration to levels above 165 meq/L. When the serum sodium exceeds 165 meq/L, urinary output typically decreases, necessitating use of more dilute fluid to continue resuscitation.[20] A minimum fluid volume appears to be necessary even when infusing hypertonic salt solution. The use of concentrated hypertonic salt solution of 1200 meq of sodium per liter results in a profound decrease and slower recovery of plasma volume and cardiac output than when solutions containing 300 meq of sodium per liter or less are used.[21] In the majority of thermally injured patients, resuscitation with hypertonic salt solution appears to offer no particular advantage and should be reserved for use in those patients with a limited cardiopulmonary reserve who are intolerant to the volumes of resuscitation fluid estimated by the various other formulas. In a group of severely burned elderly patients, Bowser-Wallace et al. have demonstrated a significant decrease in the administered volume load with no change in the administered salt load when using hypertonic saline resuscitation.[22] Laboratory studies have shown that the restorative effect upon cardiac output of 1 meq of sodium is equal to that of 13 mL of salt-free, noncolloid fluid.[23] Substitution of salt dose for volume dose in that ratio can be used to reduce the volume of resuscitation fluid given to patients lacking in physiologic reserve.

Suggested Formula

Blind adherence to any resuscitation formula will result in a number of patients being either over- or underresuscitated. Sufficient fluid should be admin-

Table 10-3 Recommendations for Fluid Administration in First 24 Hours

Adults:	2 mL/kg/% TBSB LR (rate titrated to urine output)
Children:	(<30 kg) – 3 mL/kg/% TBSB LR
	+
	Maintenance fluids (D5 ½NS)
	(rate titrated to urine output)
	a½ volume given over first 8 hours

LR = lactated Ringer's solution.

istered to minimize blood and plasma volume changes and to reduce the effects of injury on organ function. However, edema which forms in unburned tissue secondary to redistribution of the infused crystalloid should be minimized in an attempt to prevent the morbidity associated with excessive fluid administration. Individualized resuscitation is essential to prevent the morbidity associated with either under- or overresuscitation. The authors recommend the use of a balanced electrolyte solution such as Ringer's lactate during the first 24 hours of resuscitation. A modification of the Brooke formula is used in which the amount of fluid required by an adult is estimated as 2 mL/kg/% body surface area burn. Because capillary leak in the injured tissue is greatest during the first 8 hours following injury, one-half of this volume is given during this period and the second half during the ensuing 16 hours. The fluid needs of children who have a greater surface area per unit body mass are estimated as 3 mL/kg/% burn. In addition, maintenance fluid requirements of children are administered as 5% dextrose (D5) in one-half normal saline calculated as 2000 mL/m^2 body surface area (Table 10-3). Adequate documentation of the increased fluid requirements of children exists in the literature.[24,25] In a retrospective review of resuscitation data of children with massive thermal injury from this Institute, the average resuscitation volume minus maintenance requirements was 3.91 ± 2.2 mL/kg/% body surface area burn. Based upon these observations, we feel that resuscitation should commence at 3 mL/kg/% body surface area burn. Approximately 50 percent of burned children will be adequately resuscitated with this formula. In the remaining patients, it will be necessary to increase the fluid administration rate to achieve a urine output of 0.5 to 1 mL/kg/h, which serves as a readily available index of adequate resuscitation.

Monitoring

One end point of fluid resuscitation is adequate tissue perfusion, and urine output is used as an index of renal blood flow and overall perfusion. To avoid the complications of inadequate or excessive resuscitation, frequent monitoring of the patient's general condition and hemodynamic status is mandatory. In adults, a urine output of 30 to 50 mL/h is deemed adequate. In children weighing less than 30 kg, a urine output of 0.5 to 1.0 mL/kg/h is adequate. Urine output in excess of this amount which is not osmotically driven denotes excessive fluid administration and the fluid infusion rate should be decreased. Conversely, oliguria in the first 24 to 48 hours following thermal injury is almost always secondary to inadequate volume resuscitation, and the rate of fluid administration should be increased.

Changes in the rate of fluid administration when a patient's urine output is either excessive or suboptimal should be made in a systematic fashion. Intravenous (IV) rates should be changed on a magnitude of 10 to 20 percent every 1 to 2 hours until the desired effect is achieved. Rapid and excessive decreases in the IV rate should be avoided (i.e., >25 percent) lest hypovolemia and shock be precipitated secondary to the obligatory fluid losses into the burn wound. Conversely, large increases in the IV rate or bolus fluid administration may exacerbate or potentiate pulmonary injury.

EFFECT OF SMOKE EXPOSURE

Permeability Changes

Smoke exposure has been shown to result in an increase in pulmonary microvascular permeability as manifested by increased lung lymph flow and an increase in the lymph/plasma protein ratio.[26–29] Alterations in both endothelial and epithelial permeability are thought to be produced by smoke exposure.[30–33] Although these changes in permeability may result in an increase in extravascular lung water, the magnitude of the increase and the clinical consequences thereof may be blunted by protective mechanisms such as increased lung lymph clearance and decreases in perimicrovascular oncotic pressure. Peitzman et al.[34] were able to document clinically significant increases in extravascular lung water only in patients with severe parenchymal injury and not in those with airway injury alone. The increase in microvascular permeability induced by smoke exposure appears to be partially mediated by prostaglandins.[35,36] Increases in pulmonary microvascular pressures secondary to excessive fluid administration or fluid boluses may transiently overwhelm these protective mechanisms resulting in pulmonary edema. Although one should not compromise fluid resuscitation by arbitrarily restricting the volume of fluid administered, a uniform rate of fluid administration may prevent transient surges in microvascular pressures and minimize pulmonary edema in the early phase of resuscitation.

Clinical Implications

The clinical impact of inhalation injury on resuscitation requirements is unclear. Various authors have indicated that the presence of moderate to severe inhalation injury results in an increase in fluid requirements during the first 24 to 48 hours following injury.[37–40] Navar et al.,[41] in a retrospective study, concluded that the presence of inhalation injury resulted in an increase in fluid and sodium requirements necessary to maintain an acceptable urinary output of 1 mL/kg/h when compared to a group of patients without inhalation injury. Patients with inhalation injury had a mean fluid requirement of 5.76 mL/kg/% total body surface area burn and a mean sodium requirement of 0.94 meq/kg/% body surface area burn as compared to the fluid requirements of 3.9 mL/kg/% total body surface area burn and sodium requirements of 0.68 meq/kg/% total body surface area burn in a group of burned patients without inhalation injury. Those authors recommended that fluid resuscitation commence at approximately 5.5 mL/kg/% body surface area burn in patients with documented inhalation injury. A similar retrospective study from the same institution looking at fluid resuscitation of thermally injured children could not demonstrate an increased fluid requirement in those children with inhalation injury as compared to those without.[25]

Scheulen and Munster[38] reported a 37-percent increase in fluid requirements for patients with inhalation injury as compared to those without in a group of 101 adult patients with burns covering 20 to 60% of the total body surface. The two groups of patients were not comparable in respect to mean age (43 versus 33), mean burn size (38% versus 32%), and mean full thickness component (18.5% versus 13.5%). No attempt to analyze these data correcting for these differences was made. Comparison of resuscitation between the two groups showed nearly identical hourly urine outputs although the group with inhalation injury received approximately one-third more fluid during the initial 24 hours. The authors concluded that extra fluid administration may contribute to pulmonary morbidity and suggested that one should be willing to accept lower urine output volumes, i.e., 0.3 to 0.5 mL/kg/h, in patients with inhalation injury in order to minimize the infused resuscitation volumes.

The suggestion to limit resuscitation volume and accept lower urinary outputs in patients with inhalation injury prompted Herndon et al.[42] to study the effect of resuscitation on inhalation injury in an ovine model. Utilizing the lung-lymph fistula model, sheep were randomized to one of three groups: (1) sham smoke inhalation and maintenance fluids, (2) smoke inhalation plus maintenance fluids, and (3) smoke inhalation plus two times maintenance fluids. Animals that received smoke injury and only maintenance fluids demonstrated a lower Po_2, higher lung lymph flow, a higher lymph/plasma protein ratio (i.e., a greater increase in protein flux across the capillary membrane), a lower cardiac output, and higher pulmonary artery pressures as compared to those sheep which received smoke plus two times maintenance fluids. These results have been interpreted as indicating that underresuscitation following inhalation injury may be deleterious and thus speak against limiting resuscitation volumes and accepting lower urine outputs when resuscitating patients with inhalation injury.

HEMODYNAMIC RESPONSE TO RESUSCITATION

Invasive monitoring is rarely indicated in the routine monitoring of fluid resuscitation. Indications for such monitoring are: (1) failure to respond in a 4- to 6-hour period to an hourly IV rate that would result in infusion of 6 mL/kg/% body surface area burn in the first 24 hours, (2) severe inhalation injury, and (3) preexisting cardiac disease. In these patients, a Swan-Ganz catheter should be placed to assess intravascular volume status and myocardial function by measuring the pulmonary capillary occlusion pressure and cardiac output. Those patients who demonstrate compromised cardiac function in the presence of an elevated pulmonary capillary occlusion pressure should receive inotropic support with either dopamine or another inotropic agent. The use of invasive monitoring to assess the adequacy of resuscitation can be helpful in patients who show persistent signs of hypovolemia or evidence of fluid overload. The routine use of such invasive monitoring in uncomplicated patients should be avoided. Use of such monitoring to guide infusion of sufficient volume to restore pulmonary artery occlusion pressure and cardiac output to normal levels commonly results in excessive urinary output (>200 mL/h is not uncommon), little if any improvement in other vital signs, more than anticipated weight gain and greater amounts of peripheral edema, all of which may have deleterious effects and complicate subsequent management.[11]

Sphygmomanometric measurements of blood pressure are unreliable and can be particularly misleading when obtained in a burned limb. As edema forms beneath the eschar, progressive attenuation of the auditory signal may prompt an increase in the resuscitation fluid infusion rate, which in turn causes even greater edema formation. Such monitoring can result in massive fluid overload. Measurements of blood pressure obtained by intravascular cannula in peripheral arteries may also be inaccurate secondary to the elevated circulating levels of catecholamines, which may produce severe vasospasm. Thus, blood pressure measurements are undependable as an index of resuscitation adequacy.

In the second 24 hours following thermal injury the resuscitation regimen is altered to include colloid-containing solutions in order to replenish the plasma volume deficit. This is possible because the capillary permeability leak present in the first 24 hours has essentially sealed. The volume of colloid-containing fluid administered is dependent upon burn size with 0.3 mL/kg/% burn given to patients with burns of up to 50 percent of the total body surface and 0.5 mL/kg/% burn given to patients with burns of more than 70 percent of body surface. A solution of albumin diluted to physiologic concentration in lactated Ringer's or normal saline may be used. During this time, no other sodium-containing fluids are infused because the patient has been salt-loaded during the initial 24 hours of resuscitation. Additional fluid in the form of 5% dextrose in water is infused at the rate necessary to maintain a urinary output between 30 and 50 mL/h. The administration of colloid-containing fluid helps to minimize the fluid volume administered in the second 24 hours. In burned children restoration of the plasma volume deficit is accomplished in a similar manner. Salt-loading is reduced in a similar fashion, but solutions of D5 and water are to be avoided to prevent induction of symptomatic hyponatremia and possible cerebral edema. Five percent dextrose in one-half normal saline should be administered in order to maintain an adequate urine output of 0.5 to 1.0 mL/kg/h in these children (Table 10-4).

The hemodynamic response to this resuscitation schema is predictable (Fig. 10-1). Patients resusci-

Table 10-4 Recommendations for Fluid Administration in Second 24 Hours

Adults:	0.3–0.5 mL/kg/% TBSB 5% albumin in LR + D5W (titrated to urine output 50–70 mL/h)
Children:	(<30 kg) 0.3–0.5 mL/kg/% TBSB 5% albumin in LR + D5 ½NS (titrated to urine output 0.5–1.0 mL/kg/h)

tated with the modified Brooke formula will experience an early decrement in blood and plasma volume with subsequent restoration of plasma volume to predicted normal levels during the latter part of the second 24 hours following injury. Cardiac output which is initially depressed increases to predicted normal levels between the 12th and 18th hours at a time when a progressive decrease in blood and plasma volume is still occurring. Cardiac output thereafter rises to supranormal levels during the second day after injury as the plasma volume deficit is restored.[43]

On the basis of both clinical experience and laboratory studies it appears as if inhalation injury in combination with cutaneous thermal injury, particularly in patients with extensive burns increases fluid requirements during the initial resuscitation phase. More importantly, since such patients appear to be susceptible to the complications of both over- and underresuscitation, blind adherence to any resuscitation formula must be avoided. Because of the vast patient-specific differences in fluid requirements, no one formula will satisfy the resuscitation needs of all patients. Frequent monitoring of the patient's overall status and urinary output is paramount in order to prevent compounding the pulmonary effects of inhalation injury and avoid the morbidity associated with inappropriate resuscitation.

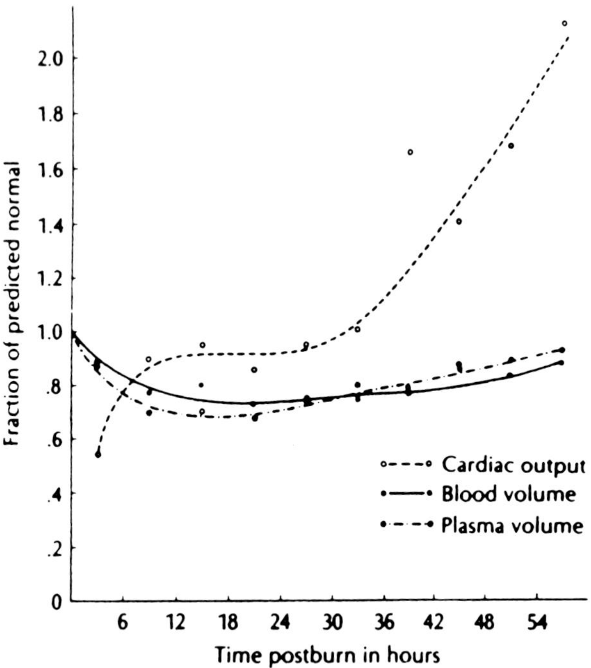

Figure 10-1 Cardiac output, initially depressed, responds promptly to fluid therapy and rises to predicted normal levels between 12 and 18 hours following injury, at a time when blood and plasma volumes are progressively decreasing. In the second 24 hours as continued resuscitation restores the plasma volume deficit, cardiac output rises to supranormal levels.

REFERENCES

1. Alexander F, Mathieson M, Teoh KHT, et al: Arachidonic acid metabolites mediate early burn edema. *J Trauma* 24:709, 1984.
2. Bjornson AB, Bjornson HS, Knippenberg RW: Temporal relationships among immunologic alterations in a guinea pig model of thermal injury. *J Infect Dis* 153:1098, 1986.
3. Gelfand JA, Donelan M, Burke JF: Preferential activation and depletion of the alternative complement pathway by burn injury. *Ann Surg* 198:58, 1983.
4. Herndon DN, Abston S, Stein MD: Increased thromboxane B_2 levels in the plasma of burned and septic burned patients. *Surg Gynecol Obstet* 159:210, 1984.
5. Kupper TS, Deitch EA, Baker CC, et al: The human burn wound as a primary source of interleukin-1 activity. *Sur-*

gery 100:409, 1986.
6. Shea SM, Caulfield JB, Burke JF: Microvascular ultrastructure in thermal injury: A reconsideration of the role of mediators. *Microvasc Res* 5:87, 1973.
7. Montero KE, Lubbesmeyer HJ, Traber DL, et al: Inhalation injury increases systemic microvascular permeability. *Surg Forum* 38:303, 1987.
8. Mason AD Jr: The mathematics of resuscitation. *J Trauma* 20:1015, 1980.
9. Carvajal HF, Lubbesmeyer HJ, Brouhard BH: Relationship of burn site to vascular permeability changes in rats. *Surg Gynecol Obstet* 189:193, 1979.
10. Pruitt BA Jr, Mason AD Jr: Hemodynamic studies of burned patients during resuscitation, in Matter P, Barclay TL, Konickova Z (eds): *Research in Burns*. Bern, Huber, 1971.
11. Goodwin CW, Dorethy J, Lam V, et al: Randomized trial of efficacy of crystalloid and colloid resuscitation on hemodynamic response and lung water following thermal injury. *Ann Surg* 197:520, 1983.
12. Goodwin CW, Lam V, Mason AD Jr, et al; Colloid and crystalloid have same effect on lung water after thermal injury. *Surg Forum* 32:294, 1981.
13. Herndon DN, Barrow RE, Traber DL, et al: Extravascular lung water changes following smoke inhalation and massive burn injury. *Surg* 102:341, 1987.
14. Tranbaugh RF, Lewis FR, Christensen JM, et al: Lung water changes after thermal injury: The effects of crystalloid resuscitation and sepsis. *Ann Surg* 192:479, 1980.
15. Miniati M, Pistolesi M, Milne ENC, et al: Detection of lung edema. *Crit Care Med* 15(12):1146, 1987.
16. Prien T, Traber LD, Herndon DN, et al: Pulmonary edema with smoke inhalation, undetected by indicator-dilution technique. *J Appl Physiol* 63(3):907, 1987.
17. Sharar SR, Heimbach DM, Winn RK, Hildebrandt J: Effects of body surface scald burn on lung fluid balance and cutaneous blood flow in goats. Abstract presented at the 19th Annual Meeting of the American Burn Association, Washington, DC, April 29–May 2, 1987.
18. Asch MJ, Feldman RJ, Walker HL, et al: Systemic and pulmonary hemodynamic changes accompanying thermal injury. *Ann Surg* 178:218, 1973.
19. Pruitt BA Jr, in Caldwell FT, Bowser BH: Critical evaluation of hypertonic and hypotonic solutions to resuscitate severely burned children: A prospective study. *Ann Surg* 198:552, 1979.
20. Shimazaki S, Yoshioka T, Tanaka N, et al: Body fluid changes during hypertonic lactated saline solution therapy for burn shock. *J Trauma* 17:38, 1977.
21. Moylan JA Jr, Reckler JM, Mason AD Jr: Hypertonic lactate saline resuscitation in thermal injury. *Surg Forum* 22:49, 1976.
22. Bowser-Wallace BH, Cone JB, Caldwell FT Jr: Hypertonic lactated saline resuscitation of severely burned patients over 60 years of age. *J Trauma* 25:22, 1985.
23. Moylan JA Jr, Mason AD Jr, Rogers PW, et al: Postburn shock: A critical evaluation of resuscitation. *J Trauma* 13:354, 1973.
24. Graves TA, Cioffi WG, McManus WF, et al: Fluid resuscitation of infants and children with massive thermal injury. *J Trauma* 28(12):656, 1988.
25. Merrell SW, Saffle JR, Warden GD, et al: Fluid resuscitation in thermally injured children. *Am J Surg* 152:664, 1986.
26. Traber DL, Schlag G, Redl H, et al: Pulmonary edema and compliance changes following smoke inhalation. *J Burn Care Rehabil* 6:490, 1985.
27. Herndon DN, Adams T Jr, Traber LD, et al: Inhalation injury and positive pressure ventilation in a sheep model. *Circ Shock* 12:107, 1984.
28. Guyton AC, Moffatt DS, Adain TH: Role of alveolar surface tension in transepithelial movement of fluid, in Robinson B, Van Golde IMG, Batenberg SS (eds): *Pulmonary Surfactant*. Amsterdam: Elsevier, 1984, pp 171–86.
29. Clark WR Jr, Nieman GF, Goyette D, et al: Effect of crystalloid on lung fluid balance after smoke inhalation. *Ann Surg* 208:56, 1988.
30. Nieman GF, Clark WR, Goyette D, et al: Increased pulmonary microvascular permeability following wood smoke inhalation. Submitted for publication.
31. Davies JWL: Toxic chemicals versus lung tissue — An aspect of inhalation injury revisited. *J Burn Care Rehabil* 7:213, 1986.
32. Emmons HW: Fire and fire protection. *Sci Am* 231:21, 1974.
33. Birky M, Malek D, Paabo M: Study of biological samples obtained from victims of MGM Grand Hotel fire. *J Anal Toxicol* 7:265, 1983.
34. Peitzman AB, Shires GT III, Corbett WA, et al: Measurement of lung water in inhalation injury. *Surgery* 90:305, 1981.
35. Kimura L, Traber D, Herndon GN, et al: Ibuprofen reduces the lung lymph flow changes associated with inhalation injury. *Circ Shock* 24:183, 1988.
36. Demling RH, Zhu D, Lalonde C: Early pulmonary and hemodynamic effects of a chest wall burn (effect of ibuprofen). *Surgery* 104(1):10, 1988.
37. O'Neill JA: Fluid resuscitation in the burned child: A reappraisal. *J Pediatr Surg* 17:604, 1982.
38. Scheulen JJ, Munster AM: The Parkland formula in patients with burns and inhalation injury. *J Trauma* 22:869, 1982.
39. Agarwal N, Petro J, Salisbury RE: Physiologic profile mointoring in burned patients. *J Trauma* 23:577, 1982.
40. Baxter CR, Shires GT: Guidelines for fluid resuscitation. Proceedings of the Second Consensus Development Conference on Supportive Therapy in Burn Care. *J Trauma* 21(suppl):687, 1981.
41. Navar PD, Saffle JR, Warden GD: Effect of inhalation injury on fluid resuscitation requirements after thermal injury. *Am J Surg* 150:716, 1985.
42. Herndon DN, Traber DL, Traber LD: The effect of resuscitation on inhalation injury. *Surgery* 100:248, 1986.
43. Pruitt BA Jr, Mason AD Jr, Moncrief JA: Hemodynamic changes in the early postburn patient: The influence of fluid administration and of a vasodilator (Hydralazine). *J Trauma* 11:36, 1971.

Chapter 11

Pulmonary Infections in the Burn Patient and Their Management

Stephen D. Sears

Infections are the leading cause of mortality in burn patients.[1-4] Prior to the use of effective topical antimicrobial therapy, infection of the burn wound, with resultant bacteremia and toxemia, was the leading cause of death in the burn unit.[5-7] More recently, pneumonia has become one of the most frequent life-threatening infections and is an important determinant of survival.[8] The majority of pneumonias are nosocomial, occurring in the burn patient after 72 hours of hospitalization, and are often associated with either an inhalation injury or endotracheal intubation with exposure to respiratory therapy equipment, or both.[9-12] Although pneumonia may develop earlier, either from prior colonization with pathogenic microorganisms, such as *Streptococcus pneumoniae* or *Haemophilus influenzae,* or from aspiration of gastric or oropharyngeal contents, this is the exception rather than the rule. These "early pneumonias," caused by community-acquired pathogens, are often quite responsive to therapy. A nosocomial pneumonia, on the other hand, is an infection of the lower respiratory tract that develops in hospitalized patients and that is typically caused by "hospital flora" and is often more difficult to treat. According to a recent Centers for Disease Control (CDC) study,[13] the lung is the third most common site for hospital-acquired infections, accounting for 15 to 20 percent of all nosocomial infections. However, in contrast to more common nosocomial infections (i.e., urinary tract and wound infections) that have relatively low attendant mortality, nosocomial pneumonias are disproportionately associated with increased mortality and may cause as much as 15 percent of all deaths occurring in patients.[14,15] This makes hospital-acquired pneumonias the most common fatal nosocomial infection in this country. This is especially true in the modern burn unit, in which pulmonary infections extract a significant toll of morbidity and mortality. The intent of this review is to identify current concepts of the risk factors, pathogenesis, etiology, diagnosis, therapy, and prevention of pulmonary infections, especially nosocomial pneumonia in the hospitalized burn patient.

PNEUMONIA

Risk Factors

The likelihood of developing pneumonia is increased when certain conditions are present (Table 11-1). One of the most important risk factors predisposing to pneumonia in the hospitalized burn patient is endotracheal intubation.[14,16] The incidence of pneumonia developing is estimated to be four times higher for intubated than nonintubated patients, and tracheostomy increases this risk even more.[11–13] Clearly, intubated patients tend to be more ill and are therefore potentially more susceptible to infections, but the presence of an endotracheal tube increases the likelihood of infection by eliminating the natural host defense mechanisms. In the intubated patient, the filtration system of the upper airways is bypassed, colonization of the upper airways is facilitated, and colonizing bacteria have easy access to the lower respiratory tree. The source of the bacteria remains controversial, but bacteria may originate from the patient's own flora, from the burn wound either hematogenously or by aerosolization during dressing changes, or from the immediate environment. Once bacterial colonization is established, the risk of pneumonia increases dramatically, especially if the patient remains intubated for more than 72 hours.

Exposure to respiratory therapy equipment adds an increased risk of pneumonia above and beyond the risk associated with endotracheal intubation.[17–19] Shortly after the use of nebulization equipment in respiratory care became common, several epidemics of nosocomial pneumonia were reported.[19–21] The risk of ventilator-associated pneumonia was significant but has now decreased with a better understanding of the necessity to decontaminate and maintain respiratory equipment.[22,23] Intubated patients receiving respiratory therapy may be at an even increased risk of pneumonia because of coincident exposure to other procedures such as suctioning, which may injure the mucosa and thereby reduce resistance to infection or allow increased colonization of the airway with pathogenic bacteria.[24] Respiratory therapy equipment, if not properly cared for, may also provide a source of exogenous organisms that can contaminate the patient's respiratory tract, the personnel caring for the patient, and the immediate environment.[25]

Smoke inhalation with resultant pulmonary injury is another major risk factor associated with the development of pneumonia in the burned patient.[26,27] Serious pulmonary compromise is often observed when inhalation injury is present. Inhalation injury is covered more fully in Chap. 9. Briefly, when an inhalation injury is present, the airway may be injured directly by the heat from superheated air, as well as by the products of incomplete combustion. The heat injury to the upper airway may cause edema and result in a marked increase in the work of breathing.[28] Pulmonary compromise also may occur when compounds, such as potent acids and aldehydes, present in the smoke are inhaled. This can result in severe tracheobronchitis, with loss of normal ciliary action, often not evident for 24 to 48

Table 11-1 Risk Factors for Nosocomial Pneumonia

Host specific
Advanced age
Burn wound
Immunosuppression
Impaired consciousness
Obesity
Serious underlying illness
Smoke inhalation
Hospital specific
Antibiotics
Aspiration (oropharyngeal or gastric)
Colonization (oropharyngeal or gastric)
Intubation
Respiratory therapy
Surgery (especially abdominal and thoracic)

hours. This may lead to the development of mucous and cellular debris in the bronchi and bronchioles which favors the proliferation of bacteria. Atelectasis may be severe, dynamic lung compliance decreases, and shunting and hypoxemia increase.[29–31]

The use of antibiotics in the hospitalized patient has also been associated with an increased incidence of nosocomial pneumonia.[32,33] The presumed reason for this is that antibiotics either select for or promote the growth of more resistant bacteria during therapy, which then may either become colonizing or infecting pathogens. Consequently, *prophylactic usage of antibiotics should be discouraged unless clearly indicated.* Many other commonly used pharamacologic agents are capable of disrupting normal pulmonary defenses and therefore may be associated with an increased risk of pneumonia. Drugs such as ethanol, hypnotics, narcotics, and neuroleptics predispose a patient to aspiration by altering consciousness and by depressing the gag and cough reflexes.[34] In healthy persons, lung defenses, which include the alveolar macrophages and the peripheral polymorphonuclear (PMNs) leukocytes, are usually adequate. Even so, these defenses can be overwhelmed by a large inoculum of bacteria. In hospitalized patients, the defenses may be inadequate due to the underlying disease process and are often altered by certain medical interventions that diminish the inflammatory response. Drugs, such as aspirin, corticosteroids, aminophylline, and calcium channel blockers, can impair alveolar-macrophage function.[35] Similarly, many agents can interfere with pulmonary inflammatory responses by decreasing PMN function, although the clinical relevance of this is not certain.

Major surgery, which is very common in burn patients, constitutes another important risk for the development of pneumonia.[14] Very high rates of pneumonia, up to 50 percent, have been reported with emergency surgery, but even elective procedures have an appreciable rate, as much as 12 percent.[36] This is not surprising, since intubation and antibiotic usage, which have already been described as major risks, are commonly used in surgical patients. Certain host characteristics, including age, obesity, and the severity of underlying diseases, are all associated with an increased likelihood of pneumonia. The burn itself can be considered a risk factor for the development of pneumonia. In patients without inhalation injury but with large burns, hyperventilation, due to pain from either the burn or the topical antimicrobial agent mafenide, with subsequent decreases in tidal volume, may lead to atelectasis and then pneumonia. Circumferential full thickness chest burns may lead to a decrease in compliance and make pulmonary toilet difficult. Also, of presumed importance is the profoundly altered host defenses common in burn patients. Many complex alterations in both cellular and humoral components of the immune systems of burn patients have been described and may well influence the epidemiology of pulmonary infections.[3,4,37]

CASE 1

A 72-year-old woman was hospitalized at Francis Scott Key Medical Center Burn Unit with a 32% total body surface burn suffered in a house fire. On admission, she was dyspneic and mildly confused and had inspiratory stridor. She had burns on the chest, back, and both legs. She received standard fluid resuscitation and was intubated. She had a previous history of mitral stenosis, with a porcine mitral valve replacement 8 years earlier. She had underlying, chronic obstructive pulmonary disease, was a heavy cigarette smoker, was obese, and had a type II diabetes, for which she took oral hypoglycemic agents.

Her first 48 hours after burn were marked by wide swings in blood pressure, pulse, and temperature. She was given morphine for pain control, and on the third hospital day, she had the first of multiple surgeries. On the fifth hospital day, the patient became febrile, and diffuse rales were noted on examination; copious amounts of frothy sputum were suctioned from her endotracheal tube. On the following day, her sputum became thicker and more tenacious. Her temperature rose to 103.2°F, her white blood cell count was elevated to 19,000/mm.^{3} Her chest x-ray, which had previously been clear, now revealed bilateral pulmonary edema and patchy infiltrates (Fig. 11-1). Sputum Gram stain showed many PMNs and many gram-negative bacilli. Therapy was begun with piperacillin sodium and amikacin sulfate, and the sputum cultures subsequently grew *Enterobacter cloacae,* which was susceptible to this antibiotic regimen. She became

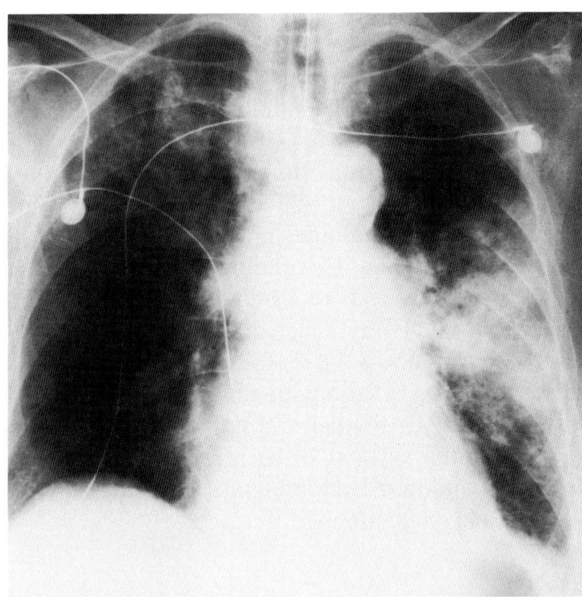

Figure 11-1 Chest x-ray from a 72-year-old woman with a 32 percent body burn showing bilateral pulmonary infiltrates.

more alert by the tenth hospital day, and her respiratory status improved and she was extubated. Subsequently, she recovered uneventfully from her pneumonia and was eventually discharged from the hospital.

This patient had multiple risk factors for nosocomial pneumonia, including advanced age, obesity, underlying cardiopulmonary disease and diabetes, and she required intubation and mechanical ventilation. She received pain medicine which can decrease the gag reflex, had an inhalational injury and underwent excisional surgery. It is therefore not surprising at all that she developed a gram-negative, hospital-acquired pneumonia.

For patients developing pneumonia early in the hospital course (generally less than 72 hours), several factors that alter normal host defenses and predispose to infection usually exist. Alterations in the level of consciousness from any cause can compromise normal swallowing mechanisms and lead to aspiration of oropharyngeal flora into the lower respiratory tree. If this occurs in a host with an underlying illness such as chronic parenchymal pulmonary disease, especially a cigarette smoker, the likelihood of a pneumonia developing increases. Previous colonization with known respiratory pathogens is likewise a risk for the early development of pneumonia.

CASE 2

The patient was a 27-year-old white man admitted to the Baltimore Regional Burn Center on 2/1/88, with an inhalation injury, and an 8% total body surface area burn. The burn occurred while he was driving a forklift when a liquid propane tank exploded. He was treated initially in a local emergency room, was intubated because of the possible inhalation injury, and was flown via helicopter to the burn center. On exam, he had 8% body burn to his head, face, neck, bilateral hands and bilateral knees. On admission, his blood gases were unremarkable. On the second hospital day, his blood gases deteriorated significantly and he required increasing positive end-expiratory pressure (PEEP) and increasing F_{IO_2}'s to maintain adequate oxygenation. He developed a fever and had an increasing respiratory rate, and physical exam was consistent with consolidation. A lobar infiltrate on chest x-ray was noted (Fig. 11-2). Clinically, he had a pneumonia and was producing purulent sputum. The Gram stain showed PMNs, gram-positive diplococci, and pleomorphic gram-negative rods. The culture grew out *S. pneumoniae* and *H. influenzae*. He was started on cefuroxime and did well. His course stabilized and his temperature returned to normal. He had resolution of his pulmonary symptoms with decrease in sputum production. He was extubated 2 days later. He received a 10-day course of cefuroxime, at which time he was discharged to home.

This case illustrates the typical course and etiology of pneumonia that may develop in the first few days after a burn. The pathogens *S. pneumoniae* and *H. influenzae* are typical outpatient pathogens and reflect colonization with these organisms prior to the burn injury. It is likely that the inhalation injury and the endotracheal intubation were the major risk factors in the development of pneumonia in this patient.

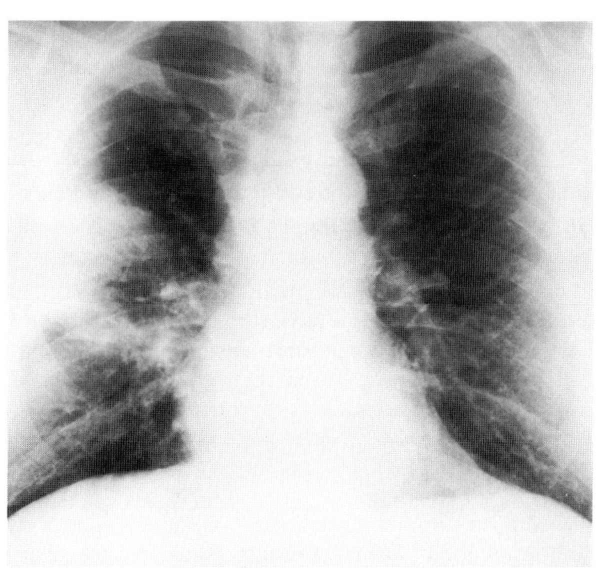
A

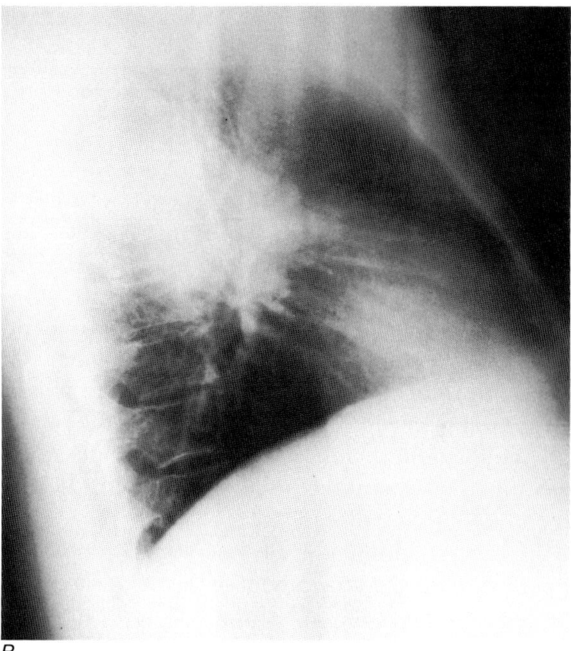
B

Figure 11-2 Chest x-ray from a 27-year-old man with an infiltrate that developed 2 days after admission to the burn unit. The PA film on the left and lateral film on the right clearly show a dense consolidation in the right lung. Cultures of the sputum grew *S. pneumoniae* and *H. influenzae.*

Pathogenesis

Pneumonia results from the aspiration of oropharyngeal flora, inhalation of airborne pathogens, or direct spread from a contiguous source or via hematogenous spread.[38] The majority of pneumonias appear to result from aspiration of potential pathogens which have colonized the mucosal surfaces of the upper airways. Aspiration occurs commonly in patients with depressed consciousness and is increased by a diminished or absent gag or cough reflex and by both nasogastric and endotracheal intubation.[39] For a further discussion of aspiration, see Chap. 16. Pharyngeal secretions are aspirated in the majority of healthy persons during sleep, but clearly not everyone who aspirates bacteria from prior colonization develops pneumonia.[40] Pneumonia develops if the defense mechanisms, including the integrity of the cellular and humoral defenses, are overcome by either the volume or virulence of the infecting organisms.[41–43]

Pneumonia occurs when pathogenic organisms bypass the airway defenses, are aspirated in secretions, and escape from lung defense mechanisms. A key process in this chain of events is the initial colonization of the oropharynx with pathogenic bacteria.[44–46] Multiple risk factors for colonization have been described (Table 11-2). The "normal" bacteria in the oropharynx of healthy persons consist predominantly of anaerobic bacteria and streptococci and only rarely are gram-negative bacilli (GNB) found.[47] Several factors have been identified that may increase the likelihood of upper airway colonization with GNB in the hospitalized patient. In a classic study,[48] 213 patients admitted to the hospital were monitored with frequent cultures of the oro-

Table 11-2 Risk Factors for Oropharyngeal Colonization

Alcoholism	Malnutrition
Antibiotic therapy	Intubation
Coma	Leukopenia
Gastric colonization	Nasogastric tubes
Hypotension	Underlying illness

pharynx. Ninety-five patients (45%) became colonized with aerobic gram-negative bacilli by the end of the first week in the hospital. Pneumonia subsequently developed in 22 (23%), compared to only 4 of 118 noncolonized patients (3.3%). The risk of airway colonization with gram-negatives increased with time and was directly correlated with the degree of underlying illness.

The crucial initiating event in colonization of the upper airway is the attachment of the bacteria to the epithelial or mucosal cell surface.[49] Typically, the "normal" flora occupy the available attachment sites.[50] In contrast, the oropharyngeal flora in colonized patients contain few gram-positive cocci and many gram-negative bacilli per epithelial cell.[51] In vitro bacterial adherence assays using buccal cells have confirmed this altered colonization pattern.[52] Gram-negative organisms clearly become the organism predominant on cells from seriously ill patients. The mechanisms by which aerobic gram-negative bacilli become more adherent to airway mucosa in hospitalized patients is felt to be determined by an interplay of specific bacterial adhesions and changing host cellular receptors. The microbial composition of the oropharyngeal flora is partly determined by the ability of each bacterial species to adhere to the epithelial cells.[52] Bacterial lectins such as the pili on cell membranes of *Pseudomonas aeruginosa* have been identified as important in adherence to airway mucosa.[53] Also, considerable data have been collected suggesting that the mucosal cell surface glycoprotein, fibronectin, plays an integral part in controlling oropharyngeal bacterial interactions.[54] Under normal circumstances, buccal cells are coated with fibronectin, which promotes binding of gram-positive organisms, thereby preventing adherence of gram-negative bacilli.[55] Fibronectin also appears to prevent adherence of *P. aeruginosa* to buccal cells.[56] Of even more interest are recent studies documenting increased levels of salivary protease in seriously ill hospitalized patients.[57] This increased level of protease was associated with increased degradation of fibronectin with a concomitant increase in adherent gram-negative bacilli. Fibronectin levels in patients may also be related to nutritional status.[58] Starvation is associated with increased adherence of *P. aeruginosa* to buccal cells, and this reverts to normal with nutritional supplementation. Interestingly, several studies have documented decreased levels of plasma fibronectin in both trauma and major burns.[59,60] The implications of these observations are presently uncertain but might well be used in new strategies in the prevention of airway bacterial colonization.

Potential sources of gram-negative bacilli in seriously ill patients are multiple and include the flora of the upper airway, stomach, and colon; hands of hospital personnel; inhalation therapy equipment and solutions; the hospital environment; and dietary supplements. Fecal-oral transmission of bacteria to the airways is considered to occur commonly in the hospitalized patient, but this route does not adequately explain the frequency of colonization by such nonfecal organisms as *P. aeruginosa, Serratia marcescens,* and *Acinetobacter* species, which typically are environmental organisms.[61] Enterobacteriaceae (fecal flora) can be cultured from the hypopharynx and rectum prior to the trachea, but this is not true for the non-Enterobacteriaceae.[62] It is, therefore, likely that environmental sources exist for non-Enterobacteriaceae and that colonizing Enterobacteriaceae originate primarily in the patient's flora. Other studies have implicated transmission of pathogenic bacteria via the hands of health care personnel as an important source of colonizing organisms.[63] But even with strict adherence to hand washing and other infection control measures, colonization often occurs.

Recent evidence has implicated gastric alkalinization, used for the prevention of stress ulceration, as a significant risk factor for gastric colonization with pathogenic bacteria.[64] The rise in gastric pH increases the risk of bacterial gastric colonization which in turn, via retrograde movement of bacteria, has been shown to increase tracheal colonization.[65] Two recent studies have now shown that this increases the risk of nosocomial pneumonia.[66,67] It appears that non-pH-altering agents such as sucralfate may be preferable to agents that alter pH and allow overgrowth.[11] Similarly, enteral feedings have been recently shown to increase the likelihood of gastric bacterial colonization and hence the possibility of tracheal colonization.[68]

Airborne transmission is probably of little importance in the epidemiology of nosocomial bacterial pneumonia. Small particles or aerosols that are generated by coughs and sneezes, as well as nebulization equipment, may remain airborne for long periods, may disseminate widely in the local environment, and may potentially infect large numbers of persons.[69] This rarely occurs, though, because the bacterial density in the air in hospitals is quite low. Likewise, hematogenous spread of organisms from a primary focus of infection is an uncommon cause of pneumonia.[3,4] Prior to the use of topical burn wound antibiotics, hematogenous pneumonia resulting from septicemia from a distant focus of infection was more common.[5] The burn wound was usually the source, but suppurative thrombophlebitis or visceral infection could also serve as the nidus for bacteremia. Bronchopneumonia developing from aspiration of colonized secretions is now the most common form of pneumonia in burn patients. Bronchopneumonia more commonly occurs earlier in the postburn period (typically in the first 2 weeks) than does hematogenous pneumonia (seen often after the third postburn week), although there may be significant overlap.[4] Of note is that the mortality rate appears to be higher with hematogenous pneumonia, but this may reflect the primary bacteremia and underlying infection. Practically speaking, it is difficult to differentiate between bacteremic bronchopneumonia and bacteremia-associated pneumonia, and therapy should be aimed at both the pulmonary process as well as any underlying infection.

Etiology

Almost any microbiologic agent can cause pneumonia. In the adult patient admitted to the burn unit who develops pneumonia in the first 3 days, the organisms isolated will almost always be "community acquired" (Table 11-3). The large majority of these cases of community-acquired purulent pneumonia will be due to *S. pneumoniae* or mixed anaerobic-aerobic organisms associated with gastric aspiration.[70] Occasionally, the agents of the atypical pneumonia syndrome, such as *Mycoplasma pneumoniae*, *Legionella pneumophila*, rickettsia, and viruses, can be causative, but this is unusual. In the winter, influenza A virus may be found. It is estimated that 2 to 18 percent of acute community-acquired pneumonias in adults may be caused by *H. influenzae*, but the true incidence is unknown since isolation of this organism may represent coloniza-

Table 11-3 Comparison of the Causes of Community and Nosocomial Pneumonia in Adults

Pathogen	Community-acquired, %	Nosocomial, %
Bacterial	70–80	>90
S. pneumoniae	60–75	3–9
H. influenzae	4–5	?
S. aureus	1–5	10–20
Gram-negative bacilli	Rare	>50
Anaerobes	Rare	30
Legionella sp.	2–5	0–25
M. tuberculosis	2	?
Atypicals	10–20	Rare
M. pneumoniae	5–18	
C. psittaci	2–3	
Viruses	10–20	Rare
Influenza	8	
Other viruses	2–8	

SOURCE: Adapted from MacFarlane JT: Treatment of lower respiratory infections. *Lancet* 2:1447, 1987.

tion and not infection.[71] Occasionally, *Staphylococcus aureus* and gram-negative pathogens such as *Klebsiella pneumoniae* may also be associated with outpatient pneumonias. Although other microbiologic agents such as mycobacteria, fungi, and parasites can quite clearly cause community-acquired pneumonia, they do so rarely. In contrast to community-acquired pneumonia in adults, viruses such as influenza A, parainfluenza, and respiratory syncytial virus, are important causes of pneumonias in children. Bacterial pneumonia with *H. influenzae* is also an important cause in this age group.

Aspiration of gastric or oropharyngeal secretions and resulting infection may also be seen in the first 3 days after burn. (For a complete discussion, see "Lung Abscess," below.) The bacteriologic findings in aspiration pneumonia reflect the flora of the oropharynx. Anaerobic bacteria occur alone in approximately 50 percent of cases, and in a combination with aerobes in 45 to 50 percent. The predominant anaerobic organisms isolated are *Bacteroides melaninogenicus, Fusobacterium* species, and anaerobic cocci. *Streptococcus* species are the most common aerobic isolates.

There is little prospective data on the likely etiologic agents causing pneumonia in burn patients. Since the majority of pneumonias occur after 3 days in the hospital, gram-negative bacilli and *S. aureus* predominate.[72] In the majority of hospital-acquired cases, single pathogenic isolates have been identified, but polymicrobial gram-negative pneumonia is also common.[73] The National Nosocomial Infections Study (NNIS),[13,74] a nationwide database collected by the Centers for Disease Control, has consistently shown that in hospitals in the United States, the majority of pathogens causing nosocomial pneumonias are gram-negative bacilli (Table 11-4). Very few anaerobic bacteria and viruses were reported, probably because of the difficulty in isolating and identifying these agents. However, it is believed that anaerobes may actually be involved in one-third of all nosocomial pneumonias (Table 11-5) and may even be the sole agent in some cases.[75]

Other bacteria associated with nosocomial pneumonias may require special conditions for accurate identification or may be associated with specific host characteristics. In patients with chronic obstructive pulmonary disease (COPD), *H. influenzae* is a common colonizing as well as infecting pathogen. In certain geographic areas, *L. pneumophila* is endemic and has been clearly shown to cause nosocomial pneumonia.[76] Importantly, patients treated

Table 11-4 Most Frequently Isolated Pathogens Causing Nosocomial Pneumonias in the United States

Pathogen	Frequency, %
Pseudomonas species	16.9
S. aureus	12.9
Klebsiella species	11.6
Enterobacter species	9.4
E. coli	6.4
Serratia species	5.8
Proteus species	4.2

SOURCE: Data from Centers for Disease Control, National Nosocomial Infections Study Report, Annual Summary, 1984.

Table 11-5 Polymicrobial Etiology of Nosocomial Pneumonia

Organism	% pure culture (n = 73)	% total (n = 159)
Aerobes	96	93
Gram-positive		
S. pneumoniae	30	31
S. aureas	22	26
S. faecalis	—	7
Gram-negative		
H. influenzae	7	17
E. coli	5	14
Klebsiella spp.	25	23
P. mirabilis	0	11
P. aeruginosa	5	9
Other	—	7
Anaerobes	4	35
Peptostreptococcus	—	14
B. fragilis	—	8
Fusobacterium	—	10
Other	—	20

SOURCE: Adapted from Bartlett JG, O'Keefe P, Tally FP, et al: Bacteriology of hospital-acquired pneumonia. *Arch Intern Med* 146:868, 1986.

with broad-spectrum antibiotics have an increased risk of developing pneumonia with "super-infecting" organisms, such as group D streptococci and fungi.[77] Viral infections may also cause pneumonia and be difficult to diagnose. In a recent prospective study of nosocomial pneumonia on a pediatric service, viral infections were found to be responsible for 20 percent of the cases.[78] The incidence of these unusual pathogens in the burn patient with pneumonia is unknown, but it is likely to be low.

The majority of pneumonia in burn patients is caused by hospital flora; *it is therefore, absolutely vital that the epidemiology and ecology of the local nosocomial pathogens be known.* The bacterial flora associated with nosocomial infections may vary between hospitals, between different areas in the same hospital, and over time. For example, Table 11-6 shows the distribution of bacterial species isolated from the sputum of patients at the Baltimore Regional Burn Center between 1985 and 1987. It would appear from these data that *P. aeruginosa* was the predominant gram-negative pathogen causing pneumonia, but careful inspection of these data (Table 11-7) reveals a somewhat different picture.

Table 11-6 Sputum Cultures* from the Baltimore Regional Burn Center, 1985–87

Bacterial species	No. of isolates	% of total
Gram-negative		
Pseudomonas sp.	30	21
Serratia sp.	21	15
Klebsiella sp.	17	12
Enterobacter sp.	11	8
H. influenzae	8	6
Proteus sp.	5	4
Citrobacter sp.	5	4
E. coli	3	2
Acinetobacter sp.	1	1
	101	73
Gram-positive		
S. aureus	33	23
S. pneumoniae	4	3
Group D streptococcus	2	1
	39	27

*All sputum cultures were judged as adequate by screening for >10 PMNs per high-power field (hpf).

Table 11-7 Sputum Cultures* from the Baltimore Regional Burn Center, Yearly Totals for 1985–87

	No. of isolates		
Bacterial species	1985 (%)	1986 (%)	1987 (%)
Pseudomonas sp.	13 (34)	12 (18)	5 (13)
Serratia sp.	0	16 (25)	5 (13)
Enterobacter sp.	6 (16)	2 (3)	3 (8)
Klebsiella sp.	5 (13)	6 (9)	6 (16)
Haemophilus sp.	1 (3)	3 (4)	4 (10)
Proteus sp.	0	3 (4)	2 (5)
Acinetobacter sp.	0	0	1 (3)
E. coli	2 (5)	0	1 (3)
Citrobacter sp.	0	5 (7)	0
All gram-negatives	27 (71)	47 (72)	27 (71)
S. aureus	10 (26)	14 (22)	9 (24)
S. pneumoniae	1 (3)	2 (3)	2 (5)
Group D streptococcus	0	2 (3)	0
All gram-positives	11 (29)	18 (28)	10 (29)
Total no. of isolates	38	65	37
Total no. of patients	20	23	20
Isolates per patient	1.9	2.8	1.9

*All sputum cultures were judged as adequate by screening for >10 PMNs/hpf.

Although *P. aeruginosa* was the most common gram-negative isolate in 1985, there was an outbreak of *S. marcescens* in 1986, and *K. pneumonia* was a major pathogen in 1987. Importantly, the *Serratia* in 1986 was restricted to the burn unit and was not associated with nosocomial infections in the rest of the hospital. If hospital-wide microbiologic monitoring was relied on, these trends may have been overlooked. If microbiologic monitoring does not exist in an individual hospital, the NNIS provides descriptive data that can be used as a general guide. In all cases, though, surveillance data collected in an individual institution analyzing the prevalence of antibiotic resistance among bacterial isolates should be obtained if at all possible.

Clinical Manifestations and Diagnosis

The diagnosis of pneumonia in the critically ill burn patient with an inhalation injury may be one of the most difficult in clinical medicine. The classic signs of pneumonia, such as the presence of pulmonary infiltrates and sputum production, may be seen in the burn patient without pneumonia. Symptoms may be unreliable or unobtainable in critically ill patients, and fever and leukocytosis secondary to the burn wound itself may simulate infection. In addition, the presence of an inhalation injury may be associated with an increase in tracheobronchial secretions, making the differentiation between tracheobronchitis and pneumonia unclear.[79,80] Similarly, cough and sputum production may be seen in the intubated patient, without pneumonia being present.[81] Also, in patients with adult respiratory distress syndrome, common in severe burns, the diagnosis of pulmonary infection is particularly difficult to determine.

Even finding pathogenic bacteria in pulmonary secretions does not allow one unequivocally to make the diagnosis of pneumonia. Gram-negative bacilli and *S. aureus* are frequently found to colonize the airways of critically ill patients.[82] As many as 75 percent of positive sputum cultures represent airway colonization rather than invasive infection.[83] Likewise, a significant minority of infections may also be mistaken for colonization. Therefore, it may be impossible to determine whether patients with inhalational injury and respiratory distress have pneumonia. This will inevitably lead to some errors in management and makes clinical experience coupled with a careful physical examination essential. When one is examining a critically ill patient to determine whether pneumonia is present, the following questions should be considered: (1) Has there been a change in clinical status unexplained by other events? (2) Has there been a sudden change in fever pattern, an increase in a lung infiltrate, a drop in arterial Po_2, or other significant change in ventilator requirements? (3) Has there been a significant change in either the quantity or purulence of respiratory secretions? If the answer to these questions is yes, it is likely that a pneumonia does indeed exist. While such criteria for diagnosing nosocomial pneumonia lack sensitivity and specificity, they usually are the most reliable primary indicators for the clinician.

Once the diagnosis of pneumonia has been entertained or established, the next hurdle is to determine the precise etiology. This may be extremely difficult since microbiologic evaluation does not always yield usable information.[84] Even so, it is important that expectorated sputum or respiratory secretions obtained by endotracheal aspiration be examined microscopically by Gram stain and be sent to the laboratory for culture. If sputum is not readily obtainable, chest physiotherapy, and ultrasonic nebulization can be used. Typical morphologic features on Gram stain can be used to identify bacterial species (Table 11-8). Sputum specimens, unfortunately, are often contaminated with upper airway flora, making the interpretation potentially inaccurate. Because of this, the reliability of sputum cultures for bacteriologic diagnosis has been challenged as having little sensitivity and specificity.[85,86] Gram stain grading has been proposed as a method to determine the extent of oropharyngeal contamination and the acceptability of a specimen for bacterial culture. Specimens with fewer than 25 squamous epithelial cells and more than 10 PMNs per low-power field tend to be representative of purulent sputum and are suitable for bacterial culture.[87] Unfortunately, in patients with tracheostomies or endotracheal tubes, there may be an abundance of leukocytes because of the inflammatory reaction to the device itself.[88] This makes even a grading technique difficult to interpret. Investiga-

Table 11-8 Morphologic Features — Pathogenic Bacteria Commonly Found by Gram-Stain Examination

Morphology	Likely pathogen
Gram-positive cocci in clusters	*S. aureus*
Gram-positive cocci in chains and in pairs	*S. pneumoniae*
Gram-negative cocci in pairs	*Branhamella catarrhalis*
Gram-negative cocco-bacilli	*H. influenzae*
Gram-negative bacilli	Enterobacteriaceae *Pseudomonas* species
Mixed organisms	Anaerobes

tors have proposed that serial examination of tracheal aspirates in patients with endotracheal tubes should be evaluated for elastin fibers, and higher Gram stain grading for neutrophils should be used.[89] In one study, the presence of elastin fibers in patients with endotracheal tubes preceded the development of pulmonary infiltrates and occurred more frequently during infection with gram-negative bacilli.[89] Although sputum culture alone may not give a definitive answer, if obtained properly, the results may be helpful in providing antimicrobial susceptibility data.

Because of the difficulties in interpreting sputum specimens, blood cultures should be drawn from all patients with presumed pneumonia. Organisms isolated from blood, pleural fluid, lung bronchial washings, and transtracheal aspirates should be considered pathogenic, and therefore of significance.[90] Since the microbiologic evaluation of contaminated respiratory specimens may be misleading, a number of invasive techniques have been developed in order to obtain noncontaminated specimens for diagnostic evaluation[91] (Table 11-9). Many of these methods are not particularly practical for widespread use but occasionally may be helpful in individual patients. Transtracheal aspiration, which is not recommended in intubated patients, is occasionally useful for obtaining specimens below the carina, which can be Gram stained and then cultured for anaerobic bacteria.[92] Another method, which has been used to obtain uncontaminated specimens, is percutaneous-needle lung aspiration, but this is not advised for patients on positive pressure breathing devices.[93] Recently, shielded bronchoscopic sampling of lower airway secretions has also been suggested as a method for obtaining lower airway specimens without contamination from upper airway respiratory organisms.[94] Open lung biopsy is the most accurate method to obtain a specimen but is rarely indicated in this population. Although these invasive methods may be useful in individual patients, they often are not well tolerated by critically ill patients with suspected pneumonia. Knowledge of the advantages and disadvantages of each is therefore imperative and these procedures should only be used if appropriate expertise exists and the samples obtained can be processed immediately.

Table 11-9 Comparison of Procedures for Obtaining Microbiologic Specimens for Diagnosis of Nosocomial Pneumonias

Procedure	Sensitivity	Specificity	Morbidity
Expectorated sputum	High	Almost nil	Nil
Transtracheal aspiration	High	Low	Low
Fiberoptic bronchoscopy			
Standard catheter brush	High	Low	Low
Washings	Moderate	Low	Low
Protected specimen brush	High	High	Low
Transbronchial biopsy	Moderate	High	Moderate
Transthoracic needle aspiration	Low	High	High
Open lung biopsy	High	High	High

SOURCE: Adapted from Sanford JP: Lower Respiratory Tract Infections, in Bennett JV, Brachman PS (eds): *Hospital Infections*. Boston, Little Brown, 1986, p 385–422.

Although chest x-rays may be occasionally misleading, they can be useful indicators of bacterial pneumonia. Findings suggestive of pneumonia include segmental, patchy, or lobar infiltrates or cavitation which may be accompanied by a pleural effusion. In the intensive care unit, it may be necessary to perform serial x-rays to evaluate infiltrates over time, which is often much more helpful than a single x-ray film view. The classic physical findings of pulmonary consolidation, including rales and bronchial breath sounds especially if associated with fever and dyspnea, are often seen in patients with infection in the lung. But, unfortunately, the spectrum of specific diseases presenting with fever and new pulmonary infiltrates in hospitalized patients encompasses both a variety of infectious and noninfectious causes. Common noninfectious causes of pulmonary infiltrates such as atelectasis, congestive heart failure, pulmonary embolism, pulmonary hemorrhage, and the adult respiratory distress syndrome need to be differentiated from nosocomial pneumonia.

Treatment

Treatment of pneumonia may be empiric when the etiologic agent has not been identified, or it may be specific when the etiologic agent is known. Intravenous antibiotics remain the mainstay of treatment for pneumonia, but a number of investigational therapies have been proposed, including endotracheal antibiotics and passive immunization.[16] Systemic antibiotics should be used wisely because injudicious use not only will fail to be beneficial to the patient but may also produce harmful effects either through toxicity directly or by contributing to the emergence of resistant strains of microorganisms.[95] No single agent or combination of agents can destroy all the organisms to which a burned patient is exposed, and multiagent therapy may have the untoward effect of predisposing to superinfection by yeast, fungi, or resistant organisms. Dosages must be adjusted based on serum concentrations when serum assays are available.[96] Antibiotics should be used for a long enough period to produce the appropriate effect but not long enough to allow for the emergence of resistance. Above all, active surveillance and monitoring of the burned patient should be a mandatory component of effective therapy. Since burn patients with a hospital-acquired pneumonia will be severely ill, it is also imperative to pay strict attention to oxygenation and ventilation.[97] Intubation and artificial ventilation should be considered early in the course of the illness if respiratory failure is present or if the patient cannot be managed adequately by lesser means.

Empiric therapy should be selected after a careful microscopic examination of the sputum or tracheal aspirate since this may help provide a tentative etiology. Empiric therapy requires a thorough understanding of the likely pathogens as well as the efficacy, safety, and cost profiles of the antibiotics selected. It is therefore important to consider the clinical setting and host characteristics prior to selecting appropriate presumptive antibiotic therapy. It is often useful to answer the following questions when considering the likely etiology of pneumonia: (1) Has the patient recently received antibiotics? (2) Does the patient have an underlying illness that would increase the risk of colonization with certain organisms (i.e., bronchitis and *H. influenzae*)? (3) Have recent surveillance cultures of the patient's sputum been consistently positive for a particular organism? (4) Does the patient have underlying organ failures or allergies which will guide selection of an antimicrobial agent? Of equal importance are such things as the recent experience with nosocomial pathogens in a given hospital intensive care unit. Certain hospitals may have a particularly high incidence of pneumonias caused by multiantibiotic-resistant *P. aeruginosa, Acinetobacter* sp., or *Serratia* sp. After carefully evaluating the available microbiologic data, examining the patient, and investigating the local epidemiology, a reasonable "guess" at the infecting pathogen can be made.

The empiric treatment of nosocomial pneumonia should usually include coverage for aerobic gram-negative bacilli, specifically resistant organisms, and should also have activity against *S. aureus*. Based upon these considerations, several antibiotic regimens have been employed for empiric therapy of nosocomial pneumonia. Probably one of the more commonly used combinations is a semisynthetic penicillin plus an aminoglycoside, but in certain situations a cephalosporin plus an aminoglycoside or clindamycin plus an aminoglycoside may be very useful.[98,99] In the presence of a known large aspiration, the antibiotic selected should have activity against the anaerobic flora. Table 11-10 lists empiric therapy for nosocomial pneumonia. This table is meant to serve only as a very general guide to the selection of specific antibiotics, because no one regimen will be successful in all situations. It is always necessary to obtain as much epidemiologic and clinical information as possible prior to the selection of an empiric regimen.

Generally combination therapy, usually with an

Table 11-10 Classification and Therapy of Pneumonia

Treatment	Treatment
Community-acquired pneumonia	Initial therapy: ampicillin/penicillin. Additional considerations: erythromycin for penicillin-sensitive patients (also active against agents of atypical infections; add antistaphylococcal penicillin (e.g., oxacillin, nafcillin) to primary therapy if pneumonia is postinfluenzal or likely to be due to *S. aureus*.
Nosocomial pneumonia	Initial therapy: third-generation cephalosporin plus aminoglycoside in severe infection. Additional considerations: where pseudomonal infection is likely give antipseudomonal cephalosporin or penicillin plus an aminoglycoside.
Community-acquired aspiration anaerobic pneumonia	Clindamycin or benzylpenicillin
Nosocomial aspiration pneumonia	Initial therapy: aminoglycoside or third generation cephalosporin plus clindamycin or benzylpenicillin

SOURCE: Adapted from MacFarlane JT: Treatment of lower respiratory infections. *Lancet* 2:1447, 1987.

aminoglycoside and a B-lactam drug, as the initial selection has been recommended.[95,99,100] Although combinations of antimicrobials may be synergistic or additive, this can not be determined without sophisticated laboratory studies. Recently, there have been reports of single B-lactam therapy for serious gram-negative rod infections.[101–103] Although these reports are encouraging, the reliability of single-agent therapy to treat infections due to *P. aeruginosa* and *S. marcescens* pneumonia is yet to be fully confirmed. Thus, in the initial empiric stages of therapy, most clinicians still would include an aminoglycoside in the regimen.

Once an etiologic agent is identified and the antimicrobial susceptibilities are known, therapy should be altered to an antibiotic regime that minimizes toxicity and maximizes efficacy by maintaining levels of drug that are inhibitory for the organism. Whether combination chemotherapy is necessary to treat pneumonia is an unresolved issue.[104] Combinations of antibiotics may suppress the emergence of resistance and be synergistic and therefore more effective in treating nosocomial pneumonia than a single antibiotic active against the isolate. But combination therapy may increase toxicity, clearly costs more, and may be associated with an increased rate of superinfections.[105] Currently available clinical data suggest that infections caused by *S. aureus* can usually be managed with single agents such as nafcillin sodium, oxacillin sodium, cefazolin sodium, or vancomycin hydrochloride.[106] When pneumonia is caused by enteric gram-negative pathogens, most authorities recommend combination therapy with the possible exception of infection due to either *Escherichia coli* or *Proteus mirabilis*. For pneumonias caused by these pathogens, monotherapy with an agent such as ampicillin should usually suffice. Whether infections caused by *K. pneumoniae* require two active agents as compared to only one remains controversial.[99] Cephalosporins are extremely active against *K. pneumoniae* and should be included in the therapeutic regimen if these organisms are present. For other gram-negative organisms, a wide variety of antibiotic combinations have been used, but a B-lactam–aminoglycoside combination has been the most extensively studied and has been documented to be efficacious.[107] There is no clear advantage to one combination over another as long as the organisms are susceptible to both agents. In infections caused by *P. aeruginosa,* an extended spectrum penicillin and aminoglycoside are generally used.[108]

While many consider aminoglycosides to be the cornerstone of therapy for serious gram-negative respiratory infections, their role in these infections has recently been questioned.[109] The narrow toxic-to-therapeutic ratios for aminoglycosides and the low serum levels make these difficult drugs to use. In addition, the penetration of aminoglycosides into infected respiratory tissues is poor and may result in local drug concentrations insufficient to treat infecting organisms.[110] Despite these problems, evidence exists that aminoglycosides may be more active than B-lactams against certain resistant gram-negative bacilli.[111] If aminoglycosides are used, it is important to follow some basic rules to maximize their effectiveness and to minimize toxicity. Renal failure is a known toxicity, is defined by a rise in serum creatinine of at least 0.5 mg%, and is related to the total dose of aminoglycoside. Toxicity is best avoided by carefully monitoring the peak and trough levels. Desired troughs for gentamicin and tobramycin are 2 μg/mL or less, and for amikacin is less than 10 μg/mL.[112,113] Although renal failure is often reversible, it can prolong hospital stay, requires frequent monitoring, and can be a significant problem in dosing other therapeutic agents. For efficacy, it is important to achieve peak levels of gentamicin and tobramycin between 6 μg/mL and 12 μg/mL and peak levels for amikacin between 24 μg/mL and 30 μg/mL.[114]

The availability of newer antimicrobial agents with a broad spectrum of activity, reasonable safety profiles, and increased efficacy offers an alternative approach to the aminoglycosides. These agents make the possibility of single-drug therapy very appealing. If proven successful, these agents could decrease the number of adverse drug reactions and ultimately decrease costs. All third-generation cephalosporins have expanded activity against enteric gram-negative bacilli.[101] These agents, which include cefoperazone sodium, cefotaxime sodium, ceftizoxime sodium, ceftriaxone sodium, and moxalactam disodium, are all useful against most strains of *E. coli, Klebsiella, Serratia,* and *Proteus*. These agents may be less active against *Enterobacter* and are unreliable against *P. aeruginosa,* and *Acinetobacter* species. Two recently released agents that should have important usage in the management of gram-negative bacillary pneumonia are ceftazadime and imipenem/cilastatin.[102,103] Ceftazidime, a third generation cephalosporin, possesses broad-spectrum activity against a wide variety of gram-negative pathogens, including *P. aeruginosa, Serratia,* and *Enterobacter* and most strains of *Proteus, Citerobacter, Klebsiella,* and *E. coli.* Of the cephalosporins, it appears to be the most active against *P. aeruginosa*. However, ceftazidime has marginal activity against *S. aureus* and anaerobic bacteria. Imipenem has the broadest spectrum of activity of any antimicrobial agent currently available. It is highly active against gram-positive cocci such as *S. aureus,* most streptococci, most gram-negative rods including *Pseudomonas* and *Acinetobacter,* as well as most anaerobes. Although, the third-generation cephalosporins and imipenem have significant activity against the organisms that cause nosocomial pneumonia, resistance has already been reported to occur with the use of these agents alone.[115] So although monotherapy in the treatment of nosocomial pneumonia appears promising, until well designed, carefully controlled, randomized trials evaluating these agents have been performed, combination therapy will remain the standard.

To avoid the systemic toxicity of the aminoglycosides, several other approaches have been utilized to improve drug delivery into infected lung tissue.[116] It has been noted that the levels of antibiotics within bronchial secretions are approximately 10 percent of those found in serum, and these may be too low to treat infections caused by the more resistant gram-negative pathogens.[110] To overcome these difficulties, direct instillation of aerosolized aminoglycosides into the respiratory tract via the endotracheal tube has been studied.[117–121] In a European trial, patients with nosocomial gram-negative pneumonia were treated with systemic antibiotics plus 25 mg of sisomicin instilled into the respiratory tract every 8 hours.[116] More patients in the group receiving local aminoglycoside treatment experienced improvement, and superinfections with resistant flora were no different between the two groups. Another trial using gentamicin instilled directly in the endotracheal tube did not find results as encouraging.[120]

In addition to antibiotics, there exists considerable interest in immunologic methods of treatment of gram-negative pneumonia.[122–124] Gamma globulins, including the J5-cross-protective antisera and hyperimmune *Pseudomonas* globulin, may be a potentially valuable aid for the treatment of gram-negative pneumonias.[125–128] These therapies are currently being evaluated, and clinical and experimental data are presently insufficient to establish their direct therapeutic usefulness.

Until newer methods of treating pneumonia become established, systemic antibiotics will remain the first choice of therapy in the burned patient. Because of this, it is extremely important that antibiotics be used properly. In the past, as a result of antibiotic pressure and the emergence of resistant bacteria, burn units became the site of virulent microorganisms. This has resulted in the closing of individual burn units. To avoid this, active surveillance of burn patients and the burn unit should be routine, and careful selection and proper use of antibiotics essential. The ideal antimicrobial agent does not exist. If it did, it would rapidly penetrate into the site of the infecting organisms, in this case the lung, would be nontoxic and bactericidal, and would not be associated with superinfections and resistance. Because therapy is not perfect, it is imperative that the choice of an antimicrobial agent be made with a thorough knowledge of the side effects, toxicity, and potential benefits of the agent. Burn patients will be exposed to microorganisms regardless of effective infection control procedures, and no single or combination of antimicrobial agents will be effective against all known microorganisms. Since combination therapy may be associated with the emergence of resistant organisms or a superinfection by yeast, fungi or resistant bacteria, antibiotics should be used only long enough to produce the desired effect and no longer. The pharmacokinetics, including the distribution, metabolism, and excretion of systemic antibiotics are altered in burn patients.[129,130] Therefore the dosages must be adjusted on the basis of serum concentrations, and renal function should be monitored.[131] Increasing numbers of new antimicrobial agents leaves the clinician with a tremendous armamentarium with which to treat infections. If used wisely, these agents will remain useful for the foreseeable future.

Prevention

The primary objective in preventing pneumonia in the burn patient is to reduce the acquisition of bacterial pathogens in the upper airways and thus to reduce the potential for the aspiration of these organisms into the lower respiratory tract (Tables 11-11 and 11-12). Approaches to the control of nosocomial bacterial pneumonia have emphasized the following: (1) the prevention of colonization, (2) the prevention of postoperative pneumonia, (3) the prevention of aspiration, (4) the maintenance of respiratory therapy equipment, (5) the usage of proper aseptic techniques for the patients whose respiratory tract is at risk, and (6) the alteration of host susceptibility. Although it is probably impossible to completely prevent hospital-acquired pneumonia, there nevertheless are a number of "commonsense" recommendations that can be made to help decrease the incidence.

Table 11-11 Prevention of Nosocomial Pneumonias

Environment
Equipment maintenance
Maintenance of medications for nebulization
Appropriate design and staffing of critical care areas
Patient
Avoidance of unnecessary ventilation or intubation
Cough and deep-breathing exercises
Compliance with suctioning techniques
Prophylactic antibiotics (only in unique circumstances)
Vaccination (investigational)
Personnel
Hand washing between patient contacts
Reporting of communicable diseases
Adherence to isolation policies

SOURCE: Brown RB, Ryczak M, Sands M: Management of nosocomial pneumonia. *Hosp Form* 21:1208, 1986.

Table 11-12 Strategies to Prevent Nosocomial Pneumonia

Colonization
Infection control measures (hand washing, ventilator circuit changes)
Preserve normal gastric pH
Topical antibiotics
Maintain normal salivary proteolytic activity
Local fibronectin replacement
Administer bacterial adhesion or epithelial cell receptor analogs
Aspiration
Avoidance of central nervous system depressants
Elimination of the endotracheal tube as a reservoir
Host defense
Prompt therapy for underlying medical disorders
Nutritional support (appropriate administration and route)
Judicious use of medications
Active and passive immunization
Immunomodulators

Prevention of Colonization The initial step in the development of nosocomial pneumonia is the colonization of the respiratory tract with pathogenic bacteria.[132,133] Presently, little of practical application is available to decrease pharyngeal colonization with gram-negative bacilli, but several areas of research hold promise. Endobronchial prophylactic antibiotics have been given in an attempt to reduce colonization and to affect the rate of nosocomial pneumonia.[121] Aerosolized gentamicin has been given to burn patients with inhalation injury.[134] Unfortunately, pulmonary and septic complications were not reduced and the prophylactic gentamicin aerosol was associated with the isolation of gentamicin-resistant bacteria. In another study, the installation of endotracheal gentamicin in patients with tracheostomies was associated with a decrease of purulent sputum and a decrease in documented lung infiltrates but again was associated with a slight increase in gentamicin resistance.[122] In another study, a combination of an aminoglycoside and polymyxin B was given.[118] Bronchial irritation was noted with this regimen. Another study of polymyxin B aerosol given to patients in a respiratory intensive care unit originally found encouraging results, but in the final phases of that study, antibiotic-resistant respiratory pathogens emerged, and increased pneumonia-related mortality was observed.[119] Therefore, presently the routine use of prophylactic endobronchial antibiotics cannot be recommended. Neither should routine systemic administration of prophylactic antibiotics be used to prevent nosocomial pneumonia, since this approach is not effective and it has also been shown to be associated with the emergence of resistant microorganisms.[135]

Fibronectin appears to be protective of colonization in the upper respiratory tract.[54] Increases in salivary proteolytic enzyme activity are thought to reduce the concentrations of fibronectin. Investigations are under way to elucidate the mechanism for this increase and to develop techniques to either reduce the production or neutralize it with cxogenous antiproteases.[57] Another approach under investigation is the local administration of fibronectin. Other approaches include the possibility of using epithelial receptor analogues or possibly bacterial pili analogues to block bacterial adherence and thus colonization of the upper respiratory tract.[136]

Recently, two different research groups have published reports that suggest pH-altering agents in the gastrointestinal (GI) tract are associated with an increased likelihood of the development of pneumonia in the intubated intensive care unit patient.[66,67] Although more data are clearly needed, it may be prudent at this point to consider using non-pH-altering agents such as sucralfate rather than histamine type 2 (H_2) blockers or antacids for stress ulcer prophylaxis.

Preventing Postoperative Pneumonia Patients who have recently undergone surgery are at increased risk for developing nosocomial pneumonia.[13,14] They often have impaired swallowing, decreased respiratory clearance mechanisms due to the influence of narcotics or sedatives, and may be immobilized because of postoperative pain. This is especially true in the postoperative burn patient. These high-risk patients should benefit from postoperative interventions that try to expand the lungs and assist with the removal of secretions.[137] It is important to try to prevent the development of atelectasis, which may serve as a first step in the development of a pneumonia. Since many patients do not voluntarily expand their lungs after surgery because of pain, especially if the burn involves the thoracic cage, it is necessary to encourage deep breathing and lung expansion. If a patient is not intubated, then an incentive spirometer, chest physical therapy with postural drainage, and percussion may be useful.[98] In the intubated patient, it is necessary to use meticulous care in maintaining the patency of the airway using pulmonary toilet, frequent suctioning, and the avoidance of contamination of the endotracheal (ET) tube. Although endotracheal suctioning is currently recommended to minimize the volume of secretions, this procedure may run the risk of inoculating the lungs by dislodging bacterial aggregates often found in the lumens of ET tubes.[138,139] Recently, it has been determined that the ET tube itself may serve as a reservoir for persistent contamination of the tracheobronchial tree.[138,139] The tube, often made of polyvinyl chloride, may have binding characteristics that facilitate the adherence of aggregates of pathogenic bacteria. These aggregates may be dislodged by the routine care of the ET tube.[138] Although currently the standard care of the intubated patient is to remove secretions with frequent suctioning, it might be that in the future more frequent changes of ET tubes rather than routine suctioning will be used. This approach is currently being studied.

Preventing Aspiration Although no effective technique exists to eliminate the aspiration of small quantities of pharyngeal secretions, certain nonspecific measures may be useful. In the nonintubated patient, such things as feeding patients with the heads of their beds elevated, giving small frequent feedings rather than large ones, and positioning patients on their sides rather than on their backs may be useful. Patients who are at risk of aspirating oropharyngeal secretions are also at risk of aspirating gastric contents. These patients may require tracheal intubation or feeding by methods that reduce this risk. One such method is the use of a gastrostomy feeding tube, but such a tube does not entirely eliminate the possibility of aspiration. Presently, there is little effective prevention for the aspiration of small aggregates of bacterial colonies from the oropharynx and ET tube into the lower airways. Because of this, it is extremely important to adhere to appropriate infection control guidelines to minimize colonization and cross contamination of patients with bacteria and to maintain respiratory equipment in as sterile a manner as possible.

Maintenance of Respiratory Therapy Equipment Respiratory therapy equipment should be meticulously maintained. Careful monitoring, decontamination after usage, and adherence to the CDC guidelines should help decrease the incidence of nosocomial pneumonia.[13,74,140–142] These guidelines though, are largely empiric, based more on common sense than on controlled observations. More recently several research groups have begun to critically evaluate accepted guidelines. For instance, a study in intensive care unit patients found that ventilatory circuit changes only need to be changed every 48 hours as opposed to the routine changing every 24 hours.[143] Similarly, mechanical ventilators with cascade humidifiers which maintain temperatures high enough to be inhibitory to bacterial growth only need to be changed every 48 hours. Numerous filters and traps have been developed for use on the inspiratory and expiratory sides of the ventilatory circuits, but the effectiveness of these in preventing pneumonia has not been demonstrated. Most of the published guidelines that pertain to respiratory therapy equipment contain many other "commonsense" recommendations such as the washing of hands between patient contacts, wearing sterile gloves for endotracheal suctioning, and avoiding contact between hospital personnel and high-risk patients. Other seemingly important but unvalidated procedures include using sterile water rather than tap water to fill respiratory equipment reservoirs since this practice may decrease the likelihood of colonization with organisms such as *L.*

pneumophila. Clearly, compulsive care of the ventilatory apparatus is always indicated. Care should be taken to ensure that medications and other materials used for respiratory support are sterile. Disposable substances should be used when feasible and disposable equipment should not be reused. Finally and probably most importantly, patients should be maintained on ventilators for the shortest possible time.

Infection Control — Aseptic Technique Appropriate infection control guidelines have been published and should be routinely followed.[22,140] Infection control recommendations intended to decrease the incidence of pneumonia in high-risk patients have been primarily aimed at minimizing cross contamination of the patient. Although it is known that decontamination of respiratory therapy equipment can reduce the risk of nosocomial pneumonia and that adherence to CDC infection control guidelines can decrease all nosocomial infections, there is little controlled data on the role of infection control practices in reducing the risk of bacterial colonization of the upper airway, and therefore, pneumonia.[144,145] Again, common sense should prevail, since following established practices should decrease infection rates. Asepsis refers to practices that reduce the number of microorganisms and prevent or reduce transmission from person to person or both. According to the CDC guidelines, items that will touch normally sterile tissues are to be sterilized.[22,140] Aseptic techniques should be used for procedures that involve contact with mucous membranes such as suctioning or manipulation of the airway.

Although environmental bacterial contamination has been documented to be associated with outbreaks of nosocomial pathogens, person-to-person transmission is considered the most likely and important means of bacterial spread.[63,146,147] The hands of health care personnel giving direct patient care have been consistently implicated as a source of transmission of pathogenic bacteria between patients. During outbreaks of bacterial pneumonia, colonized or infected patients may serve as secondary reservoirs of the epidemic organisms and the health care personnel serve inadvertently as the vector. Therefore, frequent and appropriate hand washing is essential for effective infection control.[22,63] Hand washing with an antiseptic rather than a nonantiseptic hand washing agent has been found to be associated with a lower rate of infection and should be encouraged, although most authorities feel that the mechanical action of hand washing is probably all that is necessary.[140] In any case, hand washing should be a mandatory routine in the care of the burn patient.

The recent advent of "body substance isolation," or what is generally referred to as Universal Precautions, is likely to also help prevent cross contamination of patients. The use of barriers, i.e., the wearing of gloves, routinely for contact with secretions may provide additional protection for the patient from the hands of colonized personnel. Visitors need to follow the same precautions and access to patient care areas should be limited. Patients colonized or infected with highly resistant bacteria may need to be placed in special isolation rooms, and staff-patient ratios may need to be adjusted. The routine use of gloves, or gown-and-glove combination, with patients in intensive care has been found to reduce the overall incidence of nosocomial infections and is especially important in the burn unit. Important additional measures that might be used for the control of nosocomial pneumonia include surveillance and staff education. The Centers for Disease Control Senic Project found that postoperative pneumonia rates could be reduced by 27 percent with the establishment of high-intensity surveillance programs.[13,74] Surveillance of respiratory cultures may be quite valuable in allowing the appropriate selection of antibiotics while awaiting definitive results of cultures.

Altering Host Susceptibility As an alternative to antibiotic prophylaxis, immunization against bacterial pathogens has been examined as a means of preventing nosocomial pneumonia. Studies in experimental animal models have demonstrated that active immunization with cell wall lipopolysaccharides of *P. aeruginosa* provide significant protection against bacterial colonization, but clinical trials of vaccination have demonstrated only limited efficacy.[148] The development of a hyperimmune anti-*Pseudomonas* globulin offers the potential for rapid immunization using passive administration of type-specific antibodies, but presently clinical data are limited.[123] Pneumococcal pneumonia is predominantly a community-acquired infection, but immunization of hospitalized patients can occasionally be useful, although there are limited data on the efficacy of this vaccine and antibody response in patients in the intensive care or burn units. Another immunologic approach is to confer protection against a wide range of potential gram-negative bacterial pathogens of the human respiratory tract. So-called cross-protective vaccines or antisera, such as the J5 mutant of *E. coli,* might be candidate immunogens. Recent studies with the J5 antiserum suggest a protective role against gram-negative septicemia, but the degree of protection by this serum in pulmonary infections has not been determined.[126]

It is clear from the above discussion that our ability to prevent pneumonia in the critically ill burn patient has not kept pace with our understanding of the pathogenesis, risk factors, and transmission of this important infection (Table 11-12). As we learn more about oropharyngeal colonization and understand more of the biochemical and immunologic reactions of the host, it may become easier to interrupt the series of events that lead to the development of pneumonia. In the meantime, it is exceedingly important to maintain a continued vigilance of the patients' hospital environment, to follow the available infection control guidelines, and to keep abreast of new data on infection prevention as they become available.[149] General measures such as proper hand washing, sufficient space and personnel for each hospitalized patient, and isolation of selected ill or high-risk patients remain extremely important and cannot be overemphasized.

OTHER INFECTIOUS PROCESSES

Lung Abscess

A lung abscess is a suppurative, destructive pulmonary infection that most often follows aspiration of oropharyngeal contents. It begins as a necrotizing pneumonia and without effective therapy soon develops into a cavity, typically with an air-fluid level.

Pathogenesis Aspiration of oral secretions with bacteria is the most important predisposing event in the development of an abscess.[150] In lung abscesses that develop outside of the hospital, aspiration is usually related to altered consciousness from diverse causes including cerebral vascular accidents, seizure disorders, alcoholism, drug overdose, and dysphagia. In the hospitalized patient, aspiration is likely due to one or more of the following: general anesthesia, endotracheal intubation, the presence of a nasogastric tube, sedation, and tracheostomies. Aspiration is a common event. In studies using radioactive tracers, 70 percent of patients with depressed consciousness and 40 percent of normal healthy subjects have been documented to aspirate small volumes of secretions while sleeping.[40] If the normal lung clearance mechanisms are impaired or a large volume of aspirated secretions reaches the pulmonary parenchyma, then a pulmonary infection is likely to ensue. Untreated this infection may progress and become cavitary. Other less common underlying processes associated with the development of a lung abscess include carcinomas, septic embolization, secondary infections of a bland infarction, bronchiectasis, bacteremia, inhalation of infected aerosols, vasculitis, and unusual pathogens such as nocardia, mycobacteria, and fungi.

The dependent segments of the lung are the most likely locations for aspirated material to lodge. Because of this the primary site of a lung abscess is the posterior segment of the right upper lobe. The next most frequent site is the apical segment of the lower lobes. These segments are dependent when the subject is in the horizontal position. Subdiaphragmatic infection may extend to the lung or to the pleural space by way of the lymphatics, directly through the diaphragm or defects in it, or by way of the bloodstream. Septic emboli from bacterial endocarditis of the tricuspid valve or from pelvic vein thrombophlebitis may result in metastatic lung abscesses located throughout the lung.

The pathology of a lung abscess involves necrosis

resulting from inflammation, with the development of cavitation and abscess formation. The cavity may become partially lined with regenerating epithelium. There is usually no significant vascular involvement, but localized emphysema and bronchiectasis may develop. Some microorganisms, especially *P. aeruginosa,* may cause a localized arteritis resulting in infarction, necrosis, and cavitation.

Etiology Most lung abscesses are caused by multiple organisms (average, 3.1). Lung abscesses occurring in the outpatient setting are caused by endogenous bacteria (normal flora) of the upper respiratory tract, predominantly anaerobes.[151] Nosocomial abscesses may involve multiple pathogens, but gram-negative enteric bacilli, such as *Klebsiella* sp., nonfermenters, such as *P. aeruginosa,* and gram-positive organisms, such as *S. aureus,* are commonly found.[152] In the hospitalized patient, anaerobes still play a role but rarely are they the primary pathogen isolated. The most commonly encountered anaerobes are gram-negative rods and cocci, such as *Bacteroides* sp. and *Fusobacterium* sp.

Necrotizing pneumonia, often caused by *S. aureus, K. pneumonia,* and *P. aeruginosa,* is a common precursor to the development of a lung abscess in the hospitalized patient. Infrequently, pneumococci (type 3) and gram-negative bacilli, such as *E. coli, L. pneumophila,* and *Proteus* sp., may cause enough pulmonary necrosis to cavitate. Unusual but important pathogens that cause abscess formation are *Nocardia* and *Actinomyces*. Tuberculosis may also cause necrotizing pneumonia and abscess formation, and rarely fungal infection (aspergillus, mucormycosis, histoplasmosis, and coccidiomycosis) can be associated with lung abscess, but these are unlikely in the hospital setting.

Metastatic lung abscesses may occur and are usually due to septic emboli from subacute bacterial endocarditis (SBE) or bacteremia from a distant source. Multiple abscesses are most likely secondary to a hematogenous source. The most characteristic hematogenous lung abscess is due to *S. aureus,* which is commonly associated with superficial skin or soft tissue infections and is the leading cause of infections in intravenous catheters, but hematogenous pulmonary infection with gram-negative enteric bacilli occurs also, especially in association with urinary tract infection, bowel surgery, or other nosocomial infections. Although unusual organisms may cause pulmonary abscesses, anaerobes, *S. aureus,* and gram-negative bacilli remain the predominant etiologic bacteria.

Clinical Manifestations In patients admitted to the hospital with primary lung abscesses, symptoms will have been present for at least 2 weeks but sometimes as long as several months. Typically, low-grade fever (101 to 102°F) with weight loss and sputum production are seen. Although foul-smelling sputum is considered to be a hallmark of an anaerobic infection, it is only present 50 percent of the time. In infections occurring in the hospital with organisms such as *S. aureus, Klebsiella,* and *P. aeruginosa,* the symptoms are those of a severe pneumonia. The patients generally are quite ill with spiking fevers (102 to 103°F), leukocytosis, and possibly signs of impending shock. As the pneumonia progresses, lung destruction ensues with the rapid development of necrosis and cavitation. Empyema is seen in approximately one-third of lung abscesses. Brain abscess is seen less often but remains a very serious complication. Bacteremia may occur with necrotizing pneumonia, but it is less common after abscess formation. When bacteremia occurs, seeding of other organs can occur. Local bronchiectasis is common, and pulmonary volume loss is a likely sequela.

Diagnosis A lung abscess is suspected on clinical grounds and is diagnosed by a chest x-ray. A cavity with an air-fluid level or a pneumonitis with multiple small excavations is typically seen. Although the diagnosis is relatively simple, determining a specific etiology may be much more difficult. Anaerobic bacteria comprise much of the "normal" flora of the oropharynx of outpatients. Likewise, *S. aureus* and *K. pneumoniae* are common colonizers of the mouth or upper respiratory tract of hospitalized patients. It is therefore necessary to obtain specimens other than expectorated sputum to accurately determine the etiology of most lung abscesses. Empyema fluid, if available, is an appropriate specimen for bacteriologic analysis. Blood cultures may occasionally be positive, especially in necrotizing pneumonia or abscesses from secondary causes, and if positive, are very useful. If neither blood cultures nor empyema fluid is available or diagnostic, it may be necessary to perform percutaneous transtracheal aspiration.[91] This procedure is relatively safe, reliable, and dependable but should be avoided in patients with a bleeding diathesis or poor oxygenation and is not useful in intubated patients. Percutaneous transthoracic aspiration may also be useful but has a higher rate of complications.[93] Recently, fiberoptic bronchoscopy with a "protected" bronchial brush has been used to obtain specimens free of oropharyngeal contamination, but the reliability of this method is controversial.[94] In the practical case, it is often difficult to perform any of these procedures, and etiologic diagnosis is "guessed" by examining the epidemiology of the situation, the host factors, the known etiologic agents, and any other descriptive data unique to the clinical situation.

Therapy An extended course (2 to 4 months) of antimicrobial drugs is usually needed for the therapy for lung abscess. The selection of an appropriate antimicrobial should be guided by the culture and sensitivity of the etiologic agent, if it is available. When the etiology is unavailable, therapy will be empiric and, in primary lung abscess, should always contain an agent active against anaerobic bacteria. Unfortunately, the anaerobic organisms involved in lung abscess and necrotizing pneumonia are becoming increasingly resistant to penicillin G. Reports of penicillin failure have been increasing.[153] Recent reports have even described some frank penicillin failures.[154] Penicillin is still favored in patients who are mildly or moderately ill but should not be the sole therapy in patients acutely ill with a necrotizing anaerobic infection. When using penicillin, higher doses (10 to 20 million units/day intravenous [IV]) are necessary. After there has been good clinical response, the dosage can be lowered and oral therapy employed. Other penicillins are less active against anaerobes, and oral cephalosporins should be avoided. Likewise, a significant percentage of anaerobes are resistant to tetracyclines. Clindamycin is active against most anaerobic isolates with the exception of some strains of *Peptostreptococcus, Bacteroides ureolyticus, Fusobacterium varium,* and some strains of clostridia and can usually be used as single-agent therapy of anaerobic lung abscesses. Metronidazole is active against all gram-negative anaerobes but is not effective against the oropharyngeal flora, such as microaerophilic streptococci and other anaerobic cocci. Therefore, metronidazole is usually combined with penicillin G or another agent (if it is used) in the treatment of anaerobic pulmonary infections. Several newer agents have good activity against anaerobic bacteria including cefoxitin, the carboxyl penicillins (carbenicillin, ticarcillin), and the piperazine and ureido penicillins (azlocillin, mezlocillin, piperacillin). The third generation cephalosporins and related new compounds have less activity against anaerobes, except for the carbapenam imipenem which has broad antianaerobic activity. Also, chloramphenicol, a less widely used agent because of associated aplastic anemia, is active against almost all anaerobic bacteria.

For the acutely ill hospitalized burn patient with a necrotizing pneumonia and/or cavitation in whom precise etiology is not yet known, broad-spectrum antimicrobial agents are essential. For staphylococcal infections, a penicillinase-resistant penicillin is preferable, but an antistaph cephalosporin or vancomycin can be used in the allergic patient. For infections due to *K. pneumoniae, P. aeruginosa,* or other gram-negative bacilli, combination therapy with an extended spectrum penicillin and/or cephalosporin and an aminoglycoside is often necessary. Empiric therapy should always be readjusted as more information becomes available. A reasoned approach using narrow-spectrum directed antibiotics based on the known data is preferable to broad-spectrum "shotgun" therapy. Certain nonspecific measures, such as postural drainage, are also very important in the management of the patient with a lung abscess.[155] Bronchoscopy may be useful to secure drainage, although surgical resection of a lung abscess is rarely required. Generally, surgery should be avoided because of the hazard of the spread of infection.

The prognosis of a lung abscess varies with the underlying condition and the speed with which appropriate therapy is begun. Primary community-acquired lung abscess has a mortality rate approaching 15 percent, whereas anaerobic necrotizing pneumonia approaches 25 percent. The mortality may be significantly higher in acute cavitating pneumonias caused by *S. aureus, K. pneumoniae* and *P. aeruginosa*. In the intubated burn patient with a necrotizing pneumonia that cavitates, the prognosis is poor despite aggressive therapy.

Empyema

Empyema is a purulent inflammatory exudate of the pleural cavity that is usually secondary to infection in the lung but can arise from other nearby or distant foci of infection.

Pathogenesis Although a parapneumonic effusion is seen in up to 44 percent of patients with community-acquired acute bacterial pneumonia, empyema occurs much less commonly. Empyema more likely occurs in association with a lung abscess or a bronchopleural fistula and is commonly seen in rupture of the esophagus and after esophageal surgery.[156] Empyema also occurs from hematogenous spread of infection and commonly from embolization from right-sided endocarditis. Bacteria can also be directly introduced into the pleural space during surgery, trauma, or thoracentesis or by extension from a contiguous focus. A localized intraabdominal infection such as a subphrenic abscess may also be associated with an empyema. In the critically ill, intubated, intensive care unit patient, an empyema can develop in conjunction with a nosocomial pneumonia or by the development of a pneumothorax secondary to barotrauma.

There are three phases to the pathologic response of an empyema: the exudative phase, the fibropurulent phase, and the organizing phase.[157] The exudative phase results from the early outpouring of thin fluid in response to the infecting organism. As this fluid begins to accumulate increasing numbers of PMNs, fibrin, and cellular debris, it becomes increasingly inflammatory and loculations may develop. Clinical symptoms usually are apparent during this phase. Without therapy, fibroblasts will grow into the exudate during the organizing phase and produce a membrane referred to as the "peel." During this phase, the lung may become fixed and often needs to be treated by surgical resection. Occasionally, the empyema may drain spontaneously through the chest wall (empyema necessitatis) or into the lung.

Etiology Prior to the age of antibiotics, empyema was usually secondary to pneumonia, with either *S. pneumoniae* or *S. pyogenes,* or associated with aspiration pneumonia.[158] An empyema that develops in the hospital is usually secondary to nosocomial pneumonia or thoracic surgery.[159]

The organisms most commonly isolated usually reflect the predominant flora of the individual hospital but are likely to include *S. aureus,* group D streptococci, and enteric gram-negative bacilli. Anaerobic bacteria are commonly found, and if special care is taken in the transport of specimens, anaerobes can also be frequently isolated in hospital-acquired empyema. Other less common microorganisms isolated in empyemas include mycobacteria, fungi, actinomyces, and nocardia. Cultures of empyema fluid may be sterile if prior antibiotic therapy had been instituted or transportation and culturing methods had not been optimal.

Clinical Manifestations and Diagnosis The clinical presentation of community-acquired empyema is insidious with fever, dyspnea, weight loss, chills, hemoptysis, and chest tenderness. Symptoms of a hospital-acquired empyema are nonspecific and usually are masked by the underlying process, such as pneumonia or prior thoracic surgery. Physical findings usually reveal the presence of pleural fluid.

The diagnosis requires aspiration and examination of pleural fluid. Prior to this, several diagnostic studies may be very helpful in defining and localizing pleural fluid collections. The chest x-ray is an important first step and can identify fluid collections of 250 cc or greater on an erect film. Lateral decubitus films can identify as little as 50 to 100 cc and are useful to determine if the fluid is freely movable. A very useful sign is an air-fluid level in a nonmovable fluid collection. This is virtually diagnostic of an empyema. If the appearance of the chest film is suggestive of pleural fluid (blunting of the costophrenic angle or a concave meniscus along the chest wall), but the fluid is not movable, a diagnostic ultrasound may be very useful.[160] Ultrasound can often differentiate fluid from fibrosis and can be used to accurately locate the pleural fluid to guide the thoracentesis needle. Recently computed tomography (CT) scans have also been used to localize pleural fluid and have been useful in guiding thoracentesis into small collections of fluid.[161]

In all cases, diagnosis is made after aspirating and examining the pleural fluid for volume, color, consistency, odor, total protein content, glucose, lactic acid dehydrogenase (LDH), pH, and complete blood count. The fluid should be sent for specific microbiologic tests, including Gram and acid-fast stains, wet mount for fungi, and culture for anaerobic and aerobic bacteria as well as mycobacteria and fungi. Typically, inflammatory exudates have protein concentrations above 3.0 g/100 mL and LDH levels about 500 units and are purulent.[162] Foul-smelling fluid suggests anaerobic infection.

Parapneumonic effusions typically consist of serous fluid with a pH greater than 7.2. There may be a small number of neutrophils, and the protein and LDH tend to be low. If the PMNs become numerous and the fluid has the appearance of pus, it is considered to be an empyema. In this situation, Gram stain is often positive, pH is less than 7.2, protein and LDH are high, glucose is low, and the culture is positive. In culture-negative empyema — low fluid pH (less than 7.2), low glucose concentration, and high protein and LDH — special tests for the identification of bacteria may be necessary. Sterile empyema fluid is often due to prior antibiotic therapy, but special techniques may still identify microorganisms. Pleural biopsy for *Mycobacterium tuberculosis* and counter immunoelectrophoresis for pneumococcus or hemophilus may be necessary. Recently, pleuroscopy has helped in establishing the etiology of pleural effusions, and this technique may also be useful for patients with empyema.[163]

Therapy Treatment of an empyema requires antimicrobial therapy and adequate drainage of the pleural space. The empiric choice of antibiotics should be guided by the clinical setting and the presumptive etiology which can be based on Gram stain morphology. Once culture and sensitivity data are available, antibiotics can be adjusted. Antibiotics may need to be given for a prolonged period but usually are necessary only for a short time after adequate tube drainage. Empyemas almost always require tube drainage. Repeated thoracentesis in the early exudative phase of empyema may give adequate drainage, but tube drainage should be promptly instituted if clinical resolution is slow or fluid reaccumulates. The water seal intercostal drainage is usually maintained for 10 to 14 days. The chest tube is gradually withdrawn if the empyema space is small and the cavity is allowed to fill with granulation tissue. In a quarter of patients with empyema, especially those with large cavities and loculations, open drainage with rib resection may be necessary. Decortication, i.e., removal of the entire empyema "peel," may be preferred in younger patients, since this can avoid the long period of wound irrigation and dressings needed with open drainage.[164]

Empyema usually responds quite well to the early institution of appropriate therapy. As with many diseases, aged patients and those with chronic underlying diseases have a poorer prognosis. Polymicrobial empyema and gram-negative bacterial empyema have a poorer prognosis than infection with a single bacterial species. Hospital-acquired empyema has a much higher mortality than community-acquired empyema.

SPECIFIC ETIOLOGIC AGENTS

The principles outlined in the preceding sections can be used for the management of pulmonary infections regardless of the etiology, while the following overview of selected etiologic agents provides specific information on causes of pneumonia. Table 11-13 should be viewed as a quick reference guide for therapy of selected pathogens.

Staphylococcus aureus

The development of staphylococcal lower respiratory tract infection may be either from aspiration of previously colonized pulmonary secretions or via hematogenous dissemination from a peripheral site.[165] Aspiration is felt to be the most common mechanism, since staphylococci very commonly colonize the upper respiratory tract of hospitalized patients.[107] Once staphylococci become established on the respiratory mucosa, spread to the bronchial tree occurs readily, provided the inoculum of organisms aspirated is sufficient and that the bronchial pulmonary defenses are compromised or both. Staphylococcal pneumonia in adults is often associated with a previous viral respiratory tract infection, such as influenza[166] but is also very common in the burned patient. This is most likely due to rapid colonization of the burn wound and the upper respiratory tract in burn patients, especially those suffering inhalation injuries.

Once staphylococcal pneumonia develops, it rapidly progresses. Symptoms include tachypnea, dyspnea, and severe toxemia. Consolidation, abscess formation, pneumatoceles, empyema, pneumothorax, and pyopneumothorax are often seen. Pulmonary lesions appear confluent, progress rapidly, and may form an abscess. Untreated, increasing respiratory distress, abdominal distention, pallor, cyanosis, prostration, and death occur quite rapidly. Characteristically, there is a leukocytosis, and the sputum Gram stain shows PMNs and both intracellular and extracellular gram-positive cocci in clusters.

Because of the rapid progression and high morbidity and mortality, therapy with an effective antistaphylococcal agent must be instituted promptly if staphylococcal pneumonia is suspected. In areas where the incidence of methicillin-resistant staphylococcal (MRSA) infections is low, initial empiric therapy should include the parenteral administration of a penicillinase-resistant semisynthetic penicillin such as nafcillin. Patients allergic to penicillin can be treated with either a first generation cephalosporin or vancomycin. If MRSA infections are prevalent, empiric therapy should be with vancomycin, not a first-generation cephalosporin, since this will be ineffective. It is rarely necessary to use combination antimicrobial therapy for the treatment of staphylococcal infections. Therapy is usually continued for 2 to 3 weeks.

Streptococcus pneumoniae

S. pneumoniae cause approximately 5 to 10 percent of all hospital-acquired pneumonias.[167] *S. pneumoniae* is a normal inhabitant of the human respiratory tract in up to 60 percent of the population and carriage rates are higher in the winter and early spring. Most cases of pneumonia occur from small aspirations of organisms from the oropharynx. The onset of pneumococcal pneumonia is generally abrupt, with a sudden shaking chill, a rapid rise of temperature, and a corresponding tachycardia. Pleuritic pain, cough productive of a pinkish or rusty sputum, and prostration are quite common. Patients appear acutely ill. Although a lobar pneumonia is considered a classic clinical presentation, almost all radiographic presentations have been described.

Pneumococcal pneumonia usually improves promptly when an appropriate antimicrobial agent is used. Although many patients will respond within 12 to 36 hours after the initation of treatment with penicillin, in approximately half of the patients, the temperature may require up to 4 days or longer to become normal. Therefore, failure of the patient's

Table 11-13 Antimicrobial Selection Based on Organisms

Organisms	Drug of choice	Alternative drugs
Gram-positive cocci		
S. aureus		
Non-penicillinase-producing	Penicillin G	A cephalosporin Erythromycin
Penicillinase-producing	A penicillinase-resistant penicillin	A cephalosporin Vancomycin
Methicillin-resistant	Vancomycin	
S. pyogenes		
Groups A, C, G	Penicillin G	A cephalosporin Erythromycin
Enterococcus	Ampicillin or penicillin G plus an amino-glycoside	Vancomycin plus an aminoglycoside
Pneumococcus	Penicillin G	A cephalosporin Erythromycin Clindamycin Vancomycin
Anaerobic bacteria	Penicillin G	Clindamycin Metronidazole Chloramphenicol
Gram-negative bacilli	An amino-glycoside	Ampicillin
E. coli		Extended-spectrum penicillin A cephalosporin
K. pneumoniae	An amino-glycoside	A cephalosporin Extended-spectrum penicillin
Enterobacter	An amino-glycoside	Third-generation cephalosporins Extended-spectrum penicillin
Serratia	An amino-glycoside	Extended-spectrum penicillin Third-generation cephalosporins
		Trimethoprim-sulfamethoxazole
P. mirabilis	Ampicillin	An aminoglycoside A cephalosporin Extended-spectrum penicillin
Proteus, indole-positive	An amino-glycoside	Extended-spectrum penicillin Third-generation cephalosporins
P. aeruginosa	An amino-glycoside	Extended-spectrum penicillin
H. influenzae	Ampicillin	Chloramphenicol Second or third generation cephalosporins Timethoprim-sulfamethoxazole
Acinetobacter	An amino-glycoside	Extended-spectrum penicillin Trimethoprim-sulfamethoxazole
Actinomycetes		
Actinomyces isreali	Penicillin G	A tetracycline
Nocardia	A sulfonamide	Trimethoprim-sulfamethoxazole
Fungi		
C. albicans	Amphotericin B	Flucytosine Ketoconazole
Viruses		
Herpes simplex		
Herpex zoster	Acyclovir	
Influenza A	Amantadine	
CMV	None	
Others		
M. pneumoniae	Erythromycin	A tetracycline
C. psittaci	A tetracycline	Chloramphenicol
L. pneumophila	Erythromycin	Rifampin

temperature to reach normal within 24 to 48 hours should not prompt a change in the antibacterial therapy. The chest x-ray may take up to 6 to 8 weeks for resolution. Importantly, pneumococcal pneumonia is associated with bacteremia 20 percent of the time, and 20 percent of these bacteremic episodes are estimated to be fatal.[168]

The treatment of choice for infections caused by *S. pneumoniae* continues to be penicillin G. The usual recommended dose is 600,000 units of aqueous penicillin G intramuscularly twice daily. This regimen provides a wide margin of safety, minimizes the antibiotic pressure on the normal microbial flora, and minimizes the likelihood of superinfection. If the patient is allergic to penicillin, erythromycin, cephalosporins, and clindamycin can be used. Until very recently, resistance to penicillin was an unusual event. In 1977, strains of *S. pneumoniae* that were highly resistant to penicillin G as well as to a score of other antimicrobials were isolated from several locations of the Republic of South Africa.[169] These strains were found to respond to vancomycin. Recently, isolates similar to the South African strains have been recovered in the United States, although these remain uncommon. Even so, for serious pneumococcal infections, it is now recommended to test all isolates for sensitivity to penicillin.

Haemophilus influenzae Infections

H. influenzae is a small, fastidious gram-negative rod which is frequently recovered from the upper respiratory tract of healthy adults and children. The majority of these isolates do not have the typical polysaccharide capsule and are referred to as nontypeable strains. Of the six capsular sero-types, *H. influenzae* type B has been responsible for nearly all cases of invasive disease in both adults and children. *H. influenzae* has long been recognized as a major cause of childhood infections, especially in patients between 6 months and 3 years of age. For many years, isolated cases of infections with these organisms in adults have also been documented, but these were generally considered rarities. More recently, *H. influenzae* has been associated with bronchitis in adults with chronic pulmonary disease, and the clear pathogenic role of these organisms is no longer controversial.[71] Of all the serious *H. influenzae* infections in adults, pneumonia is the most common as well as one of the most difficult to diagnosis. Pneumonia caused by this organism is a life-threatening illness, and estimates of mortality from bacteremic pneumonia with *H. influenzae* are up to 30 percent.

The clinical presentation of *H. influenzae* pneumonia is not distinguishable from that of other bacterial pneumonias. There are two groups of patients that acquire infection with *H. influenzae*. One resembles that of pneumococcal pneumonia (i.e., 60 percent are over 50 years old, 30 to 40 percent are alcoholics, and 30 to 40 percent have preexisting chronic lung disease or some other associated chronic illness), and the other is young children. The true frequency of primary *Haemophilus* lung infections cannot be determined with any accuracy because routinely processed sputum cultures are unreliable and it is often difficult to determine whether *H. influenzae* is a colonizing or infecting pathogen. As in all bacterial pneumonias, collecting a representative sputum specimen and examining it properly can give very helpful and often diagnostic information. In more than 60 percent of patients with bacteremic *H. influenzae* pneumonia, careful examination of Gram stain smears of initial sputum specimens will reveal the thin pleomorphic gram-negative coccobacillary forms. Other adjunctive diagnostic methods include counterimmunoelectrophoresis of latex agglutination methods that detect the capsular antigen.

Prompt diagnosis and early treatment with an effective antimicrobial drug is necessary. The treatment of *H. influenzae* infections has become more complicated in recent years because strains resistant to ampicillin are now prevalent. These strains produce a β-lactamase, which is capable of inactivating ampicillin.[71] The incidence of ampicillin-resistant strains varies between 4 and 10 percent nationwide and may be as high as 25 to 35 percent in some communities. It appears to be slowly but steadily rising. Because of this, the empiric therapy of presumed *H. influenzae* infections may need to contain either chloramphenicol or a β-lactamase–stable drug. Trimethoprim-sulfamethoxazole (TMP-SMX) is also generally effective against *H. influenzae* strains. Treatment of pneumonia should be for at least 1 week beyond the resolution of fever and usually about 2 weeks overall. If the patient has a complicated disease, it may be necessary to treat for an additional week. Prompt recognition of *H. in-*

fluenzae infections is vital to ensure the best therapeutic results.

Streptococcus pyogenes Infections

Prior to the penicillin era, group A β-hemolytic streptococci were often associated with lower respiratory infections. Now this is uncommon. Pneumonia caused by streptococci account for less than 5 percent of all cases of nosocomial pneumonia, although streptococci have been associated with burn wound infections. Pneumonia often arises secondarily to an infection in the upper part of the respiratory tract or in the burn wound itself. Occasionally, other β-hemolytic streptococci, such as groups C and G, may be associated with the development of pneumonia.

The onset of streptococcal pneumonia tends to be abrupt with symptoms of chills, fever, anorexia, and vomiting. Cough, rusty sputum, chest pain, high intermittent fevers, and signs of severe prostration are common. A characteristic feature is the development of a rapidly progressing, large empyema. The antimicrobial agent of choice is penicillin G. Doses of 600,000 units of aqueous penicillin administered intramuscularly twice daily is sufficient, although patients with streptococcal pneumonia are often treated with 1 million units of penicillin G IV q 4–6 h.

Endogenous Aerobic Gram-Negative Bacilli

Aerobic gram-negative bacilli, such as *K. pneumoniae, Enterobacter* species, *E. coli,* and *Proteus* sp., are part of the endogenous flora of the gastrointestinal tract in normal subjects and rarely colonize the oropharynx. In contrast, chronically or severely ill individuals, especially those hospitalized, rapidly become colonized with these organisms.[38] Pneumonias caused by these organisms are responsible for at least one-quarter to one-third of all hospital-acquired pneumonias.[74] The clinical features of pneumonia due to aerobic gram-negative bacilli are characterized by early prostration, often with productive cough, dyspnea, fever, and hypotension. Sputum tends to be tenacious and purulent, and hemoptysis is often seen. Gram stain evaluation typically reveals many PMNs with sheets of gram-negative bacilli. Involvement of more than one lobe is frequent; with *Klebsiella,* there is a predilection for the upper lobes, whereas with *E. coli,* infiltrates are more common in the lower lobes. *Proteus* produces a clinical picture very similar to that of *Klebsiella,* with fever, chills, dyspnea, pleuritic chest pain, and a purulent productive cough. Generally, infections due to *Proteus* and *Klebsiella* are more likely to cavitate and form lung abscesses and empyemas than ones due to *E. coli.*

Empiric therapy is usually necessary until the results of sputum cultures and antibiotic susceptibility studies are available. Empiric therapy should be based on microbiologic surveillance data. Typical empiric therapy includes both a B-lactam and an aminoglycoside antibiotic. When the results of cultures and sensitivities are available, empiric regimens should be modified by discontinuing unneeded or ineffective drugs and using the least toxic and most effective agents. Duration of therapy should be continued until the patient has been afebrile for at least 7 days. Meticulous measures directed at supportive care, including the maintenance of airways, adequate ventilation and oxygenation, and adequate fluid and electrolyte replacement, are essential.

Exogenous Aerobic Gram-Negative Bacilli

Hospital-acquired pneumonias may be caused by exogenous aerobic gram-negative bacilli, such as *Pseudomonas* sp., *S. marcescens,* and *Acinetobacter* sp. These organisms are more commonly found in the hospital environment than in the endogenous gastrointestinal flora of patients.[170–172] Collectively, these organisms are responsible for approximately one-fifth of hospital-acquired pneumonias, and infections due to these organisms are frequently life-threatening.[173]

In the burned patient, pneumonia due to *P. aeruginosa* is probably the most commonly described and the most serious of these infections.[3,4] Typically, patients with pseudomonal infections have apprehension, toxicity, confusion, and progressive deterioration in their clinical status. *Pseudomonas* may cause an endarteritis with necrosis and tissue destruction, so that nodular infiltrates that rapidly become necrotic and cavitate are common. Development of empyema is also common and may occur in 20 to 80 percent of cases.[109] Untreated, pneumonias caused by these pathogens are some of the most rapidly progressive and fatal.

The antimicrobial regimen of choice must be selected according to the antimicrobial susceptibilities anticipated in a given hospital. In general, *P. aeruginosa* is susceptible to the newer penicillins, some of the third-generational cephalosporins, especially ceftazidime and imipenem, as well as the newer aminoglycosides. In contrast, other pseudomonads such as *P. cepacia* may be susceptible only to chloramphenicol and TMP-SMX. Likewise, *S. marcescens* may be resistant to many antimicrobial agents, although it tends to be relatively susceptible to aminoglycosides.

Tuberculosis

Hospital-acquired infections due to *M. tuberculosis* are exceedingly unusual but can occur due to reactivation disease or via secondary spread to other patients from the primary case.[174] In the past, airborne spread of tuberculosis (TB) was a recognized occupational hazard in the hospital.[175,176] This risk has lessened with the development of effective preventive programs and the overall decrease in the prevalence of tuberculosis. Even so, it is often customary in burn units located in areas of higher prevalence of TB to place patients with large burns on chemoprophylaxis if the chest x-ray shows signs of old tuberculosis. Also of note is that TB appears to be more prevalent secondary to the increase in AIDS patients. How this will affect practices in the burn unit is unclear at present.

The clinical presentation of tuberculosis is protean. Typical reactivation disease involves diffuse, often cavitary pulmonary infiltrates, especially in the upper lobes. It must be remembered, though, that primary infections may present as a typical pneumonia in any lobe and isolated pleural effusions can be seen. With the advent of modern antituberculosis drugs, the therapy of TB has been simplified and is well described in many authoritative texts.

Legionella pneumophila

Nosocomial outbreaks of *L. pneumophila,* the cause of legionnaires' disease, have been described.[177] These outbreaks tend to be geographically clustered and have occurred predominantly in immunocompromised patients. *Legionella* are hydrophilic and have been associated with contaminated water supplies.[178,179] The male-to-female case ratio in legionnaires' disease is 3 to 1; attack rates increase progressively with age and are positively correlated with a history of smoking, presence of lung disease, diabetes, cancer, renal disease, and exposure to water systems, especially showers. The diagnosis of legionnaires' disease is difficult, so it is likely that the true number of infections is underreported.[180]

Acute legionnaires' disease typically presents as a pulmonary infection with major extrapulmonary manifestations, including central nervous system, hepatic, gastrointestinal, and renal disease. There are no distinctive clinical or radiologic features; therefore, the diagnosis must be based on laboratory findings. The optimal detection depends on the use of direct fluorescent antibody (DFA) staining of secretions or tissues, as well as culture and serologic testing. Culture of the organism is not widely available, and DFA staining on sputum is very nonspecific. The detection of antibodies by the indirect fluorescent antibody (IFA) test remains the mainstay of diagnosis, but although it is very useful for retrospective analysis of cases, it is not useful when making an acute diagnosis. A presumptive diagnosis is usually based on the occurrence of a compatible illness and a single acute-phase serum titer of at least 1 to 256. A sensitive urinary antigen assay is not yet readily available.

There are few controlled clinical trials of therapy in legionnaires' disease, but erythromycin is considered to be the drug of choice.[181] Because legionella are facultative intracellular organisms that can replicate in pulmonary macrophages in vitro, antibiotic susceptibilities have little clinical relevance. Treatment should be continued for several weeks, and if erythromycin therapy is not successful or tolerated, therapy with either a tetracycline, such as doxycycline, or with rifampin may be considered. Relapses after a 2-week course of therapy have occurred, so most people treat for at least 3 weeks. Other therapies that have been used include TMP-SMX and ciprofloxacin.

Fungi

Candida, Aspergillus, and *Mucor* have been isolated from burn wounds and have been documented to cause burn wound infection, but these organisms rarely cause pulmonary infections in the burn patient.[182,183] This is somewhat surprising since *Aspergillus* and *Mucor* have been documented to cause pulmonary infections in other severely compromised patients. Of the fungal organisms, *C. albicans* has been associated with the greatest number of invasive infections.

Mycotic infections generally occur in patients with burns of greater than 30 percent. Clinical signs include fever, swelling, and conversion of the burn wound. Hyphal invasion of viable tissue is diagnostic of a fungal burn wound infection. Invasion may be identified by the microscopic examination of incisional biopsy specimens. Effective therapy of invasive fungal disease in burn patients must be begun promptly and may sometimes be empiric. Therapy consists primarily of debridement of the involved area followed by early aggressive therapy with amphotericin B.[3,4] Although *Candida* infections are responsive to amphotericin B, those infections due to *Aspergillus* and *Mucor* are often fatal even with appropriate therapy.

Viral Infections

Viral infections causing pulmonary disease in burn patients are very uncommon.[184] Foley et al. first reported on viral infections in the burn wound due to herpes viruses,[185] and later that same group published a case report on cytomegalovirus infections.[186] There have been only sporadic reports of viral infections since then, which is in part due to the inability to diagnose viral infections in general. This is most likely the reason that infections due to influenza A virus have been rarely documented in burn patients, even though they have clearly caused outbreaks of nosocomial pneumonia in other clinical settings.

Many of the infections described due to herpes simplex virus have been systemic without involvement of the burn wound.[187] Herpetic lesions typically are seen a week to a month after the burn and involve the face, neck, and chest. Lesions were usually found in areas of healing second-degree burns or donor sites. Often, secondary bacterial infection is superimposed on the primary viral process, and this in turn could be associated with the conversion of partial-thickness to full-thickness skin loss. Most infections, though, due to herpes simplex virus in burn patients are not obvious clinically. In a prospective study by Kagan et al.,[188] 40 percent of their burn patients developed infection due to herpes simplex with a mean time of infection of 2.2 weeks after burn. Both primary and reactivation infections were observed. Facial burns seem to be more associated with herpetic infection, most likely because the trigeminal ganglion is the site of the latent herpes simplex virus. Significant risk factors in this study for herpes simplex infections were age greater than 50 years, tracheal intubation, facial burns, smoke inhalation, and hospitalization longer than 3 weeks, as well as full-thickness burns. In none of these reports, though, was primary pulmonary involvement with herpes viruses described.

In a prospective evaluation of burn patients, Linnemann and MacMillan found that a third of their patients developed infections due to cytomegalovirus.[78] It should be noted that the majority of these patients were on the pediatric service. Kagan et al. also found that approximately one-third of their burn patients developed cytomegalovirus (CMV) infection, which occurred at a mean of 3.8 weeks after admission.[188] In these studies, both primary and reactivation infections were documented. The clinical picture of CMV infections in burn patients is typically one of an unexplained fever which lasts from 1 to 4 weeks in a patient whose burn wound is healing well without signs of infection. Occasionally, lymphocytosis may occur and hepatitis is seen in a minority of patients. Other common manifestations of CMV that are seen in the immunocompromised host, such as myalgias, arthralgias, pneumonia, and retinitis, have not been observed in burn patients. The reasons for this are unclear. The burn wound does not appear to be directly involved by CMV infection, and infections due to CMV in burn patients have not clearly been associated with a higher mortality. In summary, cytomegalovirus infections in burn patients may be both primary or reactivation and typically appear 1 to 4 months after burn. They occur in patients with the most severe burns, do not involve the burn itself, may be associated with fever and lymphocytosis, and may be difficult to diagnose. It is important to recognize CMV infections so that unnecessary administration of antibiotics or the performance of invasive procedures may be avoided.[189]

SUMMARY

Pneumonia in the burn patient continues to be a major cause of morbidity and mortality. The ability to prevent or treat bacterial pneumonias in the critically ill burn patient has not kept pace with our understanding of the pathogenesis of this infection. Pneumonia is often difficult to diagnose as well as to treat because of the problems associated with recognizing and differentiating infectious and noninfectious causes of pulmonary infiltrates as well as identifying etiologic agents. Patients with serious underlying illness seem to have an especially high risk of infection. Aspiration of bacteria that have colonized the oropharynx appears to be the major responsible factor for the majority of cases of nosocomial bacterial pneumonia. Important priorities for reducing the risk of pneumonia include the prevention of colonization and aspiration; adherence to established infection control practices, such as hand washing between patient contacts; the use of barriers, such as gloves, during procedures; and meticulous maintenance of respiratory therapy equipment as well as routine epidemiological surveillance of the burn unit. Clearly, more research is needed, and practical trials of interventional strategies are awaited.

REFERENCES

1. Herndon DN, Langer F, Thompson P, et al: Pulmonary injury in burned patients. *Surg Clin North Am* 67:31, 1987.
2. Demling RH: Improved survival after massive burns. *J Trauma* 23:179, 1983.
3. Luterman A, Dacso CC, Curreri WP: Infections in burn patients. *Am J Med* 81(supp 1A):45, 1986.
4. Pruitt BA Jr: The diagnosis and treatment of infection in the burn patient. *Burns* 11:79, 1984.
5. Pruitt BA, O'Neill JA, Moncrief JF, et al: Successful control of burn-wound sepsis. *JAMA* 203:1054, 1968.
6. Shirani KZ, Pruitt BA, Mason AD: The influence of inhalation injury and pneumonia on burn mortality. *Ann Surg* 205:82, 1986.
7. Anous MM, Heimbach DM: Causes of death and predictors in burned patients more than 60 years of age. *J Trauma* 26:135, 1986.
8. Pruitt BA, Flemma RJ, DiVincenti FC, et al: Pulmonary complications in burn patients. *J Thorac Cardiovasc Surg* 59:7, 1970.
9. Foley DF, Concrief JA, Mason AD: Pathology of the lung in fatally burned patients. *Ann Surg* 167:251, 1968.
10. Moylan JA, Chan C: Inhalation injury — An increasing problem. *Ann Surg* 188:34, 1978.
11. Craven DE, Kunches LM, Kilinsky V, et al: Risk factors for pneumonia and fatality in patients receiving continuous mechanical ventilation. *Am Rev Respir Dis* 133:792, 1986.
12. Cross AS, Roup B: Role of respiratory assistance devices in endemic nosocomial pneumonia. *Am J Med* 70:681, 1981.
13. Centers for Disease Control: National Nosocomial Infections Study Report, Annual Summary 1983. *MMWR* 33 (25 S):9SS, 1983.
14. Garibaldi RA, Britt MR, Coleman ML, et al: Risk factors for post operative pneumonias. *Am J Med* 70:677, 1981.
15. Sanford JP: Lower respiratory tract infections, in Bennett JV, Brachman PS (eds): *Hospital Infections*. Boston, Little Brown, 1986, pp 385–422.

16. Pennington JE: Hospital acquired pneumonias, in Wenzel RP (ed): *Prevention and Control of Nosocomial Infections*. Baltimore, Williams and Wilkins, 1987, pp 321–24.
17. Schwartz SN, Dowling JN, Benkovic C, et al: Sources of gram-negative bacilli colonizing the tracheae of intubated patients. *J Infect Dis* 138:227, 1978.
18. Pierce AK, Edmonson EB, McGee G, et al: An analysis of factors predisposing to gram-negative bacillary necrotizing pneumonia. *Am Rev Respir Dis* 94:309, 1966.
19. Reinarz JA, Pierce AK, Maysa BB, et al: The potential role of inhalation therapy equipment in nosocomial pulmonary infections. *J Clin Invest* 44:831, 1965.
20. Ringrose RE, McKown B, Felton FG, et al: A hospital outbreak of *Serratia marcescens* associated with ultrasonic nebulization. *Ann Intern Med* 69:719, 1968.
21. Mertz JJ, Scharer L, McClement L: A hospital outbreak of *Klebsiella pneumoniae* from inhalation therapy with contaminated aerosol solution. *Am Rev Respir Dis* 94:954, 1966.
22. Simmons BP, Wong ES: CDC guidelines for the prevention and control of nosocomial infections: Guideline for prevention of nosocomial pneumonia. *Am J Infect Control* 11:230, 1983.
23. Rhame F: The inanimate environment, in Bennett JV, Brachman PS (eds): *Hospital Infections*. Boston, Little Brown, 1986, pp 223–50.
24. Madden MR, Finkelstein JL, Goodwin CW: Respiratory care of the burn patient. *Clin Plast Surg* 13:29, 1986.
25. Kelsen SG, McGuckin M: The role of airborne bacteria in the contamination of fine particle nebulizers in the development of nosocomial pneumonia. *Ann NY Acad Sci* 353:218, 1980.
26. Demling RH: Smoke inhalation injury. *Postgrad Med* 82:63, 1987.
27. Pruitt BA, Erickson DR, Morris A: Progressive pulmonary insufficiency and other pulmonary complications of thermal injury. *J Trauma* 15:369, 1975.
28. DiVencenti FC, Pruitt BA, Reckler JM: Inhalation injuries. *J Trauma* 11:109, 1971.
29. Stephenson SF, Esrig BC, Polk HC, et al: The pathophysiology of smoke inhalation injury. *Ann Surg* 182:652, 1975.
30. Skornik WA, Dressler DP: Lung bacterial clearance in the burned rat. *Ann Surg* 172:837, 1970.
31. Putman CE, Loke J, Matthay RA, et al: Radiographic manifestations of acute smoke inhalation. *Am J Roentgenol* 129:865, 1977.
32. Louria DB, Kaminski T: The effects of four antimicrobial drug regimens on sputum superinfection in hospitalized patients. *Am Rev Respir Dis* 85:649, 1962.
33. Graybill JR, Marshall LW, Charache P, et al: Nosocomial pneumonia. *Am Rev Respir Dis* 108:1130, 1973.
34. Esposito AL: The effect of common pharmacologic agents on pulmonary antibacterial defenses — implications for the geriatric patient. *Clin Chest Med* 8:373, 1987.
35. Green GM, Jakab GJ, Low RB, et al: Defense mechanisms of the respiratory membrane. *Am Rev Respir Dis* 115:479, 1977.
36. Eickhoff JC: Pulmonary infections in surgical patients. *Surg Clin North Am* 60:175, 1980.
37. Alexander JW, Ogle CK, Stinnett JD, et al: A sequential prospective analysis of immunologic abnormalities and infection following severe thermal injury. *Ann Surg* 188:809, 1976.
38. Levison ME, Kay D: Pneumonia caused by gram-negative bacilli: An overview. *Rev Infect Dis* 7:S656, 1985.
39. Pierce AK, Sanford JP: State of the art: Aerobic gram-negative bacillary pneumonias. *Am Rev Respir Dis* 110:674, 1974.
40. Huxley EJ, Viroslaw J, Gray WR, et al: Pharyngeal aspiration in normal adults and patients with depressed consciousness. *Am J Med* 64:565, 1978.
41. McCrae W, Wallace P: Aspiration around high volume low pressure endotracheal cuffs. *Br Med J* 2:1220, 1981.
42. Toews GB, Gross GN, Pierce AK: Relationship of inoculum size to lung bacterial clearance and phagocytic cell response in mice. *Am Rev Respir Dis* 120:559, 1979.
43. Rehm SR, Gross GN, Pierce AK, et al: The relationship of inoculum size to lung bacterial clearance and phagocytic cell response in rats. *J Clin Invest* 66:194, 1980.
44. Rose HD, Babcock JB: Colonization of intensive care unit patients with gram-negative bacilli. *Am J Epidemiol* 101:495, 1975.
45. Johanson WG Jr: Prevention of respiratory tract infection. *Am J Med* 76:69, 1984.
46. Johanson WG Jr, Pierce AK, Sanford JP, et al: Nosocomial respiratory infection with gram-negative bacilli: The significance of colonization of the respiratory tract. *Ann Intern Med* 77:701, 1972.
47. Rosenthal S, Tager IB: Prevalence of gram-negative rods in the normal pharyngeal flora. *Ann Intern Med* 83:355, 1975.
48. Johanson WG Jr, Pierce AK, Sanford JP: Changing pharyngeal bacterial flora of hospitalized patients: The emergence of gram negative bacilli. *N Engl J Med* 281:1137, 1969.
49. Johanson WG Jr, Woods DE, Chaudhuri T: Association of respiratory tract colonization with adherence of gram-negative bacilli to epithelial cells. *J Infect Dis* 139:667, 1979.
50. Murray PR, Rosenblatt JE: Bacterial interference of oropharyngeal and clinical isolates of anaerobic bacteria. *J Infect Dis* 134:281, 1976.
51. Johanson WG Jr, Pierce AK, Sanford JP: Changing pharyngeal bacterial flora of hospitalized patients. *N Engl J Med* 281:1137, 1969.
52. Johanson WG Jr, Higuchi JH, Chaudhuri TR, et al: Bacterial adherence to epithelial cells in bacillary colonization of the respiratory tract. *Am Rev Respir Dis* 121:55, 1980.
53. Ramphal R, Sadoff JC, Pyle M, Silipigul JD: Role of pili in adherence of *Pseudomonas aeruginosa* to insured tracheal epithelium. *Infect Immun* 44:38, 1984.
54. Woods DE: Role of fibronectin in the pathogenesis of gram-negative bacillary pneumonia. *Rev Infect Dis* 9:S386, 1987.
55. Proctor RA: Fibronectin: A brief overview of its structure, function, and physiology. *Rev Infect Dis* 9:S317, 1987.
56. Woods DE, Straus DC, Johanson WG Jr, et al: Role of fibronectin in the prevention of adherence of *Pseudo-*

monas aeruginosa to buccal cells. *J Infect Dis* 143:784, 1981.
57. Woods DE, Straus DC, Johanson WG Jr, et al: Role of salivary protease activity in adherence of gram-negative bacilli to mammalian buccal epithelial cells in vivo. *J Clin Invest* 68:1435, 1981.
58. Martin TR: The relationship between malnutrition and lung infections. *Clin Chest Med* 8:359, 1987.
59. Saba TM, Jaffe E: Plasma fibronectin (opsonic glycoprotein): Its synthesis of vascular endothelial cells and role in cardiopulmonary integrity after trauma as related to reticuloendothelial function. *Am J Med* 68:577, 1980.
60. Zhi-yong S, Shi-hoe X, Xiao-ming J, et al: Changes in plasma fibronectin levels in burn patients. *Burns* 13:114, 1987.
61. Pollack M, Neiman RE, Reinhardt JA, et al: Factors influencing colonization and antibiotic-resistance patterns of gram-negative bacteria in hospital patients. *Lancet* 1:668, 1972.
62. LaForce FM: Hospital-acquired gram-negative rod pneumonias: An overview. *Am J Med* 70:664, 1981.
63. Larson EL: Persistent carriage of gram-negative bacteria on hands. *Am J Infect Control* 9:112, 1981.
64. Atherton ST, White DJ: Stomach as a source of bacteria colonizing respiratory tract during artificial ventilization. *Lancet* 2:968, 1978.
65. DuMoulin GC, Hedley-Whyte J, Peterson DG, et al: Aspiration of gastric bacteria in antacid treated patients. *Lancet* 1:242, 1982.
66. Driks MR, Craven DE, Celli BR, et al: Nosocomial pneumonia in intubated patients given sucralfate as compared with antacids or histamine type 2 blockers: The role of gastric colonization. *N Engl J Med* 317:1376, 1987.
67. Tryba M: Risk of acute stress bleeding and nosocomial pneumonia in ventilated intensive care unit patients: Sucralfate vs. antacids. *Am J Med* 83(suppl 3B):117, 1987.
68. Pingleton SK, Hinthorn DR, Liv C: Enteral nutrition in patients receiving mechanical ventilation: Multiple sources of tracheal colonization include the stomach. *Am J Med* 80:827, 1986.
69. Schwartz SN, Dowling JN, Benkovic C, et al: Sources of gram-negative bacilli colonizing the tracheae of intubated patients. *J Infect Dis* 138:227, 1978.
70. Donowitz GR, Mandell GL: Acute pneumonia, in Mandell GL, Douglas RG, Bennett JE (eds): *Principles and Practices of Infectious Diseases,* 2d ed. New York, Wiley, 1985, pp 394–404.
71. Simon HB, Southwick FS, Moellering RC, et al: *Haemophilus influenzae* in hospitalized adults: Current perspectives. *Am J Med* 69:219, 1980.
72. Mylotte JM, Beam TR Jr: Comparison of community-acquired and nosocomial pneumococcal pneumonia. *Am Rev Respir Dis* 123:265, 1981.
73. Berger R, Arango L: Etiologic diagnosis of bacterial nosocomial pneumonia in seriously ill patients. *Crit Care Med* 13:833, 1985.
74. Haley RW, Hooton TM, Culver DH, et al: Nosocomial infections in U.S. hospitals, 1975–76: Estimated frequency by selected characteristics of patients. *Am J Med* 70:947, 1981.
75. Bartlett JG, O'Keefe P, Talley FP, et al: Bacteriology of hospital-acquired pneumonia. *Arch Intern Med* 146:868, 1986.
76. Meyer RD, Edelstein PH: *Legionella* pneumonias, in Pennington JEE (ed): *Respiratory Infections: Diagnosis and Management*. New York, Raven Press, 1983, pp 283–97.
77. Tillotson JR, Finland M: Bacterial colonization and clinical super-infection of the respiratory tract complicating antibiotic treatment of pneumonia. *J Infect Dis* 119:597, 1969.
78. Linnemann CC Jr, MacMillan BG: Viral infections in pediatric burn patients. *Am J Dis Child* 135:750, 1981.
79. Shook CD, MacMillan BG, Altemeier WA: Pulmonary complications of the burn patient. *Arch Surg* 215:97, 1968.
80. MacMillan BG, Edmonds P, Hummel RP, et al: Epidemiology of *Pseudomonas* in a burn intensive care unit. *J Trauma* 13:627, 1973.
81. Lund T, Goodwin CW, McManus WF, et al: Upper airway sequelae in burn patients requiring endotracheal intubation or tracheostomy. *Ann Surg* 201:374, 1985.
82. Johanson WG Jr, Pierce AK, Sanford JP, et al: Nosocomial respiratory infections with gram negative bacilli. *Ann Intern Med* 77:701, 1972.
83. Andrews CP, Coalson JJ, Smith JD, et al: Diagnosis of nosocomial bacterial pneumonia in acute diffuse lung injury. *Chest* 80:554, 1981.
84. Lentino JR, Lucks DA: Nonvalue of sputum culture in the management of lower respiratory tract infections. *J Clin Microbiol* 25:758, 1987.
85. Guzzetta P, Toews GB, Robertson KJ, et al: Rapid diagnosis of community-acquired bacterial pneumonia. *Am Rev Respir Dis* 128:461, 1983.
86. Murray PR, Washington JA II: Microscopic and bacteriologic analysis of expectorated sputum. *Mayo Clin Proc* 50:339, 1975.
87. Washington JA II: Techniques for noninvasive diagnosis of lower respiratory tract infections. *J Crit Illness* 22:97, 1988.
88. Niederman MS, Ferranti RD, Ziegler A: Respiratory infections complicating long term tracheostomy: The implications of persistent gram-negative tracheobronchial colonization. *Chest* 85:39, 1984.
89. Salata RA, Lederman MM, Schlaes DM, et al: Diagnosis of nosocomial pneumonia in intubated, intensive care unit patients. *Am Rev Respir Dis* 135:426, 1987.
90. Washington JA II: Noninvasive techniques for lower respiratory tract infections, in Pennington JE (ed): *Respiratory Infections: Diagnosis and Management*. New York, Raven Press, 1983, pp 41–54.
91. Bartlett JG: Invasive diagnostic techniques in respiratory infections, in Pennington JE (ed): *Respiratory Infections: Diagnosis and Management*. New York, Raven Press, 1983, pp 55–77.
92. Davidson M, Tempest B, Palmer DL Bacteriologic diagnosis of acute pneumonia: Comparison of sputum, transtracheal aspirates, and lung aspirates. *JAMA* 235:158, 1976.
93. Lambert SC, George RB: Diagnosing nosocomial pneu-

monia in mechanically ventilated patients. *J Crit Illness* 2:37, 1987.

94. Broughton WA, Bass JB, Kirkpatrick MD: The technique of protected brush catheter bronchoscopy. *J Crit Illness* 2:63, 1987.
95. Dacso CC, Luterman A, Curreri WP: Systemic antibiotic treatment in burned patients. *Surg Clin North Am* 67:57, 1987.
96. Sawchuk RJ, Rector TS: Drug kinetics in burn patients. *Clin Pharmacokinet* 5:548, 1980.
97. Graham WGB, Bradley DA: Efficacy of chest physiotherapy and intermittent positive-pressure breathing in the resolution of pneumonia. *N Engl J Med* 299:624, 1978.
98. Rusnak MG, Drake TA, Hackbarth CJ, et al: Single versus combination antibiotic therapy for pneumonia due to *Pseudomonas aeruginosa* in neutropenic guinea pigs. *J Infect Dis* 149:980, 1984.
99. Eliopoulos GM, Moellering RC Jr: Antibiotic synergism and antimicrobial combinations in clinical infections. *Rev Infect Dis* 4:282, 1982.
100. Haburchak DR, Pruitt BA: Use of systemic antibiotics in the burned patient. *Surg Clin North Am* 58:1119, 1978.
101. Thornsberry C: Review of in vitro activity of third-generation cephalosporins and other newer B-lactam antibiotics against clnically important bacteria. *Am J Med* 79(suppl 2A):14, 1985.
102. Yost RL, Ramphal R: Ceftazidime review. *Drug Intell Clin Pharm* 19:509, 1985.
103. Salata RA, Gebhart RL, Palmer DL, et al: Pneumonia treated with imipenem/cilastatin. *Am J Med* 78(suppl 6A):104, 1985.
104. Quenzer RW: A perspective of cephalosporins in pneumonia. *Chest* 92:531, 1987.
105. Sanders CC, Watanakunakorn C: Emergence of resistance to lactams, aminoglycosides and quinolones during combination therapy for infection due to *Serratia marcescens*. *J Infect Dis* 153:617, 1986.
106. Waldvogel FA: *Staphylococcus aureus* (including toxic shock syndrome), in: Mandell GL, Douglass RG Jr, Bennett FE, (eds): *Principles and Practice of Infectious Disease*, 2nd ed. New York, Wiley, 1985, chap 156, pp 1097–1171.
107. MacFarlane JT: Treatment of lower respiratory infections. *Lancet* 2:1446, 1987.
108. Pennington JE, Reynolds HY, Carbone PP: *Pseudomonas aeruginosa* pneumonia: A retrospective study of 36 cases. *Am J Med* 55:155, 1973.
109. Flint LM, Gott J, Short L, et al: Serum level monitoring of aminoglycoside antibiotics: Limitations in intensive care unit–related bacterial pneumonia. *Arch Surg* 120:99, 1985.
110. Pennington JE: Penetration of antibiotics into respiratory secretions. *Rev Infect Dis* 3:67, 1981.
111. Neu HC: Clinical use of aminoglycosides, in Whelton A, Neu HC (eds): *The Aminoglycosides. Microbiology, Clinical Use and Toxicology*. New York, Dekker, 1982, pp 611–28.
112. Louria DB, Young L, Armstrong D, et al: Gentamicin in the treatment of pulmonary infections. *J Infect Dis* 119:483, 1969.
113. Trenholme GM, McKellar PP, Rivera N, et al: Amikacin in the treatment of gram-negative pneumonia. *Am J Med* 62:949, 1977.
114. Moore RD, Smith CR, Lietman PS: Association of aminoglycoside plasma levels with therapeutic outcome in gram-negative pneumonia. *Am J Med* 77:657, 1984.
115. Culbertson GR, McManus AT, Conarro PA: Clinical trial of imipenem/cilastatin in severely burned and infected patients. *Surg Gynecol Obstet* 165:25, 1987.
116. Klastersky J, Carpentier-Meunier F, Kahan-Coppens, et al: Endotracheally adminstered antibiotics for gram-negative pneumonia. *Chest* 75:586, 1979.
117. Greenfield S, Teres D, Bushnell LS, et al: Prevention of gram-negative bacillary pneumonia using aerosol polymyxin as prophylaxis: I. Effect on the colonization pattern of the upper respiratory tract of seriously ill patients. *J Clin Invest* 52:2935, 1973.
118. Feeley TW, du Moulin GC, Hedley-Whyte J, et al: Aerosol polymyxin and pneumonia in seriously ill patients. *N Engl J Med* 293:471, 1975.
119. Klick JM, DuMoulin GC, Hedley-Whyte J, et al: Prevention of gram-negative bacillary pneumonia using polymixin aerosol as prophylaxis: II. Effect on the incidence of pneumonia in seriously ill patients. *J Clin Invest* 55:514, 1975.
120. Klatersky J, Huysmans E, Weerts D, et al: Endotracheally administered gentamicin for the prevention of infections of the respiratory tract in patients with tracheostomy: A double-blind study. *Chest* 65:650, 1974.
121. Klatersky J, Hensgens C, Noterman J, et al: Endotracheal antibiotics for the prevention of tracheobronchial infections in tracheotomized unconscious patient: A comparative study of gentamicin and aminosidin–polymixin B combination. *Chest* 68:302, 1975.
122. Baumgartner JD, Glauser MP: Controversies in the use of passive immunotherapy for bacterial infections in the critically ill patients. *Rev Infect Dis* 9:194, 1987.
123. Pennington JE, Pier GB, Sadoff JC, et al: Active and passive immunization strategies for *Pseudomonas aeruginosa* pneumonia. *Rev Infect Dis* 8:S426, 1986.
124. Stamm WE, Martin SM, Bennett JV: Epidemiology of nosocomial infections due to gram-negative bacilli: Aspects relevant to development and use of vaccines. *J Infect Dis* 136:S151, 1977.
125. Collins MS, Roby RE: Protective activity of an intravenous immune globulin (human) enriched in antibody against lipopolysaccharide antigens of *Pseudomonas aeruginosa*. *Am J Med* 76:168, 1984.
126. Ziegler EJ, McCutchan JA, Fierer J, et al: Treatment of gram-negative bacteremia and shock with human antiserum to a mutant *Escherichia coli*. *N Engl J Med* 307:1225, 1982.
127. Alexander JW, Fisher MW: Immunization against *Pseudomonas* in infection after thermal injury. *J Infect Dis* 130:S152, 1974.
128. Young LS, Meyer RD, Armstrong D: *Pseudomonas aeruginosa* vaccine in cancer patients. *Ann Intern Med* 79:518, 1973.
129. Zaske DE, Sawchuk RJ, Gerding DN, et al: Increased

dosage requirements of gentamicin in burn patients. *J Trauma* 16:284, 1976.
130. Loirat P, Rohan J, Baullat A, et al: Increased glomerular filtration rate in patients with major burns and its effects on the pharmacokinetics of tobramycin. *N Engl J Med* 299:915, 1978.
131. Sawchuk RJ, Zaske DE: Pharmacokinetic of dosing regimens which utilize multiple intravenous infusions: Gentamycin in burn patients. *J Pharmacokinet Biopharm* 4:183, 1976.
132. LaForce FM, Hopkins J, Trow R, et al: Human oral defenses against gram-negative rods. *Am Rev Respir Dis* 114:929, 1976.
133. Toews GB: Nosocomial pneumonia. *Am J Med Sci* 29:355, 1986.
134. Levine BA, Petroff PA, Slade CL, et al: Prospective trials of dexamethasone and aerosolized gentamicin in the treatment of inhalation injury in the burned patient. *J Trauma* 18:188, 1978.
135. Durtschi MB, Orgain C, Counts GW, et al: A prospective study of prophylactic penicillin in acutely burned hospitalized patients. *J Trauma* 22:11, 1982.
136. Nelsen S, Chidiac C, Summer WR: New strategies for preventing nosocomial pneumonia. *J Crit Illness* 3:12, 1988.
137. Valenti WM, Trudell RG, Bentley DW: Factors predisposing to oropharyngeal colonization with gram-negative bacilli in the aged. *N Engl J Med* 298:1108, 1978.
138. Sottile FD, Thomas JM, Prough DS, et al: Nosocomial pulmonary infection: Possible etiologic significance of bacterial adhesion to endotracheal tubes. *Crit Care Med* 14:265, 1986.
139. Craven DE, Goularte TA, Make BS: Contaminated condensate in mechanical ventilator circuits. *Am Rev Respir Dis* 129:625, 1984.
140. Garner JS, Fevero MS: CDC guidelines for the prevention and control of nosocomial infections: Guidelines for handwashing and hospital environmental control, 1985. *Am J Infect Control* 14:110, 1986.
141. Morris AH: Nebulizer contamination in a burn unit. *Am Rev Respir Dis* 107:802, 1973.
142. Reinarz JA, Pierce AK, Mays BB, et al: Potential role of inhalation therapy equipment in nosocomial pulmonary infection. *J Clin Invest* 44:831, 1965.
143. Craven DE, Connolly MG, Lichtenberg DA, et al: Contamination of mechanical ventilator with tubing changes every 24 or 48 hours. *N Engl J Med* 306:1505, 1982.
144. Burke JF, Quinby WC, Bondoc CC, et al: The contribution of a bacterially isolated environment to the prevention of infection in seriously burned patients. *Ann Surg* 186:377, 1977.
145. Maki DG, Alvarado CJ, Hassemer CA, et al: Relation of the inanimate hospital environment to endemic nosocomial infection. *N Engl J Med* 25:1562, 1982.
146. Shirani KZ, McManus AT, Vaughan GM, et al: Effects of environment on infection in burn patients. *Arch Surg* 121:31, 1986.
147. Haynes BW Jr, Hench ME: Hospital isolation system for preventing cross-contamination by staphylococcal and pseudomonas organisms in burn wounds. *Ann Surg* 162:641, 1965.
148. Pennington, JE: *Pseudomonas aeruginosa* pneumonia: The potential for immune intervention, in Weinstein L, Fields BN (eds): *Seminars in Infectious Diseases*. New York, Thieme-Stratton, 1983, pp 71–80.
149. Alexander JW: Control of infection following burn injury. *Arch Surg* 103:435, 1971.
150. Bartlett JG, Gorbach SL, Tally FP, et al: Bacteriology and treatment of primary lung abscess. *Am Rev Respir Dis* 19:510, 1974.
151. Bartlett JG, Fineguld SM: Anaerobic infections of the lung and pleural space. *Am Rev Respir Dis* 110:56, 1974.
152. Poe RH, Marcus HR, Emerson GL: Lung abscess due to *Pseudomonas cepacia*. *Am Rev Respir Dis* 115:861, 1977.
153. Panwalker AP: Failure of penicillin in anaerobic necrotizing pneumonia. *Chest* 82:500, 1982.
154. Levison ME, Mangura CT, Lorber B, et al: Clindamycin compared with penicillin for the treatment of anaerobic lung abscess. *Ann Intern Med* 98:466, 1983.
155. Bartlett JG, Fineguld SA: Anaerobic pleuropulmonary infections. *Medicine* 51:413, 1972.
156. Snider GL, Saleh SS: Empyema of the thorax in adults: Review of 105 cases. *Dis Chest* 54:410, 1968.
157. American Thoracic Society: Management of nontuberculous empyema: A statement of the committee on surgery. *Am Rev Respir Dis* 85:935, 1962.
158. Denfield GFP: Recent trends in empyema thoracis. *Dr J Dis Chest* 75:358, 1981.
159. Weese WC, Shindler ER, Smith IM, et al: Empyema of the thorax there and now. *Arch Intern Med* 131:516, 1973.
160. Sandweiss DA, Hanson JC, Goslink BB: Ultrasound in diagnosis, localization and treatment of located pleural empyema. *Ann Intern Med* 82:50, 1975.
161. Vix VA: Roentgenographic manifestations of pleural disease. *Semin Roentgenol* 12:277, 1977.
162. Chandrasekhar AJ, Palatao P, Dubin A, et al: Pleural fluid lactic acid dehydrogenase activity and protein content. *Arch Intern Med* 123:48, 1969.
163. Weissberg D, Kaufman M: Diagnostic and therapeutic pleuroscopy. *Chest* 78:732, 1980.
164. Mayo P, Saha SP, McElvein RB: Acute empyema in children treated by open thoracotomy and decortication. *Ann Thorac Surg* 34:401, 1982.
165. Hausmann W, Karlish AJ: Staphylococcal pneumonia in adults. *Br Med J* 2:845, 1956.
166. Martin CM, Kunin CM, Gottlieb LS, et al: Asian influenza A in Boston, 1957–1958: II. Severe staphylococcal pneumonia complicating influenza. *Arch Intern Med* 103:532, 1959.
167. Ort S, Ryan JL, Borden G, et al: Pneumococcal pneumonia in hospitalized patients. *JAMA* 249:214, 1983.
168. Austrian R, Gold J: Pneumococcal bacteremia with especial reference to bacteremic pneumococcal pneumonia. *Ann Intern Med* 60:759, 1964.
169. Dajani AS: Antibiotic-resistant pneumococci. *Pediatr Infect Dis* 1:143, 1982.
170. Buxton AE, Anderson RL, Werdegar D, et al: Nosocomial respiratory tract infection and colonization with

Acinetobacter calcoaceticus: Epidemiologic characteristics. *Am J Med* 65:507, 1978.
171. Olson B, Weinstein RA, Nathan C, et al: Epidemiology of endemic *Pseudomonas aeruginosa:* Why infection control efforts have failed. *J Infect Dis* 150:808, 1984.
172. MacMillan BG, Edmonds P, Hummel RP, et al: Epidemiology of *Pseudomonas* in a burn intensive care unit. *J Trauma* 13:627, 1973.
173. Horan TC, White JW, Jarvis WR, et al: Nosocomial infection surveillance, 1984. *MMWR* CDC Surveill Summ 35:1755, 1986.
174. Catanzaro A: Nosocomial tuberculosis. *Am Rev Respir Dis* 125:559, 1982.
175. Craven RB, Wenzel RP, Atuk NO: Minimizing tuberculosis risk to hospital personnel and students exposed to unexpected disease. *Ann Intern Med* 82:628, 1975.
176. Ehrenkranz NJ, Kicklighter JL: Tuberculosis outbreak in a general hospital: Evidence of airborne spread of infection. *Ann Intern Med* 77:377, 1972.
177. Kirby BD, Snyder KM, Meyer RD, et al: Legionnaires' disease: Report of sixty-five nosocomially acquired cases and review of the literature. *Medicine* 59:188, 1980.
178. Cordes LG, Wiesenthal AM, Gorman GW, et al: Isolation of *Legionella pneumophila* from hospital shower heads. *Ann Intern Med* 94:195, 1981.
179. Arnow PM, Chou T, Weill D, et al: Nosocomial legionnaires disease caused by aerosolized tap water from respiratory care devices. *J Infect Dis* 146:460, 1982.
180. Muder RR, Yu VL, McClure JK, et al: Nosocomial legionnaires disease uncovered in a prospective pneumonia study: Implications for underdiagnosis. *JAMA* 249:3184, 1983.
181. Edelstein PH: Control of *Legionella* in hospitals. *J Hosp Infect* 8:109, 1986.
182. Grube BA, Marvin JA, Heimbach DM: Candida: A decreasing problem for the burned patient. *Arch Surg* 123:194, 1988.
183. Bruck HM, Nash G, Stein JM, et al: Studies on the occurrence and significance of yeasts and fungi in the burn wound. *Ann Surg* 176:108, 1972.
184. Matthews SCW, Levick PL, Coombes EJ, et al: Viral infections in a group of burned patients. *Burns* 6:55, 1978.
185. Foley FD, Greenawald KA, Nash G, et al: Herpesvirus infection in burned patients. *N Engl J Med* 282:652, 1970.
186. Nash G, Asch J, Foley FD, et al: Disseminated cytomegalic inclusion disease in a burned adult. *JAMA* 214:587, 1970.
187. Matthews SC, Levick PL, Coombes EJ, et al: Viral infections in a group of burned patients. *Burns* 6:55, 1978.
188. Kagan RJ, Naraqoi S, Matsuda T, et al: Herpes simplex virus and cytomegalovirus infections in burn patients. *J Trauma* 25:40, 1985.
189. Deepe GS Jr, MacMillan BG, Linnemann CC Jr: Unexplained fever in burn patients due to cytomegalovirus infection. *JAMA* 248:2299, 1982.

Chapter 12

Surgical Considerations

Andrew M. Munster

This chapter is not intended to be an overview of burn wound management, which is well covered by chapters in current textbooks.[1,2] Accordingly, initial debridement, topical therapy, control of burn wound sepsis, and the indications and techniques of escharotomy and fasciotomy will not be dealt with here.

What is specifically relevant to the clinician managing a patient with burns and smoke inhalation is a thorough understanding of the evolution and the current status of excisional therapy, its benefits and hazards, and its timing. There is probably no area of burn therapy that is more controversial than the operative management of the burn wound in patients with pulmonary injury, and none where precise prospective data are so lacking. This area will therefore be extensively discussed. Since tracheostomy is an integral part of this discussion, the role of tracheostomy will be considered as well.

EARLY EXCISION AND CLOSURE OF THE BURN WOUND

Historically, there was some experimentation with the technique of early wound excision and closure in the era before the advent of effective topical chemotherapy.[3–9] During this era, excision of *large* burns was rare, but Bennett and Thompson reported in 1969 a review of 20 cases in the literature with survival of excisions of burns of larger than 60 percent, to which they added 6 cases of their own.[10]

Further early reviews by Artz and Thompson[11] and Hendren et al.[12] stressed the benefits of early excision of large burns and pediatric burns. The introduction of effective topical chemotherapy in the 1960s[13] reduced the mortality from burn wound sepsis to such a degree that enthusiasm for hazardous early excision and wound closure waned for a few years. As burn units accumulated experience and began to report their results, it came to be appreciated that even with the use of effective topical chemotherapy, mortality could be reduced further by early aggressive closure of the burn wound.[14,15] The reduction of mortality as a result of early closure of the wound has now been well documented.[16,17] Recently, the Brooke group reported on 210 patients with burns over 30 percent with a 56 percent incidence of inhalation injury as diagnosed by history, physical examination, bronchoscopy, and xenon scan. Mortality in this group was 44.3 percent. The average waiting time to initial excision was 13.5 days following the injury in survivors and 12.5 in nonsurvivors, but excision was only possible in 40 (43 percent) of nonsurvivors, with pulmonary insufficiency being a contraindication. These authors conclude that apparent advantages of excision as reported in the literature may be due only to patient selection, since complications of the injury itself may preclude surgery.[18] Obviously, this approach is not yet free of controversy.

In patients with small burns, early excision and grafting reduces the length of hospitalization, lowers costs, and shortens time away from work.[19] There is also evidence that the length of surgery and the additional anesthesia involved in an operation of a sufficient magnitude to excise a large burn early are not directly related to mortality. Foy et al.[20] analyzed 197 procedures in 62 patients and found no differences in complication rate in patients who had the procedures in under 3 hours, compared with procedures exceeding 3 hours in length. However, these investigators did not analyze patients with smoke inhalation separately.

There appears to be no contraindication to excising burns in special at-risk age groups, such as the elderly.[21]

There may be other benefits to early closure of the burn wound as well. In 30 patients with a mean 42.8 percent burns, surgical excision and skin grafting improved postoperative lymphocyte function for a period of 5 days.[22]

The trend toward early excision and wound closure has been international rather than restricted to the United States. As an example, in the People's Republic of China, where much experience has accumulated with this procedure over the last 30 years, areas up to 40 percent of the burn surface are routinely excised at the first sitting, and in fact, even infected burn wounds are aggressively attacked surgically.[23]

By contrast, there has been substantial opposition to the concept of early excision and closure in patients who are at potential anesthetic and surgical risk even by those surgeons who are proponents of early excision. As late as 1969, in an authoritative textbook on burn management, it was stated that "inhalation injury is . . . an absolute contraindication to excision" and "inhalation injury detectable by the third or fourth day after burn by clinical signs, derangements in ventilatory function studies, or aberrations in blood gas measurements prohibit excision."[24] Pulmonary dysfunction has been well recognized as a complication of excision of the burn wound[25] perhaps because of the bacteremia commonly associated with burn surgery.[26] An increase in pulmonary complications has been reported, particularly in elderly patients, following excision, especially in the presence of preexisting lung problems.[27]

More recent evidence suggests strongly that endotoxin generated at the time of wound excision is deleterious to pulmonary function and that this phenomenon is correlated with the release of arachidonic acid metabolites in the lungs.[28,29] In this latter report, the authors document that pulmonary dysfunction correlated with wound thromboxane release is lowest very early after burn in an experimental model and increases from day 1 through day 7 after injury. There is additional evidence that age-related cardiac changes, which may affect the susceptibility of patients to general anesthesia, are refractory to the effects of adequate resuscitation. Aged guinea pigs have decreased myocardial contractibility, compared with young, and this cannot be corrected by resuscitation.[30]

We have recently attempted to abrogate perioperative pulmonary dysfunction caused by endotoxin release by the perioperative administration of polymyxin B, a known neutralizer of circulating endotoxins. While the endotoxemia was effectively controlled, we could find no evidence of improvements in perioperative pulmonary parameters as a result of this therapy.[31]

There is some evidence that if excision and wound closure fail to save the patient's life, these procedures do not alter the pathology of the cause of death. In the review of 95 deaths over 5 years, Peck and Heimbach[32] found that the actual cause of death was not altered in patients who died following early excision.

In summary, there is strong evidence that in small and moderate-size burns the complication rate is reduced, hospitalization time is shortened, and function improved by excision and closure of the wound within 5 to 7 days of the injury. There is also convincing indirect evidence that the mortality rate of very large burns can be improved by the same procedure. It must be remembered, however, that there are very few prospective randomized studies and most large reports use historical controls over a period of years, thereby potentially neglecting other advances in burn care during the same period of time such as improvements in nutrition, resuscitation, anesthesia, and nursing team care. Furthermore, these reports on the improvement of mortality from early wound excision and closure do not usually address specific subgroups of patients, such as patients with underlying medical conditions or pulmonary injury.

EARLY EXCISION IN THE PATIENT WITH INHALATION INJURY

The contribution of inhalation injury to the mortality rate of burn patients has only recently become truly appreciated. For many years, if a patient had sustained inhalation injury, 20 percent was "empirically" added to the mortality rate as predicted by various age and burn size–related formulas. Not only did a landmark publication in 1986[33] report that mortality due to inhalation injury was substantially greater than 20 percent additional to the age and burn size–related rate (in that series the mortality of patients without smoke inhalation was 4.1 percent, mortality of those with inhalation injury was 56 percent) but it also for the first time conclusively showed that the mortality rate of inhalation injury was *burn size–related*. Patients with burns over 20 percent with smoke inhalation had a mortality of 60.1 percent. At or under 4 years of age, patients with smoke inhalation had a mortality rate of 44 percent, while at age 59 or over the mortality rate increased to 92 percent.

In addition to the hazard posed to a surgical patient by inhalation injury, there are also some technical considerations relevant to anesthesia in this group of patients. For example, it has been shown that compliance falls from a normal 0.13 L/cm to 0.05 L/cm, and work of breathing increases from 0.04 to 2.26 kgm/min in patients with inhalation injury.[34]

Demling[35] measured pulmonary function in 37 patients undergoing 70 burn procedures. Twenty-two of these patients had significant impairment in lung function. Demling noted only a transient decrease in compliance and oxygenation from the operative procedure; however, he eliminated patients who were too unstable to transport. Demling laid out criteria for surgery as follows: (1) fascial excision and tourniquet wherever possible, (2) total burn size to be excised not to exceed 25 percent of the total body surface, (3) length of the operative procedure not to exceed 2 hours, (4) blood requirement to be held to under 4 units, and (5) the operating room environment to be maintained at 80°F. This limit on the size of excision was extended by Chicarilli et al.,[36] who increased "traditional" excision size to 30 to 70 percent of the total body surface in one sitting, either tangential or fascial. There were no controls in this report, but the authors did note a 71 percent survival in 17 patients with burns over 30 percent. The entire group had a mortality rate predicted to be above 50 percent. They also noted that three patients with well-developed adult respiratory distress syndrome whose peak airway pressures exceeded 50 to 60 mmHg showed dramatic improvement after surgery. Similar improvements following massive excision on burns were reported by Herndon et al.[37] In this report of 1057 cases, the total incidence of inhalation injury was 11 percent, but 46 percent of nonsurvivors had injury. These authors performed very prompt surgery for massive burns (for survivors, the first visit to the operating room took place within 22.8 hours, and for nonsurvivors, within 25.3 hours from the time of injury) and suggest that adequate prehospital resuscitation is critical and that early operation is an acceptable method of treatment, provided resuscitation is adequate. This finding is supported by experimental reports which link the pathology of smoke inhalation to time.[38] In an animal model, these authors demonstrate that mild smoke exposure shows pathologic changes peaking at 24 hours, after which a healing process begins; following severe smoke exposure, the pathologic findings continue to deteriorate after the first 24 hours. Obviously, the timing of surgery is critical in patients with inhalation injury.

In an initial report in 1987 and a more extensive report in 1989, the Galveston group addressed the problem of excisional surgery in patients with smoke inhalation.[39,40] In this latter painstaking study, which required almost 8 years to complete, the authors could demonstrate a reduction in mortality from early excision only in patients between 17 and 30 years of age with *no inhalation injury* but could not demonstrate a significant benefit in either adults with inhalation injury or in children. The practice of this group of authors, as pointed out previously, is excision of the entire or almost entire burn wound initially, rather than the sequential excision of 15 to 20 percent at each sitting, which is the more common practice of most centers. This report on the effect of surgical intervention on the mortality of patients with smoke inhalation does, however, match the general clinical experience of most burn surgeons, although further prospective data are urgently needed.

The overall mortality of burns is now under 10 percent at most centers. Among patients who succumb, the incidence of smoke inhalation is so high that it would be extremely difficult to demonstrate the superiority of a management technique such as early burn wound excision over another method such as less aggressive excision in this particular subgroup of patients, without requiring a multicenter study of several thousand patients.

In conclusion, early excision and closure of the burn wound are a desirable objective which can be expected to reduce the morbidity of burn patients and perhaps the mortality of burn patients without severe smoke inhalation. By extension, it is also appropriate for patients with inhalation injury *provided* that certain elementary criteria for the trip to the operating room and tolerance of operation and general anesthesia can be met. In addition, there is some experimental evidence that the sooner after admission this procedure can be undertaken the better.

PERIOPERATIVE MANAGEMENT

Fluid and Electrolyte Management

It is well documented that smoke inhalation brings about an increased requirement for resuscitation.[41,42] In patients who are resuscitated with lactated Ringer's solution, there is experimental evidence that the increased need for fluid resuscitation increases extravascular lung water.[43] In dogs, extravascular lung water increases by 42 percent when exposure to smoke is combined with intravenous lactated Ringer's solution at 10 percent of body weight, compared to an increase of only 2 percent when lactated Ringer's is given alone, or 28 percent when experimental smoke inhalation is administered alone. Therefore, intraoperative management such as is customary with sodium-containing solutions is unusually hazardous in burn patients with respiratory injury. It is common practice today to replace blood loss with packed red cells and make up the colloid portion of blood with lactated Ringer's or saline solutions. While this practice is theoretically sound, the patient who has been well resuscitated is already in positive sodium and water balance perhaps by as much as 15 to 20 L of water and 2000 to 3000 meq of sodium, and further administration of massive amounts of crystalloid solution during surgery may well lead to pulmonary decompensation in the postoperative period. Therefore, the administration of salt-containing fluids during and around the time of surgery to these patients must be kept to an absolute minimum.

Respirator Management

As noted previously, patients with smoke inhalation have not only diminished compliance but also an element of bronchospasm and increased airway resistance.[44] Bronchospasm may be treatable in the operating room. It has been recommended that, if possible, the patient's own respirator might be used in the operating room, since many operating room respirators are not capable of developing the adequate minute volumes required by these patients.

Transportation is a serious problem in units where the clinical service is at some distance from the operating room itself. In our center, patients with a minute volume requirement in excess of 18 L/min, an inspired oxygen concentration requirement in excess of 60 percent, and a need for higher than 8 or 10 mm of positive end-expiratory pressure (PEEP) are considered to be at the limit of transportability, although extraordinary measures can be taken to resolve this difficulty, as discussed in Chap. 13.

Cardiovascular Stability and Monitoring

In patients with a history of myocardial disease and in patients with very extensive third degree burns, inhalation injury poses additional hazards. The requirements for intraoperative monitoring by central venous catheter, arterial line, Swan-Ganz catheter, and electrocardiogram are even more stringent than usual and are dealt with in Chap. 13. It is imperative that blood replacement be accurate and saline or lactated Ringer's solution replacement be kept to a minimum during the operative period. The blood loss of most burn patients is quite predictable, and several handy formulas for the estimation of blood loss exist. Replacement should begin immediately after induction rather than after blood loss has progressed.[45]

In summary, in the patient with burns and significant smoke inhalation, the following questions need to be answered prior to excisional surgery. The answers to some of these questions do not appear in the literature; they are gleaned mostly from experience.

1. Does the procedure *have* to be done? If the patient is stable, has extensive second degree burns, most of which may heal within a week or two, and has severe respirator-dependent smoke inhalation, would it not be better to wait a few days?
2. What are the chances of getting good quality wound coverage? Are most of the deep sites to be excised in unfavorable sites (back, buttocks, breasts) or favorable sites (anterior trunk, extremities)?
3. What are the patient's current respirator settings and oxygen requirements? Is the patient stable for transportation and likely to remain stable in the operating theater?
4. Is there enough help in the operating room to reduce total operating time to reasonable length? We agree with the recommendations of Demling[35] to keep the total excision time under 2 hours and the area usually under 15 to 20 percent of the total body surface. If one is to do very extensive surgery in a reasonable length of time, an operating team must consist of at least four surgeons, preferably five. In the People's Republic of China, impressive total body excisions are expeditiously accomplished by the prompt availability of expert surgical personnel.
5. Last but not least, is the anesthesia team familiar with the specific problems of burns and smoke inhalation? Have they followed the patient since admission and know the resuscitation patterns, has a member of the anesthesia team been involved in the patient's care, and is the same team going to be available for the administration of anesthesia?

It has been our experience that only a few institutions have "dedicated" anesthesiologists for the management of burn patients. Clearly, in such institutions procedures with much bigger scope can be undertaken, earlier and with greater safety, than in others where the administration of anesthesia is part of a general service with daily random assignments.

TRACHEOSTOMY

Most patients with burns and smoke inhalation undergoing tracheostomy have a preexisting endotracheal tube in place. Since most complications of tracheal intubation are due to the balloon rather than the tube and since the balloons of both tracheostomy and endotracheal tubes are approximately in the same place, it becomes very difficult to distinguish between complications due purely to one or another method of intubation. For this reason, the literature contains no clear guidelines on which patients should have a tracheostomy in contrast to continued endotracheal intubation; it is unlikely that clear indications will ever emerge. As so much else in burn management, the issue becomes one of judgment. The problem of tracheal stenosis is discussed in some detail in Chap. 16.

Until quite recently, tracheostomy was held to be a treatment method of the last resort for burn patients. As recently as 1986, Robinson and Miller[46] held that early tracheostomy was indicated only rarely in burn patients because of increased mortality and morbidity. Similarly, Lund et al.,[47] reviewing 41 patients requiring endotracheal intubation or tracheostomy, concluded that endotracheal, preferably nasotracheal, intubation should be the initial modality of treatment in patients needing respiratory support for the first 3 weeks after admission. Other authors[48] prefer nasotracheal intubation because of nonoperative placement, ease of discontinuation, minimal bacterial contamination, and easy access to the treatment of burns of the neck. However, in an extensive review of over 3000 patients with 99 tracheostomies, Jones et al.[49] found that neither the sepsis rate nor the mortality rate was increased when endotracheal tubes were converted to tracheostomies. Similarly, Calhoun et al.[50] in a review of 1092 patients admitted to the Shriners Burns Institute in Galveston found that no predictive factors could be identified that could indicate which patients would develop long-term airway sequelae following endotracheal intubation or tracheostomy. Similarly, in a review of 88 tracheostomies over a 48-month period, where inhalation injury was present in 59.6 percent of patients, Hunt et al.[51] found that the decision to perform a tracheostomy should be individualized rather than put down to an arbitrary number of days.

Since many patients with inhalation injury, and certainly most patients with severe inhalation injury, will require respirator support, the question of whether to perform tracheostomy will commonly face the clinician. Based on our own experience and the literature, we currently recommend the following guidelines:

Absolute Indications

1. Patient remains unextubatable after 3 weeks of respirator support.
2. Intubated patient has persistent upper airway obstruction after 3 weeks of endotracheal intubation.

Relative Indications

1. Patient with difficult airway has required intubation over a fiberoptic bronchoscope and requires several operative procedures for burn wound coverage.
2. Patient with massive burns >60 percent is intubated and still hypoxemic or requires high levels of respirator support at 7 to 10 days after burn.
3. Patient is difficult to manipulate because of massive obesity or associated injuries and will require repeated prone operative procedures.
4. Patient has repeated atelectasis or pneumonia due to inability to suction left main stem bronchus adequately through endotracheal tube.
5. Patient has repeated mechanical complications of endotracheal tube, e.g., plugging.

In removing the tracheostomy tube from a patient with inhalation injury and burns, we recommend one of two methodologies. Patients who have been on respirator support but who appear to have an intact upper airway (this can be confirmed by nasopharyngoscopic inspection while intubated) may have the tracheostomy tubes simply removed and a dressing placed over the incision. Patients who have problems with upper airway injury, edema, or granulomata and who are thought to be at risk of upper airway obstruction may be "weaned" through the successive use of downscaled fenestrated tubes, the size of the tube being changed downward every 2 to 3 days until the patient demonstrates a competent upper airway, at which time the entire system may be removed.

Technical considerations in the performance of a tracheostomy are the same in patients with inhalation injury as in burn patients without smoke inhalation. These will not be considered in detail here except to mention that neck edema, tracheal deviation, and edema of the thyroid isthmus as well as engorgement of the neck veins, particularly the anterior jugular veins, can create unusual technical hazards in this group of patients.

REFERENCES

1. Boswick JA Jr (ed): *The Art and Science of Burn Care*. Rockville, Md, Aspen, 1987.
2. Cameron JL (ed): *Current Surgical Therapy—3*. Toronto, Decker, 1989.
3. Taylor PH, Moncrief JA, Pugsley LQ, et al: The management of extensively burned patients by staged excision. *Surg Gynecol Obstet* 115:347, 1962.
4. Cramer LM, McCormack RM, Carroll DD: Progressive partial excision and early grafting in lethal burns. *Plast Reconstr Surg* 30:595, 1962.
5. Jackson D, Toplex E, Carson JS, Towburg, EJL: Primary excision and grafting of large burns. *Ann Surg* 152:167, 1960.
6. Moncrief JA, Switzer WE, Rose RL: Primary excision and grafting in the treatment of third degree burns of the dorsum of the hand. *Plast Reconstr Surg* 33:305, 1964.
7. MacMillan BG: Early excision of burns. *J Trauma* 7:74, 1967.
8. Haynes BW Jr: Early excision and grafting in third degree burns. *Ann Surg* 169:736, 1969.
9. Janzekovic Z: A new concept in the early excision and immediate grafting of burns. *J Trauma* 10:1103, 1970.
10. Bennett JE, Thompson JE: The role of aggressive surgical treatment in the severely burned patient. *J Trauma* 9:776, 1969.
11. Artz CP, Thompson NJ: Early excision of large areas in burns. *Surgery* 63:868, 1968.
12. Hendren WH, Constable JD, Zawacki BE: Early partial excision of major burns in children. *J Pediatr Surg* 3:445, 1968.
13. Artz CP, Moncrief JA: *The Treatment of Burns*. Philadelphia, Saunders, 1969, chap 6, p 142.
14. Feller I, Thalen D, Dornell RG: Improvements in burn care, 1965–1979. *JAMA* 244:2074, 1980.
15. Wolfe RA, Roi LD, Flora JD, et al: Mortality differences and speed of wound closure among specialized burn care facilities. *JAMA* 250:763, 1983.
16. Burke J: Prompt eschar excision: A treatment system contributing to reduced burn mortality. *Ann Surg* 204:272, 1986.
17. Tompkins RG, Remensnyder PJ, Burke JF, et al: Significant reductions in mortality for children with burn injuries through the use of prompt eschar excision. *Ann Surg* 208:577, 1988.
18. McManus WF, Mason AD Jr, Pruitt BA Jr: Excision of the burn wound in patients with large burns. *Arch Surg* 124:718, 1989.
19. Engrav LH, Heimbach DM, Reus JL, et al: Early excision and grafting vs. nonoperative treatment of burns of indeterminant depth: A randomized prospective study. *J Trauma* 23:1001, 1983.
20. Foy HM, Pavlin E, Heimbach DM: Excision and grafting of large burns: Operation length not related to increased morbidity. *J Trauma* 26:51, 1986.
21. Heimbach DM: Early Burn Wound Excision and Grafting, in Boswick JA Jr (ed): *The Art and Science of Burn Care*. Rockville, Md, Aspen, 1987.
22. Stratta RJ, Saffle JR, Ninneman JL, et al: The effect of surgical excision and grafting procedures on postburn lymphocyte suppression. *J Trauma* 25:46, 1985.
23. Yang CC, Hsu WS, Shih TS (eds): *The Treatment of Burns*. Berlin, Springer-Verlag, 1982, chap 3.
24. Baxter CR: Early surgical excision and immediate grafting, in Artz CP, Moncrief JA, Pruitt BS Jr (eds): *Burns: A Team Approach*. Philadelphia, Saunders, 1979, chap 15.
25. Demling RH: Effect of early burn excision on pulmonary function. *J Trauma* 24:830, 1984.
26. Beard C, Ribeiro C, Jones D: The bacteremia associated with burns and surgery. *Br J Surg* 62:638, 1975.
27. Curreri PW, Luterman A, Brown D, et al: Burn injury: Analysis of survival and hospitalization time for 937 patients. *Ann Surg* 192:472, 1980.
28. Demling RH, Wenger H, Hechtman HB, et al: Role of sub-

cutaneous tissue endotoxin in the production of prostanoid-induced lung injury. *Circ Shock* 17:147, 1985.

29. Katz A, Ryan P, Lalonde C, Demling RH: Pulmonary dysfunction after burn wound excision correlation with wound thromboxane release and bacterial content. *Surg Forum*, 36:89, 1985.
30. Horton JW, Baxter CR, and White DJ: Differences in cardiac responses to resuscitation from burn shock. *Surg Gynecol Obstet* 168:201, 1989.
31. Munster AM, Xiao GX, Guo Y, et al: Control of endotoxemia in burn patients by use of Polymyxin B. *J Burn Care Rehabil*, in press.
32. Peck MD, Heimbach DM: Does early excision of burn wounds change the pattern of mortality? *J Burn Care Rehabil* 10:7, 1989.
33. Thompson PB, Herndon DN, Traber DL, Abston DL: Effect on mortality of inhalation injury. *J Trauma* 26:163, 1986.
34. Garzan AA, Seltzer B, et al: Respiratory mechanics in patients with inhalation burns. *J Trauma* 10:57, 1970.
35. Demling RH: Effect of early burn excision and grafting on pulmonary function. *J Trauma* 24:830, 1984.
36. Chicarilli ZN, Cuono CN, Heinrich JJ, et al: Selective aggressive burn excision for high mortality subgroups. *J Trauma* 26:18, 1986.
37. Herndon DN, Gore D, Cole M, et al: Determinants of mortality in pediatric patients with greater than 70% full thickness total body surface area thermal injury treated by early total excision and grafting. *J Trauma* 27:208, 1987.
38. Shimazu T, Yukioka T, Hubbard GB, et al: A dose-responsive model of smoke inhalation injury. *Ann Surg* 206:89, 1987.
39. Thompson P, Herndon DN, Abston S, Rutan T: Effect of early excision on patients with major thermal injury. *J Trauma* 27:205, 1987.
40. Herndon DN, Barrow RE, Rutan RL, et al: A comparison of conservative versus early excision: Therapies in severely burned patients. *Ann Surg* 209:547, 1989.
41. Navar PD, Saffle JR, Warden GD: Effect of inhalation injury on fluid requirements after thermal injury. *Am J Surg* 150:716, 1985.
42. Scheulen JJ, Munster AM: The Parkland formula in patients with burns and inhalation injury. *J Trauma* 22:869, 1982.
43. Clark WR, Nieman GF, Goyelte D, Gryboski D: Effects of crystalloid in lung fluid balance after smoke inhalation. *Ann Surg* 208:56, 1988.
44. Pavlin EG, Strakeljohn C: Operating room considerations, in Boswick JA (ed): *The Art and Science of Burn Care*. Rockville, Md, Aspen, 1987, chap 12.
45. Moran KG, O'Reilly TJ, Furman W, Munster AM: A new algorithm for calculation of blood loss in excisional burn surgery. *Am Surg* 54:207, 1988.
46. Robinson L, Miller RH: Smoke inhalation injuries. *Am J Otolaryngol* 7:375, 1986.
47. Lund T, Goodwin CW, McManus WF, et al: Upper airway sequelae in burn patients requiring endotracheal intubation or tracheostomy. *Ann Surg* 201:374, 1985.
48. Herndon DN, Barrow RE, Linares HA, et al: Inhalation injury in burned patients: Effects and treatment. *Burns Incl Therm Inj* 14:349, 1988.
49. Jones WG, Madden M, Finkelstein J, et al: Tracheostomies in burn patients. *Ann Surg* 209:471, 1989.
50. Calhoun KH, Deskin RW, Garza C, et al: Long-term airway sequelae in a pediatric burn population. *Laryngoscope* 98:721, 1988.
51. Hunt JL, Purdue GF, Gunning T: Is tracheostomy warranted in the burn patient? Indications and complications. *J Burn Care Rehabil* 7:492, 1986.

Chapter 13

Anesthetic Aspects

Michael J. Sendak
William R. Furman

The clinical course of burned patients may be considered to have three phases: the early resuscitative phase, the subsequent debridement and grafting phase, and the late reconstructive phase.[1] Airway and respiratory problems often occur in each phase. This chapter will discuss the airway management of patients with thermal burns of the face and/or inhalational injuries, and perioperative anesthetic care of the burn patient with respiratory failure.

AIRWAY MANAGEMENT OF INHALATIONAL INJURIES

Types of Inhalational Injuries

Respiratory failure during the first few hours to days after burn injury can be caused by asphyxia due to carbon monoxide poisoning, by upper airway obstruction due to edema of the tissues of the pharynx and/or larynx, by lower airway damage in the form of tracheobronchitis or small airway and parenchymal damage,[2–5] or by any combination of these three disorders. The exact pattern and severity of the injury is determined by the type, temperature, and concentration of gases inhaled, the solubility characteristics of these gases, the presence or absence of superheated particulates in the inhaled smoke, and the duration of exposure.[5–7] The most severe inhalational injuries are incurred when victims are trapped in an enclosed space (either physically or because of unconsciousness) and when the fire involves plastic materials.[5,8–11] Details of noxious gases emitted in fires may be found in Chap. 3.

Asphyxia When victims are trapped in burning structures such as buildings or vehicles, they become hypoxic from breathing a gas mixture which contains carbon monoxide (CO) and is deficient in oxygen. Although the low inspired-oxygen (O_2) concentration contributes to tissue hypoxia, the effect of CO poisoning is far more important. Carbon monoxide binds to hemoglobin 200 times more readily than does O_2, decreasing the amount of hemoglobin available for oxygen transport. In addition to decreasing the arterial content of oxygen, CO also increases the stability of the oxyhemoglobin molecule, inhibiting release of oxygen to the tissues,[12,13] and ultimately causing hypoxic organ dysfunction and cell death in the brain, heart, and abdominal viscera.

Because the consequences are so dire, CO poisoning must be suspected and treated promptly in any fire victim, especially those who have been trapped in confined spaces. They may complain of headache, nausea, angina pectoris, or shortness of breath and may appear tachypneic, irritable, or delirious, or have an altered level of consciousness, but not appear cyanosed.

The degree of carbon monoxide poisoning and attendant tissue hypoxia may be quantified by measuring the carboxyhemoglobin level, expressed as the percent saturation of hemoglobin in arterial blood (Sa_{CO}). Saturations greater than 15 percent are usually toxic, and those over 50 percent are nearly always lethal. It is also possible to measure the Sa_{CO} noninvasively via pulse oximetry using a special three-wavelength oximeter; however, the standard (two-wavelength) pulse oximeters which are now in widespread use cannot differentiate oxyhemoglobin from carboxyhemoglobin.[14]

Once the victim has been removed from the fire and begins to breathe room air (21% oxygen, 0% carbon monoxide), CO elimination begins to take place and tissue oxygenation starts to improve. Since the half-time of elimination of CO can be shortened from 4 hours (breathing room air) to 40 minutes if 100% oxygen is administered,[1,15] any patient with a suspected (or documented) elevation of Sa_{CO} should receive as high an inspired concentration as possible. Many victims of carbon monoxide poisoning require endotracheal intubation to accomplish this.

Upper Airway Obstruction Upper airway injury (above the true vocal cords) may result from inhalation of hot air, flames, and toxic chemicals.[16,17] Early recognition of the risk of development of this problem is essential, as swelling may rapidly become so extreme that successful laryngoscopy and intubation are impossible and emergency tracheostomy is required. There is often erythema, blistering, and necrosis of the surface epithelium,[18] with edema becoming significant after a latent period of 4 to 48 hours.[19–21] Upper airway edema parallels the generalized extravascular fluid deposition that occurs during volume resuscitation.[22] The distribution of edema in the upper airway is not uniform;[2,11,22,23] the tongue and laryngeal surface of the epiglottis are fairly resistant, while the pharyngeal epiglottic surface and laryngeal ventricles are quite susceptible. The mucosa over the false cords, the aryepiglottic folds, and the arytenoid eminences may become severely edematous and can prolapse and produce partial or complete airway occlusion.

Upper airway obstruction occurs in 20 to 30% of burn victims with inhalation injury[24] and poses a dire emergency. The possibility of upper airway obstruction should be anticipated in all victims of closed-space fires, particularly when there are facial burns, an injected tongue, sooty oral or nasal secretions or if hoarseness develops. Early intubation is recommended for any patient with significant intraoral or pharyngeal burns, as progressive edema may make intubation extremely hazardous or impossible. This is a conservative approach and requires endotracheal intubation in a number of patients who would not progress to significant airway compromise.[24,25]

An alternative approach is to evaluate these patients with either pulmonary flow-volume curves or nasopharyngoscopy.[22,26–29] Both techniques require a cooperative patient, and serial evaluations are often necessary. These should be performed at intervals more frequent than dictated by the victim's symptoms, for the upper airway may become impaired gradually, provoking little or no change in the patient's clinical appearance until nearly complete obstruction has occurred.[30]

Flow-volume loops, discussed in Chap. 7, offer a noninvasive means of evaluating a patient for the presence of inspiratory obstruction, but these may at first appear normal during the course of development of severe edema, and are therefore no substitute for direct examination of the larynx whenever there is clinical suspicion of an upper airway injury. The use of the fiberoptic nasopharyngoscope is a means of direct examination of the airway which is relatively comfortable for the patient and can be repeated at frequent intervals if necessary. Nasopharyngoscopes have a much smaller diameter than fiberoptic bronchoscopes (3 to 4 mm compared to 5 to 6 mm) and are usually tolerated well by the awake patient, even if topical anesthesia is not used. When it is not feasible to repeatedly examine the airway, the most prudent course is to secure it early (intubate) if serious clinical suspicion of upper airway injury exists.[12,15] Additional discussion of airway management in patients with inhalational injury may be found in Chap. 9.

Pulmonary Insufficiency Respiratory failure due to pulmonary insufficiency may develop at any time from 3 hours to 3 days after smoke inhalation.[6,19,20,31,32] The inciting injury is chemical in nature, as true thermal damage to the lower respiratory tract does not occur unless steam or burning gases have been inhaled. This is because the heat associated with inhalation of hot air is dissipated in the pharynx and supraglottic areas and because the heat involved evokes reflex closure of the epiglottis.[11,25,33,34]

No such mechanisms inhibit the inhalation of toxic chemicals contained in smoke, however, and thus the lungs are generally exposed to caustic products of combustion. Smoke inhalation causes the cessation of ciliary function,[35] impairs clearance of mucus and debris, and results in loss of surfactant activity;[36] the release of chemotactic substances such as histamine, serotonin, and kallikreins;[8] and extensive mucosal edema.[6] Regional atelectasis, bronchospasm, and air trapping[37] follow, and after several hours, there is sloughing of epithelium and formation of a mucopurulent membrane (pseudomembranous tracheobronchitis).[2,25,35] Eventually there is formation of hyalin membranes, deposition of fibrin, intra-alveolar hemorrhage, and finally, interstitial and alveolar pulmonary edema.[2,35]

In patients with a combination of smoke inhalation and cutaneous burns these changes may be even more dramatic. Animal studies have demonstrated that thermal injury alone results in pulmonary dysfunction.[38–44] The mechanism for this may include complement activation, formation of oxygen free radicals or prostanoids, alterations in pulmonary vascular resistance, and changes in colloid oncotic or hydrostatic pressures (either intravascular or interstitial). A consistent feature in these models is an increase in lung lymph flow, suggesting a component of altered microvascular permeability and an increase in pulmonary transvascular fluid flux. These factors may explain why patients with both smoke inhalation and cutaneous injury demonstrate significant compromise in pulmonary function at an early stage in their disease. This is discussed further in Chap. 4.

Survival later into the clinical course carries considerable risk for the development of bacterial bronchopneumonia.[34,45] This results from alterations in immunologic function (both cellular and humoral), disruption of normal anatomic barriers, and loss of peripheral airway patency.[34,45–56] These are discussed in Chap. 11.

Techniques of Intubation for Patients with Inhalational Injuries

Asphyxia Asphyxia requires rapid, aggressive therapy to maintain or restore both cerebral and myocardial tissue oxygenation and viability. Whenever a burn victim is stuporous, confused, or comatose upon admission to hospital, the alteration of mental status should be assumed to be due to cerebral tissue hypoxia. Arterial blood gases and carboxyhemoglobin determination should be obtained, and intubation should be performed without delay to improve oxygenation of the brain.

Because of the urgency, this usually takes place at the time of admission of the patient in the hospital emergency room or burn unit. In this situation, the main anesthetic considerations are those which apply to any trauma victim with respiratory failure at the time of arrival. As with other trauma patients, the airway must be controlled via endotracheal intubation in order to ensure oxygenation and ventilation and to prevent aspiration of gastric contents.

Pharmacologic Considerations While neuromuscular blocking agents are generally not required during airway management of comatose burn victims, those who are stuporous or delirious tend to resist manipulation and may therefore require muscle relaxation to facilitate intubation, especially if the orotracheal route is chosen. Although delirious patients almost invariably suffer memory loss, many anesthesiologists prefer to administer a sedative-hypnotic agent during intubation when they give a muscle relaxant to an awake but confused patient. This prevents unpleasant memories of the laryngoscopy and helps the patient tolerate the subsequent discomfort of remaining intubated afterward. Narcotic analgesics are also used in this situation to relieve the pain of laryngoscopy and endotracheal intubation.

When selecting agents for this purpose, the possibility of intravascular volume depletion or hypoxic myocardial depression must be considered (see Table 13-1). Thiobarbiturates such as thiamylal and thiopental have a rapid onset of action but possess myocardial depressant properties and are usually best used in reduced doses or avoided in favor of agents less likely to cause hypotension, such as the benzodiazepines midazolam and diazepam or ketamine.[57] The use of the depolarizing muscle relaxant is not contraindicated at this early stage (see below).

Aspiration Prevention Aspiration is associated with a mortality rate of approximately 30 percent (ranging from 3 to 70 percent)[58–63] and continues to be a significant cause of anesthetic-related mortality and morbidity.[64–67] The inhalation of gastric contents in a patient already compromised by smoke-induced pulmonary dysfunction may prove to be an overwhelming insult. Since gastric emptying is known to cease at the time of significant injury, it must be assumed that every burn victim has a full stomach and that active or passive regurgitation during intubation carries a significant risk for the aspiration of gastric contents. Accordingly, whenever intubation is facilitated by pharmacologic agents, a rapid-sequence protocol is essential during laryngoscopy and intubation.

The rapid-sequence protocol minimizes aspira-

Table 13-1 Pharmacologic Agents Used in Airway Management of Burn Patients

Generic name	Dose	Indication	Problems
Thiopental	1 mg/kg increments 4–5 mg/kg	Sedation Rapid sequence	Myocardial depression
Diazepam	2.5–5 mg increments	Amnesia	Scleroses veins; 24-h time action
Midazolam	0.5–1 mg increments	Amnesia	
Ketamine	1-mg/kg increments	Anesthesia for wound care	Tachycardia; hypertension; increased secretions; hallucinations on awakening
Morphine	5–10 mg increments	Analgesia	Histamine release
Fentanyl	50-μg increments	Analgesia	
Succinylcholine	1–1.5 mg/kg	Paralysis	Potassium release; *only used in first 24 hours postburn*
NDMRs*			
Pancuronium	0.1–0.4 mg/kg	Paralysis; long-acting	Slow onset; large doses required for rapid sequence; effect may last for 2–3 hours
Vecuronium	0.1–0.4 mg/kg	Paralysis; shorter-acting	Same as pancuronium, with shorter length of effect (1.5 hours)

*Atracurium, metocurine, and *d*-tubocurarine are omitted because each has the potential to cause histamine release in the high doses usually required for burn patients. The two agents listed should serve most needs.

tion risk by physically blocking the pathway from the stomach to the lungs and limiting the amount of time which elapses from when the patient is weakened by muscle relaxants and sedatives to when the orotracheal tube is in place with the cuff inflated. If the patient is conscious and cooperative, it may be feasible to administer oral antacids prior to intubation and thus reduce the risk that aspirated gastric contents will damage the lungs. One ounce of sodium citrate, given orally, has been demonstrated to adequately neutralize gastric acidity.[68] This clear antacid mixes well with the stomach contents, and it is virtually harmless in the event of aspiration.[69,70] In contrast, particulate antacids are less effective because they tend to layer out within the stomach, and if aspirated, they evoke a significant pneumonitis.[71] The insertion of nasogastric tubes prior to intubation is not indicated because these devices are not capable of completely emptying the stomach and have the added disadvantage of rendering the gastroesophageal sphincter incompetent, promoting regurgitation.

Prior to intubation, 100% oxygen should be administered by mask, but positive pressure ventilation, which can cause insufflation of air into the stomach, should be avoided. Cricoesophageal compression (Sellick maneuver) is begun before administration of muscle relaxants or sedatives and maintained until the endotracheal tube is inserted and its position has been confirmed.[72] To perform this maneuver, the thumb and index finger are placed over the anterior aspect of the circular cricoid cartilage and pressure is exerted directly toward the cervical spine, in order to temporarily obliterate the esophageal lumen (Fig. 13-1). Intraesophageal pressures at least as high as 100 cm of water cannot overcome this type of esophageal compression. Thus, aspiration resulting from pas-

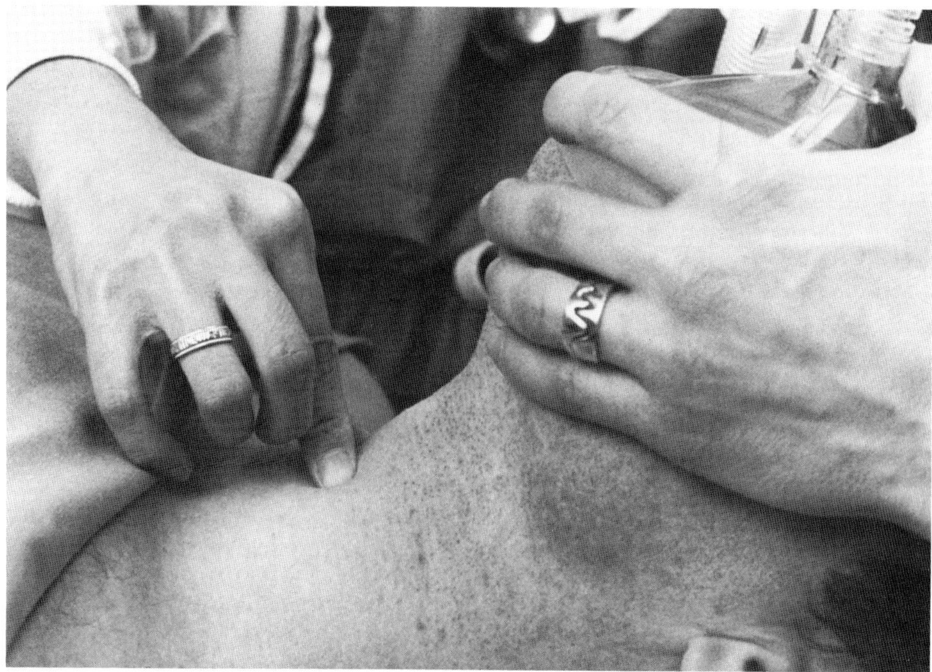

Figure 13-1 Technique of cricoesophageal compression to obliterate the esophageal lumen before and during rapid-sequence induction of anesthesia.

sive regurgitation will not occur. If laryngoscopy should induce active retching or vomiting, cricoid pressure should still be maintained, despite concerns (mostly theoretical) of possible esophageal rupture.[73,74] If difficulties of any type should arise during the process of tracheal intubation, it is crucial that cricoesophageal pressure be maintained, for this is precisely the time when regurgitation and aspiration are most likely to occur.

Technique of Intubation When there is no contraindication to do so, the oral route under direct vision is preferred for intubation of victims of CO poisoning because it is the fastest option. However, if combativeness on the part of the patient necessitates the use of a muscle relaxant, and it is likely that oral intubation will be technically difficult, the nasal approach offers an opportunity to control the airway without first making the patient apneic. Thus, the nasal route may be slower but safer, as it avoids the potential risk of prolonged apnea during the time from muscle paralysis to ultimate airway control if oral intubation proves difficult. The key to safety in this situation is the ability to correctly recognize, in advance, patients who will be difficult to intubate orally, such as massively obese or facially traumatized victims.

In addition, if the stability of the cervical spine is in doubt because a history is unobtainable, or when there is a history of a deceleration injury, such as jumping from a height or a motor vehicle accident, it is necessary to maintain the patient's neck in a neutral position during intubation in order to prevent spinal injury. This makes it more difficult to visualize the larynx with a laryngoscope because the head may not be positioned optimally for intubation. Ideally during laryngoscopy, the head should be lifted into the "sniffing position" by flexing the spine at the level of the lower cervical vertebrae and extending it at the atlantoaxial joint, bringing the axes of the mouth, pharynx, and larynx into alignment and permitting a clear view of the glottis. When the head must be kept in a neutral position, direct visualization of the vocal cords is harder to achieve, and a nasal intubation is often preferable.

Like the oral route, the nasal approach to intubation has some disadvantages. It usually takes longer to perform, requires some cooperation from the patient, and may provoke epistaxis. The latter two problems may be ameliorated by preparing the nasal passages with topical anesthesia and a vasoconstrictor. Lidocaine 4% mixed in equal amounts with phenylephrine 1% is suitable for this purpose, as is cocaine 4%. A disadvantage of cocaine is the fact that it is potentially cardiotoxic, and many burn victims incur their injuries while in a state of intoxication by cocaine and other drugs.

Cotton-tipped applicators can be placed in the nose (on both sides, in case the side first selected proves obstructed by a deviated septum) to anesthetize the nasal mucosa. After anesthetizing the nasal passages, it is helpful to dilate them by inserting a lubricated nasal airway of sufficient size to gently displace the turbinates and reduce the risk of trauma during the passage of the endotracheal tube. The use of a series of successively larger nasal airways is a good way to do this. In this manner effective preparation for a nasal intubation can be accomplished in about 5 minutes.

Another disadvantage of the nasal route is the fact that the blind nasal approach is often simply impossible, and the alternative technique of inserting a nasotracheal tube over a bronchoscope requires the availability of an individual with the special technical training and skill to manipulate the fiberoptic instrument. The small, 3- to 4-mm nasopharyngoscopes, which are so useful for serial airway examinations (see above), are unsuitable for this purpose because they are too short and lack an adequate suction channel for removing secretions during the procedure; the larger, 5- or 6-mm bronchoscopes are usually required.

Inability to Intubate One disadvantage of the rapid-sequence intubation technique is the fact that, occasionally, the larynx proves unforeseeably difficult to visualize on the first attempt. Since the pa-

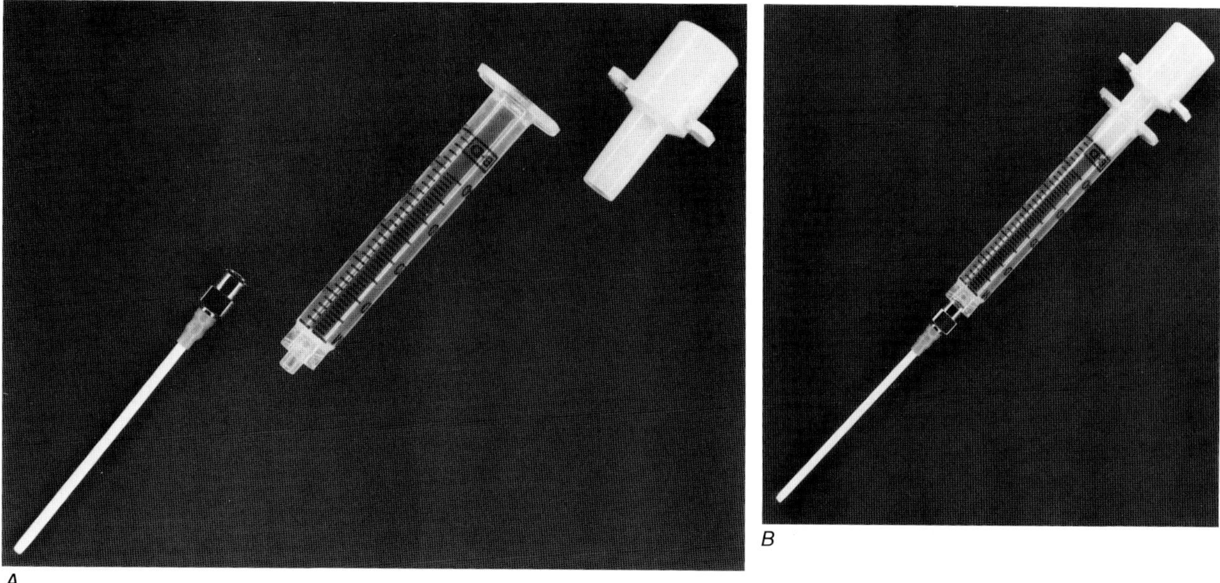

Figure 13-2 Equipment required for emergency cricothyroidotomy, shown unassembled (*A*) and assembled (*B*).

tient has been given a muscle relaxant and is apneic, positive pressure ventilation with oxygen is necessary, despite the risk of insufflation of air into the stomach. During this period of controlled ventilation, cricoesophageal pressure must be maintained. The currently available manual resuscitators, fitted with O_2 reservoirs, and a tightly fitting face mask, allow ventilation with high inspired-oxygen concentrations. With flow rates of 15 L/min, nearly 100% O_2 can be delivered[75] before a repeat attempt to intubate.

If mask ventilation also proves impossible, hypoxia and hypercarbia will rapidly ensue, and the only remaining remedy is emergency transtracheal oxygenation via cricothyroidotomy and subsequent tracheostomy.[76] The equipment required for emergency cricothyroidotomy is shown in Fig. 13-2. A large bore intravenous cannula (10 or 14 gauge) is used to puncture the cricothyroid membrane. A 3-mL syringe with the plunger removed is attached to this cannula, and the connector from a 7.0-mm endotracheal tube is inserted into the syringe to allow attachment of the resuscitation bag.[77] In this manner, oxygenation can be quickly reestablished before either a repeat attempt at laryngoscopy or a tracheostomy. Although they are able to provide adequate oxygenation, transtracheal cannulas are generally ineffective for removing CO_2.

Upper Airway Obstruction Upper airway edema requiring endotracheal intubation usually becomes manifest during the first 24 to 48 hours. In addition to the anesthetic considerations discussed above, altered responses to neuromuscular blocking agents and a much increased risk of inability to either ventilate by mask or visualize the larynx if edema is diagnosed late become prime concerns.

Early recognition of the potential for upper airway obstruction should lead to serial examinations of the airway and therefore allows intubation to be performed before life-threatening airway compromise occurs. If upper airway swelling is diagnosed early enough, intubation may be performed as discussed above in the treatment of asphyxia by either an oral or nasal technique. As in the case of asphyxia, a rapid-sequence protocol is preferred when the degree of swelling is known to be mild and there are no other anatomic concerns (such as massive obesity or facial or cervical trauma). Late recognition of upper airway swelling seriously constrains the choices of technique and greatly increases the risks to the patient (see below).

Neuromuscular Blocking Agents Burn victims develop sensitivity to succinylcholine (and other depolarizing muscle relaxants) and resistance to all nondepolarizing neuromuscular blocking agents during the first few days postburn. Succinylcholine provokes a massive release of potassium from the muscle of burned patients, especially if the burn exceeds 10 percent of the body surface area (BSA).[78–81] While normal patients experience a small elevation of the serum potassium (average of 0.5 meq/L) after receiving succinylcholine, burn victims are at risk for suffering elevations to arrhythmogenic levels. This response seems most likely to occur from 5 days to 3 months postburn, with a peak effect between 20 and 60 days. Although it is probably safe in the first few days, many authors recommend abjuring succinylcholine after the first 8 to 12 hours. Exactly when this drug is once again safe to use is controversial. Some authors suggest that the drug may be used after 6 months if all the burns have healed, while others recommend that it not be used for 2 years.[78–81]

If a rapid-sequence technique is selected for intubation after the first 8 to 12 hours, a nondepolarizing muscle relaxant (NDMR) should be used. Burn victims develop resistance to NDMRs at about the same time that they become sensitive to depolarizing agents, especially if the burn exceeds 40 percent of the body surface area. Accordingly, during the first 2 days, when upper airway obstruction usually develops, little resistance to NDMRs should be expected, and the standard dosages for rapid-sequence induction may be used. Later, especially in patients with larger burns, doses may have to be increased to achieve relaxation in a patient of the same age and size. The mechanism for this is not fully understood, but an increase in receptor number is believed to play a major role, and neither drug metabolism nor the ability to competitively antagonize their effects is significantly altered.[78–86]

Late Diagnosis If the diagnosis of airway compromise is reached late, opportunities for a blind or fiberoptic nasal intubation are usually lost because the introduction of topical anesthetics may produce severe coughing or laryngospasm. These in turn can result in damage to the protruding and friable pharyngeal mucosa and ultimately lead to bleeding or lethal swelling. During intubation, the bronchoscope itself may occlude the diminished airway passage and result in a hypoxic cardiac arrest.

Similarly, the risks of inability to visualize the larynx or even ventilate by mask preclude the use of sedatives or muscle relaxants and require an awake oral intubation despite the obvious discomfort to the patient. At the worst, the condition may be analogous to that of acute epiglottitis and may need to be managed similarly. The best solution then might be to transport the patient to the operating room, perform a slow inhalational anesthetic induction using halothane and 100% O_2, and intubate if possible under deep inhalational anesthesia. Prior to the induction, preparations should be made for an emergency cricothyroidotomy or formal tracheostomy, to be performed if oral intubation is not possible.

Pulmonary Insufficiency Respiratory failure due to chemical pneumonitis, bacterial pneumonia, or cardiogenic pulmonary edema may occur at any time after burn injury. Anesthetic concerns in such cases may encompass any and all of the issues discussed above. If the upper airway is known to be unaffected, a standard rapid-sequence induction is usually chosen in order to protect the lungs from aspiration of gastric contents, with care taken to not depress cardiovascular function. If the patient has had a nasogastric tube inserted, it may be removed, however it is also acceptable to leave it in place, as cricoesophageal pressure will still occlude the esophagus, and the nasogastric tube will serve as a vent to relieve intragastric pressure.[87]

The choice of muscle relaxant depends on how much time has elapsed since the burn injury. As discussed above, if more than 8 to 12 hours have passed, a nondepolarizing muscle relaxant is required. In patients with large burns who are several days postburn, it might be predicted that a rapid-sequence induction would require even larger doses of NDMRs than those used in the general population; however, this issue has yet to be completely studied.

Certainly the risk of prolonged muscle relaxation caused by a very large dose of drug would generally be an acceptable side effect if the large dose allowed the airway to be secured expeditiously. The standard NDMR for rapid-sequence intubation is the relatively long acting agent pancuronium (0.15 mg/kg). While curare, metocurine, and atracurium are shorter-acting, they are less desirable because they lead to histamine release. Vecuronium is an alternative, shorter-acting NDMR with no cardiovascular side effects. In the case of vecuronium, it is known that a dose of 0.4 mg/kg (four times the standard intubating dose) produces no adverse reactions in a healthy population and allows intubation to be performed within 80 seconds of administration. This is one-half the time required after a dose of 0.1 mg/kg and results in a tripling of the time to spontaneous recovery of 75 percent of neuromuscular function (from 42 to 115 minutes).[88]

Once endotracheal intubation has been completed, the tube may be secured to the face by means of adhesive tape or umbilical tape or even wired to the teeth.[89] There are also commercially available attachments with Velcro straps that are effective in providing tube stabilization. These rapidly become soiled with the patient's secretions and are quite expensive but do not allow the endotracheal tube to slide out of position as adhesive or umbilical tape may do when wet.

Protecting intubated burn patients from inadvertent extubation is a difficult problem. Nasotracheal tubes are much easier than oral ones to maintain in position during movement of the patient. Consideration should be therefore be given to electively changing any orotracheal tube to a nasal one whenever it appears that prolonged intubation will be required, especially if the patient is combative. If the patient has sustained facial trauma, or the risk of paranasal sinusitis is deemed too great for a nasal intubation, or if it is simply clinically obvious that intubation for more than 2 or 3 weeks will be required, an early elective tracheostomy should be considered. While this is an aggressive approach, the benefit lies in secure access to and protection of the airway throughout a prolonged intensive care and operative course.

PERIOPERATIVE MANAGEMENT

It is often necessary to proceed with anesthesia in burn patients despite severe pulmonary dysfunction and hemodynamic instability because aggressive surgical excision and grafting of burn wounds is viewed as an important measure in the control of life-threatening burn would infection. Frequently, these patients are taken to the operating room for debridement and grafting as early as within 48 hours of their initial injury.[90–94] When this occurs, the anesthesiologist becomes an integral component of the medical team caring for the burn patient with respiratory failure, acquiring responsibility for oxygenation, ventilation, fluid therapy, metabolic homeostasis, cardiovascular support, and monitoring, a responsibility which is acquired at the time of transport from the intensive care unit (ICU) and continues through the operative procedure and the transport back to the ICU. This section discusses the preoperative evaluation, care during transport, and intraoperative care of burn patients who have been intubated because of respiratory failure.

Preoperative Evaluation

In general, the preoperative anesthesia evaluation consists of a review of the patient's history, physical exam, and laboratory findings and a consideration of the surgical plan. With regard to critically ill burn patients, a detailed study of the postburn hospital course is a vital part of the history because the patient's condition can change very rapidly.

History and Hospital Course As with any preanesthetic evaluation, it is important to determine the patient's past medical and surgical history, with specific emphasis on allergies, prior anesthetics, and cardiopulmonary disease. Due to the overwhelming nature of the injury, the patient is often unable to provide much data. As a result, a thorough review of the events since the time of hospital admission may be the principle source of information. This review should concentrate on the following areas: fluid resuscitation, monitoring and intravenous access, cardiovascular and renal function, medications, and pulmonary function.

All burn victims require large volumes of sodium-containing fluids. In the first 24 hours, depending upon which formula is used, between 2 and 4 mL of intravenous crystalloid per kilogram are given for every 1 percent of the body surface area burned. Most formulas prescribe colloid at some point during the first 48 hours.[95,96] Secure intravenous access is required to achieve this, and often the anticipated needs for fluid or blood product administration or for a more invasive level of monitoring during surgery dictate the placement of additional catheters. This decision should be made at the time of the preoperative visit, with the choice of lines and their insertion sites being made jointly with the burn care team.

The clinical response to fluid administration should be reviewed to determine if the efforts to maintain the intravascular volume have been successful (vital signs, evidence of prerenal azotemia, rising hematocrit, or falling weight) and to evaluate the myocardial response to the stress of burn injury and its therapy. When signs of myocardial ischemia or pump failure develop during this period, arterial, central venous, and pulmonary artery catheters are usually inserted. The data obtained from the direct measurement of cardiac pressures and outputs can then be used to guide further resuscitative measures, as well as anesthetic technique. When fluid requirements exceed the amounts absorbed, renal failure may develop. The state of renal function is important because decreases in renal function lead to decreases in the clearance of electrolytes, free water, and drugs excreted by the kidney and to increases in overall mortality.[97–100]

The preoperative evaluation should include a review of all the patient's medications and a note of any known drug allergies. Among the agents commonly required by patients with major burns are antibiotics (intravenous and topical), total parenteral nutrition, antacids, histamine blockers (H_2 blockers), analgesics, vasopressors, inotropes, and bronchodilators. Usually, these medications and their dosages should be noted and continued through the perioperative period unless some specific drug-anesthetic interaction poses a potential problem. The potential for drug-drug interactions[78,101] and the capacity for significant protein loss from the burn would to lead to sensitivity to highly protein bound medications[44,102] should also be considered.

The topical antimicrobials used in care of the burn wound can produce complications. Silver nitrate can cause absorption of large quantities of distilled water and loss of significant amounts of sodium, potassium, calcium, and chloride through the burn wound, resulting in hyponatremia and metabolic alkalosis. Also, gram-negative bacteria within the burn wound can reduce nitrates to nitrites, which diffuse into the patient's bloodstream, causing the formation of methemoglobin, which can compromise tissue oxygen delivery. As with carboxyhemoglobin, neither an arterial blood gas nor a standard pulse oximeter will detect this problem.[103,104] In patients with large burns treated with silver nitrate dressings, a direct spectrophotometric measurement of the methemoglobin percentage may be obtained.

Other topical agents which can affect anesthetic management are mafenide and povidone-iodine. Mafenide is readily absorbed into the systemic circulation and inhibits the enzyme carbonic anhydrase, resulting in metabolic acidosis. Povidone-iodine ointment can produce metabolic acidosis via direct nephrotoxicity. In addition, the high osmolality of this ointment causes substantial free water loss into the burn wound leading to hypernatremia and intravascular volume loss.[105]

Respiratory failure in the burn patient may be multifactorial (see above). While smoke inhalation is an obvious cause of some of this dysfunction, it is also true that burn injury itself, even when the burn does not involve the chest wall, can cause respiratory sequellae. This is likely to be the result of complement activation, prostanoid production, and/or release of oxygen free radicals and can be complicated by chest wall edema due to generalized changes in capillary permeability, which occur during the resuscitation phase.[38–43] The magnitude of the restrictive ventilatory defect caused by chest wall edema is significantly increased by chest wall burns and eschar formation. Further compromise may occur if diaphragmatic excursion is impaired by ileus, pain, or abdominal eschar.

Smoke inhalation can injure the respiratory system by causing a variety of problems, including chemical tracheobronchitis with mucosal sloughing; diminished surfactant activity, which can lead to micro- and macroatelectasis; bronchoconstriction; intraalveolar hemorrhage; deposition of platelets, fibrin microaggregates, and microthrombi in the pulmonary vasculature; altered pulmonary capillary permeability and increased transpulmonary fluid flux; interstitial pulmonary edema; and the adult respiratory distress syndrome. The adverse physiologic effects of these processes that can be predicted include diminished lung volumes, reduced lung compliance, and compromised expiratory flow rates.[36,106–108] The work of breathing, airway resistance, venous admixture, pulmonary artery pressure and pulmonary vascular resistance all increase.[109,110] Mismatches in ventilation and perfusion result in dead space ventilation and shunting.[111,112]

At the time of the preoperative visit, the degree of pulmonary disease should be determined, the current level of respiratory support should be noted, and an assessment of the adequacy (blood gas values) of this support should be made. Because of the additional respiratory depression caused by anesthetic agents, it is almost a certainty that the patient's pulmonary status will be no better in the immediate postoperative period than it was just prior to surgery. The utility of evaluating the level and adequacy of respiratory support before surgery lies in the fact that successful preoperative ventilatory settings are the best guide for intraoperative and postoperative management. Burn patients are hypermetabolic[113,114] and exhibit increased levels of oxygen consumption and carbon dioxide production (in addition to elevated systolic and diastolic pressures, pulse rate, cardiac output, core temperature, and minute ventilation). These factors make it difficult to predict the correct ventilator settings in any given patient and force the anesthesiologist to rely on those which have been demonstrated to result in satisfactory uptake of oxygen and elimination of carbon dioxide.

The integrity of the endotracheal tube (ETT) should be ensured before surgery. In the interest of patient safety, all members of the burn care team should be informed of the ideal location of the ETT. A useful practice is to prominently display in the patient's room a sign indicating the size of the tube and its correct depth (referenced in centimeters to the incisors, gums, or nares, as appropriate) after radiographic confirmation of satisfactory placement. This allows immediate recognition if the ETT is dislodged during nursing care, dressing changes, or transport to the operating room, and minimizes the interval of either extubation or endobronchial intubation.

Physical Examination and Laboratory Data Documentation of a current physical examination is always indicated before anesthesia, with an emphasis on the cardiopulmonary and neurologic systems. It is important to auscultate for murmurs that may indicate valvular or papillary muscle dysfunction and for the presence of an early diastolic gallop which may be the initial sign of congestive heart failure in a patient without a pulmonary artery catheter. Adventitious breath sounds are likely to be present in any burn patient, but wheezing may indicate a reversible component of airway obstruction, which requires postoperative or intraoperative bronchodilators. The identification of impairments of neurologic function is important both for postoperative comparison and, where the level of consciousness is already depressed, as an indication of a decreased need for anesthetic agents.

A review of the patient's current laboratory data is necessary because critically ill patients change very rapidly. Abnormalities of standard laboratory blood tests (electrolytes, glucose, hematocrit, coagulation studies, and renal and hepatic function measurements) need to be accurately noted prior to anesthesia, even though they usually do not necessitate a delay in surgery. Arterial blood gases and a chest x-ray should be evaluated close to the time of operation. Either of these may reveal an unexpected deterioration in pulmonary function, such as might be caused by a collapsed lobe or a small pneumothorax, and might require treatment before surgery can proceed. A recent preoperative electrocardiogram should also be reviewed.

Surgical Plan At the time of the preoperative anesthesia visit, inquiry should be made concerning which areas are to be debrided and grafted, approximately what percentage of the BSA will be affected, and whether any or all of the procedures will be performed with the patient in a position other than supine. This allows the anesthesiologist to plan in advance the placement of monitoring equipment, the magnitude of fluid and blood products to be required, and the placement of additional intravenous access or invasive monitoring devices, if indicated. The overall purpose of the preanesthetic visit is emphasized in this inquiry: to maximize communication among the burn team members and plan all aspects of the operative procedure in advance as much as possible. Doing so eliminates time-consuming last minute surprises in the operating room and results in better, more efficient patient care.

Transport to and from the Operating Room

Transfer of the intubated patient with burns and inhalational injury from the ICU to the operating room can be extremely hazardous. It entails removal of a critically ill patient from the relatively safe and controlled ICU environment and transportation through hallways and corridors. Measures must be taken to ensure the patient's safety in areas where little if any help may be available. In some institutions, transfer necessitates the use of an elevator, a situation which completely separates the transport team from the rest of the world for some period of time. This team should be able to provide emergency medical care in isolation and therefore must be prepared to perform reintubation and advanced cardiac life support. At least two anesthesia personnel are usually required to manage the airway, observe the monitors, and administer medications in such emergency situations. In preparation for transport, consideration should be given to establishing monitoring for use during transfer and to how ventilatory support is to be continued during this difficult interval. If the patient is combative, the use of sedatives and muscle relaxants should also be contemplated.

Monitoring Critically ill patients do not require less intense monitoring in hallways and elevators than they do in the ICU; therefore, consideration should be given to the use of continuous displays of ECG, arterial pressure, and arterial oxygen saturation (Sa_{O_2}) by using portable, battery-powered instruments during transport. Sa_{O_2} monitoring is especially valuable for intubated patients as it can assist in identification of a dislodged endotracheal tube (extubation or endobronchial intubation).

The metabolic rate in patients with major burns is markedly elevated,[113,115] especially when these patients are receiving nutritional support.[116] Because of this, it can be difficult to accurately estimate ventilatory requirements, and a capnometer can be useful; however, portable, battery-powered capnometers are not yet widely available. Finally, continuous auscultation of the heart and breath sounds should be performed by means of a precordial or esophageal stethoscope.

Temperature monitoring is not usually performed during transfer to the operating room. Both evaporative and convective heat loss should be expected during this period, because the ambient temperature is low, and burn patients have suffered loss of cutaneous insulation. To ameliorate this potential problem, the patient should be covered with plastic wraps and warm blankets before initiating transfer.

Ventilatory Support Special attention must be paid to the means by which oxygenation and ventilation will be accomplished during transport because of the severe nature of pulmonary dysfunction occurring in patients with both inhalational injury and surface burns. It is often necessary to use a system which is capable of delivering 100% oxygen, positive end-expiratory pressure (PEEP), and very high inspiratory pressures and doing so for an extended period of time. Special care may be required in the selection of a breathing apparatus and oxygen supply for these patients.

Most of the standard bag-valve systems do not provide 100% oxygen unless high flow rates are used and a reservoir component is added to the system. Also, most of these systems cannot provide PEEP and contain a rather inconveniently bulky nonrebreathing valve located immediately proximal to the patient, through which inspired gas must flow.[117] The location of this valve adds considerable respiratory resistance,[118] and the valve can become dysfunctional from the condensation of respiratory moisture.[117] Other potential problems with these devices include a tendency for respiratory obstruction to occur when minute ventilation exceeds inspiratory flow and the possibility that very high fresh gas flows may jam the valve in the inspiratory position. Because of these drawbacks, this type of breathing system is often unsuitable for the support of burn patients with elevated ventilatory requirements.

A better alternative for the transport of critically ill patients is the use of an anesthesia gas delivery apparatus, such as the Mapleson D system. The system does not suffer from the problems encountered in the standard manual resuscitators because the expiratory valve is not interposed between the fresh gas flow and the patient.[119] In addition, fresh gas (oxygen) is introduced close to the patient, so that during controlled ventilation the flushing effect of fresh gas flow forces alveolar and dead space gas out the expiratory valve, and rebreathing is twice the minute ventilation.[120,121] Additionally, the universal arm utilized with the Mapleson D system provides an airway pressure manometer, and PEEP can be obtained through adjustments in the expiratory valve and the manual pressure applied to the reservoir bag.

One oxygen tank may be inadequate for transfer of a burn patient to the operating room. The oxygen container most commonly used during patient transport is an E cylinder, which contains approximately 620 liters of oxygen when filled (regulator reads 2200 psi). The multiplication product of the expected length of time required for transport and the oxygen flow required for manual ventilation is the total volume of oxygen needed. This total can be compared to the 620 liters in a full tank, and the number of tanks needed for transfer (including emergency spares) can be determined.

It is not uncommon for a burn patient to require as much as 30 L/min of fresh gas flow to support ventilation. To provide such a high flow, two tanks may be yoked together, as the standard regulators are limited at 15 to 20 L/min. In such cases, it may be helpful to perform a trial of no less than 5 minutes of oxygenation and ventilation using the breathing system that will be employed during transport, while the patient is still attached to all the monitoring systems in the ICU. If there is any doubt about the adequacy of the portable breathing system at that point, arterial blood gases can be obtained for confirmation. Occasionally, the degree of pulmonary dysfunction will be so great that respiratory function simply cannot be supported during transfer to the operating room, and surgery will remain impossible until clinical improvement occurs. If a trial period in the ICU is not attempted, hypoxemia, hypertension, and arrhythmias will rapidly develop in the hallway or elevator, and will most likely lead to the patient's death unless mechanical ventilation is reinstituted.

At times, the patient is so combative as to impede effective ventilation and oxygenation, and safe transfer to the operating room can only be effected if sedatives and muscle relaxants are administered. Benzodiazepines are safe in these patients if amnesia is desired, and only nondepolarizing muscle relaxants should be used (see above).

Diazepam is effective, but its half-life is shortened in burn patients due to their hypermetabolism. With repeated dosing, however, active metabolites accumulate because of impaired hepatic function, and prolonged sedation results.[78,122] The concomitant use of cimetidine further reduces diazepam clearance, a property not shared by ranitidine. Ranitidine, however, has been shown to potentiate the soporific effect of midazolam.[123]

It is usually acceptable to produce long-term sedation around the time of surgery in patients with respiratory failure because they will require continued mechanical ventilatory support after the operative procedure. Likewise, delayed recovery from NDMRs is rarely disadvantageous, hence large doses may be given to ensure complete relaxation during transfer. For example, some burn patients may require and receive in excess of 0.4 mg/kg of pancuronium to achieve the desired effect.

Operating Room Care

When the patient arrives in the operating room, the initial tasks are to switch from the portable ventilatory support and monitoring systems to the operating room equipment. Next, any additional monitoring devices are applied, and other intravascular lines, if needed, are started. Further muscle relaxant and anesthetic agents are added, and the patient is positioned for surgery. Thereafter, anesthetic agents are administered and pulmonary and cardiovascular support are provided for the duration of the operative procedure. At the conclusion of the operation, the process is reversed, and the portable ventilation and monitoring systems are again utilized during transfer back to the ICU. During the intraoperative period, the aspects of anesthetic care which are unique in burn patients with respiratory failure are monitoring, temperature control, and alterations in pulmonary and cardiovascular function.

Monitoring Monitoring of hemodynamics and gas exchange during anesthesia is standard in all patients and of great value in burn patients, especially those with respiratory failure. Burn injury and the means to treat it often makes the application of ECG leads, blood pressure cuffs, and pulse oximeters difficult. When the burn involves the limbs or chest, the only way to achieve ECG contact may be via needle electrodes, and measurements of blood pressure by cuff may not be possible at all. The treatment of respiratory failure usually includes the insertion of an arterial catheter. If this has not been done before surgery and if no limb is free of injury, a femoral arterial line is usually required for blood pressure monitoring. An axillary artery is an alternative site.

Noninvasive estimation of the efficacy of gas exchange by the use of oximeters and capnometers is becoming standard practice in anesthetic care. Oximeters are generally accurate for saturations in the range of 22 to 100%[124] if an adequate signal can be achieved. Unfortunately, burns of the face and extremities often preclude satisfactory placement of an oximeter probe. Burn injury does not lead to technical difficulties with the use of a capnometer, which is a useful device because it may provide early detection of a disconnected breathing circuit or a dislodged, misplaced or obstructed endotracheal tube.[125] The capnometer also reflects trends in the adequacy of ventilation as a means of removal of carbon dioxide. Auscultation of heart tones and breath sounds and measurement of temperature and urine output are also not affected by burn injury.

Temperature Control Intraoperative heat loss by convection, conduction, radiation, and evaporation is incurred by all patients undergoing surgery and anesthesia.[126,127] Convective loss is caused by the high rate of airflow peculiar to operating rooms, conductive loss by direct contact of body tissues with cold surfaces and solutions, and radiation of heat by the low environmental temperatures. Evaporative cooling occurs in the skin and respiratory tree, especially if there are large areas of disruption or loss of skin coverage.[128,129]

For the burn patient, the significance of heat loss is compounded by the hypermetabolic state which follows burn injury and results in a need to maintain a higher than normal core temperature. During surgery the body temperature falls because the anesthetic agents prevent homeostatic mechanisms from counteracting heat loss. General anesthetics reduce peripheral and central receptor sensitivity to cold, depress the thermoregulatory center, and produce peripheral vasodilatation.[126,130,131] Skeletal muscle relaxants eliminate shivering, thereby impeding thermogenesis.[132,133] After recovery from anesthesia, homeostatic mechanisms once again become functional, and there is intense shivering, which greatly increases the consumption of oxygen and calories.[134–136]

The best remedy for intraoperative heat loss is prevention. The most effective means for heat conservation is through the elimination of evaporative losses from the lung. The anesthesia circuit can be adapted to provide heated and humidified gas inflow to the patient.[137] To reduce radiant, conductive, and convective heat loss, the ambient temperature in the operating room should be maintained above 25°C, and a heating blanket or a radiant heat lamp used. Intravenous and topical solutions should be warmed, and all areas of the patient not included in the surgical field should be covered and insulated.

Pulmonary Function While the inhalation of large amounts of smoke appears to have no major effects on pulmonary mechanics and perfusion in the early postinjury period,[138] this is not the case several days later (see above). Clinically, many of these patients develop the adult respiratory distress syndrome (ARDS) accompanied by tracheobronchitis. Abdominal or chest wall burns may add a superimposed restrictive ventilatory defect.[139] Thus, there may be restrictive and obstructive defects present along with an impairment of diffusion of gases.

The administration of general anesthesia to these patients generally worsens their deficits. In healthy subjects, the functional residual capacity (FRC) and compliance (C_L) are reduced, airway resistance (R_{aw}) is increased, and ventilation-perfusion (V/Q) matching is impaired. All of these effects are seen in burn victims.

FRC is reduced during anesthesia in healthy subjects by a mean value of 15 to 20 percent.[140–142] This is probably due to a decrease in diaphragmatic muscle tension and an increase in abdominal expiratory muscle tension[143,144] at end expiration. These alterations in muscle function allow ascent of the diaphragm into the chest, thereby diminishing lung volumes.[145,146] In some ventilatory units, where the closing capacity lies within the tidal volume, this decline in FRC leads to airway closure.[147] Compliance of the lung is reduced during anesthesia,[145,148–150] but it is unclear whether this is a direct effect of the anesthetics on pulmonary surfactant or secondary to the reduced FRC.[151] The removal of pulmonary secretions is hindered, and this may potentiate the loss of lung volume and atelectasis.[147]

The reduction in lung volumes also results in reduced airway caliber, which increases airway resistance and promotes airway collapse.[141,152–154] This effect is partially offset by the bronchodilatation that results from anesthetic gases.[154–156] Anesthetics increase ventilation/perfusion mismatching and worsen venous admixture[157] by increasing the alveolar component of physiologic dead space.[158] They may also impede the tendency of the lungs to correct V/Q mismatching through hypoxic pulmonary vasoconstriction.[159]

The best initial ventilator settings during surgery are those which were successful in achieving adequate oxygenation and carbon dioxide removal in the ICU. Deteriorations in both parameters may be expected during the operative procedure. Increases in inspired oxygen concentration and in PEEP are the usual means to improve oxygenation, while alterations in respiratory rate and tidal volume are required to improve carbon dioxide excretion.

When oxygenation is severely compromised, 100% oxygen is usually required. This may lead to absorption atelectasis,[160] a condition in which areas of the lung are converted from a condition of low ventilation relative to perfusion (low V/Q), into areas of atelectasis (V/Q = 0), with right-to-left shunting.[161] PEEP is often successful in preventing closure of some of these areas of the lung, and thus may improve oxygenation. It may enlarge alveolar size, recruit collapsed alveoli, increase lung volumes, reduce airway resistance, and improve compliance.[162–164]

In some instances, however, PEEP may compromise tissue O_2 delivery. While it has been the presumption that low lung compliance in acute lung injury limited airway pressure transmission to the pleural space and thereby protected against the untoward hemodynamic effects of PEEP therapy,[160] it has recently been suggested that this is not the case.[165] PEEP applied to poorly compliant lungs caused a significant reduction in cardiac output, stroke volume, mean arterial pressure, left ventricular and diastolic pressure, and oxygen delivery, while increasing both pulmonary and systemic vascular resistances.

Removal of carbon dioxide is impeded by the increases in dead space ventilation which occur in patients with smoke inhalation.[45,112,166] Additionally, CO_2 production increases proportionally with size of the cutaneous burn,[167] and is affected by the composition of the nutritional support the patient receives. Both factors further increase ventilatory requirements.

Large glucose loads have been demonstrated to increase CO_2 production.[168,169] Replacing glucose with intravenous lipid emulsions is helpful, but lipid infusions may contribute to hypoxemia in patients with damaged lungs. This was previously attributed to increased triglyceride levels, but it is now believed that the observed decreases in arterial oxygen tension result from ventilation-perfusion inequalities caused by increases in prostaglandin production.[170–174]

Increases in ventilation can be accomplished with either higher tidal volumes, faster respiratory rates, or both. Large tidal volumes delivered at slow rates are usually successful if the diseased region of lung is composed primarily of units with prolonged time constants. This condition is characterized by ventilatory obstruction with elevated airway resistance, low expiratory flow rates, and the need for a prolonged expiratory time (slow respiratory rate). On the other hand, when the diseased lung units have shortened time constants, they fill and empty rapidly but usually have diminished compliance. This reduction in compliance, characteristic of restrictive lung disease, is responsible for very high ventilatory pressures and a risk of barotrauma if large tidal volumes are attempted. With small tidal volumes, this problem is avoided.[175,176]

Smoke inhalation produces a diffuse injury with varying degrees of both obstruction and restriction, making it difficult to predict in advance whether increases in P_{CO_2} will be best treated with an increase in respiratory rate or in tidal volume. Sometimes, when expiratory airflow obstruction is prominent, increasing the inspiratory flow rate is beneficial because it shortens inspiratory time while increasing the time for exhalation. However, the high inspiratory flow rate often requires a high pressure, which can be harmful to the patient, and may be unobtainable by the operating room ventilator.

High levels of minute ventilation, especially in the presence of increased airway resistance, can also lead to barotrauma by causing a condition called intrinsic or auto-PEEP.[177] At high respiratory rates and tidal volumes, the expiratory phase may become too short to allow the lungs to deflate before the next inspiratory phase begins. When this happens, alveolar pressure remains positive throughout the breathing cycle and intrathoracic pressures are elevated. Venous return and cardiac output can also be impaired by auto-PEEP.

Cardiovascular Function Profound alterations in the cardiovascular system occur after thermal injury. Cardiovascular performance during the burn surgery is determined by whatever cardiac disease the patient had before injury and influenced by the burn injury itself, the anesthetic agents used, the degree of respiratory dysfunction, and the operative blood loss.

Immediately post burn, there is an increase in vascular permeability in the area of the burn. For burns greater than 30 percent total BSA, this permeability becomes generalized and results in a massive loss of intravascular volume, and cardiac output is reduced far more than would be anticipated solely on the basis of the diminished plasma volume.[178] The reason for this exaggerated fall in cardiac output is believed to be a circulating myocardial depressant factor.[179–182] The systemic vascular resistance (SVR) is significantly elevated for the first 24 hours after the burn, becomes normal by 24 hours, but is significantly reduced by 72 hours following the burn.[183] Cardiac output also normalizes by 36 hours and then rises to supernormal levels, indicating the onset of a hypermetabolic state.

A consistent hemodynamic change observed during surgery and anesthesia is a decrease in cardiac output.[184] All of the intravenous and inhalational anesthetics currently in use are potential myocardial depressants,[185] an effect which is usually potentiated in diseased or injured hearts. The volatile anesthetics halothane, enflurane, isoflurane, and nitrous oxide are widely recognized to produce dose-related myocardial depression,[186–190] antagonism of sympathetic vasoconstriction, and direct vasodilatation. Ketamine is often used as an alternative because it is known to produce sympathetic stimulation in healthy subjects.[57,191] In burn patients, ketamine often supports the blood pressure and cardiac output well; however, it too has been shown to be a direct myocardial depressant.[192] In catecholamine-depleted patients and in patients dependent upon a high level of sympathetic activity, ketamine can reduce sympathetic stimulation and cause cardiovascular collapse.[185,193] For a patient whose myocardium cannot even tolerate ketamine, an amnestic agent such as scopolamine may be the only recourse.

The functions of the pulmonary and cardiovascular systems are so intertwined that deterioration of one often dramatically effects the other.[194] Positive pressure ventilation influences systemic venous return, pulmonary vascular resistance, pulmonary venous return, and right and left ventricular output.[194,195] PEEP, increased minute ventilation, and elevated airway and alveolar pressures have been demonstrated to reduce systemic venous return and diminish output from both ventricles.[196]

Hypovolemia compounds this impairment of circulatory flow. Hemorrhage is an anticipated complication with the surgical debridement of burns, but both the volume and suddenness of blood loss can be overwhelming. For each 1 percent of BSA excised, approximately 3 to 4 percent of the total blood volume may be rapidly lost,[197–199] especially if the surgical team debrides the burn and harvests the donor site simultaneously. Secure intravenous access of adequate caliber and readily available blood products are mandatory as hypovolemia often results in a profound depression of cardiac output and blood pressure. For many patients, the first unit of intraoperative blood transfusion should begin at the time of surgical incision, for visual estimates of blood loss are often inaccurate, and the ultimate need to transfuse during the procedure is ensured.

CONCLUSION

Inhalational injuries and associated major burns place their victims in a life-threatening condition which may last for many months. The technical and physiologic problems which complicate the anesthetic management of these patients require meticulous attention to every detail of medical care as well as coordination of the efforts of the various members of the burn care team.

REFERENCES

1. Welch GW: Anesthesia for the thermally injured patient, in Artz CP, Moncrief JA, Pruitt BA (eds): *Burns: A Team Approach*. Philadelphia, Saunders, 1979, pp 299–306.
2. Mallory TB, Brickley WJ: Pathology: With special reference to the pulmonary lesions. *Ann Surg* 117:865, 1943.
3. Horovitz JH: Abnormalities caused by smoke inhalation, editorial. *J Trauma* 19(suppl):915, 1979.
4. Horovitz JH: Diagnostic tools for use in smoke inhalation, editorial. *J Trauma* 21(suppl):717, 1981.
5. Crapo RO: Smoke-inhalation injuries. *JAMA* 246:1694, 1981.
6. Herndon DN, Langner F, Thompson P, et al: Pulmonary

injury in burned patients. *Surg Clin North Am* 67:31, 1987.

7. Cahalane M, Demling RH: Early respiratory abnormalities from smoke inhalation. *JAMA* 251:771, 1984.
8. Herndon DN, Thompson PB, Traber DL: Pulmonary injury in burned patients. *Crit Care Clin* 1:79, 1985.
9. Dyer RF, Esch VH: Polyvinyl choloride toxicity in fires. *JAMA* 235:393, 1976.
10. Moylan JA: Inhalation injury. *J Trauma* 21(suppl):720, 1981.
11. Moritz AR, Henriques FC, McLean R: The effects of inhaled heat on the air passages and lungs. *Am J Pathol* 21:311, 1945.
12. Lamb JD: Anaesthetic considerations for major thermal injury. *Can Anaesth Soc J* 32:84, 1985.
13. Dreisbach RH: *Handbook of Poisoning: Diagnosis & Treatment*, Los Altos, Lange Medical Publishing, 1974.
14. Barker SJ, Tremper KK: The effect of carbon monoxide inhalation on pulse oximetry and transcutaneous P_{O_2}. *Anesthesiology* 66:677, 1987.
15. Demling RH: Postgraduate course: Respiratory Injury Part III. *J Burn Care Rehabil* 7:277, 1986.
16. Skold G, Brunk U: Respiratory tract inflammation after exposure to fire smoke. *Acta Pathol Microbiol Immunol Scand* 52:19, 1961.
17. Alpert S, Levenson SM: Respiratory tract injury associated with burns. *NY J Med* 70:1633, 1970.
18. Reed GF, Camp HL: Upper airway problems in severely burned patients. *Ann Otol Rhinol Laryngol* 78:741, 1969.
19. Beal DD, Conner GH: Respiratory tract injury: A guide to management following thermal and smoke injury. *Laryngoscope* 80:25, 1970.
20. Webster JR, McCabe MM, Karp M: Recognition and management of smoke inhalation. *JAMA* 201:287, 1967.
21. Beecher HK: Resuscitation and sedation of patients with burns which include the airway: Some problems of immediate therapy. *Ann Surg* 117:825, 1943.
22. Haponik EF, Meyers DA, Munster AM, et al: Acute upper airway injury in burn patients. *Am Rev Respir Dis* 135:360, 1987.
23. Foley FD: The burn autopsy: Fatal complications of burns. *Am J Clin Pathol* 52:1, 1969.
24. Haponik EF, Munster AM, Wise RA, et al: Upper airway function in burn patients: Correlation of flow-volume curves and nasopharyngoscopy. *Am Rev Respir Dis* 129:251, 1984.
25. Heimbach D: Inhalation injury, in Wachtel TL, Frank DH (eds): *Burns of the Head and Neck*. Philadelphia, Saunders, 1984, pp 15–23.
26. Jung RC: Respiratory tract burns after aspiration of hot coffee. *Chest* 72:125, 1977.
27. Wanner A, Cutchavaree A: Early recognition of upper airway obstruction following smoke inhalation. *Am Rev Respir Dis* 180:1421, 1973.
28. Moylan JA, Adib K, Birnbaum M: Fiberoptic bronchoscopy following thermal injury. *Surg Gynecol Obstet* 140:541, 1975.
29. Hunt JL, Agee RN, Pruitt BA: Fiberoptic bronchoscopy in acute inhalation injury. *J Trauma* 15:641, 1975.
30. Wachtel TL, Long WB, Frank HA: Thermal injuries of the upper respiratory tract, in Wachtel TL, Frank DH (eds): *Burns of the Head and Neck*. Philadelphia, Saunders, 1984, pp 7–14.
31. Wroblewski DA, Bower GC: The significance of facial burns in acute smoke inhalation. *Crit Care Med* 7:335, 1979.
32. Zawacki BE, Jung RC, Joyce J, et al: Smoke, burns, and the natural history of inhalation injury in fire victims: A correlation of experimental and clinical data. *Ann Surg* 185:100, 1977.
33. Moncrief JA: Tracheostomy in burns. *Arch Surg* 79:45, 1959.
34. Stone HH, Rhame DW, Corbitt JD, et al: Respiratory burns: A correlation of clinical and laboratory results. *Ann Surg* 165:157, 1967.
35. Trunkey DD: Inhalation injury. *Surg Clin North Am* 58:1133, 1978.
36. Nieman GF, Clark WR, Wax SD, et al: The effect of smoke inhalation on pulmonary surfactant. *Ann Surg* 191:171, 1980.
37. Aub JC, Pittman H, Brues AM: The pulmonary complications: A clinical description. *Ann Surg* 117:834, 1943.
38. Demling RH, Will JA, Belzer FO: The effect of major thermal injury on the pulmonary microcirculation. *Surgery* 83:746, 1978.
39. Demling RH, Wong C, Jin LJ, et al: Early lung dysfunction after major burns: Role of edema and vasoactive mediators. *J Trauma* 25:959, 1985.
40. Demling RH, Wenger H, Lalonde CC, et al: Endotoxin-induced prostanoid production by the burn wound can cause distant lung dysfunction. *Surgery* 99:421, 1986.
41. Katz A, Ryan P, Lalond C, et al: Topical ibuprofen decreases thromboxane release from the endotoxin-stimulated burn wound. *J Trauma* 26:157, 1986.
42. Till GO, Beauchamp C, Menapace D, et al: Oxygen radical dependent lung damage following thermal injury of rat skin. *J Trauma* 23:269, 1983.
43. Till GO, Hatherill JR, Tourtellotte WW, et al: Lipid peroxidation and acute lung injury after thermal trauma to skin. *Am J Pathol* 119:376, 1985.
44. Demling RH, Kramer G, Harms B: Role of thermal injury-induced hypoproteinemia on fluid flux and protein permeability in burned and non-burned tissue. *Surgery* 95:136, 1984.
45. Stephenson SF, Esrig BC, Polk HC, et al: The pathophysiology of smoke inhalation injury. *Ann Surg* 182:652, 1975.
46. Stone HH, Martin JD: Pulmonary injury associated with thermal burns. *Surg Gynecol Obstet* 129:1242, 1969.
47. Luterman A, Dasco CC, Curreri PW: Infections in burn patients. *Am J Med* 81:45, 1986.
48. Chu CS: New concepts of pulmonary burn injury. *J Trauma* 21:958, 1981.
49. Bartlett RH: Types of respiratory injury. *J Trauma* 19(suppl):918, 1979.
50. Achauer BM, Allyn PA, Furnas DW, et al: Pulmonary complications of burns: The major threat to the burn patient. *Ann Surg* 177:311, 1973.

51. Alexander JW: Burn care: A specialty in evolution — 1985 presidential address, American Burn Association. *J Trauma* 26:1, 1986.
52. Moore FD, Davis C, Rodrick M, et al: Neutrophil activation in thermal injury as assessed by increased expression of complement receptors. *N Engl J Med* 314:948, 1986.
53. Fick RB, Paul ES, Merrill WW, et al: Alterations in the antibacterial properties of rabbit pulmonary macrophages exposed to wood smoke. *Am Rev Respir Dis* 129:76, 1984.
54. Demarest GB, Hudson LD, Altman LC: Impaired alveolar macrophage chemotaxis in patients with acute smoke inhalation. *Am Rev Respir Dis* 119:279, 1979.
55. Stratta RJ, Warden GD, Ninnemann JL, et al: Immunologic parameters in burned patients: Effect of therapeutic interventions. *J Trauma* 26:7, 1986.
56. Moran K, Munster AM: Alterations of the host defense mechanism in burned patients. *Surg Clin North Am* 67:47, 1987.
57. White PF, Way WL, Trevor AJ: Ketamine — Its pharmacology and therapeutic uses. *Anesthesiology* 56:119, 1982.
58. Mendelson CL: The aspiration of stomach contents into the lungs during obstetric anesthesia. *Am J Obstet Gynecol* 52:191, 1946.
59. Arms RA, Dines DE, Tinstman TC: Aspiration pneumonia. *Chest* 65:136, 1974.
60. Awe WC, Fletcher WS, Jacob SW: The pathophysiology of aspiration pneumonitis. *Surgery* 60:232, 1966.
61. Cameron JL, Mitchell WH, Zuidema GD: Aspiration pneumonia: Clinical outcome following documented aspiration. *Arch Surg* 106:49, 1973.
62. Dines DE, Titus JL, Sessler AD: Aspiration pneumonitis. *Mayo Clin Proc* 45:347, 1970.
63. Cameron JL, Caldini P, Toung JK, et al: Aspiration pneumonia: Pathophysiologic data following experimental aspiration. *Surgery* 72:238, 1972.
64. Hatton F, Tiret L, Vourch'h G, et al: Morbidity and mortality associated with anesthesia — French survey: Preliminary results, in Vickers MD, Lunn JN (eds): *Mortality in Anesthesia*. Berlin, Springer-Verlag, 1983, pp 25–38.
65. Rosen M: Maternal mortality associated with anaesthesia in England and Wales, in Vickers MD, Lunn JN (eds): *Mortality in Anesthesia*. Berlin, Springer-Verlag, 1983, pp 39–44.
66. Norlander O, Hallen B: Anesthetic mortality and pulmonary function, in Vickers MD, Lunn JN (eds): *Mortality in Anesthesia*. Berlin, Springer-Verlag, 1983, pp 59–68.
67. Giesecke AH, Egbert LD: Anesthesia for trauma surgery, in Miller RD (ed): *Anesthesia*. New York, Churchill Livingstone, 1986, pp 1819–1835.
68. Gibbs CP, Banner TC: Effectiveness of Bicitra as a preoperative antacid. *Anesthesiology* 61:97, 1984.
69. Eyler SW, Cullen BF, Murphy ME, et al: Antacid aspiration in rabbits: A comparison of Mylanta and Bicitra. *Anesth Analg* 61:288, 1982.
70. Holdsworth JD, Johnson K, Mascall G, et al: Mixing of antacids with stomach contents: Another approach to the prevention of acid aspiration (Mendelson's) syndrome. *Anaesthesia* 35:641, 1980.
71. Gibbs CP, Schwartz DJ, Wynne JW, et al: Antacid pulmonary aspiration in the dog. *Anesthesiology* 51:380, 1979.
72. Sellick BA: Cricoid pressure to control regurgitation of stomach contents during induction of anesthesia. *Lancet* 2:404, 1961.
73. Sellick BA: Rupture of the oesophagus following cricoid pressure? *Anaesthesia* 37:213, 1982.
74. Notcutt WG: Rupture of the oesophagus following cricoid pressure? *Anaesthesia* 36:911, 1981.
75. Carden E, Friedman D: Further studies of manually operated self-inflating resuscitation bags. *Anesth Analg* 56:202, 1977.
76. Tunstall ME, Sheikh A: Failed intubation protocol: Oxygenation without aspiration. *Clin Anaesth* 4:171, 1986.
77. Myers RA, Linberg SE, Cowley RA, et al: Carbon monoxide poisoning: The injury and its treatment. *JACEP* 8:479, 1979.
78. Martyn JAJ: Clinical pharmacology and drug therapy in the burned patient. *Anesthesiology* 65:67, 1986.
79. Gronert GA, Theye RA: Pathophysiology of hyperkalemia induced by succinylcholine. *Anesthesiology* 43:89, 1975.
80. Schaner PJ, Brown RL, Kirksey TD, et al: Succinylcholine-induced hyperkalemia in burned patients. *Anesth Analg* 48:764, 1969.
81. Martyn JAJ, Goldhill DR, Goudsouzian NG: Clinical pharmacology of muscle relaxants in patients with burns. *J Clin Pharmacol* 26:680, 1986.
82. Martyn JAJ, Mattel RS, Greenblatt DJ, et al: Pharmacokinetics of *d*-tubocurarine in patients with thermal injury. *Anesth Analg* 61:241, 1982.
83. Dwersteg JF, Pavlin EG, Heimbach DM: Patients with burns are resistant to atracurium. *Anesthesiology* 65:517, 1986.
84. Hagen J, Martyn JAJ, Szyfelbein SK, et al: Cardiovascular and neuromuscular responses to high-dose pancuronium-metocurine in pediatric burned and reconstructive patients. *Anesth Analg* 65:1340, 1986.
85. Martyn JAJ, Goudsouzian NG, Matteo RS, et al: Metocurine requirements and plasma concentrations in burned paediatric patients. *Br J Anaesth* 55:263, 1983.
86. Mills A, Martyn JAJ: Evaluation of vecuronium neuromuscular blockade in pediatric patients with thermal injury. *Anaesth Analg* 66:S119, 1987.
87. Satiani B, Bonner JT, Stone HH: Factors influencing intraoperative gastric regurgitation: A prospective random study of nasal gastric tube drainage. *Arch Surg* 113:721, 1978.
88. Tullock WC, Diana P, Cook DR, et al: High dose vecuronium: Onset and duration. *Anesth Analg* 67:S235, 1988.
89. Pavlin EG: Anesthetic considerations, in Heimbach DM, Engrav LH (eds): *Surgical Management of the Burn Wound*. New York, Raven Press, 1984, pp 139–46.

90. Munster AM: *Burn Care for the House Officer.* Baltimore, Williams & Wilkins, 1980.
91. Burdge JJ, Katz B, Edwards R, et al: Surgical treatment of burns in elderly patients. *J Trauma* 28:214, 1988.
92. Chicarilli ZN, Cuono CB, Heinrich JJ, et al: Selective aggressive burn excision for high mortality subgroups. *J Trauma* 26:18, 1986.
93. Foy HM, Pavlin E, Heimbach DM: Excision and grafting of large burns: Operation length not related to increased morbidity. *J Trauma* 26:51, 1986.
94. Engrav LH, Heimbach DM, Rues JL, et al: Early excision and grafting vs non-operative treatment of burns of indeterminate depth: A randomized prospective study. *J Trauma* 23:1001, 1983.
95. Demling RH: Burns. *N Engl J Med* 313:1389, 1985.
96. Moncrief JA: Replacement therapy, in Artz CP, Moncrief JA, Pruitt BA (eds): *Burns: A Team Approach*. Philadelphia, Saunders, 1979, pp 169–92.
97. Cameron JS: Acute renal failure in the intensive care unit today. *Intensive Care Med* 12:64, 1986.
98. Coffi WG, Ashikaga T, Gamelli RL: Probability of surviving post operative acute renal failure: Development of a prognostic index. *Ann Surg* 200:205, 1984.
99. Butkus DE: Persistant high mortality in acute renal failure. *Arch Intern Med* 143:209, 1983.
100. Eklund J, Granberg PO, Liljedahl SO: Studies on renal function in burns. *Acta Chir Scand* 136:627, 1970.
101. Watkins WD, Leslie JB, DeBruijn NP: Pharmacologic principles, in Miller RD (ed): *Anesthesia,* 2d ed. New York, Churchill Livingstone, 1986, pp 55–73.
102. Martyn JAJ, Abernethy DR, Greenblatt DJ: Plasma protein binding of drugs after severe burn injury. *Clin Pharmacol Ther* 35:535, 1984.
103. Yelderman M, Corenmen J: Realtime oximetry, in Prakash O (ed): *Computing in Anesthesia and Intensive Care*. Boston, Martinus and Nijhoff, 1983, pp 328–41.
104. Barker SJ, Tremper KK, Hyatt J: Effects of methemoglobinemia on pulse oximetry and mixed venous oximetry. *Anesthesiology* 70:112, 1989.
105. Peterson HD: Topical antibacterials, in Boswick JA (ed): *The Art and Science of Burn Care*. Rockville, Md., Aspen, 1987, pp 181–87.
106. Whitener DR, Whitener LM, Robertson KJ, et al: Pulmonary function measurements in patients with thermal injury and smoke inhalation. *Am Rev Respir Dis* 122:731, 1980.
107. Nishimura N, Hiranuma N: Respiratory changes after major burn injury. *Crit Care Med* 10:25, 1982.
108. Petroff PA, Hander EW, Clayton WH, et al: Pulmonary function studies after smoke inhalation. *Am J Surg* 132:346, 1976.
109. Garzon AA, Seltzer B, Song IC, et al: Respiratory mechanics in patients with inhalation burns. *J Trauma* 10:57, 1970.
110. Asch MJ, Feldman RJ, Walker HJ, et al: Systemic and pulmonary hemodynamic changes accompanying thermal injury. *Ann Surg* 178:218, 1973.
111. Luce EA, Su CT, Hoopes JE: Alveolar-arterial oxygen gradient in the burn patient. *J Trauma* 16:212, 1976.
112. Robinson NB, Hudson LD, Robertson HT, et al: Ventilation and perfusion alterations after smoke inhalation injury. *Surgery* 90:352, 1981.
113. Wilmore DW: Nutrition and metabolism following thermal injury. *Clin Plast Surg* 1:603, 1974.
114. Popp MB, Friedberg DL, MacMillan BG: Clinical characteristics of hypertension in burned children. *Ann Surg* 191:473, 1980.
115. Wilmore DW, Long JM, Mason AD, et al: Catecholamines: Mediators of the hypermetabolic response to burn injury. *Ann Surg* 180:653, 1974.
116. Allard JP, Jeejheebhoy KN, Whitwell J, et al: Factors influencing energy expenditure in patients with burns. *J Trauma* 28:199, 1988.
117. Orkin FK: Anesthetic systems, in Miller RD (ed): *Anesthesia,* 2d ed. New York, Churchill Livingstone, 1986, pp 117–60.
118. Orkin LR, Siegal M, Rovenstine EA: Resistance to breathing by apparatus used in anesthesia: II. Valves in machines. *Anesth Analg* 36:19, 1957.
119. Conway CM: Anesthetic circuits, in Scurr C, Feldman S (eds): *Scientific Foundations of Anesthesia*. Chicago, Year Book Medical Publishers, 1974, pp 509–15.
120. Sykes MK: Rebreathing circuits: A review. *Br J Anaesth* 40:666, 1968.
121. Mapleson WW: The elimination of rebreathing in various semiclosed anaesthetic systems. *Br J Anaesth* 26:323, 1954.
122. Martyn JAJ, Greenblatt DJ, Quinby WC: Diazepam kinetics in patients with severe burns. *Anesth Analg* 62:293, 1983.
123. Kirsch W, Hoensch H, Janisch HD: Interactions and non-interactions with ranitidine. *Clin Pharmacokinet* 9:493, 1984.
124. Sendak MJ, Harris AP, Donham RT: Accuracy of pulse oximetry during arterial oxyhemoglobin desaturation in dogs. *Anesthesiology* 68:111, 1988.
125. Swedlow DB: Capnometry and capnography: An anesthesia disaster warning system. *Semin Anesth* 5:194, 1986.
126. Benazon D: Hypothermia, in Scurr C, Feldman S (eds): *Scientific Foundations of Anaesthesia*. Chicago, Year Book Medical Publishers, 1974, pp 344–57.
127. Stephen CR: Postoperative temperature changes. *Anesthesiology* 22:795, 1961.
128. Cork RC: Temperature monitoring, in Boitt CD (ed): *Monitoring in Anesthesia and Critical Care Medicine*. New York, Churchill Livingstone, 1985, pp 441–57.
129. Wilson RD: Anesthesia and the burned child. *Int Anesthesiol Clin* 13:203, 1975.
130. Theye RA, Michenfelder JD: The effect of halothane on canine cerebral metabolism. *Anesthesiology* 29:1113, 1968.
131. Foregger R: Surface temperatures during anesthesia. *Anesthesiology* 4:392, 1943.
132. Ham J, Miller RD, Benet LZ, et al: Pharmacokinetics and pharmacodynamics of *d*-tubocurarine during hypothermia in the cat. *Anesthesiology* 49:324, 1978.
133. Miller RD, Agoston S, Van der Pol F, et al: Hypothermia

in the pharmacokinetics and pharmacodynamics of pancuronium in the cat. *J Pharmacol Exp Ther* 207:532, 1978.
134. Wilmore DW, Mason AD, Johnson DW, et al: Effect of ambient temperature on heat production and heat loss in burn patients. *J Appl Physiol* 38:593, 1975.
135. Crabtree JH, Bowser BH, Campbell JW, et al: Energy metabolism in anesthetized children with burns. *Am J Surg* 140:832, 1980.
136. Caldwell FT, Bowser BH, Crabtree JH: The effect of occlusive dressings on the energy metabolism of severely burned children. *Ann Surg* 193:579, 1981.
137. Shelly MP, Lloyd GM, Park GR: A review of the mechanisms and methods of humidification of inspired gases. *Intensive Care Med* 14:1, 1988.
138. Prien T, Traber DL, Richardson JA, et al: Early effects of inhalation injury on lung mechanics and pulmonary perfusion. *Intensive Care Med* 14:25, 1988.
139. Demling RH, Crawford G, Lind L, et al: Restrictive pulmonary dysfunction caused by the grafted chest and abdominal burn. *Crit Care Med* 16:743, 1988.
140. Don HF, Robson JG: The mechanics of the respiratory system during anesthesia. *Anesthesiology* 26:168, 1965.
141. Brismar B, Hedenstierna G, Lundquist H, et al: Pulmonary densities during anesthesia with muscle relaxation — A proposal of atelectasis. *Anesthesiology* 62:422, 1985.
142. Hedenstierna G, Strandberg A, Brismar B, et al: Functional residual capacity, thoracoabdominal dimensions and central blood volume during general anesthesia with muscle paralysis and mechanical ventilation. *Anesthesiology* 62:247, 1985.
143. Don HF, Wahba M, Cuadrado L, et al: The effects of anesthesia in 100 percent oxygen on the functional residual capacity of the lungs. *Anesthesiology* 32:521, 1970.
144. Freund F, Roos A, Dodd RB: Expiratory activity of the abdominal muscles in man during general anesthesia. *J Appl Physiol* 19:693, 1964.
145. Westbrook PR, Stubbs SE, Sessler AD, et al: Effects of anesthesia and muscle paralysis on respiratory mechanics in normal man. *J Appl Physiol* 34:81, 1973.
146. Marsh HM, Southorn PA, Rehder K: Anesthesia, sedation, and the chest wall. *Int Anesthesiol Clin* 22(4):1, 1984.
147. Foltz BD, Benumof JL: Mechanisms of hypoxemia and hypercapnia in the perioperative period. *Crit Care Clin* 3:269, 1987.
148. Rehder K, Sessler AD, Marsh HM: General anesthesia and the lung. *Am Rev Respir Dis* 112:541, 1975.
149. Marsh HM, Rehder K, Knopp JJ: Analgesia, anesthesia, and chest wall motion. An editorial. *Anesthesiology* 55:493, 1981.
150. Schmidt ER, Rehder K: General anesthesia and the chest wall. *Anesthesiology* 55:668, 1981.
151. Nunn JF: Respiratory aspects of anesthesia, in: *Applied Respiratory Physiology,* 3d ed. London, Butterworths, 1987, pp 350–78.
152. Mead J, Agostoni E: Dynamics of breathing, in Fenn WO, Rahn H (eds): *Handbook of Physiology, Respiration,* vol 1. Baltimore, Williams and Wilkins, 1964, pp 411–27.
153. Tokics L, Hedenstierna G, Strandberg A, et al: Lung collapse and gas exchange during anesthesia: Effects of spontaneous breathing, muscle paralysis, and positive end-expiratory pressure. *Anesthesiology* 66:157, 1987.
154. Lehane JR: The effect of anesthesia on airway caliber. *Int Anesthesiol Clin* 22(4):29, 1984.
155. Lehane JR, Jordan C, Jones JG: Influence of halothane and enflurane on respiratory airflow resistance and specific conductance in anaesthetized man. *Br J Anaesth* 52:773, 1980.
156. Heneghan CPH, Bergman NA, Jordan C, et al: Effect of isoflurane on bronchomotor tone in man. *Br J Anaesth* 58:24, 1986.
157. Nunn JF: Oxygen — Friend or foe. *J R Soc Med* 78:618, 1985.
158. Nunn JF, Hill DW: Respiratory dead space and arterial to end-tidal CO_2 tension difference in anesthetized man. *J Appl Physiol* 15:383, 1960.
159. Marshall BE, Marshall C: Anesthesia and pulmonary circulation, in Covino BG, Fozzard HA, Rehder K, Strichartz G (eds): *Effects of Anesthesia*. Bethesda, American Physiologic Society, 1985, pp 121–36.
160. Chapin JC, Downs JB, Douglas ME, et al: Lung expansion and airway pressure transmission, with positive end-expiratory pressure. *Arch Surg* 114:1193, 1979.
161. Wagner PD, Saltzman HA, West JB: Measurement of continuous distributions of ventilation-perfusion ratios: Theory. *J Appl Physiol* 36:588, 1974.
162. Nunn JF: Artificial ventilation, in *Applied Respiratory Physiology,* 3d ed. London, Butterworths, 1987, pp 392–422.
163. Tobin MJ, Dantzker DR: Mechanical ventilation and weaning, in Dantzker DR (ed): *Cardiopulmonary Critical Care*. Orlando, Fla, Grune and Statton, 1986, pp 203–62.
164. Shapiro BA, Cane RD, Harrison RA: Positive end-expiratory pressure therapy in adults with special reference to acute lung injury: A review of the literature and suggested clinical correlations. *Crit Care Med* 12:127, 1984.
165. Venus B, Cohen LE, Smith RA: Hemodynamics and intrathoracic pressure transmission during controlled mechanical ventilation and positive end-expiratory pressure in normal and low compliant lungs. *Crit Care Med* 16:686, 1988.
166. Suwa K, Hedley-Whyte J, Bendixen HH: Circulation and physiologic dead space changes on controlling the ventilation of dogs. *J Appl Physiol* 231:1855, 1966.
167. Saffle JR, Medina E, Raymond J, et al: Use of indirect calorimetry in the nutritional management of burned patients. *J Trauma* 25:32, 1985.
168. Nordenstrom J, Jeevanandam M, Elwyn DH, et al: Increasing glucose intake during total parenteral nutrition increases norepinephrine excretion in trauma and sepsis. *Clin Physiol* 1:525, 1981.
169. Askanazi J, Nordenstrom J, Rosenbaum SH, et al: Nutrition for the patient with respiratory failure: Glucose vs fat. *Anesthesiology* 54:373, 1981.
170. Hageman JR, McCulloch K, Gora P, et al: Intralipid al-

terations in pulmonary prostaglandin metabolism and gas exchange. *Crit Care Med* 11:794, 1983.
171. Hageman JR, Hunt CE: Fat emulsions and lung function. *Clin Chest Med* 7:69, 1986.
172. McKeen CR, Brigham KL, Bowers RE, et al: Pulmonary vascular effects of fat emulsion infusion in unanesthetized sheep. *J Clin Invest* 61:1291, 1978.
173. Greeley WJ, Leslie JB, Reves JG: Prostaglandins and the cardiovascular system: A review and update. *J Cardiothorac Anesth* 1:331, 1987.
174. Demling RH: The role of mediators in human ARDS. *J Crit Care* 3:56, 1988.
175. Tuxen DV, Lane S: The effects of ventilatory pattern on hyperinflation, airway pressures, and circulation in mechanical ventilation of patients with severe air-flow obstruction. *Am Rev Respir Dis* 136:872, 1987.
176. Hubmayr RD, Gay PC, Tayyab M: Respiratory system mechanics in ventilated patients: Technics and indications. *Mayo Clin Proc* 62:358, 1987.
177. Truwit JD, Marini JJ: Evaluation of thoracic mechanics in the ventilated patient: Part 1. Primary measurements. *J Crit Care* 3:133, 1988.
178. Moncrief JA: Burns. *N Engl J Med* 288:444, 1973.
179. Horton JW, White J, Baxter CR: The role of oxygen-derived free radicals in burn-induced myocardial contractile depression. *J Burn Care Rehabil* 9:589, 1989.
180. Moati F, Sepulchre C, Miskulin M, et al: Pharmacologic properties of a cardiotoxic factor isolated from the blood serum of burned patients. *J Pathol* 127:147, 1979.
181. Baxter C, Cook W, Shires GT: Serum myocardial depressant factor of burn shock. *Surg Forum* 17:1, 1966.
182. Raffa J, Trunkey D: Myocardial depression in acute thermal injury. *J Trauma* 18:90, 1978.
183. Aikawa N, Martyn JAJ, Burke JF: Pulmonary artery catheterization and thermodilution cardiac output determination in the management of critically burned patients. *Am J Surg* 135:811, 1978.
184. Lappas DG, Powel WM, Daggett WM: Cardiac dysfunction in the perioperative period: Pathophysiology, diagnosis, and treatment. *Anesthesiology* 47:117, 1977.
185. Barker SJ, Gamel DM, Tremper KK: Cardiovascular effects of anesthesia and operation. *Crit Care Clin* 3:251, 1987.
186. Brown BR, Crout JR: A comparative study of the effects of five general anesthetics on myocardial contractility: Isometric conditions. *Anesthesiology* 34:236, 1971.
187. Wolf WJ, Neal MB, Mathew BP, et al: Comparison of the in vitro myocardial depressant effects of isoflurane and halothane anesthesia. *Anesthesiology* 69:660, 1988.
188. Sahlman L, Henriksson BA, Martner J, et al: Effects of halothane, enflurane, and isoflurane on coronary vascular tone, myocardial performance, and oxygen consumption during controlled changes in aortic and left atrial pressure. *Anesthesiology* 69:1, 1988.
189. Seifen E, Seifen AB, Kennedy RH, et al: Comparison of cardiac effects of enflurance, isoflurane, and halothane in the dog heart-lung preparation. *J Cardiothorac Anesth* 1:543, 1987.
190. Gregoretti S, Gelman S, Dimick A, et al: Total body oxygen supply-demand balance in burned patients under enflurane anesthesia. *J Trauma* 27:158, 1987.
191. Chodoff P: Evidence for central adrenergic action of ketamine. *Anesth Analg* 51:247, 1972.
192. Berry DG: Effect of ketamine on the isolated chick embryo heart. *Anesth Analg* 53:919, 1974.
193. Weiskoph RB, Bogetz MS, Roizen MF, et al: Cardiovascular and metabolic sequelae of inducing anesthesia with ketamine or thiopental in hypovolemic swine. *Anesthesiology* 60:214, 1984.
194. Jin L, Lalonde C, Demling RH: Effect of anesthesia and positive pressure ventilation on early post burn hemodynamic instability. *J Trauma* 26:26, 1986.
195. Robotham JL, Scharf SM: The effects of positive and negative pressure ventilation on cardiac performance. *Clin Chest Med* 4:161, 1983.
196. Pinsky MR: Cardiopulmonary interaction — The effects of negative and positive pleural pressure on cardiac output, in Dantzker DR (ed): *Cardiopulmonary Critical Care*. Orlando, Fla, Grune and Stratton, 1986, pp 89–121.
197. Moran KT, O'Reilly TJ, Furman WR, et al: A new algorithm for calculation of blood loss in excisional burn surgery. *Am Surg* 54:207, 1988.
198. Snelling CF, Shaw K: Quantitative evaluation of blood loss during debridement and grafting of burns. *Can J Surg* 25:416, 1982.
199. Canizaro PC, Sawyer RB, Switzer WE: Blood loss during excision of third-degree burns. *Arch Surg* 88:800, 1964.

Chapter 14

Pharmacologic Considerations during Treatment of Respiratory Dysfunction of Thermal and/or Inhalation Injury

J. A. Jeevendra Martyn

Respiratory dysfunction following thermal injury can be the result of direct damage to the respiratory tract due to the inhalation of toxic products or the result of the secondary effects of cutaneous burns. The presence of inhalation injury and/or pneumonia in addition to a cutaneous burn can have significant, independent, and profound effects on burn mortality. These effects vary with age and burn size in a predictable manner.[1,2] The management of respiratory dysfunction in the presence of thermal injury demands a multifaceted approach, including the treatment of the inhalation injury, the cutaneous burn, and the complications that occur in association with these conditions. The scope of this chapter is to demonstrate how thermally injured patients behave differently than normal subjects in the handling of (pharmacokinetics) and the response to (pharmacodynamics) administered drugs.

In this chapter burn injury to the lung or skin is assumed to induce similar pharmacologic responses, since there are no studies to date as to how inhalation injury in the absence of cutaneous burn may affect drug kinetics and dynamics, that is, pharmacologic studies performed following burns have not discriminated between the confounding effects of inhalation injury and those of cutaneous burn injury. However, it should be stated that the metabolic, cardiovascular, and inflammatory responses to direct inhalation injury are not too different from the responses to cutaneous burn.[3–5] Prior to the discussion of the individual drugs and how their pharmacology is altered in burn patients, a general overview of the systemic changes occurring after burn trauma and how these may influence the pharmacologic responses to drugs is relevant.

SYSTEMIC RESPONSES TO BURN INJURY

Blood Flow Changes

A dramatic decrease in cardiac output[6,7] is the immediate effect of a cutaneous burn injury. The causes of this decrease are multifactorial and include a decrease in circulating volume, an increase in systemic vascular resistance due to the release of vasoactive hormones,[8] and myocardial depression.[7] Treatment of just one of these derangements, such as decreasing afterload by the use of vasodilators or increasing the preload by volume infusion, will not be sufficient to restore cardiac output to normal levels. This period of hypodynamic circulation continues for approximately 24 to 36 hours after burn injury.[7] During the subsequent period, following repletion of circulating volume to normal levels, cardiac output reaches normal levels and then becomes hyperdynamic.[7–10] Cardiac outputs exceeding 20 L/min have been observed in young healthy patients. This response persists until either inflammation decreases or burn wounds are completely closed. Increased cardiac output results in increased blood flow not only to the burn wound but also to the splanchnic organs, including the kidney and the liver.[11–13] In the presence of sepsis, cardiac output and the hypermetabolic state can further increase or decrease depending on whether the patient is compensated or decompensated.[11]

These changes in blood flow can have marked effects on the absorption, distribution, and elimination of drugs. During the hypodynamic phase, because of poor blood flow to the muscle tissue, skin, and intestines, drugs administered via intramuscular, subcutaneous, or enteral routes will not be absorbed because of the poor perfusion of these tissues. In these instances, if repeated doses of drugs are administered by these routes to overcome poor drug response, when perfusion is reestablished in the post resuscitation period, rapid absorption of these drugs will sometimes result in toxicity; therefore, small incremental doses of intravenous medication are the preferred method of administration. During the hyperdynamic state, where perfusion is restored to normal or even increased, there is no evidence to indicate that absorption via the gut is impaired or increased. On the other hand, elimination by renal or hepatic routes can be enhanced. Increased splanchnic blood flow results in an increased glomerular filtration rate with very rapid elimination of drugs filtered through the glomerulus; these include antibiotics and some of the H_2-receptor antagonists.[14,15] Similarly, because of the increased blood flow through the liver, flow-dependent drugs may have an enhanced elimination, although definitive studies have not been performed. Drugs that are dependent on hepatic blood flow for their elimination include lidocaine, meperidine, morphine, and propanolol.

Organ Function following Burns

Functional changes in the eliminating organs (liver, lung, and kidney) can be caused by either cutaneous burns or inhaled toxins. Such functional changes, if present, can affect drug pharmacokinetics. Of particular importance in regard to inhaled toxins are the effects of carbon monoxide and cyanide, which can cause histotoxic hypoxia in all organs including the liver and the kidney.[16,17] In addition to organ toxicity, ischemia due to hypovolemia also can lead to organ dysfunction. In the most severe forms of ischemia, acute tubular necrosis of the kidney occurs,[18] while in the liver this injury manifests as elevations of liver enzymes.[19] Myoglobineamia due to muscle damage also can cause renal dysfunction.[20] Despite the presence of enhanced glomerular function in patients who have been adequately resuscitated, disturbed renal osmolal regulation is present in patients with severe burns.[18] Even during hyperosmolal states, marked antidiuresis is uncommon, suggesting an inadequate renal response to antidiuretic hormone or an impaired ability of the renal tubules to concentrate urine. Thus, elimination of drugs by tubular secretion may be impaired. Enhanced glomerular function, reduced concentrating capacity, and tubular rejection of sodium are correlated positively with the severity of trauma.[15,18] Thus, adequate urine flow may be present with hypovolemia and/or during renal failure.

In the liver, clinical and laboratory evidence of hepatic injury exists as early as 24 hours after burn.[19] Liver changes observed in clinical and experimental studies include increased metabolic activity (protein synthesis and breakdown),[11] swelling of hepatocyte nuclei, focal hepatic necrosis, and fatty liver.[21] Other laboratory indicators of liver dysfunction include elevations of SGOT, SGPT, and alkaline phosphatase levels. The early occurrence of hepatic injury suggests that acute hemodynamic alterations may play a role in the etiology of hepatic dysfunction. The effect of these alterations in liver function on drug metabolism has not been completely characterized.

Plasma Protein Binding Changes

Severe (more than 25 percent body surface area) burn injury is associated with alterations in plasma protein concentrations.[22] Two major drug-binding projteins have been identified in human plasma: albumin[23] and alpha-1-acid glycoprotein.[24] Concentrations of albumin and alpha-1-acid glycoprotein frequently deviate from normal levels during disease states; albumin concentrations generally decrease, while alpha-1-acid glycoprotein concentrations increase in chronic, subacute, and acute inflammatory processes (e.g., trauma, burns, renal failure, infection, and liver disease). The decrease in albumin concentrations results in decreased plasma protein binding (increased free fraction) of drugs such as anticoagulants, antiepileptics, sulfonylureas, and benzodiazepenes.[25,26] On the other hand, the increased concentrations of alpha-1-acid glycoprotein in these instances result in increased plasma protein binding (decreased free fraction) of drugs such as lidocaine, propranolol, neuromuscular relaxants, tricyclics, and narcotics (Fig. 14-1).[25,26]

Alterations in plasma protein binding of drugs as such do not change the absolute concentration of free drug — and hence its clinical activity — at steady state, as long as the free clearance and dosing rates remain unchanged.[25] Binding changes, however, will alter the interpretation of plasma drug concentrations reported by most clinical laboratories because they report total (free + bound) concentrations. Thus, when there are disease-induced changes in binding and laboratories report drug concentrations (e.g., lidocaine, phenytoin, digoxin), it will not be evident whether the fraction or concentration is subtherapeutic, therapeutic, or toxic. True therapeutic concentration will be evident only if the free fraction is also measured during this time. Clinically, the high doses of narcotics and muscle relaxants required in burn patients are partly related to the increased binding of these drugs to alpha-1-acid glycoprotein. Finally, alterations in binding can also affect the elimination of drugs by the kidney and the liver.[25]

PHARMACOLOGIC STUDIES IN BURNED PATIENTS

Pharmacologic studies of several major groups of drugs have important implications for their therapeutic uses in burned patients with and without inhalation injury.

Systemic Antimicrobial Therapy

Despite the significant advances of the last 40 years in the treatment of burned patients, infections continue to present a serious problem. Up to 75 percent of critically ill burned patients who survive the initial resuscitation period but develop a burn wound infection will subsequently die from sepsis despite intensive local and systemic antibiotic therapy.[27] Accordingly, the primary role in the management of burn wound infection is to prevent the development of infection and to effectively treat those infections which evolve. In the lung, infections can occur either because of a hematogenous spread from the burn wound or as a result of inhalation injury.[1–3,27]

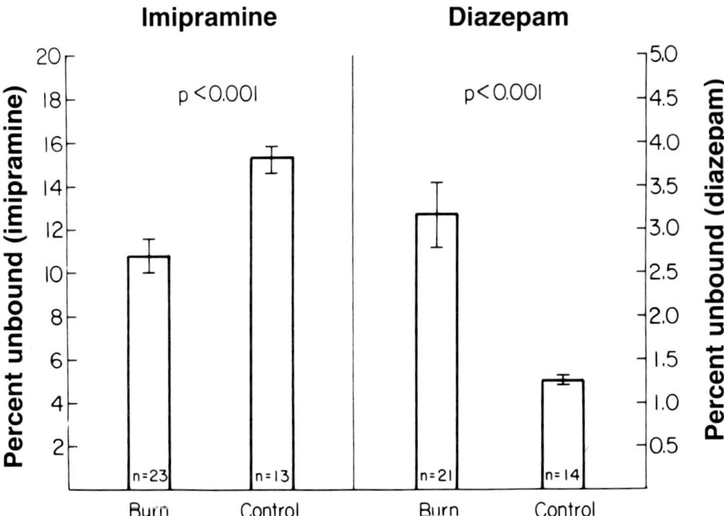

Figure 14-1 Protein binding of drugs following burn injury. Free fraction of imipramine in burned patients (left) is lower in comparison to healthy controls. The percent of unbound diazepam in plasma in all burn patients is higher than that of healthy controls. The changes are related to increases and decreases in plasma levels of alpha-1-acid-glycoprotein and albumin, respectively. (*Martyn et al.*[25])

Prior to the advent of topical antimicrobial therapy and effective surgical wound management, secondary pulmonary infections were most commonly the result of the former. Other common sources of secondary bacterial contamination of the lung include suppurative thrombophlebitis, soft tissue abscesses, and intraperitoneal infection.

Systemic antibiotics should be used only in patients with documented infection. The choice of agent should be based on cultures and sensitivity tests. There is no clinical value in using either prophylactic or aerosolized antibiotics in burned patients with pulmonary infections[28]; these may actually induce the emergence of multiple drug-resistant microorganisms. The use of parenteral antibiotics in the burned patient should be reserved for the treatment of all uncontrolled infections. In the burned patient sepsis commonly occurs in the absence of positive blood culture; a positive blood culture, however, should be treated immediately by the administration of parenteral antibiotics to prevent bacterial dissemination from the burn wound. Unfortunately, the penetration of systemic antibiotics into the area of infection is not predictable. This is especially true of full-thickness wounds and in burn-wound infections that may be associated with occlusive vasculitis. Irrespective of the etiology of the infection, the choice of systemic antibiotic should be based on results of culture material from infected tissue such as blood, urine, and wound, the species of infecting organism, the pattern of sensitivity, the status of the patient, and the impact of the drug on the flora endogenous to the unit. In other words, antibiotic therapy for treatment of infection must be individualized.

It is well established that generally higher-than-normal doses of certain antibiotics are required in burned patients in order to maintain adequate therapeutic levels.[14,29] The major reasons for the increased dose requirements include enhanced drug elimination by the kidney resulting from burn-induced increases in the glomerular filtration rate[14,15] and loss of drug through the burn wound.[30] For drugs with minimal protein binding, creatinine clearance may give an indirect estimate of the capacity of the burned patient to excrete antibiotic drugs by glomerular filtration. The elimination half-life of tobramycin, which was directly correlated with creatinine clearance, exemplifies this situation.[14] Most antibiotics have minimal protein-binding; thus, measured plasma concentrations will reflect true therapeutic concentrations. This contrasts with drugs that predominantly bind to albumin or alpha-1-acid glycoprotein, where measured plasma drug concentrations do not reflect therapeutic free concentrations.[25]

Chemoprophylaxis of Stress Ulceration

Acute stress ulceration of the stomach and duodenum is the most common life-threatening gastrointestinal complication of burn injury.[7,31] A prospective study in adults found that gastric erosion occurred within 72 hours of injury in 86 percent of adults with burns covering more than 40 percent body surface area; 28 percent of these erosions progressed to gastric or duodenal ulceration.[31] The incidence of life-threatening hemorrhage was about 5 percent. The incidence of ulceration, which appears twice as frequently in children as in adults,[32] has markedly diminished over the last 5 years, probably because of early tube feeding, which buffers gastric acid secretion, better methods of resuscitation, and coadministration of antacids.[33] The presence of sepsis and respiratory failure tends to play a significant role in the pathophysiology of stress ulcer and hemorrhage.[34,35] Thus, even patients with minimal cutaneous burns but with respiratory dysfunction due to inhalation injury are more prone to stress ulceration of the stomach.[34]

Therapy of stress ulceration should be directed initially at preventing conditions favoring its development.[33] These include physiologic support, correction of hypovolemia, shock, acidosis, and the control of pain.[34,35] Subsequent control of stress ulceration and bleeding in critically ill patients includes early enteral feeding and the administration of oral antacids (e.g., Mylanta) and/or H_2-receptor antagonists.[36,37] Although hypersecretion of gastric acid probably does not play a role in stress ulceration of burns,[38] acid neutralization offers protection against the development of Curling's ulcer.[7] The usual antacid regimen consists of the aspiration of the nasogastric contents at hourly intervals and the administration of antacids and feeds through the nasogastric tube to neutralize the acidity of the stomach to a pH $\geq$ 4.0. In a retrospective study in burned patients, bleeding occurred in 30 percent of patients fed with a usual diet but only in 3 percent of patients receiving Vivonex.[39]

Although antacids (e.g., Mylanta) and feeding have been found to be more effective than cimetidine in the elevation of gastric pH, certain conditions preclude the institution of these regimens, including sepsis or burn-induced gastrointestinal ileus and perioperative fasting. Feeding or oral antacid administration during this time can result in pulmonary aspiration of gastric contents. In these states, therefore, parenterally administered H_2-receptor antagonists such as cimetidine or ranitidine are useful chemoprophylactic agents for control of stress ulceration. Numerous studies have documented that burn injury is associated with alterations in the pharmacokinetic as well as pharmacodynamic responses to cimetidine. The pharmacokinetic alterations include an enhanced clearance and shorter elimination half-life compared to nonburned patients.[15,40] Enhanced elimination kinetics in burned patients were directly related to increased glomerular filtration, since a good correlation was found between cimetidine and creatinine clearance (Fig. 14-2).[15] Pharmacodynamic alterations were evident in children as a higher plasma cimetidine concentration requirement to achieve effective control of gastric pH compared to adults with similar size burns. In adult burn patients, plasma cimetidine concentrations of 0.5 to 1.0 μg/mL achieved gastric pH $\geq$ 4.0[15]; pediatric burn patients required concentrations higher than 1.0 μg/ml.[40] Although studies in nonburned intensive care unit (ICU) patients have indicated that continuous infusion of cimetidine results in better and sustained control of gastric pH,[41] continuous infusion of cimetidine in burned patients using higher bolus doses and high infusion rates have not con-

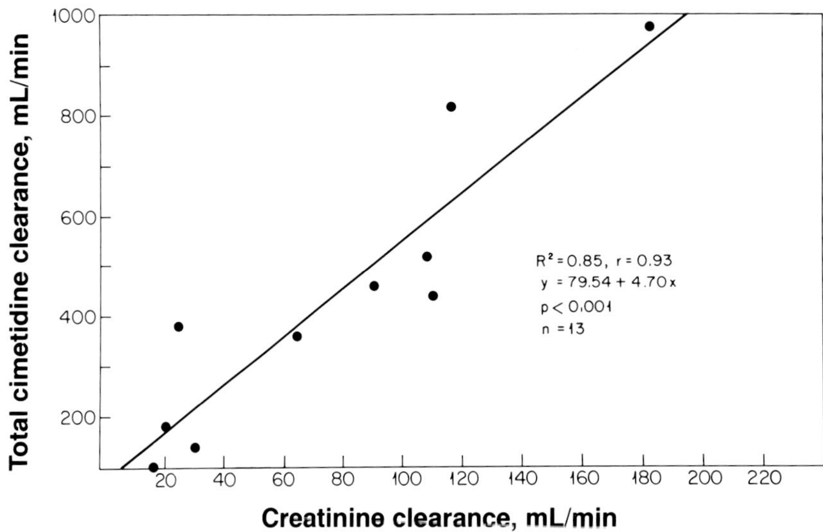

Figure 14-2 Correlation of cimetidine clearance with creatinine clearance in burned children. There is a significant positive correlation between the two (R_2 = 0.85, r = 0.93), as well as a positive correlation (R_2 = 0.78, r = 0.88) between burn size and creatinine clearance (not shown in figure), that is, as burn size increased, creatinine clearance (glomerular filteration rate) increased. (*Martyn et al.*[15,40])

firmed this.[42] Preliminary studies with ranitidine are promising.[43]

Complications occur with the administration of both antacids and H_2-receptor antagonists. Aspiration of antacid is a potential problem, particularly in patients with gastric ileus. Antacids also require excessive nursing time, since gastric pH is monitored every 1 to 2 hours. Additional complications related to the use of antacids include diarrhea, hypercalcemia, hypermagnesemia, and other metabolic disturbances.[36] The reported adverse effects of H_2-receptor antagonists include inhibition of liver metabolizing enzymes, neutropenia, and altered immunologic response.[44] Such effects are potentially serious for burn patients, but the relationship of clinical toxicity to elevated plasma levels of H_2-receptor antagonists has not been established. An important side effect of antacid or H_2-receptor antagonist therapy is the colonization of the gastric lumen by gram-negative bacteria. An increased incidence of nosocomial infection, transferred from the gastric mucosa to the lung, has been documented.[45] The usefulness of sucralfate, which prevents stress ulceration without increasing gastric pH, has not been tested in burn patients.

Neuromuscular Relaxants

Burn injury alters the pharmacokinetics and pharmacodynamics of all neuromuscular relaxants presently in clinical use.[46,47] Clinical studies performed in recent years have documented the magnitude and direction of these alterations, resulting in improved therapeutic guidelines for the use of these drugs.

The administration of succinylcholine, a depolarizing muscle relaxant that is structurally similar to acetylcholine, can induce a massive potassium release from muscle cells which may result in lethal hyperkalemia[46] (Fig. 14-3). This hyperkalemic response is related to the dose of succinylcholine, time elapsed since injury, and the severity of burn injury.[46,48,49] In normal muscle, depolarization with succinylcholine causes an increase in membrane permeability and the release of potassium from the

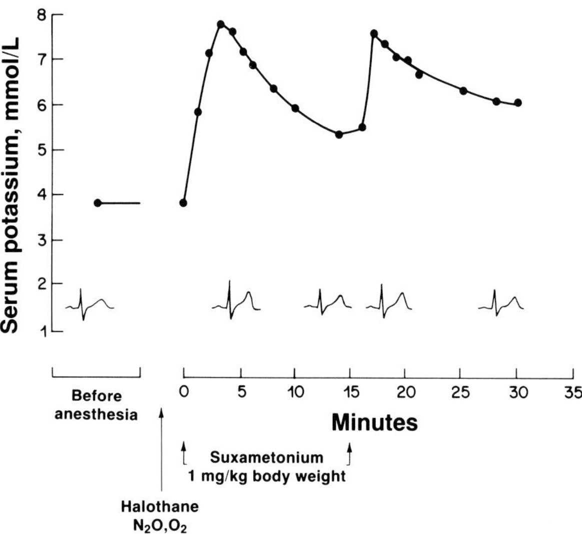

Figure 14-3 Changes in plasma potassium levels in a burned patient after succinylcholine administration. Potassium levels reached lethal levels with associated ECG changes. The high potassium levels persist for a considerable period of time. (*Viby-Mogensen et al.*[48])

cell at discrete end-plate areas. This depolarization by succinylcholine and egress of potassium does not result in significant elevations of plasma potassium levels. Following burn injury a denervation-like phenomenon occurs with increases in acetylcholine receptor number in the muscle membrane.[50] Thus, instead of the discrete end-plate areas releasing potassium following the administration of succinylcholine, increased acetylcholine receptors induced by burn injury release potassium, causing hyperkalemia.[47] The factors and/or mediators that induce the receptor changes at the neuromuscular junction have not been characterized.

If succinylcholine has been administered inadvertently and cardiac arrest develops, calcium chloride or calcium gluconate should be administered in incremental doses until the peaked T waves on the electrocardiogram return to normal. Ventricular fibrillation and/or tachycardia will not resolve even with defibrillation until the high potassium levels are antagonized with calcium. Although one might anticipate potassium levels to normalize fairly rapidly because of redistribution and tissue uptake, hyperkalemia lasting for over 25 minutes has been recorded. During the period of cardiac arrest, cardiopulmonary resuscitation should be instituted in order to maintain vital organ function. Therapeutic maneuvers to reduce potassium levels include the administration of bicarbonate, glucose with insulin, or epinephrine, which will support the cardiovascular system in addition to driving the potassium intracellularly.[51]

In contrast to the hypersensitivity to depolarizing relaxants, burn patients are resistant (hyposensitive) to the effects of nondepolarizing relaxants such as *d*-tubocurarine and pancuronium.[47] All of the nondepolarizing neuromuscular relaxants presently in clinical use, including the recently introduced atracurium and vecuronium, have been documented to require a higher intravenous dose and/or plasma concentration for effective paralysis in patients with burns compared to those without burns (Fig. 14-4). The shift in the dose-response curves for these relaxants is related to both time after burn and magnitude of burn.[47] The resistance to the neuromuscular relaxants peaks at 7 to 10 days post burn and is maintained at this level for some time, depending on the burn size. Thus, initial doses of *d*-tubocurarine, metocurine, pancuronium, atracurium, and vecuronium would be 1.8, 0.8, 0.13, 2.0, and 0.13 mg/kg, respectively, for burned patients compared with 0.51, 0.3, 0.05, 0.25, and 0.05 mg/kg, respectively, in patients without burns.[47] One-half to one-fourth of the initial doses may be required every 30 to 60 minutes to maintain effective paralysis.

Resistance reverts to normal over several weeks or months while burn wounds heal. Altered pharmacokinetics, including enhanced renal excretion, play a minor role in the increased dose requirement of these drugs.[52] Increased plasma protein binding to alpha-1-acid glycoprotein also plays a role in the increased dose requirement.[53] Changes in binding alone, however, cannot totally explain shifts in the dose-response curves. Using the rodent model of burn injury, the effective dose of *d*-tubocurarine was shown to correlate significantly with increased

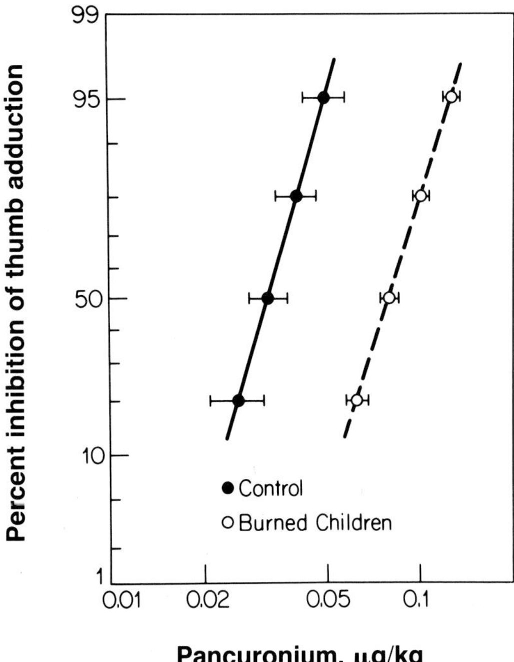

Figure 14-4 Pancuronium dose-response curves for muscle paralysis in control and burn patients. Burn patients have significant rightward shifts in the dose requirement. The effective dose in controls was 0.05 mg/kg, compared to 0.13 mg/kg in burn patients. Shifts of similar or greater magnitude were seen for other relaxants as well. (*Martyn et al.*[47])

acetylcholine receptor number ($R^2 = 0.65$).[54] Thus, it seems that the higher dose requirement for nondepolarizing muscle relaxants is related to changes in receptor number (pharmacodynamics) and to changes in protein binding, as well as pharmacokinetics.[52–54]

Muscle relaxants have important uses not only in the operating room but also in the intensive care unit. In patients who are mechanically ventilated, especially those receiving high levels of positive end-expiratory pressure, muscle relaxants are used to reduce total thoracic compliance and improve ventilation.[55] In addition to improved gas exchange, there is evidence for the faster recovery of lung function following acute respiratory distress syndrome with the use of muscle relaxants.[56,57] The mechanisms operative in improving lung function and recovery have yet to be defined. Thus, it is not an uncommon practice to use muscle relaxants in burned patients who require complete control of ventilation; however, it must be emphasized that muscle relaxants should never be used alone but always in conjunction with sedatives and narcotics, as it is imperative to avoid awake but paralyzed patients.

Sedatives and Narcotics

Control of pain and anxiety is an important aspect of the care of the burn patient. Recently, efforts have been made to understand the physiologic significance of the hypermetabolic (stress) response to trauma, and techniques to modify these responses have been suggested.[58,59] The afferent responses to increased metabolism can be accentuated by the brain, particularly in the presence of pain and anxiety.[5,58,59] The question has been raised whether the persistent presence of pain increases the circulating levels of catecholamines and other catabolic hormones, decreases the blood flow to organs, and increases the catabolic process.[58] The fact that severe protracted pain and anxiety can cause immunodeficiency has now been recognized and may be an important consideration particularly for the burn patient.[60] Preliminary studies by Demling and others indicate that inadequate sedation and pain control might result in increased morbidity and mortality.[58]

The problem of pain and anxiety control becomes even more critical to artificially ventilated patients because of their inability to communicate or in very young children because of their inability to express themselves adequately. If muscle relaxants are used to enhance the ventilatory effects of the respirator, the result may be a paralyzed and immobilized patient who is unable to convey his or her feelings but is experiencing a great deal of pain. Despite these important issues, no precise guidelines are available for the management of anxiety and pain in burn patients. The reasons for these deficiencies have been addressed and include concerns about the possibility of addiction and the inability of patients to eliminate administered drugs.[61,62] These concerns are now proved to be unfounded.[61]

Inhalation Agents Inhalation of methoxyflurane (self-administered or otherwise) for control of pain has been discontinued in burn centers because of the potential for nephrotoxicity.[63] Nitrous oxide-oxygen mixtures are quite popular in the United Kingdom and have been used in some burn centers in the United States, although the nitrous oxide–oxygen mixture alone is not sufficient for adequate analgesia and must be combined with other intravenous narcotics and sedatives.[64] Two advantages of nitrous oxide usage is that it can be self-administered and that its effects are short-lived; with the discontinuation of this agent, effects wear off in 2 to 3 minutes. The drug's side effects include the inhibition of cell proliferation in bone marrow and leukopenia.[65] Whether the short but daily exposure to nitrous oxide during dressing changes or tubbing, especially in the burn patient who already has hematologic and immunologic abnormalities,[66] will more quickly potentiate these abnormalities is unknown. Environmental contamination with nitrous oxide can be a potential problem particularly to pregnant employees because of the possibility of miscarriage when exposed to the anesthetic drug.[67]

Benzodiazepines Benzodiazepines such as chlordiazepoxide (Librium), diazepam (Valium), and lorazepam (Ativan) are sedatives commonly used in treating burn patients. All of these drugs are eliminated by hepatic metabolism and have low metabolic clearance.[68] Prior studies have documented increased tolerance of sedatives and anesthetic drugs following burn injury.[69,70] Clinical impression suggests that sedative requirements, including those for lorazepam and diazepam, are increased in burn patients. To determine whether alterations in diazepam kinetics might explain the observed insensitivity of such patients to the effects of this drug, a clinical pharmacokinetic study was performed.[71] Diazepam elimination half-life was longer in burn patients compared to controls (Table 14-1), due mainly to a reduction in clearance of free diazepam.[71] The mechanism for the reduced clearance of free diazepam in burn patients is unknown but may be due to nonspecific impairment of hepatic drug metabolizing capacity, as suggested in some animal studies.[72] Alternatively, the mechanism may be attributable to simultaneous administration of other medications. Of particular importance in this context is cimetidine, which is known to inhibit diazepam clearance. Thus, repeated administration of diazepam to burned patients, particularly when cimetidine is coadministered may result in significant accumulations of the drug in the body. In any case, the diazepam study findings indicate that reduced diazepam sensitivity in burn patients cannot be explained on a pharmacokinetic basis.[71]

The pharmacokinetics of lorazepam have also been studied in burn patients[73] (Table 14-1), who had a significantly higher clearance, larger volume of distribution and shorter elimination half-life than did control subjects despite the fact that all burn patients were coadministered cimetidine. Thus it seems evident that clinical burn trauma does not impair the metabolism of lorazepam in contrast to di-

Table 14-1 Pharmacokinetics of Diazepam and Lorazepam (mean ± S.E.)

	Diazepam		Lorazepam	
	Controls	Burns	Controls	Burns
Volume of distribution, L/kg	1.53 ± 0.2	2.88 ± 0.6	1.39 ± 0.1	2.65 ± 0.55*
Elimination half-life, hours	36.0 ± 5.0	72.0 ± 26.0*	13.9 ± 0.8	9.59 ± 1.3*
Total clearance, mL/min/kg	0.53 ± 0.07	0.64 ± 0.11	1.16 ± 0.1	4.28 ± 1.2*

*Significantly different from controls.
SOURCE: Martyn et al.[71,73]

azepam. Diazepam is metabolized by cytochrome P-450 oxidases (Phase I reaction), which can be influenced by population characteristics such as age, disease, and the concomitant administration of drugs. On the other hand, metabolism by conjugation (Phase II reaction) is said to be far less susceptible to such factors. The study with lorazepam confirms the speculation that conjugated drugs such as lorazepam are less impaired in disease states and may be preferred in critically ill patients, especially when repeated administration is necessary.

Narcotic Agents Despite the persistence and prominence of pain in burned patients, little attention has been paid to the pharmacology of narcotic drugs in burned patients. It is generally accepted that burn patients require higher than normal doses of narcotic drugs, especially during burn dressing changes. Meperidine and morphine are the most widely used narcotic agents for control of pain.[62] Because most patients, particularly children, dislike receiving intramuscular medications, oral Percocet (5 mg oxycodone + 325 mg acetaminophen per tablet) is also used for pain control.[74] Although most of the narcotic drugs can be administered orally, their onset is hence prolonged and their bioavailability may be decreased. Therefore, the intravenous route is preferred, since a drug can be titrated for a given end point. The main disadvantages of morphine and meperidine are their prolonged duration of action (4 to 6 hours), which means that when appropriately medicated for burn dressing change, the patient might have respiratory depression at a time beyond dressing changes when pain stimulus is not present. Because of their prolonged duration of action, however, these drugs are useful for sedation of patients on respirators. The serious drawback to meperidine use is that its metabolite, normeperidine, can accumulate with repeated large doses and cause central nervous system excitation, including convulsions.[75] In the presence of renal failure the metabolites of both morphine and meperidine can accumulate in the circulation, leading to potential central effects, including sedation. Another serious side effect of these narcotics is chest wall rigidity, which often occurs when they are rapidly administered.[76]

Studies on morphine and sufentanil (a short-acting synthetic narcotic) pharmacokinetics show that clearances are similar or somewhat enhanced[77,78] compared to that of controls. On the other hand, meperidine clearance may be impaired.[75] All of these pharmacokinetic studies should be regarded as preliminary, since appropriate controls were not performed; historical controls were used for comparison. Despite the lack of adequate data relative to narcotic agents in burn patients, no pharmacokinetic reasons seem apparent for withholding at least morphine and sufentanil from burn patients. It must also be emphasized that, contrary to popular belief, the narcotic requirement is increased in burn patients in proportion to the magnitude of burn injury.[79] The multiple factors that operate to bring about this increased requirement have not been characterized.

Cardiovascular Drugs

Numerous animal studies have documented the usefulness of cardiotonic and vasoactive substances such as verapamil, nitroprusside, and digoxin to improve cardiovascular function.[10,80,81] Clinical studies, however, have not confirmed the usefulness of these drugs. Drugs clinically used to improve cardiovascular function include dopamine, epinephrine, norepinephrine (Levophed), and isoproterenol. In some instances, particularly during sepsis or in the presence of coronary artery disease, volume replacement alone is insufficient to support the cardiovascular system. If the cardiovascular system is not supported during this time, secondary respiratory dysfunction can occur. Therefore, it is imperative that volume replacement be monitored and cardiovascular function be supported appropriately.

The response of the cardiovascular system to adrenergic drugs seems to be diminished following burn injury. During the acute phase of the burn injury the use of low-dose dopamine (5 to 10 mg/kg/min) as an adjunct to volume replacement was

Table 14-2 Pulmonary and Systemic Hemodynamics to Dopamine

Dopamine dose, μg/kg/min	From 3.5	To 9.0	From 0	To 6.8
Diastolic volume, mL/m^2	110.5	128.2	99.4	90.7
Ejection fraction, %	34.0	32.0	41.0	42.0
Pulmonary arterial pressure, mmHg	26.7	30.7*	22.3	25.1*
Cardiac index, mL/min/m^2	4.0	4.3	3.9	4.0
Mean arterial pressure, mmHg	81.5	87.2	84.6	89.0
Heart rate, beats/min	110.3	113.1	108.3	111.6
Systemic vascular resistance, dyne/s/cm^3	865.4	727.9	746.9	741.6
Pulmonary vascular resistance, units	1.1	1.2	1.6	1.5

*Significantly different from controls.
SOURCE: Martyn et al.[83]

found to be ineffective.[82] The effectiveness of low-dose dopamine (3 to 9 μg/kg/min) to improve right ventricular dysfunction has also been evaluated.[83] Hemodynamic variables monitored in this study included right ventricular ejection fraction and end diastolic volume, heart rate, cardiac output, and vascular pressures (Table 14-2).[83] No significant hemodynamic advantage was observed with dopamine infusion (Table 14-2). In fact, this study documented an adverse hemodynamic effect, in that pulmonary artery hypertension was observed with the administration of dopamine. The ineffectiveness of dopamine (5 to 25 μg/kg/min) in improving systemic hemodynamics in burn sepsis has also been confirmed.[84] Thus, clinical studies of dopamine to date do not substantiate any useful alpha- or beta-adrenergic effects of dopamine in burn patients.[82–84]

Table 14-3 Plasma Epinephrine (pg/mL) following Topical Application

	Patient 1	Patient 2	Patient 3	Patient 4
Pre-anesthesia	323	280	146	343
Incision	202	82	68	668
15 minutes after topical application	4337	7653	1778	3976
Recovery room	2906	3256	1252	4688

SOURCE: Modified from Timonen et al.[85]

Other clinical studies also suggest a shift to the right in the response to adrenergic agonists such as epinephrine. Following topical application of epinephrine to decrease bleeding during burn surgery, the blood pressure and heart rate responses were monitored before and after application. Epinephrine was rapidly absorbed into the systemic circulation, reaching levels 10 times higher than normal (Table 14-3).[85] Despite these high catecholamine levels, minimal changes in heart rate and no changes in blood pressure were observed. Furthermore, although halothane anesthesia was used in some patients, no arrhythmias were noted. It seems, therefore, that systemic alpha and beta responses to epinephrine are also altered in burned patients. The etiology of the unresponsiveness to these adrenergic agents is unknown, but it may be a result of the down regulation of adrenergic receptors[86] due to chronic elevation of catecholamines in burn patients.[87] The effectiveness of drugs that improve responses in smooth and cardiac muscle by increasing adenosine 3′:5′-cyclic phosphate (cyclic AMP) levels via nonadrenergic mechanism (e.g., theophylline, dobutamine)[88] has not been studied in burn patients.

SUMMARY

Even a small burn injury reduces a systemic response which may include alterations of cardiac output, organ blood flow, protein concentrations, and hormone levels; all of these factors can acutely and chronically alter the pharmacokinetics and pharmacodynamics of drugs. These changes can be complicated by concomitant factors such as sepsis and inhalation injury. Surgery, anesthesia, pain and coadministered drugs also confound the pharmacology. In some instances, burn injury induces extreme sensitivity to drugs, as exemplified by the hyperkalemic response to succinylcholine and the pulmonary artery hypertensive response to dopamine. In other instances, higher than normal doses are required because of altered pharmacokinetics and pharmacodynamics (e.g., muscle relaxants, cimetidine). Even within the same family of drugs, metabolic clearance can be markedly varied as shown for diazepam and lorazepam. Therapeutics of burn patients with and without inhalation injury are complicated and should be individualized by the careful monitoring of objective end points.

REFERENCES

1. Thomson PB, Herndon DN, Traber DL, Abston S: Effect on mortality of inhalation injury. *J Trauma* 26:163, 1986.
2. Shirani K, Pruitt BA, Mason AD: The influence of inhalation injury and pneumonia on burn mortality. *Ann Surg* 205:982, 1987.
3. Herndon DN, Traber DL, Niehaus GD, et al: The pathophysiology of smoke inhalation injury in a sheep model. *J Trauma* 24:1044, 1984.
4. Pindor MT, Dunn RB, Nuzzarello J, Glaviano VV: Cardiovascular responses of the dog to acute smoke toxicity. *Circ Shock* 11:35, 1983.
5. Demling RH: Burns. *N Engl J Med* 313:1389, 1985.
6. Aikawa N, Martyn JAJ, Burke JF: Pulmonary artery catheterization and thermodilution cardiac output determination in the management of critically burned patients. *Am J Surg* 135:811, 1978.
7. Moncrief JA: Burns. *N Engl J Med* 288:444, 1973.
8. Morgan RF, Martyn JAJ, Philbin DM, et al: Water balance and antidiuretic hormone response following acute thermal injury. *J Trauma* 20:468, 1980.
9. Martyn JAJ, Snider MT, Farago LF, Burke JF: Thermodilution right ventricular volume: A novel and better predictor of volume replacement in acute thermal injury. *J Trauma* 21:619, 1981.
10. Stair JM, Browser BH, Marvin TH, et al: The effects of sodium nitroprusside on hemodynamics of burn shock: Results of an experimental sheep model. *J Trauma* 23:939, 1983.
11. Wilmore DW, Goodwin CW, Aulick LH, et al: Effect of injury and infection on visceral metabolism and circulation. *Ann Surg* 192:491, 1980.
12. Goodwin CW, Aulick LH, Becke RA, Wilmore DW: Increased renal perfusion and kidney size in convalescent burn patients. *JAMA* 244:1588, 1980.
13. Gump PE, Price JB, Kinney JM: Blood flow and oxygen consumption in patients with severe burns. *Surg Gynecol Obstet* 43:89, 1975.
14. Loirat P, Rohan J, Bailet A, et al: Increased glomerular filtration rates in patients with major burns and its effect on pharmacokinetics of tobramycin. *N Engl J Med* 299:915, 1978.
15. Martyn JAJ, Abernethy DR, Greenblatt DJ: Increased cimetidine clearance in burn patients. *JAMA* 258:1288, 1985.
16. Silvermann SH, Purdue GF, Hunt JL, Bost RO: Cyanide toxicity in burned patients. *J Trauma* 28:171, 1988.
17. Davies JWL: Toxic chemicals versus lung tissue — An aspect of inhalation injury revisited. *J Burn Care Rehabil* 7:213, 1988.
18. Eklund J, Gramberg PO, Liljedahl SO: Studies on renal function in burns. *Acta Chir Scand* 136:627, 1970.
19. Czaja AJ, Rizzo TA, Smith WR, Pruitt BA: Acute liver disease after cutaneous thermal injury. *J Trauma* 15:887, 1975.
20. Walsh MB, Miller SL, Kagen LJ: Myoglobinemia in severely burned patients: Correlations with severity and survival. *J Trauma* 22:6, 1982.
21. Chlumska A, Konickova A, Moserov J: Morphological changes in rat liver after burning. *Burns* 1:272, 1980.
22. Daniels JC, Larson DL, Abston S, Ritzman SE: Serum protein profiles in thermal burns: I. Serum electrophoretic patterns, immunoglobulins and transport proteins. *J Trauma* 14:137, 1974.
23. Koch-Weser J, Sellers EM: Binding of drugs to serum albumin. *N Engl J Med* 294:311, 1976.
24. Piafsky BM, Borga O, Odar-Cedarlog I, et al: Increased plasma binding of propanolol and chlorpromazine mediated by disease induced elevation of plasma alpha-1-acid glycoprotein. *N Engl J Med* 199:1435, 1987.
25. Martyn JAJ, Abernethy DR, Greenblatt DJ: Plasma protein binding of drugs after severe burn injury. *Clin Pharmacol Ther* 35:534, 1984.
26. Bloedow DC, Hansbrough JF, Hardin T, Simons M: Postburn serum drug binding and serum protein concentrations. *J Clin Pharmacol* 26:147, 1986.
27. Luterman A, Dasco CC, Curren PW: Injection in burn patients. *Am J Med* 81(SIA):45, 1986.
28. Levine BA, Petroff PA, Stade CL: Prospective trials of decamethasone and aerosolized gentamicin in the treatment of initial injury in the burned patient. *J Trauma* 18:188, 1978.
29. Sawchuck RJ, Ractor TS: Drug kinetics in burn patients.

Clin Pharmacokinet 5:548, 1980.
30. Glew RH, Moellering RC, Burke JF: Gentamicin dosage in children with extensive burns. *J Trauma* 16:819, 1976.
31. Czaja AJ, McAlhany JC, Pruitt BA: Acute gastroduodenal disease after thermal injury: An endoscopic evaluation of incidence and routine history. *N Engl J Med* 29:925, 1976.
32. Sevitt S: Duodenal and gastric ulceration after burning. *Br J Surg* 54:32, 1967.
33. Silen W: Pathogenetic factors in erosive gastritis. *Am J Med* 79:45, 1985.
34. Pingleton SK: Complications of acute respiratory failure. *Am Rev Respir Dis* 137:1463, 1988.
35. Harris (Pingleton) SK, Bone RC, Ruth WE: Gastrointestinal hemorrhage in patients in a respiratory care unit. *Chest* 72:301, 1977.
36. Munster A: The early management of thermal burns. *Surgery* 87:29, 1980.
37. McKelwee HP, Sirinek KR, Levine BA: Cimetidine affords protection equal to antacids in the prevention of stress ulceration following burns. *Surgery* 86:620, 1979.
38. O'Neill JA: The influence of thermal burns on gastric acid secretion. *Surgery* 67:267, 1970.
39. Choctow WT, Fajita C, Zawacki BE: Prevention of upper gastrointestinal bleeding in burn patients. *Arch Surg* 15:1073, 1980.
40. Martyn JAJ, Greenblatt DJ, Hagen J, Hoaglin DC: Burn injury alters pharmacokinetics and pharmacodynamics of cimetidine in children. *Eur J Clin Pharmacol* (in press).
41. Ostro MJ, Russell JA, Soldin JJ, et al: Control of gastric pH with cimetidine: Bolus versus primed infusions. *Gastroenterology* 89:532, 1985.
42. Martyn JAJ, Oliveri M, Briggs SE, Greenblatt DJ: Pharmacodynamics of continuous infusions of cimetidine (abstract). *Proc Am Burn Assoc* 21:130, 1989.
43. Oliveri M, Martyn JAJ: Rantidine kinetics and dynamics in burned patients (abstract). *Proc Am Burn Assoc* 21:157, 1989.
44. McGuigan JE: A consideration of adverse effects of cimetidine. *Gastroenterology* 80:181, 1981.
45. Driks MR, Craven DE, Celli BR: Nosocomial pneumonia in intubated patients given sucralfate as compared with antacids or histamine type 2 blockers. *N Engl J Med* 317:1376, 1987.
46. Gronert GA, Theye RA. Pathophysiology of succinylcholine hyperkalemia. *Anesthesiology* 43:89, 1975.
47. Martyn JAJ, Goldhill DR, Goudsouzian NG. Clinical pharmacology of neuromuscular relaxants in patients with burns. *J Clin Pharmacol* 26:680, 1986.
48. Viby-Mogensen H., Hand HK, Hansen E, Grace J: Serum cholinesterase activity in burned patients. *Acta Anesth Scand* 19:159, 1975.
49. Brown TCK, Bell B: Electromyographic responses to small doses of suxamethonium in children with burns. *Br J Anaesth* 59:1017, 1987.
50. Kim C, Fuke N, Martyn JAJ: Thermal injury to rat increases nicotinic acetylcholine receptors in the diaphragm. *Anesthesiology* 68:401, 1988.
51. Brown MJ, Brown DC, Murphy MB: Hypokalemia from beta 2 receptor stimulation by circulating epinephrine. *N Engl J Med* 309:1414, 1983.
52. Martyn JAJ, Matteo RD, Goudsouzian DJ, et al: Pharmacokinetics of *d*-tubocurarine in patients with thermal injury. *Anesth Analg* 61:241, 1982.
53. Leibel WS, Martyn JAJ, Szyfelbein SK, Miller KW: Elevated plasma binding cannot account for the burn related *d*-tubocurarine hyposensitivity. *Anesthesiology* 54:378, 1981.
54. Kim C, Martyn JAJ, Fuke N: Thermal injury to trunk of rat causes denervation-like responses in gastrocnemius muscle. *J Appl Physiol* 65:1745, 1988.
55. Coggeshall JW, Marini JJ, Newman JH: Improved oxygenation after muscle relaxation in adult respiratory distress syndrome. *Arch Intern Med* 145:1718, 1985.
56. Crone RK, Favorito J. The effects of pancuronium in infants with hyaline membrane disease. *J Pediatr* 97:991, 1980.
57. Pollitizer MJ, Reynolds EOR, Shaw DG: Pancuronium during mechanical ventilation speeds recovery of lungs of infants with hyaline membrane disease. *J Pediatr* 97:991, 1980.
58. Demling RH: What are the functions of endorphins following thermal injury (discussion). *J Trauma* 24(suppl):5172, 1984.
59. Kehlet H: Should regional anesthesia and pharmacological agents such as beta blockers and opiates be utilized in modulating pain response? *J Trauma* 24:5177, 1985.
60. Winkelstein A: What are the immunological alterations induced by burn injury? *J Trauma* 24:572, 1984.
61. Perry S, Heidrich G. Management of pain debridement: Survey in U.S. burn units. *Pain* 13:267, 1982.
62. Perry SW: What objective measures are available for evaluating pain (discussion)? *J Trauma* 24(suppl):5191, 1984.
63. Mazze RJ: Fluorinated anestheic/nephrotoxicity: An update. *Can Anaesth Soc J* 31:516, 1984.
64. Filkins SA, Cosgrove P, Marvin JA, et al: Self-administered anesthetic: A method of pain control. *J Burn Care Rehabil* 2:33, 1981.
65. Amos RJ, Amess JAL, Hinds CJ. Incidence and pathogenesis of acute megaloblastic bone marrow change in patients receiving intensive care. *Lancet* 2:835, 1982.
66. Altman LC, Furukawa CT, Klebonoff SJ. Depressed mononuclear leukocyte chemotaxis in thermally injured patients. *J Immunol* 119:199, 1977.
67. Buring JE, Hennekeus CH, Mayrent SL, et al: Health experiences of operating room personnel. *Anesthesiology* 62:325, 1985.
68. Greenblatt DJ, Shader RI, Abernethy DR: Current status of benzodiazepines. *N Engl J Med* 309:354, 1983.
69. Coté CJ, Goudosouzian NG, Liu LMP, et al: Thiopental induction in burned children: A dose response study. *Anesth Analg* 64:1156, 1985.
70. White PF, Way WL, Trevor AJ: Ketamine — Its pharmacology and therapeutic uses. *Anesthesiology* 56:119, 1982.
71. Martyn JAJ, Greenblatt DJ, Quinby WC: Diazepam kinetics following burns. *Anesth Analg* 62:293, 1983.
72. Ciaccio EI, Fruncillo RJ: Urinary excretion of D-acid by severely burned patients. *Clin Pharmacol Ther* 25:340, 1979.
73. Martyn JAJ, Greenblatt DJ: Lorazepam clearance unimpaired in burn trauma. *Clin Pharmacol Ther* 43:250, 1988.

74. Szyfelbein SK, Osgood PF, Carr DB: The assessment of pain and plasma beta endorphin immunoreactivity in burned children. *Pain* 22:173, 1985.
75. Bloedow DC, Goodfellow LA, Marvin J, Heimbach D: Meperidine disposition in burn patients. *Res Commun Chem Pathol Pharmacol* 54:987, 1986.
76. Hill AB, Nahrwold ML, Deroayro AM, Knight PR, et al: Prevention of rigidity during fentanyl-oxygen induction of anesthesia. *Anesthesiology* 55:452, 1981.
77. Perry S, Inturrisi CE: Analgesia and morphine disposition in burn patients. *J Burn Care Rehabil* 4:276, 1983.
78. Gregoretti S, Vinik HR: Sufentanyl pharmacokinetics in burn patients undergoing skin grafting (abstract). *Anesth Analg* 65:564, 1986.
79. Atchison NE, Osgood PE, Szyfelbein SK, Carr DB: The relationship of pain to the depth and extent of burn injury in the pediatric patient (abstract). *Proc Am Burn Assoc* 18:169, 1987.
80. Hilton J: Effects of verapamil on thermal trauma depressed cardiac output in the anesthetized dog. *Burns* 10:313, 1984.
81. Moncrief JA: Effects of various fluid regimens and pharmacologic agents on the circulatory hemodynamics of the immediate post-burn period. *Ann Surg* 166:723, 1966.
82. Cone JB, Ransom JM, Tucker WE, Petrino RA, et al: Effect of dopamine on post-burn myocardial depression. *J Trauma* 22:1019, 1982.
83. Martyn JAJ, Farago L, Burke JF: Hemodynamics of low dose dopamine in nonseptic burned patients. *Circ Shock* 9:206, 1982.
84. Drueck C, Welch GW, Pruitt BA: Hemodynamic analysis of septic shock in thermal injury: Treatment with dopamine. *Am Surg* 44:424, 1978.
85. Timonen RM, Pavlin EG, Hasche RH: Epinephrine levels pre- and post-application of topical epinephrine during burn surgery. *Anesthesiology* 57:A138, 1982.
86. Motulsky HJ, Insel PA. Adrenergic receptors in man: Direct identification of physiologic regulation and clinical alterations. *N Engl J Med* 307:18, 1982.
87. Wilmore DW, Long JA, Mason AD, et al: Catecholamines: Mediator of hypermetabolic response to thermal injury. *Ann Surg* 180:653, 1974.
88. Collucci WS, Wright RF, Braunwald E: New positive inotropic agents in the treatment of congestive heart failure. *N Engl J Med* 314:290, 1986.

Chapter 15

Inhalation Injury in Children

James A. O'Neill, Jr.

The mechanisms of injury and pathophysiology of inhalation injury in children are similar to those noted in adults, but the primary manifestations of injury and some of the therapeutic approaches differ. It is the purpose of this chapter to discuss these differences as they relate to the overall considerations pertaining to respiratory injury.

MECHANISMS OF INJURY IN THE CHILD

Most children sustain inhalation injuries when they are burned in an enclosed space, as in a house fire or an automobile. Since children are generally not cigarette smokers and since most are normal without preexisting disease, they would appear to be more resistant to inhalation injury than adults. Pulmonary ventilation and perfusion are ordinarily quite efficient by 1 month of age, but it should be noted that there is a finite limit to the extent of the work of breathing that a small child can perform. Infants and children normally have a metabolic rate as high as three times the rate measurable in adults, and when such subjects are injured, the metabolic requirements increase up to twofold. Pulmonary compensation is required under these circumstances, and the degree of reserve is limited, so the smaller the subject the more likely pulmonary decompensation is to occur. Consequently, if one adds upper airway obstruction or inhalation injury to the overall picture of burn injury, pulmonary decompensation may occur early following injury. The problem becomes even more marked in the occasional child with preexisting disease such as cystic fibrosis or congenital cardiac disease. Children who are malnourished either at the time they are injured or later as a result of a burn injury not only compensate less well to the need for increased work of breathing but, additionally, have impaired pulmonary immune defense mechanisms which predispose to additional pulmonary complications. Thus, not only factors related to the inhalation injury itself but also factors related to the age and prior condition of the child influence the degree to which the child will be affected by the process. Normally, small children have more rapid respiratory rates than adults, so their tendency to inhale noxious products of combustion will be increased in direct proportion to the minute volume of respiration which is related to age and body size. Finally, inhalation injury may occur either with or without associated skin burns, but when burns are present the considerations related to management, particularly of intravenous fluid therapy, are more complicated.

FORMS OF INHALATION INJURY

Upper Airway Obstruction

The most common form of respiratory difficulty seen in young patients with burns is upper airway obstruction related to edema of the head and neck, glottic and subglottic areas (Fig. 15-1). It would appear that laryngeal edema is probably the direct result of heat injury, and although this may be evident immediately, it may not be obvious until 24 to 48 hours following burn. With fluid resuscitation, edema of the head and neck may become extreme within 12 hours whenever burns of the head and neck are present. This factor would appear to be more marked and it would appear to occur more rapidly in the child than in the adult. The subglottic region at the level of the cricoid cartilage is more narrow relative to the rest of the larynx and trachea in children than in older subjects. Additionally, the ratio of smooth muscle to cartilage in the large airways is greater in childhood than at any other time of life. Thus, edema and laryngospasm have greater significance in the child because of the relatively small size of the airway. Whereas the lower airway is relatively resistant to the effects of heat, the larynx is susceptible to true burn injury. Finally, because of the small size of the airway, it may be more difficult to relieve upper airway obstruction in small subjects than in adults.

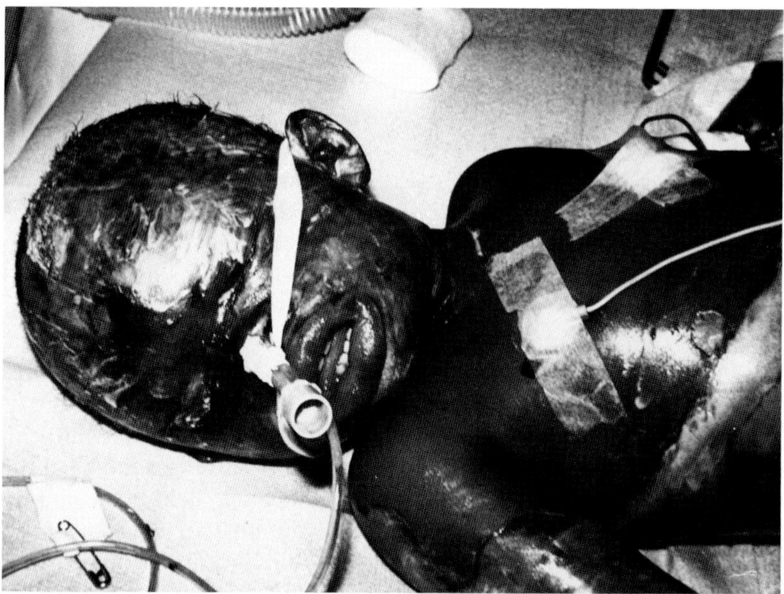

Figure 15-1 This child has an extensive burn sustained in a house fire. Nasotracheal intubation relieved upper airway obstruction, which is the most common manifestation of inhalation injury in childhood. Note the method of tube fixation and immobilization. Tracheostomy was not required.

Bronchospasm

Bronchospasm is almost as common in children as upper airway obstruction, but it is more easily relieved. Bronchospasm may be the result of irritating products of combustion which result in inflammation, or it may be stimulated by the presence of copious secretions. This smooth muscle response to injury may be manifest either at the level of the larynx or all the way to tertiary bronchi. Severe bronchospasm invariably increases the work of breathing in proportion to the degree of restriction of air exchange. Bronchospasm may also be a manifestation of distal airway injury, particularly when it is persistent over a 24-hour period following injury.

Distal Airway Damage

Distal airway injury including effects on the trachea, bronchi, and alveoli represents the most difficult challenge to management, since it results in the maximum disturbance of air exchange. Although inhalation injury to the distal airways may occur in the absence of a skin burn, if a large cutaneous injury is present, inhalation injury is complicated by hypovolemia, massive tissue destruction, the need for large-volume fluid therapy, pulmonary edema, and later infection. Studies of isolated inhalation injury have been performed analyzing the effects of heated air, flame, carbon monoxide, irritant gases, and smoke including incomplete products of combustion. While hot air and flame appear to act primarily on the larynx, the other factors exert their influence on the lower airway (Figs. 15-2 and 15-3). If severe enough at the outset, acute pulmonary edema and severe tracheobronchitis may occur, but if the individual survives the acute phase, the effect may not become evident for 24 to 48 hours.

Stone et al. performed laboratory and clinical studies related to inhalation injury and described manifestations in three time frames including pulmonary edema manifested after 8 hours following injury, respiratory insufficiency occurring in the first 24 to 36 hours after injury, and late bacterial pneumonia.[1] Shimazu and coworkers described a

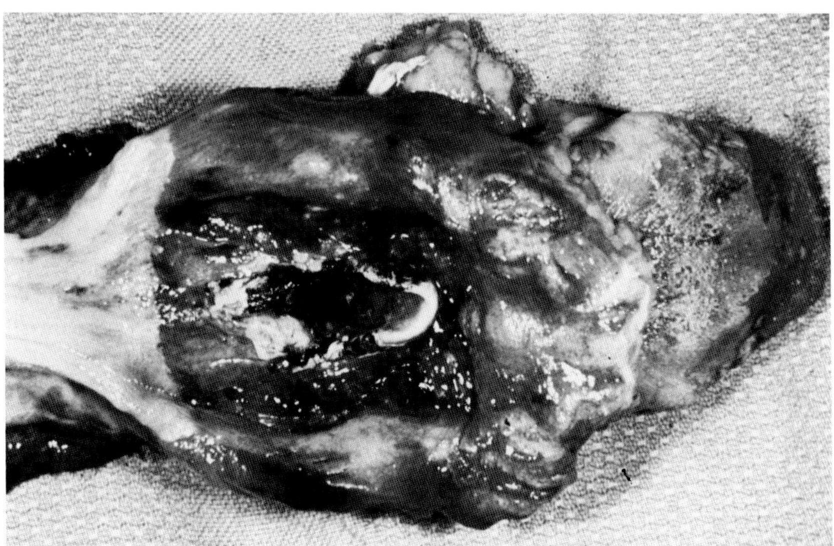

Figure 15-2 Burns of the tracheobronchial tree as shown in this postmortem specimen are primarily localized to the laryngeal region.

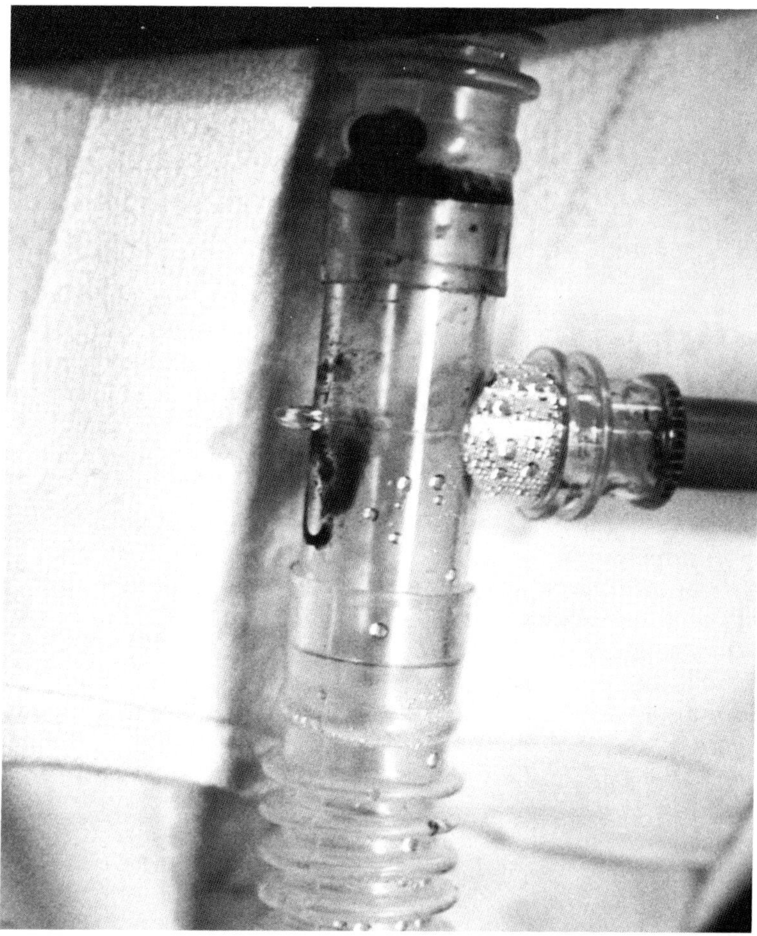

Figure 15-3 Carbonaceous tracheobronchial secretions as demonstrated in this photograph of a ventilatory T-piece indicate extensive smoke inhalation and tracheobronchitis.

dose-response model of smoke inhalation injury in sheep which closely mimicked inhalation injury seen in humans.[2] Their focus was on the physiologic effects of smoke inhalation, which indicated that with an increasing dose of smoke, significant increases in right ventricular stroke work index, P_{CO_2}, pulmonary resistance, static compliance, lung water, left ventricular stroke work index, and cardiac index occurred as well as decreases in P_{O_2}, mean blood pressure, and mean pulmonary artery pressure. Overall, the P_{O_2} demonstrated the best dose-response relationship, and these workers suggested that this might be the most reliable index for the estimation of severity of smoke inhalation injury. On the other hand, Zawacki et al. found that cardiovascular dysfunction was as profound as respiratory dysfunction in clinical and experimental studies.[3] Their studies also indicated that bacterial pneumonia was the most important factor limiting survival. However, they also demonstrated a dose-response relationship in their studies. Further confirmatory studies were performed by Stephenson et al. in a dog model where similar pathophysiologic findings to those noted by Shimazu were found.[4]

Moritz and coworkers performed experimental studies of flame and steam inhalation in dogs and described the location of injury to be the central alveoli and small bronchi.[5] Zikria and coworkers confirmed this finding and suggested that aldehydes were the main noxious substances inhaled and that they were probably more important to distal airway damage than smoke or heat. Again a dose-response relationship was found.[6]

In a classic paper, Foley et al. described the pathology of the lung in fatally burned patients.[7] Although these were primarily patients with associated skin burns and the causes of death were related to many factors, these studies of pulmonary pathology demonstrated an extremely high incidence of pneumonia in such patients. Tracheobronchitis was the most frequent finding in the lungs of these fatally burned patients, and in many instances, tracheostomy was indicted as the initiating factor in erosive tracheitis. The authors were able to clearly establish evidence for thermal and/or chemical laryngotracheitis due to the inhalation injury itself. Carbon deposition and heat necrosis of laryngeal and upper tracheal epithelium are frequently seen in patients who die in fires, but these manifestations are no longer evident after the first or second postburn day should these patients survive (Fig. 15-4).

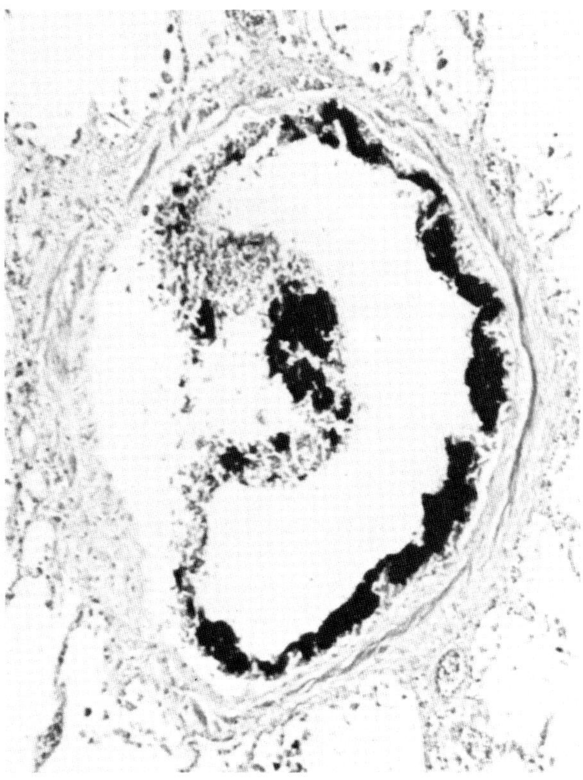

Figure 15-4 Inhalation of heated smoke may result in deposition of carbon in distal airway structures, as shown in this photomicrograph, but this clears rapidly should the patient survive the initial insult.

The location of lesions found by Foley et al. corresponded to those noted in the experimental studies of Moritz. In those patients dying of inhalation injury, the lungs tended to be edematous with spotty areas of atelectasis. They appeared to be hepatized, with large areas of bronchopneumonia and severe tracheobronchitis. All studies show that microscopic findings include capillary congestion, interstitial and intraalveolar hemorrhage, and fluid accumulation. The lining of the alveoli tends to be hyperplastic, and hyaline membranes are frequently noted. This may even extend to deposition of collagen in the same areas.

Rapaport et al. examined the effects of 30 percent body surface burns on rats and demonstrated the possibility that thermal injury may cause the release of fibrin-platelet microaggregates into the whole circulation with subsequent embolization to the pulmonary vascular tree as another factor which may be superimposed pathologically on inhalation injury.[8] On the other hand, experimental studies of Prien et al. in sheep subjected to cotton-smoke inhalation injury clearly demonstrated that the lung lesions produced were localized to the area of injury rather than being a generalized pulmonary response in a one lung inhalation model.[9] This indicated that there was a lack of hematogenous-mediated pulmonary injury with smoke inhalation, although the studies were of shorter term than the ones performed by Rapaport.

Walker et al. developed an experimental inhalation injury model in the goat and noted that inhalation injuries in this setting were usually produced by inhalation of gaseous or particulate products of incomplete combustion and were rarely due to heat alone unless steam was inhaled.[10] These workers also noted the manifestations of necrotic tracheobronchitis with broncheolitis associated with pseudomembrane and cast formation as well as multifocal atelectasis and bronchopneumonia. The time frame for recovery from these injuries in goats was 3 weeks, indicating that the jeopardy from inhalation injury, when it is severe, may last a long time. The clinical course of pediatric-age patients indicates that this also appears to be true in the young age group.

Head as well as others have analyzed the effects of inhalation injury on surfactant, and although he noted in patient studies that surfactant activity of bronchial secretions was usually within the normal range during the first week after injury, during the second week subnormal levels were noted.[11] After the third week surfactant appeared to be present in normal amounts confirming previous observations that inhalation injury appears to recover after 3 weeks.

Mason and his group have pointed out the importance of bacteria as a complicating factor in patients with inhalation injury.[12] This has also been pointed out by Achauer et al.[13] Studies by Pruitt and colleagues as well as Petroff et al. have demonstrated that control of bacteria within a burn wound has a beneficial effect on the prevention of late pulmonary complications in such patients, particularly those with inhalation injury.[14–16] The matter of bacterial complications related to inhalation injury was well demonstrated in the Achauer study in which there were three distinct groups of patients noted.[13] The first group was patients with inhalation injury presenting almost immediately with symptoms related to smoke inhalation, carbon monoxide poisoning, or problems related to airway obstruction. The second group of patients presented after 24 to 48 hours of being asymptomatic but then became tachypneic, cyanotic, and hypoxemic 1 to 5 days following injury. It was at this time that patchy bilateral pulmonary infiltrates were noted on x-ray. These patients might either go on to recover or develop progressive respiratory acidosis, high pulmonary resistance, and myocardial depression. Finally, Achauer noted a third group of patients in whom bacterial pneumonia superimposed on inhalation injury occurred late and resulted in death.

Another study by Linares et al. describes a sequence of morphologic events in experimental smoke inhalation representative of the clinical picture usually seen. They found that during the first 48 hours following inhalation injury in sheep an exudative phase occurred with accumulation of fluid and acute inflammatory cells within the alveoli and interstitial areas as well.[17] Associated with this was venular and lymphatic dilatation. Pulmonary congestion was marked, although endothelial cell damage was minimal. On the other hand, the damage to type I pneumocytes was noted to be marked and not necessarily reversible. At this early stage, the tracheobronchial epithelium also showed cytoplasmic vacuolization and focal areas of necrosis. Overlapping this first exudative phase of 48 hours was a phase noted between 12 and 72 hours following inhalation injury where there was degeneration of elements of the bronchial tree with progressive epithelial necrosis and shedding with formation of pseudomembranous casts which corresponded to those we often see coughed up by patients. These casts of the tracheobronchial tree resulted in partial or complete obstruction of the airways. There was subsequent desquamation in association with this. This latter phase, which included the formation of hyaline membranes, progressed to a proliferative phase which was noted 2 to 7 days after inhalation. There was then proliferation of type II pneumocytes with hyperplasia and mobilization of macrophages. In the upper airways, remnants of basal cells and cells from glandular ducts proliferated in order to heal the damaged epithelium. The same was true in the alveoli, where type II pneumocytes proliferated to cover the denuded basement membrane. There was atypia in these new cells, which suggested that they were not functioning normally. Finally, the last phase was that of late healing, which, as mentioned, may take as long as 3 weeks. Despite healing we know that long-standing damage may be present with the presence of bronchial polyps, bronchiolitis obliterans, and subsequent sacular bronchiectasis. Special note should be made of the fact that in the child, the small size of the airway and the degree of bronchial obstruction associated with sloughing of tracheobronchial mucosa may present much more of a problem at an earlier time than in adults.

Carbon Monoxide Poisoning

Carbon monoxide poisoning is a significant factor related to early death in patients with inhalation injury, and since it is related to the injury itself, it may present a problem whether or not the patient has an associated skin burn. The pathophysiology is that of suffocation from anoxia due to inhalation of less than normal levels of atmospheric oxygen and carboxyhemoglobinemia from inhalation of carbon monoxide. When one considers that the functional surface of the lung is in the range of 30 to 40 m^2 in a child, it is easy to envision how rapidly carbon monoxide poisoning can occur. Carbon monoxide poisoning is most apt to occur in patients burned in house fires, as demonstrated by Zikria et al.[18] Carboxyhemoglobin interferes with oxygen transport, because carbon monoxide has a greater affinity for hemoglobin than does oxygen. If patients are supersaturated with oxygen, it is possible to displace carbon monoxide from hemoglobin to a significant degree. Grube et al. have reviewed the problem of carbon monoxide toxicity and pointed out that carbon monoxide has a higher affinity for iron than does oxygen, which is responsible for its displacement of oxygen from hemoglobin and other iron-binding proteins.[19] Carbon monoxide thereby inhibits oxidative mitochondrial respiration catalyzed by cytochrome oxidase, resulting in a shift of the oxygen dissociation curve to the left. The effects of carbon monoxide toxicity in injured patients would appear to be accentuated by shock, indicating the importance of maintaining normal levels of cardiac output in such patients.

DIAGNOSIS OF INHALATION INJURY

Clinical Diagnosis

The history of a patient being trapped in an enclosed space in a house fire or automobile, with or without cutaneous burns, should suggest the possibility of inhalation injury. Burns of the head and neck associated with burns of the ala nasi, and blisters of the lips, tongue, or palate are further indications. Hoarseness, wheezing, irritative cough, and rapid respiratory rate are particularly good clinical indicators in young children. DiVincenti et al. characterized the clinical findings in adults chronologically, and we have noted the same findings except accelerated by 12 hours or more.[20] DiVincenti's group noted that early signs and symptoms were often not remarkable or were even absent and that they first appeared at times varying from 24 hours onward. The most common finding was at 48 hours, where there was productive cough with excessive tracheobronchial secretions with expectoration of carbon particles and clear fluid. By the third to fourth postburn day, sputum became purulent, and bronchial casts and necrotic epithelium were noted. Inspiratory and expiratory wheezes were evident by 48 hours, but we have noted wheezing ordinarily at 12 to 24 hours. In severe cases, cyanosis has been noted early as well. It is our feeling that clinical history and findings are usually sufficient for the diagnosis of inhalation injury and the initiation of therapy.

As mentioned above, hypoxemia is one of the best hallmarks of the severity of inhalation injury. Consequently, serial determination of blood gases is probably the most helpful as well as the simplest method of confirming one's clinical impression that inhalation injury is present as well as determining how severe it is. Hypoxemia, hypercarbia, and respiratory acidosis are the hallmarks of inhalation injury to the distal airways. As a matter of fact, hypoxemia may become evident before there are manifestations evident on chest x-ray.

Xenon 133 Lung Scan

Moylan et al. were the first to use xenon 133 lung scans for the early diagnosis of inhalation injury.[21] They used a small dose of ^{133}Xe intravenously. Since it is minimally soluble in water, it is excreted almost entirely into the alveoli on its first passage through the lungs. It is then possible using scintigraphy with a gamma camera to determine the timing of complete washout. Washout is noted to be extremely delayed in patients with inhalation injury, and additionally, there characteristically are localized areas of retention. Thus, ^{133}Xe perfusion/ventilation scanning may give one a measure of regional function in patients who have inhalation injury. It is also possible to study such patients on a serial basis because of the rapid excretion of xenon. Generally speaking there are very few false positive or false negative diagnoses with this technique, although theoretically that would be possible. Presumably, use of this technique would permit the clinician to institute early treatment, but clinical suspicion and notation of hypoxemia on blood gas determination may be just as helpful provided the clinician is aggressive enough. With regard to the child, excessive radiation is a consideration, but scanning would still appear to be safe even in this age group. Schall et al. have also pointed out the value of ^{133}Xe scanning in burn patients and have pointed out that a single scan produces an estimated radiation exposure of 100 millirads to the lungs and 2.5 millirads to the gonads, figures which are comparable to similar diagnostic x-ray studies.[22] This would be more than a single chest x-ray, of course. Xenon 133 scanning is probably the only way to make an early diagnosis in those patients who have experienced inhalation injury involving damage to the terminal bronchi and alveoli.

Bronchoscopy

In selected instances we have used fiberoptic bronchoscopy and laryngoscopy in order to make the diagnosis of inhalation injury. Obviously, laryngeal and upper airway injuries can virtually all be diagnosed with bronchoscopy, and these injuries constitute over 90 percent of the patients with inhalation airway injuries. Hunt et al. have suggested the use of fiberoptic bronchoscopy in patients burned in an enclosed space; those exposed to noxious smoke; those with facial burns; and those who are hoarse, cough up carbon, or have rales, wheezes, or hypoxemia.[23] Agee et al. in the same group studied a group of patients who had ^{133}Xe scanning as well as bronchoscopy and demonstrated that with this combination of studies essentially 100 percent of patients can be diagnosed accurately to have inhalation injury.[24] We have used fiberoptic bronchoscopy primarily for the purpose of assisting with the placement of endotracheal tubes or for therapeutic purposes in order to perform tracheobronchial toilet. In small children, we have preferred to depend on a combination of clinical impression based on physical findings as well as blood gases in order to initiate early therapy. The rationale behind performance of early bronchoscopy and lung scanning for diagnoses is to stimulate the clinician to initiate early aggressive pulmonary therapeutic measures.

Pulmonary Function Testing

Pulmonary function testing is probably best used after the first 24 hours postburn. After that interval the main manifestations of inhalation injury involve the lower airways as pneumonia and atelectasis. Certainly blood gas determinations represent one form of pulmonary function testing. Spitzer and Arnhold have described methods of studying pulmonary function in injured patients which permits determination of pulmonary mechanics in patients who are unable to cooperate.[25] One of the best methods of studying pulmonary mechanics is to use the maximum expiratory flow volume curve. Generally, patients with inhalation injury will show manifestations of diminished vital capacity and flow rate and volume and increased pulmonary resistance. Pulmonary function testing in association with blood gas determination may help to explain the reasons for the presence of ventilation/perfusion mismatch or pulmonary shunting. Also, the increases in pulmonary resistance and decreases in static lung compliance which have been noted on pulmonary function testing in patients with severe inhalation injury provide the key to the approach to treatment in terms of pulmonary toilet and ventilatory therapy.

Blood Gas Determinations

Mention has already been made of the importance of determining carboxyhemoglobin levels in patients suspected of having inhalation injury, particularly those who appear to be confused or agitated despite the lack of skin burns or shock. Mention has already been made regarding the significance of hypoxemia noted on blood gas determination, particularly performed serially. Other early indicators of pulmonary dysfunction include determination of the alveolar-to-arterial oxygen pressure difference and the arterial-oxygen-pressure-to-inspired-oxygen-fraction ratio, because these measurements estimate venous admixture across the pulmonary vascular bed using only arterial blood samples. $[P(A\text{-}a)_{O_2}]$, (Pa_{O_2}/FI_{O_2}). As with pulmonary function tests, these more sophisticated forms of blood gas utilization are probably more valuable in the determination of the severity of injury than they are from the standpoint of diagnosis.

COMPLICATIONS AND APPROACHES TO TREATMENT OF INHALATION INJURY

Upper Airway Obstruction

As mentioned, the most common manifestation of inhalation injury in childhood is obstruction of the upper airway from edema, and laryngeal or bronchial spasm. At times there is direct injury to the upper part of the larynx from the effects of heat as well. One advantage to early fiberoptic laryngoscopy and bronchoscopy is that if edema of the vocal cords is noted, early intubation can be performed. We feel that if significant respiratory distress is noted on admission or if there is any suggestion of the possibility of later compromise of the airway by edema, immediate nasal or orotracheal intubation should be performed. Our preference is for nasotracheal intubation, but if that is not possible, orotracheal intubation is satisfactory. If one delays institution of intubation, severe swelling may make insertion of the tube impossible, increasing the risk of the procedure. It is our feeling that the indications for intubation should be liberal in order to be safe. In the childhood age group, we feel that it is not only sufficient but preferable to place a noncuffed tube which is not totally occlusive, so that the tendency for subglottic stenosis can be diminished (Fig. 15-1). Fiberoptic bronchoscopy can be used to guide a nasotracheal or orotracheal tube into position. Instillation of a nasal vasoconstrictor agent is helpful. It has been our preference to intubate such patients awake, but some prefer to use paralytic agents or even general anesthesia for this purpose.

It is helpful to remember that the upper airway anatomy of the child is different from that of the adult. The child's larynx is of course smaller than the adult's and is generally more difficult to visualize because it has a more anterior position and angle than seen in the adult. In addition, the trachea is short in young children, being approximately 5 cm in length in the infant, 7 cm at 18 months of age, and proportionately longer as the child grows. It has been noted that there is a disproportion between the size of the skull and the midface in the child, and the smaller the child the more this is the case. For this reason the relatively larger occipital portion of the skull produces flexion of the cervical spine making intubation more difficult.

The other factor in the child which is more of a problem than in the adult has to do with the fact that children tend to vomit easily, so upper airway obstruction from secretions and particulate matter is more frequently a problem in young subjects. A simple technique to judge the appropriate size of the tube for intubation is to select one which is approximately the diameter of the child's nares in terms of diameter or to equate the size of the tube with the child's fifth finger. It is best to position the tube between 2 and 3 cm below the level of the cords as proven by x-ray. However, careful auscultation of both sides of the chest should be performed in order to be certain that there are good breath sounds bilaterally as a way of ruling out intubation of one of the main stem bronchi. If that occurs, it is usually the right side that has been intubated selectively. In our experience, nasal or endotracheal intubation suffices in the majority of instances, since upper airway obstruction is the primary problem in most children sustaining inhalation injury either with or without cutaneous burns. Tracheostomy has been reserved for those who have been estimated to require intubation longer than 7 to 10 days, when airway management has been difficult because of profuse secretions, or when prolonged ventilatory assistance is required. A number of studies including those of Teplitz, Slogoff, Moylan, and Lund and their coworkers have pointed out the dangers associated with the use of tracheostomy in burn patients.[26–29] The most serious problem has been the later occurrence of erosive tracheitis with bacterial seeding and subsequent bronchopneumonia. This is why we have preferred to use endotracheal tubes rather than tracheostomy whenever possible.

One of the problems which must be considered in the use of endotracheal tubes is subglottic stenosis. Unfortunately there is no reliable rule regarding how long it is safe to leave an indwelling endotracheal tube in place. However, studies performed by us in children indicate that endotracheal tubes may be left in infants for as long as 3 months without the occurrence of subglottic stenosis, but the figure is probably 2 to 3 weeks in older children.[30] The presence of bacterial pneumonia increases the potential for subglottic stenosis. In these instances, tracheostomy would then be a lesser risk.

When tracheostomy is performed, it should be performed at the level of the second and third tracheal rings rather than lower, because progressive edema of the head and neck may result in decannulation. Also, performance of tracheostomy under uncontrolled conditions may result in pneumothorax or damage to vascular structures or the esophagus.

Distal Airway and Parenchyma Injury

Patients who have severe exudative and subsequent degenerative changes in the airway with mucosal sloughing and cast formation generally require not only vigorous pulmonary toilet but also aggressive ventilatory support. While pneumothorax related to barotrauma is always a consideration in adults, it occurs more frequently in children, usually in association with accumulation of interstitial air. Depending upon the degree of pulmonary dysfunction, we generally approach mild hypoxemia with nasotracheal intubation and intermittent mandatory ventilation with continuous positive airway pressure. It is important to be certain that the child is comfortable under these conditions and does not have excessive work of breathing. Otherwise, progressive hypoxemia, hypercarbia, and significant lactic acidosis will result. An endotracheal tube is sufficient for patients requiring short-term ventilatory support, but a tracheostomy is probably preferable for those children who will require prolonged ventilatory support. Those patients who have severe manifestations of inhalation injury associated with increased pulmonary resistance and significant pulmonary edema will generally require controlled ventilation with positive inspiratory and positive end-expiratory pressure (PEEP) balanced in a fashion which will permit normalization of blood oxygen and carbon dioxide. Levels of inspired oxygen provided must be adjusted according to the demonstrated oxygen requirements of the patient. Adjunctive measures of importance include prevention of infection and aggressive tracheobronchial toilet, including serial bronchoscopies if necessary. Diuresis may also be important, particularly from the third to the seventh postburn day. When levels of PEEP are above 15 cm of water, pneumothorax frequently results. At times, high-frequency jet ventilation may be needed if excessive levels of PEEP are required and complications result. Additionally, levels above this may produce decreases in cardiac output resulting in the need for the use of inotropic drugs. Finally, maintenance of adequate nutrition is important not only from the standpoint of supporting the integrity of the respiratory musculature but also from the standpoint of maintaining the effectiveness of the patient's immune system in preventing infection. In the past, steroids have been suggested as being potentially beneficial for patients with inhalation injury. The only time we have found steroids to be of any benefit has been in patients with severe manifestations of bronchospasm, and then only temporarily. We have not been able to demonstrate any improvements in pulmonary function or outcome. In addition, we have had some reason to question whether the use of steroids has potentiated the emergence of infection.

Carbon Monoxide Poisoning

As early as 1963, Epstein et al. performed a clinicopathologic study of hypoxemia in the burned patient.[31] In their studies they noted that hypoxemia was frequently noted even though examination of the chest and chest x-ray revealed no abnormalities at the time performed. Epstein et al. were able to correlate clinical and postmortem findings with low oxygen tensions noted in patients, and their studies resulted in the recommendation that supplemental oxygen should be administered to any patient with a large total body surface burn or to those with clinical signs of pulmonary impairment or even the potential for it. This is also the best approach to patients with excessive carboxyhemoglobinemia, since the provision of 100 percent oxygen by mask may be sufficient to displace carbon monoxide molecules from the blood. At times, it is obvious that endotracheal intubation and controlled ventilation with supplemental oxygen are necessary to support the patient with carbon monoxide poisoning. This is particularly true in the child who presents with early neurologic dysfunction, because there is some evidence to suggest that early effective treatment may prevent permanent neurologic sequellae. We have tended to use hyperbaric oxygen therapy as a treatment for patients with severe smoke inhalation injuries and carbon monoxide poisoning and have not had any complications such as air embolus, seizures, or middle ear complications, but the true contribution of this form of therapy remains in question. Grube et al. analyzed hyperbaric oxygen therapy for carbon monoxide poisoning in 10 of their patients and were unable to demonstrate any benefit.[19] For this reason, we have not considered this form of therapy for patients with severe metabolic derangements or those with severe ventilatory or hemodynamic instability, since movement to the hyperbaric chamber is dangerous under these circumstances.

APPROACHES TO FLUID RESUSCITATION IN PATIENTS WITH INHALATION INJURY

Patients who have isolated inhalation injuries do not present problems with regard to fluid management. Such patients have difficulty with pulmonary edema and increased evaporative water loss associated with increased metabolic rate, but these deficits are easily covered even when diuretic therapy is necessary. On the other hand, patients with associated thermal burns, particularly those with large surface area involvement, present significant problems in this respect. Studies performed by O'Neill as well as others clearly indicate that fluid requirements are increased in patients who have inhalation injuries associated with cutaneous burns as compared with patients who have cutaneous burns alone.[32] Obviously, this complicates matters, as it is desirable to minimize the tendency to pulmonary edema. However, the prime consideration is maintenance of cardiac output and adequate organ flow so that the degree of tissue injury in the lung is not worsened by a secondary factor over and above injury itself. Studies by Navar and Merrell and their colleagues have also demonstrated that patients with inhalation injuries require volumes of resuscitation fluid in excess of those predicted by the commonly used Parkland formula.[33,34] Of even more importance is the fact that, in the study of Navar et al., the increase in fluid requirement was constant regardless of age. The mean fluid requirement in their patients with inhalation injury was 5.76 mL/kg/percent burn, whereas patients without pulmonary damage required 4 mL/kg/percent burn. In our patients the increased requirement was approximately 35 percent. In studies by Scheulen and Munster the increase was 37 percent, while it was 44 percent in the patients of Navar et al.[35] We have found it useful to monitor urine output in children as a guide to the adequacy of resuscitation in all patients, including those with inhalation injuries, with a value of 1 mL/kg/h considered adequate provided that clinical manifestations of cardiac output are also adequate. We have continued to use crystalloid resuscitation in all burn patients, including those with inhalation injuries. It has been our impression that accumulation of pulmonary edema occurs over a number of days and that it appears to be more related to the severity of the inhalation injury than to the volume of fluid required for resuscitation. In the past, it has been argued that the use of colloid in resuscitation may minimize the accumulation of extravascular lung water. However, the studies of Goodwin and coworkers have failed to show any advantage of early use of colloid in resuscitation, and actually these workers demonstrated a progressive increase in extravascular lung water over the first 7 days following injury which was not observed when crystalloid resuscitation alone was utilized.[36] For these reasons we have tended to use volumes of crystalloid resuscitation, which have supported adequate cardiac output and urine flow regardless of the degree of inhalation injury.

INFECTIOUS COMPLICATIONS IN TREATMENT

Reference has already been made to the occurrence of tracheitis seen in association with tracheostomy tubes. This indicates that scrupulous aseptic technique is vital in the management of patients with artificial airways. The risks appear to be higher in patients requiring tracheostomy, but it must be acknowledged that patients requiring this form of airway management almost undoubtedly have greater degrees of tracheobronchial injury to begin with. Because of damage to the tracheobronchial mucosa, normal ciliary and mucous clearing mechanisms are impaired. Additionally, the function of pulmonary macrophages is impaired as well, so that invasive infection is potentiated. Patients with extensive cutaneous burns become colonized with pathogenic and opportunistic organisms, and these have the potential to enter the tracheobronchial tree and pulmonary parenchyma as well. Additionally, there are blood-born factors associated with thromboembolism and infectious embolism associated with intravenous and other intravascular catheters. The key to prevention of infection is regular bacteriologic surveillance with chest x-rays and appropriate cultures of the tracheobronchial tree and all other sites of potential infection. Careful tracheobronchial toilet and prevention of atelectasis also help to minimize the chances for infection. Bacteria-specific antibiotic therapy is the most effective method of approach. Shirani et al. studied the use of immunoglobulin G (IgG) in burn patients to determine whether normal IgG levels could be achieved.[37] Their studies indicated that it is indeed possible to maintain normal IgG levels but that in patients with large burns, twice weekly infusions may be required. This is probably not a very practical method of approach, but it does provide information regarding the relationship of the patient's immune system to subsequent infection. Lalonde and Demling have suggested that complete burn wound excision and wound closure not only diminish postburn oxygen consumption but additionally diminish the chances for infection, including infection in the lung. This is consistent with the work of Dressler and Skornik, who demonstrated that the presence of eschar diminishes lung bacterial clearance, suggesting that a systemic toxin may be operative.[38,39] Studies by Shirani et al. and Merrell et al., in different burn units, have demonstrated that with better infection control and prevention of pneumonia, there has been improvement in overall mortality noted in association with inhalation injury.[40,41] This has certainly been the case in childhood. To date, no benefit has been demonstrated with the use of aerosolized antibiotics, so systemic antibiotic therapy and support of the patient's immune system would appear to be the mainstays of infection control in these patients. Regardless of these many advances in supportive therapy, mortality of severe inhalation injury remains high.

REFERENCES

1. Stone HH, Rhame W, Corbitt JD, et al: Respiratory burns: A correlation of clinical and laboratory results. *Ann Surg* 165:157, 1967.
2. Shimazu T, Yukioka T, Hubbard GB, et al: A dose-responsive model of smoke inhalation injury. *Ann Surg* 206:89, 1987.
3. Zawacki BE, Jung RC, Joyce J, et al: Smoke, burns, and the natural history of inhalation injury in fire victims: A correlation of experimental and clinical data. *Ann Surg* 185:100, 1977.
4. Stephenson SF, Esrig BC, Polk HC, et al: The pathophysiology of smoke inhalation injury. *Ann Surg* 182:652, 1975.
5. Moritz AR, Hennques FC, McLean R: The effects of inhaled heat on the air passages and lung. *Am J Pathol* 21:311, 1945.
6. Zikria BA, Ferrer JM, Flock HF: The chemical factors contributing to pulmonary damage in "smoke poisoning." *Surgery* 71:704, 1972.
7. Foley FD, Moncrief JA, Mason AD: Pathology of the lung in fatally burned patients. *Ann Surg* 167:251, 1968.
8. Rapaport FT, Nemirovsky MS, Bachvaroff R, et al: Mechanisms of pulmonary damage in severe burns. *Ann Surg* 177:472, 1973.
9. Prien T, Linares HA, Traber LD, et al: Lack of hematogenous mediated pulmonary injury with smoke inhalation. *J Burn Care Rehabil* 9:462,1988.
10. Walker HL, McLeod CG, McManus WF: Experimental inhalation injury in the goat. *J Trauma* 21:962, 1981.
11. Head JM: Inhalation injury in burns. *Am J Surg* 139:508, 1980.
12. Mason AD, McManus AT, Pruitt BA: Association of burn mortality and bacteremia. *Arch Surg* 121:1027, 1986.
13. Achauer BM, Allyn PA, Furnas DW, et al: Pulmonary complications of burns: The major threat to the burn patient. *Ann Surg* 177:311, 1973.
14. Pruitt BA, DiVincenti FC, Mason AD, et al: The occurrence and significance of pneumonia and other pulmonary complications in burned patients: Comparison of conventional and topical treatments. *J Trauma* 10:519, 1970.
15. Pruitt BA, Erickson DR, Morris A: Progressive pulmonary insufficiency and other pulmonary complications of thermal injury. *J Trauma* 15:369, 1975.
16. Petroff PA, Hander EW, Mason AD: Ventilatory patterns following burn injury and effect of Sulfamylon. *J Trauma* 15:650, 1975.
17. Linares HA, Herndon DN, Traber DL: Sequence of morphologic events in experimental smoke inhalation. *J Burn Care Rehabil* 10:27, 1989.
18. Zikria BA, Weston GC, Chodoff M, et al: Smoke and carbon monoxide poisoning in fire victims. *J Trauma* 12:641, 1972.
19. Grube BJ, Marvin JA, Heimbach DM: Therapeutic hyperbaric oxygen: Help or hindrance in burn patients with carbon monoxide poisoning? *J Burn Care Rehabil 9:249, 1988.*
20. DiVincenti FC, Pruitt BA, Reckler JM: Inhalation injuries. *J Trauma* 11:109, 1971.
21. Moylan JA, Wilmore DW, Mouton DE, et al: Early diagnosis of inhalation injury using Xenon lung scan. *Ann Surg* 176:477, 1972.
22. Schall GL, McDonald HD, Carr LB, et al: Xenon ventilation-perfusion lung scans. *JAMA* 240:2441, 1978.
23. Hunt JL, Agee RN, Pruitt BA: Fiberoptic bronchoscopy in acute inhalation injury. *J Trauma* 15:641, 1975.
24. Agee RN, Long JM, Hunt JL, et al: Use of Xenon in early diagnosis of inhalation injury. *J Trauma* 16:218, 1976.
25. Spitzer KW, Arnhold H: A valve assembly for studying pulmonary function in trauma patients. *J Thorac Cardiovasc Surg* 66:607, 1973.
26. Teplitz C, Epstein BS, Rose LR, et al: Necrotizing tracheitis induced by tracheostomy tube. *Arch Pathol* 77:14, 1964.
27. Slogoff S, Allen GW, Warden GD, et al: Tracheoesophageal fistula following prolonged tracheal intubation in a thermally injured patient. *Anesthesiology* 39:453, 1973.
28. Moylan JA, West JT, Nash G, et al: Tracheostomy in thermally injured patients: A review of five years' experience. *Am Surg* 38:119, 1972.
29. Lund T, Goodwin CW, McManus WF, et al: Upper airway sequelae in burn patients requiring endotracheal intubation or tracheostomy. *Ann Surg* 201:374, 1985.
30. O'Neill JA: Experience with iatrogenic laryngeal and tracheal stenosis. *J Pediatr Surg* 19:235, 1984.
31. Epstein BS, Hardy DL, Harrison HN, et al: Hypoxemia

in the burned patient: A clinical-pathologic study. *Ann Surg* 158:924, 1963.

32. O'Neill JA: Fluid resuscitation in the burned child — a reappraisal. *J Pediatr Surg* 17:604, 1982.
33. Navar PD, Saffle JR, Warden GD: Effect of inhalation injury on fluid resuscitation requirements after thermal injury. *Am J Surg* 150:716, 1985.
34. Merrell SW, Saffle JR, Sullivan JJ, et al: Fluid resuscitation in thermally injured children. *Am J Surg* 152:664, 1986.
35. Scheulen JJ, Munster AM: The Parkland formula in patients with burns and inhalation injury. *J Trauma* 22:869, 1982.
36. Goodwin CW, Dorethy J, Lam V, et al: Randomized trial of efficacy of crystalloid and colloid resuscitation on hemodynamic response and lung water following thermal injury. *Ann Surg* 197:520, 1983.
37. Shirani KZ, Vaughan GM, McManus AT, et al: Replacement therapy with modified immunoglobulin G in burn patients: Preliminary kinetic studies. *Am J Med* 76(3A):175, 1984.
38. Lalonde C, Demling RH: The effect of complete burn wound excision and closure on postburn oxygen consumption. *Surgery* 102:862, 1987.
39. Dressler DP, Skornik WA: Eschar: A major factor in postburn pneumonia. *Am J Surg* 127:413, 1974.
40. Shirani KZ, Pruitt BA, Mason AD: The influence of inhalation injury and pneumonia on burn mortality. *Ann Surg* 205:82, 1987.
41. Merrell SW, Saffle JR, Sullivan JJ, et al: Increased survival after major thermal injury. *Am J Surg* 154:623, 1987.

Chapter 16

Miscellaneous Pulmonary Complications

Andrew M. Munster
Leslie A. Wong

The true incidence of the complications about to be discussed is almost impossible to ascertain. Since most of the major series in the literature are retrospective, and reviewers depend on coded diagnoses, the inclusion of any one complication in the course of a patient with a major burn necessarily depends on the importance of that particular complication in the view of the person coding the chart. While clear-cut diagnoses requiring later intervention, such as subglottic stenosis, are probably accurately reported, we suspect that other diagnoses such as aspiration pneumonia are grossly underreported. Perusal of the literature, which will be referred to in more detail below, reveals a wide range in the reported incidence of these problems, which may be summarized as follows: pleural effusion 1–2.6 percent; atelectasis 2.6–8 percent; aspiration 0.3–83 percent; pulmonary embolus 0.4–29 percent; pneumothorax 0.4–8.3 percent; and tracheal stenosis 1–11 percent (of patients with tracheostomies).

The analysis to be undertaken takes into account the literature, as well as a series of 1770 patients admitted to the Baltimore Regional Burn Center over the 8-year period 1979–86. Illustrative cases will be presented for each of the major complications.

PLEURAL EFFUSION

The incidence of pleural effusion in burn patients is low. Pruitt et al.[1] reported 7 cases in 697 admissions, for an incidence of 1 percent; an autopsy series from the same authors[2] reported 1 case in 38 autopsies, 2.6 percent. In the Baltimore series, 3 patients of 1770 (0.2 percent) were diagnosed as having pleural effusion.

The effusions are usually cardiogenic and occur in elderly patients requiring massive fluid resuscitation. Diagnosis is usually made on chest roentgenogram. Because of the danger of empyema in the burn patient, small effusions should initially be treated by medical means such as diuretics. Recurrent or large effusions interfering with vital capacity should be tapped, but recurrent tapping or placement of chest tubes should be avoided. Rarely a pleural effusion will contain fluid from an extravasated subclavian catheter; these usually resolve unless they contain blood, in which case they need to be evacuated.

ATELECTASIS

Pruitt et al.[1] reported an incidence of 2.6 percent clinically apparent atelectasis; however, in a later review of radiologically diagnosed pulmonary complications, the incidence was 8 percent.[3]

CASE REPORT

A 78-year-old male sustained 20 percent total body surface burns in a house fire. His entire face and scalp had third-degree injury; he was intubated on admission because of severe smoke inhalation and required early respirator support. This third-degree burns were excised and grafted. Postoperatively, thick mucous secretions were noted and he required frequent suctioning. Nevertheless, the weaning process was proceeding well when, on the third postoperative day, he developed sudden tachypnea, hypoxemia, and hypercarbia, and chest x-ray showed complete atelectasis of the left lung. The endotracheal tube was found to be in the correct position. Bronchoscopy revealed thick mucus plugging of the left main bronchus, which was cleared. The patient required several further bronchoscopic interventions of both lungs and a tracheostomy, until final clearance and recovery 7 weeks later (Figs. 16-1 and 16-2).

The most common cause of atelectasis of a lung, in our experience, is a low-lying endotracheal (ET) tube. It is currently our recommendation that upon insertion of an ET tube, the location of the tube be checked radiologically, following which a note should be made recording the measurement of the tube at the incisor teeth. Each nursing shift checks this "reading" at the beginning of their shift. Next, inspissated secretions may actually block a tube, especially in a patient with severe inhalation injury and mucous casts (Fig. 16-3). Difficulty in passing a suction catheter through the length of a well-positioned ET tube should lead to a consideration of tube change. Both macro- and microatelectasis should be managed by aggressive pulmonary toilet, encouragement of the patient to cough, suctioning, and, if necessary, bronchoscopy. Failure to expand an atelectatic segment or lobe sets the stage for pulmonary infection. Endotracheal tube motion or slippage occurs less when the tube is inserted via the nasotracheal rather than the endotracheal route.

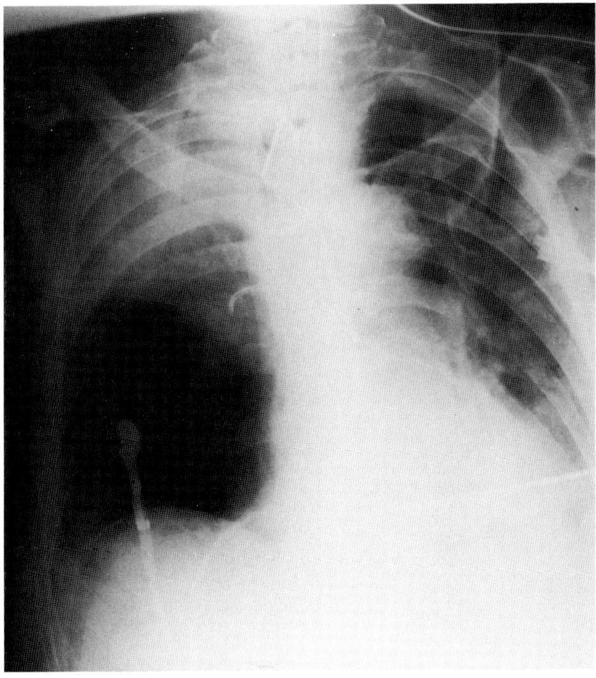

Figure 16-1 Atelectasis of the right upper lobe in a 78-year-old man.

The prevention of atelectasis is probably aided by the almost universal practice today of using continuous positive airway pressure (CPAP), although Venus et al.[4] found no difference between the mortality rate of patients who did or did not develop

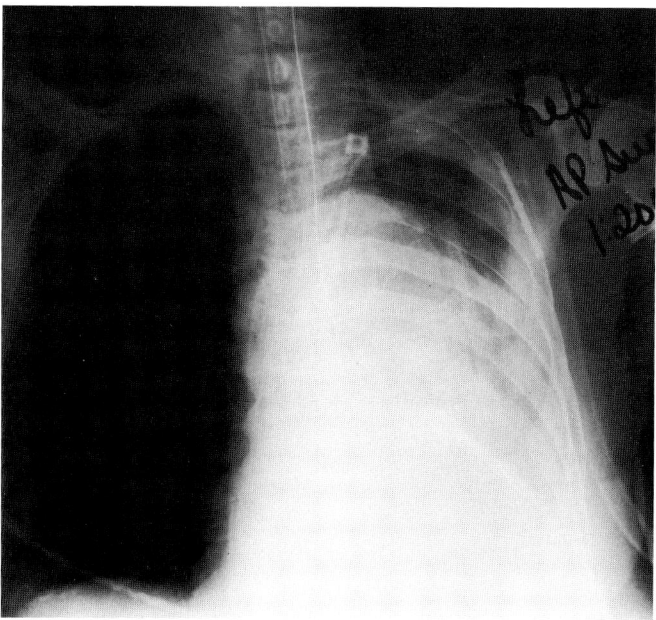

Figure 16-2 Atelectasis of the left lower lobe in the same patient as in Fig. 16-1. Both episodes led to rapid respiratory decompensation and required bronchoscopic clearing.

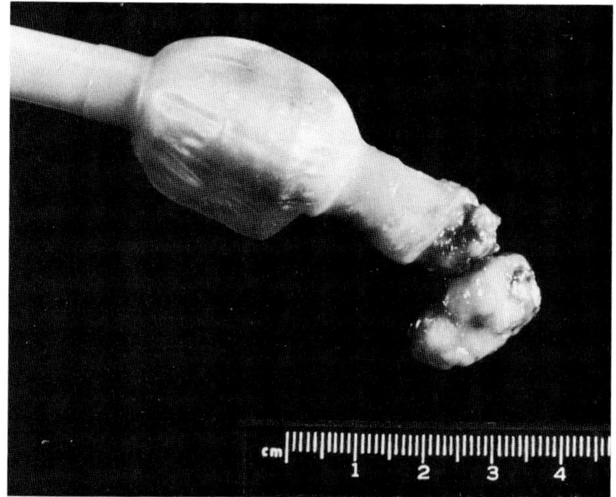

Figure 16-3 Solid plug of inspissated secretions at the end of this endotracheal tube led to respiratory arrest. Prompt replacement of the tube was followed by recovery.

atelectasis following inhalation injury. Radiologically, it has been reported that the peak incidence of atelectasis is noted at 2 to 5 days after burn,[5] but clearly, this depends on the etiology.

ASPIRATION

The incidence of aspiration pneumonia in burn patients is reported at 1 percent, but we believe this to be a gross underestimate. See Table 16-1.

The incidence of aspiration pneumonia may well be related to the increasing practice of optimizing enteral feeding rather than parenteral nutrition, to the difficulty of the recently extubated patient in swallowing, the use of small feeding tubes which do not permit accurate aspiration of gastric contents for residual measurement, and, as recently demonstrated, the growth of gram-negative pathogens in the stomachs of patients treated with antacids and histamine type 2 (H_2) blockers.

CASE REPORT

A 60-year-old male was admitted with 16 percent burns sustained in a house fire. He was intubated because of severe inhalation injury. Intubation was maintained through postburn day 5, when the patient was skin grafted. Postoperatively, the patient was successfully extubated and began on tube feedings. On the fifth postoperative day, the patient was noted to dribble tube feeding contents around the mouth and shortly thereafter required reintubation for hypoxemia. Chest films revealed a right upper as well as a left lower lobe infiltrate consistent with aspiration pneumonia. The infiltrates failed to clear. *Pseudomonas* was cultured from the sputum, and septic shock ensued despite intensive antibiotic treatment. The patient succumbed on hospital day 56 (Fig. 16-4).

Table 16-1 Aspiration Pneumonia in Burn Patients

References	Patients, no.	Aspiration, no.	%
Pruitt et al., 1970[1]	697	2	0.3
Pruitt et al., 1978[6]	1086	21	1.9
Sevitt, 1979[7]	156	2	1.2
Petroff et al., 1979[3]	60	5	8.3
Current series, 1988	1770	9	0.5
Totals	3769	39	1.0

Prevention

Aspiration pneumonia can be largely prevented by the following measures. All intubated patients receiving enteral support should be fed via a regular nasogastric tube which permits regular (q 2 h) measurement of gastric residuals, rather than a feeding tube. The balloon of an endotracheal or tracheostomy tube is *not* a safeguard against aspiration. If gastric residuals increase at any time, tube feedings *must* be stopped and the stomach emptied immediately. Patients who have been recently extubated, particularly after prolonged intubation or tracheostomy, and who are beginning oral feedings, should be closely observed by the nursing staff for adequacy of their swallowing reflex. In such patients, a lateral soft tissue tomogram of the neck will often reveal perilaryngeal edema, preventing adequate

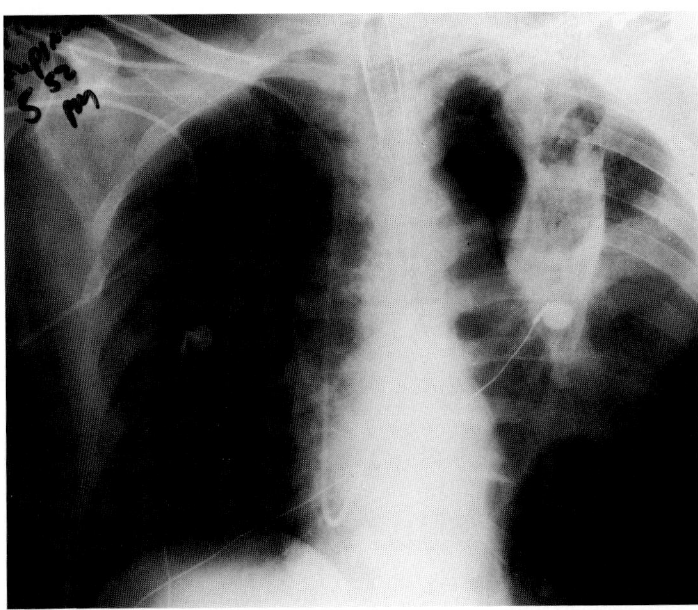

Figure 16-4 Aspiration pneumonia in a 60-year-old man leading to cavitation and, eventually, empyema.

epiglottic closure during swallowing. Contrast studies may be helpful at this stage in establishing the adequacy of the swallowing mechanism. In patients who appear to have repeated aspiration because of prolonged gastric atony, which may last several weeks particularly in elderly debilitated patients, a feeding jejunostomy may be helpful.

Finally, proven aspiration pneumonia must be considered an infective process by nosocomial enteric organisms and treated vigorously with appropriate antibiotic therapy as soon as a diagnosis is made or even suspected.

PNEUMOTHORAX

There are two common types of pneumothorax in the burn patient: iatrogenic and spontaneous, the latter being by far more dangerous. The literature tends not to differentiate between the two. The incidence of pneumothorax is difficult to ascertain because reported series show a strong case selection; however, the range is between 0.4 and 8.3 percent, as illustrated in Table 16-2. The mean incidence is 1.4 percent.

Iatrogenic pneumothorax (Figs. 16-5 and 16-6) occurs following the insertion (or attempted insertion) of a subclavian or internal jugular central venous catheter. It is commonly asymptomatic and diagnosed on the chest film taken following catheter placement. A high incidence of pneumothorax has been reported in some series following tracheostomy.[10] If such a pneumothorax is asymptomatic, small, or nonprogressive, the clinician may elect to do nothing: the air is likely to get absorbed within a few days, particularly if the patient undergoes general anesthesia for excisional surgery, in which case ventilation with an O_2-rich mixture will help absorb the nitrogen from the pleural space. Alternately, single-needle aspiration has been recommended.[6] Only if lung expansion fails to occur should tube thoracostomy be considered.

Table 16-2 Major Reports of Pneumothorax in Burn Patients

References	Patients, no.	Pneumothorax, no.	%
Foley et al., 1968[8]	233	13 (autopsy study)	5.5
Pruitt et al., 1970[1]	697	8	1.1
Moylan et al., 1972[9]	280	6 (all with tracheostomy)	2.1
Petroff et al., 1979[3]	60	5	8.3
Venus et al., 1981[4]	84	4	4.7
Lund et al., 1985[10]	217	13	5.9
Jones et al., 1988[11]	99	6 (all with tracheostomy)	6
Current series, 1988	1770	8	0.4
Totals	4270	61	1.4

Spontaneous pneumothorax in the intubated, ventilator-assisted patient is far more serious, since it can result in death within minutes,[4] particularly if the patient is on high positive end-expiratory pressure (PEEP). In prevention, consideration should be given to reducing the tidal volume and maintaining minute volume by increasing rate in any ventilator-dependent patient whose peak inspiratory pressure, because of poor compliance, begins to exceed 45 to 50 mmHg. This is particularly true in patients with staphylococcal or *Haemophilus* pneumonia, both involving organisms extraordinarily capable of rapidly necrotizing the lung parenchyma. Rapid diagnosis by auscultation and treatment by initially placing an 18-gauge needle into the second intercostal space anteriorly, followed by an appropriate chest tube, is mandatory. There may not be time to obtain a chest x-ray.

PULMONARY EMBOLISM

Considering the seriously injured relatively immobile patient population, clinically significant pulmonary embolism is surprisingly rare. However, those studies which include or concentrate on autopsy findings reveal a significant incidence of the complication. See Table 16-3.

In our experience, when pulmonary embolism does occur, it often does so in patients in whom it would be least expected, i.e., in those with small

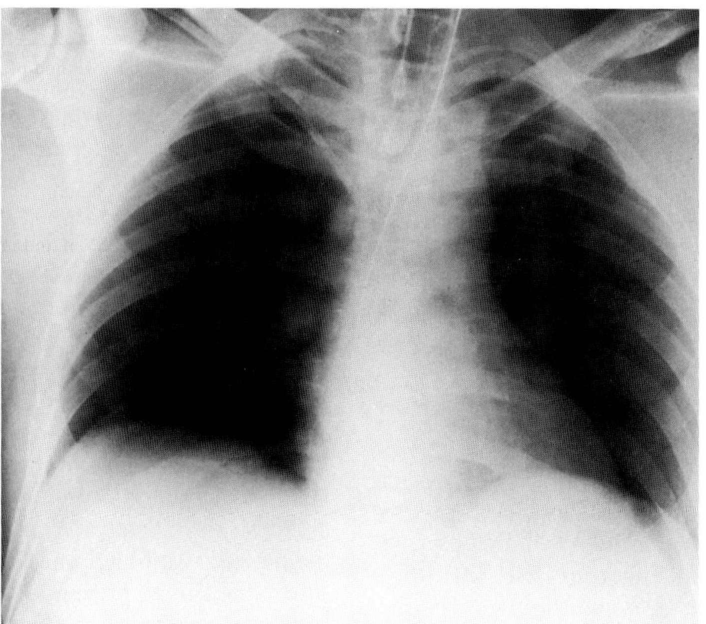

Figure 16-5 Chest roentgenogram upon admission of a 36-year-old patient with extensive burns, undergoing resuscitation, including placement of a right subclavian venous catheter. Normal film.

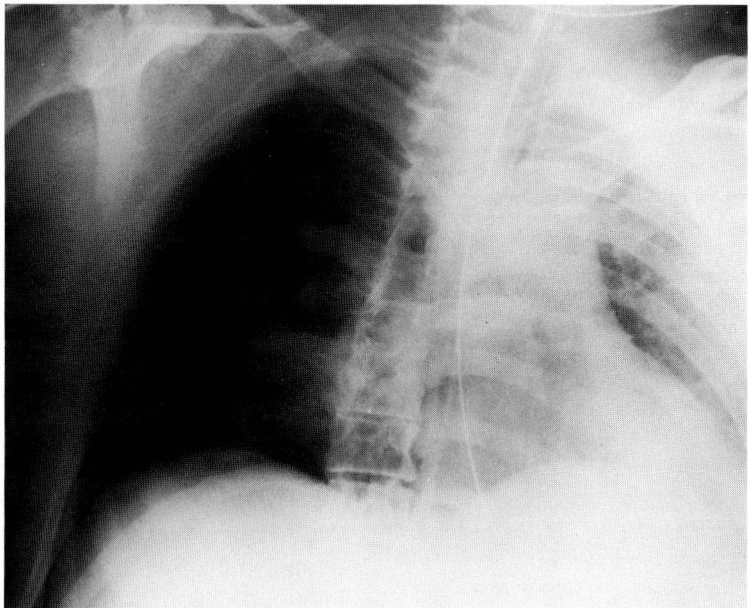

Figure 16-6 Complete right pneumothorax following attempted placement of right subclavian line. Treated by insertion of chest tube without further complications.

Table 16-3 Major Reports of Pulmonary Embolism in Burn Patients

References	Patients, no.	Pulmonary embolism, no.	Method of diagnosis	%
Foley et al., 1968[8]	817	59	Autopsy	7.2
Pruitt et al., 1970[1]	2106	6	Clinical	0.4
McDowell, 1973[12]	2258	16	Clinical and autopsy	7.1
Coleman et al., 1975[13]	24	7	Scan and autopsy	29
Munster et al., 1980[14]	1168	6	Scan and angiogram	0.5
Teixidor et al., 1983[15]	239	6	Scan and autopsy	2.5
Purdue et al., 1988[16]	2106	6	Clinical	0.4*
Total	8710	105		1.2

*NOTE: Twenty-five percent of autopsied patients were positive for findings of pulmonary embolism. In addition, two autopsy reports, in which total numbers of patients were not indicated:

Sevitt et al., 1961[17]	163	9	5.5%
Warden et al., 1973[18]	139	42	30%

burns and those who are in fact quite mobile. The following example illustrates this point.

CASE REPORT

A 27-year-old healthy male sustained 6 percent second- and third-degree burns to his upper extremities during a house fire. There was no inhalation injury. The patient underwent excision and grafting on the third postburn day and was on bed rest for 5 days following surgery. On the sixth day he was mobilized to an armchair. Later during this day he complained of right pleuritic chest pain and auscultation revealed a rub. Chest x-ray was clear, but ventilation/perfusion (V/Q) scan showed abnormalities on the right side. Pulmonary angiogram revealed multiple small scattered defects in the right upper lobe (Fig. 16-7). The patient was heparinized and remained hemodynamically stable, and repeat V/Q scan 10 days later showed complete resolution. He was placed on warfarin (Coumadin) therapy and discharged uneventfully.

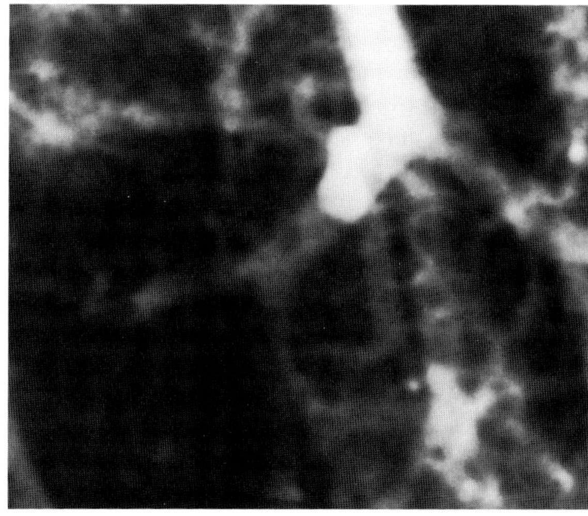

Figure 16-7 Enlargement of portion of right pulmonary angiogram showing translucency of part of the lung field and several small filling defects in a 27-year-old patient with 6 percent burns.

In our small series of six patients with proven pulmonary emboli,[14] the mean burn size was only 12.9 percent with a mean 4 percent third-degree component. There were no deaths, but the mean length of stay was prolonged because of this complication from 19.3 days for age and burn-size matched controls to 58.1 days in this group. The range of time of onset of symptoms was between 2 and 14 days after burn, and symptoms consisted of definite pleuritic pain (three patients) or vague abdominal or flank pain initially described as "muscular" in nature.

Clearly, clinicians should be alert to the possibility of pulmonary embolism and pay close attention to pain in the thorax or abdomen even in relatively mobile patients. Heparinization is the appropriate initial therapy, followed by Coumadin therapy for 3 months. Indications for ligation, clipping, or filter placement in the cava should follow standard surgical indications. We have been unable to identify a special "at risk" group for this complication, and therefore do not recommend prophylactic heparinization.

TRACHEAL STENOSIS

Tracheal complications, especially in patients with smoke inhalation, are commonly seen and consist of tracheitis, tracheal ulcerations, and granuloma formation. Very rarely, tracheal stenosis of significant degree will occur. The location of the stenosis is almost invariably subglottic and occurs at the site of the balloon of the endotracheal or tracheostomy tube. Probably because of this, even an extremely close perusal of the literature does not reveal whether the *timing* of tracheostomy in an endotracheally intubated patient has anything to do with the development of stenosis subsequently. We suspect that the occurrence of this major tracheal complication is more related to the injury of smoke inhalation and to the care with which the balloon is managed than to the absolute length of airway intubation. See Table 16-4.

CASE REPORT

A 58-year-old woman sustained 13 percent all third-degree burns to the scalp and neck while lying against a heater, intoxicated. Past medical history was significant for hypertension and emphysema. Her hospital course was complicated by poor graft takes and *Pseudomonas* pneumonia, requiring tracheostomy on postburn day 51. She remained respirator-dependent for a further month and was treated with aminophylline and corticosteroids because of severe persistent bronchospasm. By postburn day 81 she had been weaned off ventilator support but developed increasing stridor. Tracheoscopy revealed stenosis 2 cm above the carina, confirmed by computed tomography (CT) scan (Fig. 16-8). The stenosis was managed by sequential dilation to a final 6.5 mm inside diameter tube size. On postburn day 117 she underwent resection and primary anastomosis through a median sternotomy and was finally discharged from hospital approximately 5 months after burn.

In the management of intubated patients, such complications should be mostly preventible by meticulous attention to the tracheostomy or endotracheal tube cuff. Inflation of the cuff should be to the minimal pressure level consistent with preventing a leak in ventilator-dependent patients. Cuffs must be deflated every 2 hours. We have observed that sulfadiazine silver is capable of plugging the balloon valve to the point of rendering it inoperative, i.e., the balloon does not deflate; in such cases, the tube must be replaced.

Turning to other tracheal complications, granulomata in a supraglottic position occur frequently following emergency intubation with an introducer

Table 16-4 Major Reports of Tracheal Stenosis in Burn Patients

References	Patients, no.	Tracheal stenosis, no.	%
Lund et al., 1985[10]	217 (41 tracheostomies or ET tubes)	4	10
Moylan, Jr., et al., 1972[9]	280	2	1
Venus et al., 1981[4]	914	2	0.2
Stauffer et al., 1981[19]	150 ICU patients (44 tracheostomies or ET tubes)	16	36
Jones et al., 1988[11]	3246 (99 tracheostomies)	11	11
Current series, 1988	1770	3	0.2

NOTE: In addition, Majeski et al.[20] and Eliachar et al.[21] present two and three cases, respectively, but the total number surveyed is not given.

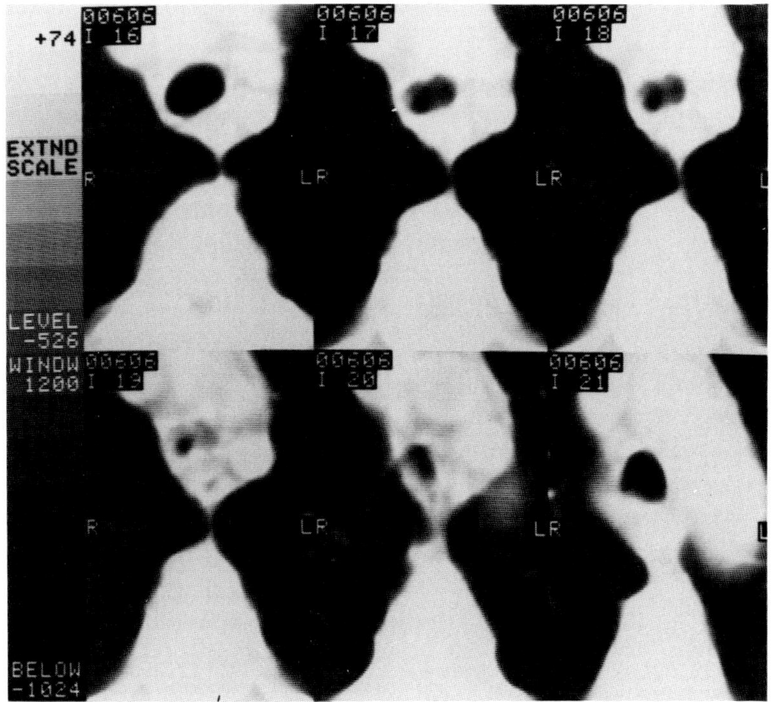

Figure 16-8 Successive cuts on the CT scan of a 58-year-old woman with 13 percent burns. At approximately 2 cm above the carina, there is an area of severe stenosis. This required surgical resection.

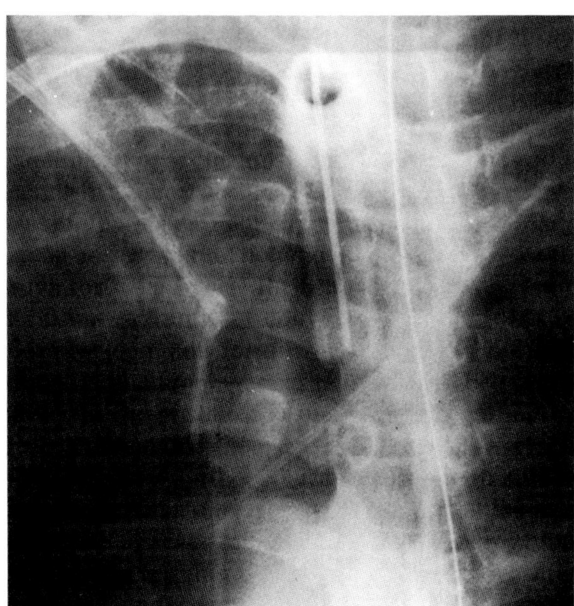

Figure 16-9 Chest roentgenogram of a patient with a non-functioning Swan-Ganz catheter clearly shows knotting.

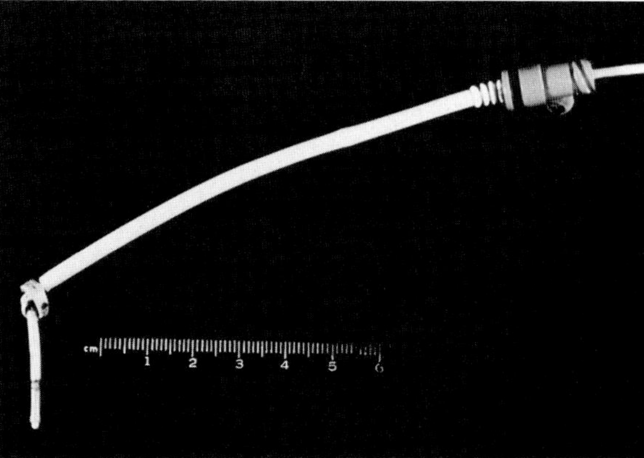

Figure 16-10 The Swan-Ganz catheter, with knot, was uneventfully removed by simple traction.

and may also give rise to stridor. These usually resolve spontaneously; if not, they can be removed by laser surgery.

OTHER COMPLICATIONS

Rare and spectacular problems can develop in burn patients with probably no greater frequency than in other serious conditions and are well reported in the literature. These include knotted Swan-Ganz catheters (Figs. 16-9 and 16-10) and shearing off of central venous lines with embolization. We have had a patient develop a massive subclavian arteriovenous aneurysm following cannulation, which eventually came to occupy the entire left thoracic outlet. It was successfully treated by angiographic embolization and eventually resected. Because of the risk of sepsis following open surgery, every effort should be made to deal with these problems radiologically.

REFERENCES

1. Pruitt BA Jr, Flemma RJ, DiVincenti FC, et al: Pulmonary complications in burn patients: A comparative study of 697 patients. *J Thorac Cardiovasc Surg* 59:7, 1970.
2. DiVincenti FC, Pruitt BA Jr, Reckler JM: Inhalation injuries. *J Trauma* 11:109, 1971.
3. Petroff PA, Pruitt BA Jr: Pulmonary disease in the burn patient, in Artz CP, Moncrief JA, Pruitt BA Jr (eds): *Burns: A Team Approach,* Philadelphia, Saunders, 1979.
4. Venus B, Matsuda T, Copiozo JB, et al: Prophylactic intubation and continuous positive airway pressure in the management of inhalation injury in burn victims. *Crit Care Med* 9:519, 1981.
5. Kangarloo H, Beachley MC, Ghahremani GC: The radiographic spectrum of pulmonary complications in burn victims. *Am J Radiol* 128:441, 1977.
6. Pruitt BA Jr, DiVincenti FC, Mason AD Jr, et al: The occurrence and significance of pneumonia and other pulmonary complications in burned patients: Comparison of conventional and topical treatments. *J Trauma* 10:519, 1970.
7. Sevitt S: A review of the complications of burns, their origin and importance for illness and death. *J Trauma* 19:358, 1979.
8. Foley FD, Moncrief JA, Mason AD Jr: Pathology of the lung in fatally burned patients. *Ann Surg* 167:251, 1968.
9. Moylan JA Jr, West JT, Nash G, et al: Tracheostomy in thermally injured patients: A review of 5 years experience. *Am Surg* 38:119, 1972.
10. Lund T, Goodwin CW, McManus WF, et al: Upper airway sequelae in burn patients requiring endotracheal intubation or tracheostomy. *Ann Surg* 201:374, 1985.
11. Jones WG, Goodwin CW, Medden M, et al: Tracheostomies in burned patients. Presented to the Twentieth Annual Meeting of the American Burn Association, Seattle, March 1988.
12. McDowall RAW: Pulmonary embolism and deep venous thrombosis in burned patients. *Br J Plast Surg* 26:176, 1973.
13. Coleman JB, Chang FC: Pulmonary embolism: An unrecognized event in severely burned patients. *Am J Surg* 130:697, 1975.
14. Munster AM, Confer S: Pulmonary embolism: A rare complication in small burns. Presented to the Annual Meeting of the American Burn Association, San Antonio, Texas, 1980.
15. Teixidor HS, Novick G, Rubin E: Pulmonary complications in burn patients. *J Can Assoc Radiol* 34:264, 1983.
16. Purdue GF, Hunt JL: Pulmonary emboli in burned patients. *J Trauma* 28:218, 1988.
17. Sevitt S, Gallagher N: Venous thrombosis and pulmonary embolism: A clinico-pathological study in injured and burned patients. *Br J Surg* 48:475, 1961.
18. Warden GD, Wilmore DW, Pruitt BA Jr: Central venous thrombosis: A hazard of medical progress. *J Trauma* 13:620, 1973.
19. Stauffer JL, Olson DE, Petty TL: Complications and consequences of endotracheal intubation and tracheostomy: A prospective study of 150 critically ill adult patients. *Am J Med* 70:65, 1981.
20. Majeski JA, Schreiber JT, Cotton R, et al: Tracheoplasty for tracheal stenosis in the pediatric burned patient. *J Trauma* 20:81, 1980.
21. Eliachar I, Moscona R, Joachims HZ, et al: The management of laryngotracheal stenosis in burned patients. *Plast Reconstr Surg* 68:11, 1981.

Chapter 17

Long-Term Respiratory Complications of Inhalation Injury

Gene L. Colice

HISTORICAL PERSPECTIVE

The Cleveland Clinic fire in 1929 and the Cocoanut Grove fire in 1942 focused attention on the potentially catastrophic risks of smoke inhalation. In both of these tragedies many of the fire victims died at the scene or soon thereafter with only minor cutaneous burns.[1,2] Similar fatalities were seen in other highly publicized fires.[3,4] Inhalation injury was indicted as the cause of these deaths and was recognized as a major killer of fire victims as early as 1962.[5] Unfortunately, translating appreciation of the risks into improvement in the outcome of inhalation injury was confounded by the many problems limiting effective management of burn victims. Burn wound sepsis was difficult to control until topical chemotherapy and refinements in surgical techniques were instituted. Acute mortality from hypovolemic shock was a serious problem until effective intravenous fluid replacement guidelines were developed for burn patients. Recognition of inhalation injury was uncertain until instruments for measuring arterial blood gases and carboxyhemoglobin levels were readily available. Supporting patients with inhalation injury for long periods was not possible until effective and reliable respiratory therapy and mechanical ventilatory equipment were developed.

By the early 1970s clinicians were better able to care for the cutaneous complications of burns and to recognize and manage smoke inhalation problems. Despite these considerable achievements, there were new and disturbing areas of confusion about smoke exposure that required clarification. Smoke seemed to be increasingly toxic. Fire fighters were noticing large amounts of smoke and noxious fumes at fires, particularly in factories dealing with plastic products. Occupational safety and health experts, recognizing the increased use of various types of plastics and other synthetics in construction materials, furniture, and fabrics, were apprehensive about the increased possibility of toxic gas generation in both industrial and house fires.[6] Catalyzed by these concerns, research efforts since the 1970s have been directed at better understanding the pathogenesis of inhalation injury. Toxins in smoke have been identified, and the histopathologic details of inhalation injury more completely described. Clinical patterns of inhalation injury have been recognized, and techniques for diagnosing smoke inhalation have been established. Again, however, these achievements have generated new questions and uncertainties. One particular concern is whether the present approach to inhalation injury is too tightly focused on the tissues of acute recognition and management and fails to adequately consider possible long-term consequences of smoke inhalation. Effective management of acute inhalation injury must be complemented by a realistic understanding of whether such injury either causes or predisposes to chronic lung disease.

INTRODUCTION

To analyze the relationship between the development of chronic respiratory disease and an acute episode of smoke inhalation, three factors will be considered. First, the nature of the toxic agents in smoke must be understood. Second, the distinctive features of the initial respiratory tract damage must be appreciated. These are determined not by the toxic effects of smoke inhalation, which appear to be nonspecific, but by the time of symptom onset following smoke inhalation and the portion of the respiratory tract involved. Four clinical patterns of inhalation injury can be characterized: asphyxiation, upper airway edema, tracheobronchitis, and lung parenchymal damage. Of these only three are possible causes of chronic pulmonary disease. Asphyxiation may be an acutely fatal event or, if timely rescue occurs, well-tolerated. Finally, the respiratory tract's ability to heal following injury must be taken into account. Given a nonspecific toxic effect, distinctive only by the portion of the respiratory tract involved, possible long-term consequences should be predictable if the reparative processes of those affected portions of the respiratory tract are understood.

TOXIC PROPERTIES OF SMOKE

Smoke is generally thought of in simplistic terms as a cloud emanating from a fire. A more rigorous definition from the American Society of Testing Materials is "a product of thermal demutation either through pyrolysis or combustion."[7] This definition expands the general notion of smoke in two important ways. It identifies a rise in temperature and not flames as the cause of substance decomposition. Ignition is not required for generation of smoke. A useful example to consider here is a "smoldering" fire. This definition also indicates that smoke consists of more than visible particles. Heat is an important component of smoke. Also present in smoke are gases. Consequently, smoke is composed of three different types of potential toxins: carbonaceous particles varying in size from microscopic to visible, heat, and gases. Smoke inhalation involves exposure to any one or combination of these constituents of smoke. Inhalation injury results from the toxicity of these three components of smoke. The severity of inhalation injury is directly related to the intrinsic toxicity and concentration of these smoke components, secondary interactions between toxins, and the duration of smoke exposure.

Heat

Heat causes immediate tissue damage. Mucosal edema, hemorrhage, and ulcerations are characteristically seen grossly, [8–10] and coagulation necrosis microscopically. The degree of thermal injury is determined by the amount of heat energy transferred from smoke to tissues. Smoke may contain air superheated to 1000°C or more,[11] but dry hot air contains surprisingly little heat energy. Steam, even though at considerably lower temperature than dry air, has a much higher heat energy content and is therefore liable to cause much more extensive tissue damage.[12,13]

The lower respiratory tract is protected to a large extent from thermal injury by the naso- and oropharynx. The upper respiratory tract is a highly efficient heat absorber.[10,12] For instance, inhaled dry air heated to between 260°C and 280°C will drop in temperature to 50°C when reaching the trachea.[14] However, in certain situations the heat absorption capacity of the upper respiratory tract can be overwhelmed. Conscious persons trapped in a closed space or comatose victims may be susceptible to heat-induced lower respiratory tract damage. Even in these cases the risks from hot dry air alone are minimal. Experimental studies in dogs indicate that, even when hot dry air is directed past the upper respiratory tract into the lungs, damage is limited primarily to the proximal tracheal mucosa. Steam, with its much higher heat content, will cause extensive bronchial and lung parenchymal injury under these conditions.[13]

Particles

Carbonaceous particles, or soot, are filtered out of inhaled smoke by the upper respiratory tract, particularly the nasopharynx. Small particles up to several μm in size generated by fires, however, can bypass these defense mechanisms and enter the lower respiratory tract.[4] Soot may be seen at bronchoscopy throughout the bronchial tree in victims of smoke inhalation. Expectoration of soot in mucus commonly occurs for days to weeks following this exposure. Fortunately, these carbonaceous particles, unless very hot, appear to cause little direct toxicity to the lungs.[15,16]

Gases

Carbon monoxide and carbon dioxide are always present in smoke and usually compose the bulk portion of the gaseous phase.[17] Ambient carbon monoxide and carbon dioxide levels may be extremely high at fire scenes.[18,19] The remainder of the gaseous phase (which will be referred to as secondary gases) varies depending on the materials burning. A variety of other physical factors, e.g., the temperature of the fire, the fire's heating rate, and ventilation, will also determine secondary gas composition.[20] It has been recognized that there are thousands of different types of gases which can be liberated by pyrolysis or combustion.[7] The more common secondary gases and their sources are listed in Chap. 3, Table 3-3. Studies performed on Boston fire fighters at actual fire scenes indicate that, of the secondary gases, acrolein is noted most frequently at levels exceeding safe short-term exposure limits.[18]

The commonly encountered secondary gases are a peculiar potpourri with distinctly different solubility characteristics (Table 3-4). Aldehydes, particularly acrolein (CH_2CHCHO) but also acetaldehyde and formaldehyde, are relatively water insoluble gases.[21] However, they are highly soluble in biologic fluids, allowing their rapid penetration of surface layers overlying epithelial cells.[22] Oxides of nitrogen (NO, NO_2), ozone (O_3), and phosgene ($COCl_2$) also have relatively low water solubility. Chlorine (Cl_2) has intermediate water solubility. Ammonia (NH_3), sulfur dioxide (SO_2), and hydrogen chloride (HCl) are all highly water soluble.[23] Water solubility is an important determinant of the secondary gas's toxicity patterns. Highly soluble gases dissolve in the water phase covering the mucous membranes of the eyes and upper respiratory tract, forming strong acids and alkalies.[24] These highly toxic substances tend to cause immediate irritation. The less-soluble secondary gases are thought to adsorb to the surface of soot, coating the carbonaceous particles and being carried by those particles into the smaller airways.[10, 24–26] Once these gases have been carried to the respiratory bronchiole, alveolar duct, and central alveolar level, they can directly damage epithelial cells.

The secondary gases cause a toxic chemical tracheobronchitis. This appears to be a direct effect, preferentially damaging the airway epithelial cells, and is reviewed in Chap. 4. Ciliated cells are particularly sensitive to these gases. Initially, ciliary function is inhibited,[12] and later, necrosis of these cells is seen.[22,27,28] Pseudomembranes, composed of sloughed necrotic epithelial cells and fibrinous exudate, cover the denuded mucosal surface and coalesce into casts of the tracheobronchial tree (Fig. 17-1).[9,10,29] The basal cells and basal lamina tend to remain intact, which may be critical for future regeneration of the surface epithelial layer (Fig. 17-2).[22] There is submucosal edema, hemorrhage, and an influx of acute inflammatory cells.[10,28,30] This pattern of tracheobronchitis is seen consistently in both animal studies[16,31,32] and autopsies of fatally burned humans.

The gaseous phase of smoke also appears to cause diffuse alveolar damage. This point was first suggested by human autopsy studies of burn victims in which extensive necrosis of alveolar type I cells and hyaline membrane formation were characteristically found. Interstitital inflammation and edema and intraalveolar edema were also seen (Fig. 17-3). Interestingly, capillary endothelial cells appeared relatively spared.[33-35] Since these observations, animal studies have shown a similar pattern of alveolar damage after acute smoke inhalation, confirming that smoke is the causative agent.[16,36,37] Many different gases have been implicated as toxic to alveolar structures. Carbon monoxide may damage alveolar type I epithelial cells.[38] At large enough exposure levels many of the secondary gases are capable of causing severe parenchymal lung damage.[23] However, both direct and indirect evidence indicates that acrolein is the secondary gas most likely to cause diffuse alveolar damage. Dogs develop extensive necrosis of alveolar type I epithelial cells after exposure to wood smoke but not kerosene smoke. Wood smoke was found to have much higher levels of acrolein than kerosene smoke.[15] Many animal studies addressing this issue have used burning cotton cloth to generate smoke,[31,32,37] which also generates acrolein. An animal smoke exposure model, carefully regulated to result in increasing acrolein exposures, caused progressively more severe lung parenchyma damage. In the same model hydrogen chloride only minimally affected smaller airways or alveoli.[16]

The secondary gases cause surface epithelial cell damage by a direct toxic effect.[23] They also seem to amplify this toxicity through interactions with pul-

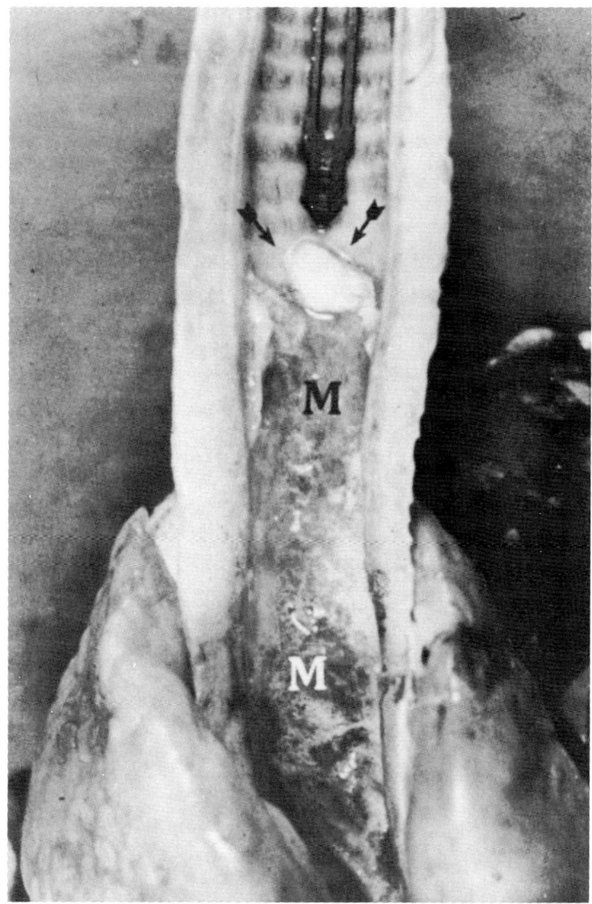

Figure 17-1 The trachea of a sheep has been removed 24 hours after smoke inhalation. A pseudomembrane (M) is shown partially separating from the tracheal epithelium (arrows). (*Used with permission from Ref. 36.*)

monary defense mechanisms. Following smoke inhalation, bronchoalveolar lavage typically reveals an acute influx of polymorphonuclear cells into the distal airspaces.[39-41] It is presumed that this acute inflammatory response is mediated by alveolar macrophage chemotactic factors.[42] The role polymorphonuclear cells play in smoke inhalation is unclear. Indirect evidence suggests they release proteolytic enzymes.[43,44] They are also thought to release free oxygen radicals.[42] There has been speculation that these enzymes and toxic oxygen forms

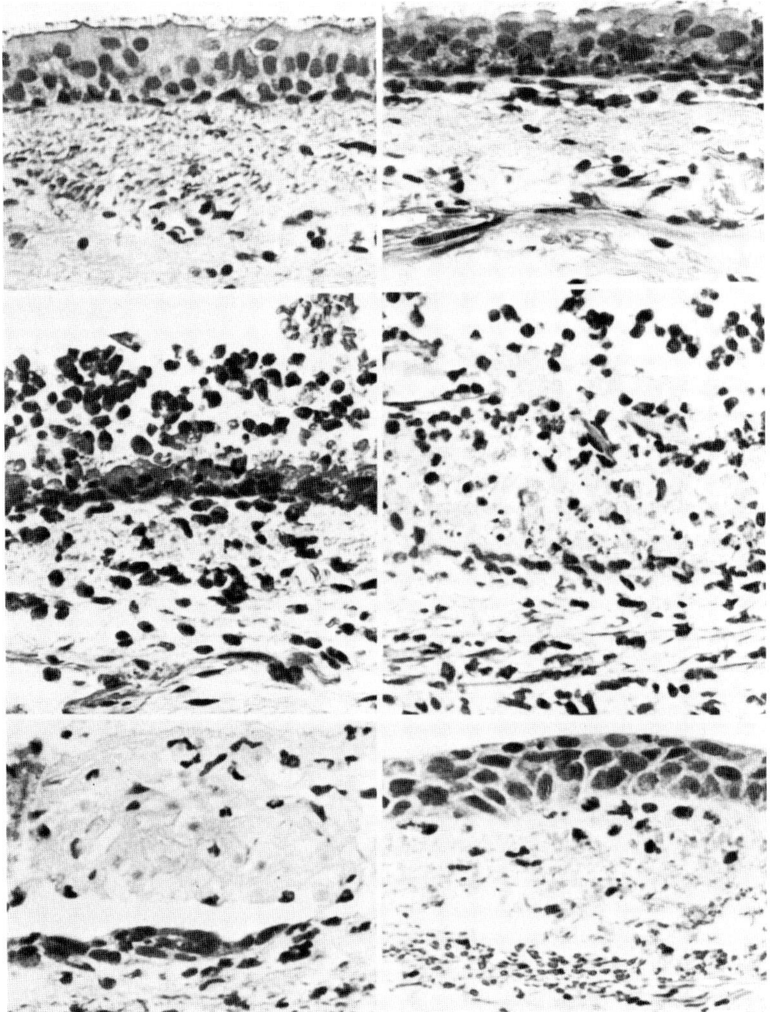

Figure 17-2 Photomicrographs (hematoxylin-eosin, $\times 700$) of tracheal epithelium from rabbits before and after smoke inhalation. Top left, control with well-defined basal layer. Top right, 6 hours after injury the epithelial lining cells are swollen. Middle left, also at 6 hours, there are focal areas of epithelial disruption with overlying pseudomembranous exudate. Middle right, by 24 hours the surface epithelial layer is destroyed, but the basal cells remain. Lower left, at 72 hours regenerating epithelium from the basal layer is seen below pseudomembranous exudate. Lower right, also at 72 hours the reparative epithelium is well seen. (*Used with permission from Ref. 22.*)

may amplify the original injury caused by smoke inhalation.[42–44]

Gases probably have multiple other adverse effects. Smoke inhalation causes diffuse atelectasis and an increased measured surface tension, attributed to a direct inhibition of functioning surfactant.[45] Smoke inhalation acutely impairs alveolar macrophage function. These cells' surface adherence, phagocytic function, and directed chemotaxis are inhibited by smoke in animal models[41] and hu-

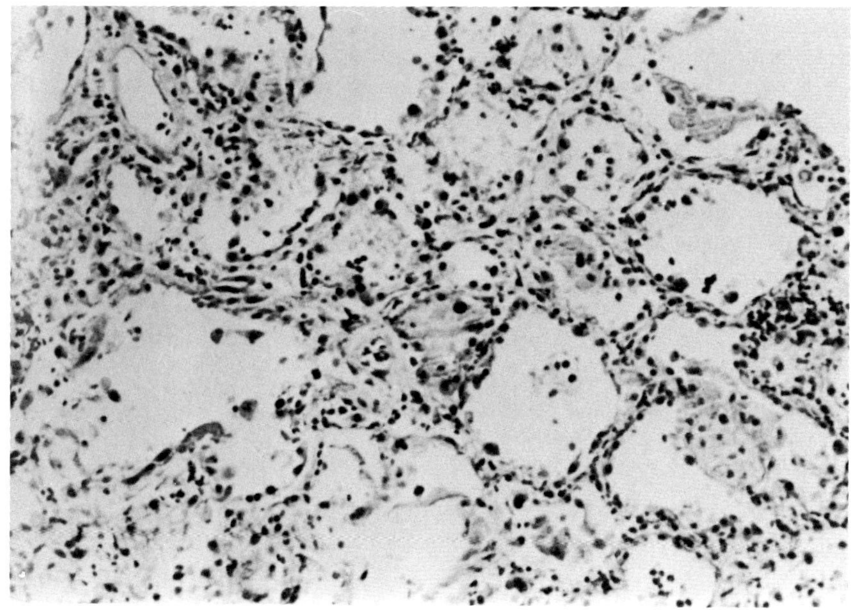

Figure 17-3 Photomicrograph (hematoxylin-eosin, ×155) of lung tissue from a patient dying of inhalation injury. Interstitial edema and inflammation are seen, along with hyaline membrane formation. (*Used with permission from Ref. 35.*)

mans.[40] These effects, in conjunction with reductions in tracheal mucus velocity[39] and ciliary function,[12] impair pulmonary bacterial defense mechanisms and may predispose patients with inhalation injury to bronchopneumonia.

PATTERNS OF INHALATION INJURY

The circumstances leading to smoke inhalation vary so markedly in clinical practice that it may be difficult to recognize distinct patterns of inhalation injury. However, for the purposes of this discussion it will be useful to categorize prototypical patterns of inhalation injury by the time of onset following smoke inhalation and the portion of the respiratory tract involved (see classification of injuries, Chap. 2). Although the mechanisms responsible for these clinical patterns have not been established entirely, insights into probable causes can be made based on the toxicity patterns of the components of smoke.

Asphyxiation

Fires consume oxygen and produce large amounts of carbon monoxide. A fire in an enclosed, poorly ventilated space may result in high ambient levels of carbon monoxide[18,19] and significantly reduced amounts of oxygen.[7] Hypoxemia and carbon monoxide poisoning are important causes of death at the fire scene or within the first few hours following smoke inhalation.[30,46,47] The secondary gases generated by fires are also potentially lethal in high concentrations. Hydrogen cyanide (HCN) is a good example of a secondary gas which may be exceedingly dangerous.[23]

Upper Airway Edema

Pharyngeal and laryngeal edema may develop within the first 12 to 36 hours following smoke inhalation.[48–50] Swelling of the aryepiglottic folds, arytenoid eminence, and interarytenoid areas is typically seen. Edema of the false and true vocal cords and the infraglottic region may also occur but is usually not as severe as the supraglottic edema.[51–53] The supraglottic area may be particularly susceptible to large amounts of fluid accumulation because of the loose attachments of its mucosa to underlying basal areas.[51,52] Large volumes of intravenous fluid given during the early resuscitative period may worsen pharyngeal and laryngeal edema.[51,52] Ulcerations of the upper respiratory tract are seen infrequently.[53] The most feared consequence of laryngeal edema is upper airway obstruction. Less well appreciated are functional abnormalities of laryngeal abduction that can be caused by upper airway injury.[51] Heat is thought to play the key role in causing upper airway swelling. The upper airway is remarkably efficient at absorbing heat and consequently is the most susceptible portion of the respiratory tract to heat injury. Secondary gases, particularly highly water soluble gases, may contribute to thermal injury of the upper airway.

Tracheobronchitis

Within the first 24 to 48 hours following smoke inhalation, wheezing and cough with expectoration of carbonaceous phlegm may develop.[9,48] Bronchospasm may be especially difficult to manage during this period. Bronchoscopy in patients with this constellation of findings usually reveals tracheobronchitis. Typically seen are erythema, mucosal edema, and soot, maximal on the carinae throughout the bronchial tree.[25,30] In severe cases patients may cough up inspissated secretions in the forms of casts of the tracheobronchial tree for up to 1 to 2 weeks after the burn. This is a worrisome sign which suggests extensive destruction of bronchial surface epithelium and an increased susceptibility to bacterial infection and secondary bronchopneumonia.[9,10] Secondary gases and steam are the most likely agents of tracheobronchial inflammation.

Lung Parenchymal Damage

Atelectasis, ventilation/perfusion mismatch, and hypoxemia with an increased alveolar-to-arterial oxygen gradient are common findings following smoke inhalation.[9,54–59] Progressive pulmonary insufficiency, characterized by severe hypoxemia, diffuse infiltrates on chest radiograph, and reduced pulmonary compliance may also develop in patients with inhalation injury. This picture is consistent with the adult respiratory distress syndrome (ARDS) and portends a poor acute prognosis, particularly if the onset of respiratory distress is quite early.[60] This syndrome is nonspecific and may be initiated by a variety of insults. Bacterial sepsis from either a cutaneous burn site or an infected intravascular catheter is a common cause of ARDS in the fire victim but usually occurs several days or longer after the initial injury. When ARDS develops within the first 72 hours following smoke inhalation, the probable causative agent is smoke toxicity. Experimental evidence indicates that secondary gases in smoke can directly cause the characteristic features of ARDS, pulmonary capillary endothelial permeability abnormalities,[31,32,37,61,62] and a histologic picture of diffuse alveolar damage.[16,37]

Always to be considered in the differential diagnosis of ARDS, or as an aggravating factor, is volume overload. Haponik et al.[63] pointed out that burn patients who developed pulmonary edema invariably also had evidence of increased circulating blood volume, i.e., an enlarged vascular pedicle width on chest radiograph. These patients also had larger amounts of fluid replacement than those who did not develop pulmonary edema. Circulatory congestion coupled with the hypoproteinemia seen in burn patients would increase fluid flux into interstitial tissues[24] and exacerbate the physiologic derangements of diffuse alveolar damage.

THE RESPIRATORY TRACT REPARATIVE PROCESS AND LONG-TERM CONSEQUENCES OF INHALATION INJURY

Just as the acute sequelae of inhalation injury can be classified according to the anatomic level of airway involvement, the chronic effects of exposure can be considered in this manner. Potential long-term respiratory complications of inhalation injury and its management are outlined in Table 17-1.

Upper Airway Edema

It has been asserted repeatedly that pharyngeal and laryngeal edema resolve spontaneously over 4 to 6 days following smoke inhalation.[9,10,64,65] However, in actuality, little is known about the long-term laryngeal consequences of inhalation injury.[66] At least one study has documented the persistence of laryngeal abnormalities for weeks following burn,[53] but a later study from the same group indicated no laryngeal abnormalities at a mean of 3 months follow-up.[67] Possible long-term effects on laryngeal function from inhalation injury are more worrisome than pharyngeal complications for several reasons. The larynx has the smallest cross-sectional area of the entire respiratory tract. Consequently, laryngeal dysfunction or pathology would be more likely to compromise the airway than pharyngeal abnormalities. The larynx also serves the important functions of protecting the lungs against aspiration and as an organ of speech. The larynx may also be subjected to trauma from translaryngeal intubation, which can cause serious chronic laryngeal abnormalities.[68–70]

Although there are important differences between the laryngeal damage caused by inhalation injury and translaryngeal intubation, patients with inhalation injury requiring translaryngeal intubation may suffer additive laryngeal insults. Consequently, these patients may be at an increased risk for developing chronic laryngeal pathology. Translaryngeal intubation causes ulceration of the posterior commissure and vocal cord mucosa.[68,71] Repair of laryngeal mucosal disruption is usually well ordered, but individual variations in granulation tissue growth and scarring may lead to granuloma formation or excessive wound contraction. These abnormal reparative processes following translaryngeal intubation have been shown to lead to vocal cord granulomas[72] and laryngeal scarring.[70] Stenosis of the posterior commissure of the larynx and functional abnormalities of the vocal cords are serious possible outcomes. Laryngeal edema is a more prominent finding than mucosal ulceration in inhalation injury.[53] Mucosal and submucosal edema without ulceration is more likely to resolve without chronic sequelae. Another important difference between these laryngeal insults is the duration of irritation. Translaryngeal intubation for short time periods, i.e., several days, may cause severe laryngeal edema and ulceration but few long-term effects.[70,72] This suggests that smoke inhalation lasting usually on the order of minutes should also be well tolerated. Longer-duration translaryngeal intubation appears to cause an increased propensity for chronic laryngeal pathology.[70] An appropriate, but unanswered, concern with prolonged translaryngeal intubation is whether underlying inhalation injury makes the larynx more susceptible to disordered healing of tube-induced mucosal ulcerations.

Table 17-1 Possible Long-Term Respiratory Complications of Inhalation Injury

Larynx
Laryngeal stenosis
Vocal cord granuloma
Laryngeal motor dysfunction
Tracheal stenosis
Bronchi
Bronchial stenosis
Bronchiectasis
Hyperreactive airways
Bronchiolitis obliterans
Chronic bronchitis and COPD
Lung parenchyma
Restrictive ventilatory defect
Reduced pulmonary capillary volume

Tracheobronchitis

The reparative process for injured tubular structures, such as the tracheobronchial tree, may result in several different types of chronic sequelae. Stricture formation and dilation are the best recognized of these complications. Another interesting response is exuberant granulation tissue overgrowth resulting in polyp formation. Individual case reports indicate that each of these chronic abnormalities may follow inhalation injury.

Tracheal stenosis may develop in either of two patterns following smoke inhalation. Long, irregular areas of tracheal stenosis are rarely seen and are probably due to severe inhalation injury.[73–75] Focal areas of tracheal stenosis may also occur when either translaryngeal intubation[76] or tracheostomy[67] is performed in patients with inhalation injury. Stenotic areas appear particularly likely to develop at the tracheal stoma site. A recent study by Lund et al.[67] found a surprisingly high incidence of tracheal stenosis. Bronchoscopy, pulmonary function tests, and radiographic studies were performed on 17 burn patients weeks to months after surviving inhalation injury requiring either translaryngeal intubation or tracheostomy. Three of the seven patients receiving tracheostomy were found to have tracheal stenosis at the stoma site following decannulation. In one case the stenosis was quite severe. Stomal stenosis formation in these cases may have been entirely due to the tracheostomy. This operation involves an incision through tracheal cartilage and scarring of this incision following decannulation is a recognized cause of tracheal stenosis.[68,69] However, some authors have suggested that underlying inhalation injury may have an interactive effect with artificial airways, promoting stricture formation.[22,34,76] The basis for this interaction is the speculation that strictures are more likely to develop when a critical amount of damage occurs to the basal lamina of the tracheal mucosa. The basal lamina may serve as an important guide to the usual mucosal repair processes. Inhalation injury alone usually appears to spare this layer.[22] Consequently, the basal lamina will facilitate normal regeneration of the tracheal mucosal layer in most cases of inhalation injury. If inhalation injury is coupled with the additional focal insult of artificial airway placement, sufficient damage to the basal lamina may occur to cause disordered repair with stricture formation. This interaction is a possible explanation for focal tracheal stenosis developing after translaryngeal intubation alone.[76] The stenosis described in these patients was found at the site of the balloon cuff seal against the tracheal mucosa (Fig. 17-4).

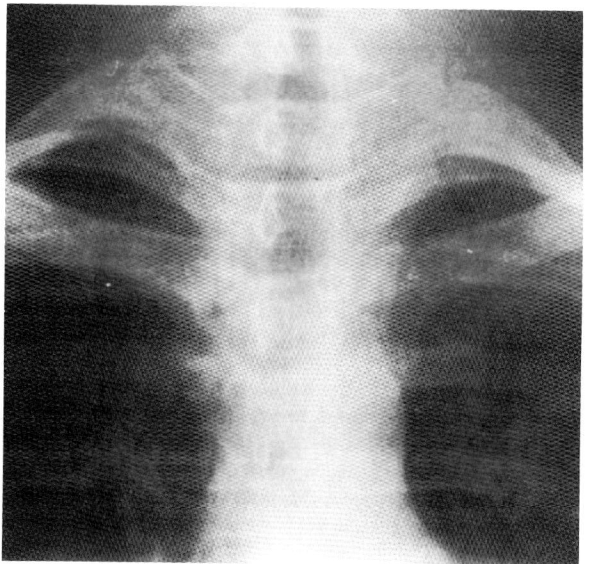

A

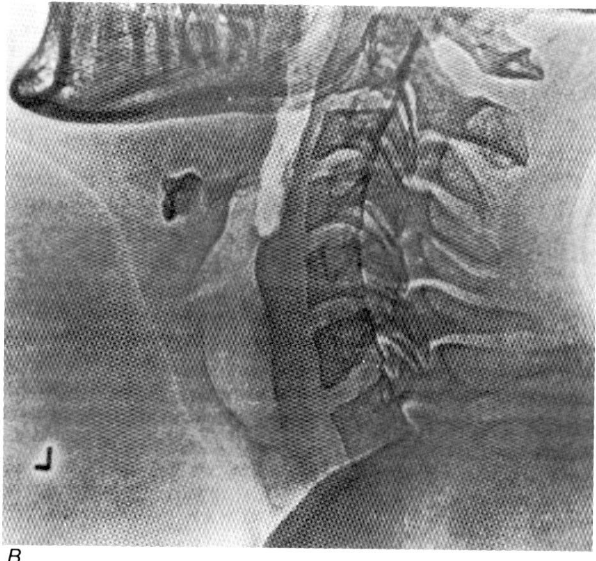

B

Figure 17-4 The chest roentgenogram (*A*) and xeroradiogram (*B*) from a patient who required translaryngeal intubation for inhalation injury. Severe tracheal stenosis is seen at the site where the balloon cuff of the tracheal tube sealed against the tracheal mucosa. (*Used with permission from Ref. 76.*)

Mechanical abrasion by the cuff of mucosa already damaged by inhalation injury was speculated to have critically damaged the basal lamina and subsequently promoted stricture formation.[76] Autopsy studies of inhalation injury patients with artificial airways have confirmed severe erosive tracheitis at the area of contact with the balloon cuff.[67]

Bronchial stenosis occurs but is less common than tracheal stenosis.[77,78] Conversely, dilatation of the respiratory tract lamina is more likely to occur at the bronchial than tracheal level because cartilaginous supports tend to maintain tracheal lumen size. Bronchiectasis is a nonspecific response to a variety of inflammatory agents.[79] Inhalation injury probably causes bronchiectasis by initiating a submucosal inflammatory reaction which weakens supporting elements of the bronchial wall. Bronchiectasis is a rare complication of inhalation injury but, when it occurs, causes diffuse and occasionally intractable disease (Fig. 17-5).[58,60,77]

In rare cases mucosal regeneration following inhalation injury appears excessive and polypoid

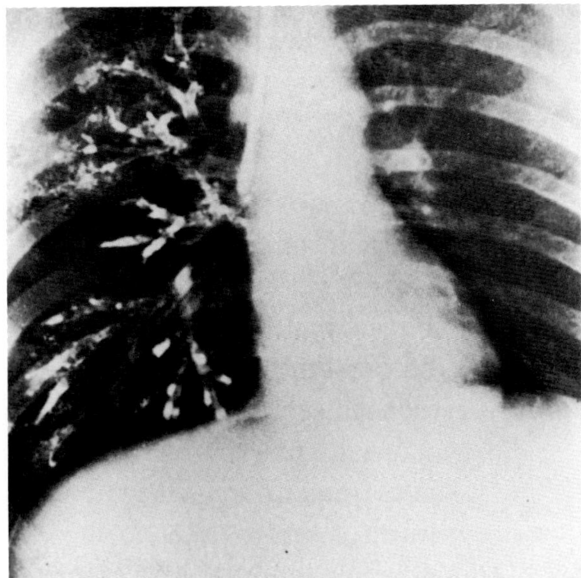

Figure 17-5 Bronchogram performed 4 months after inhalation injury showing bronchiectasis throughout right lower lobe. (*Used with permission from Ref. 110.*)

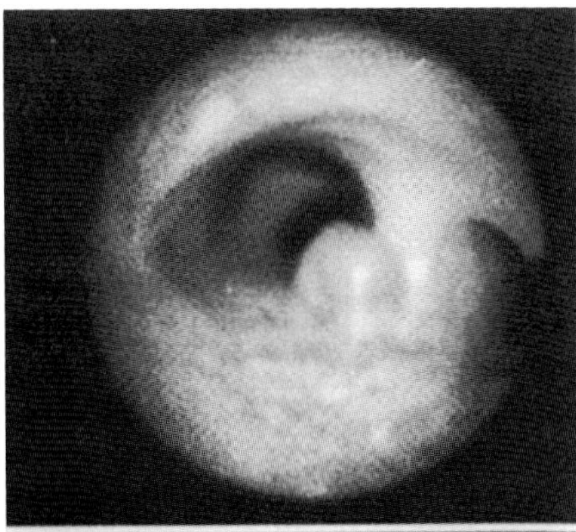

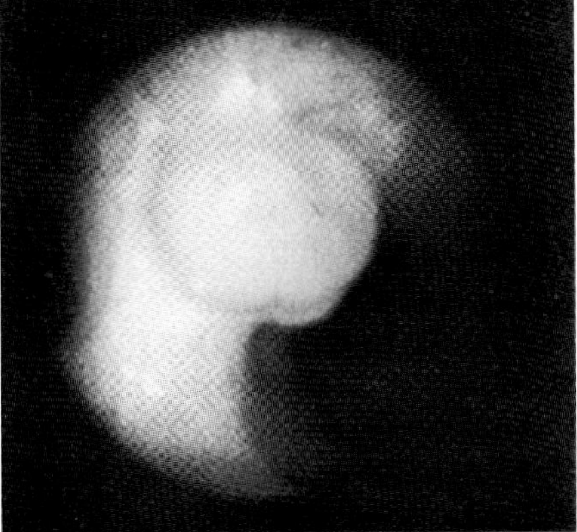

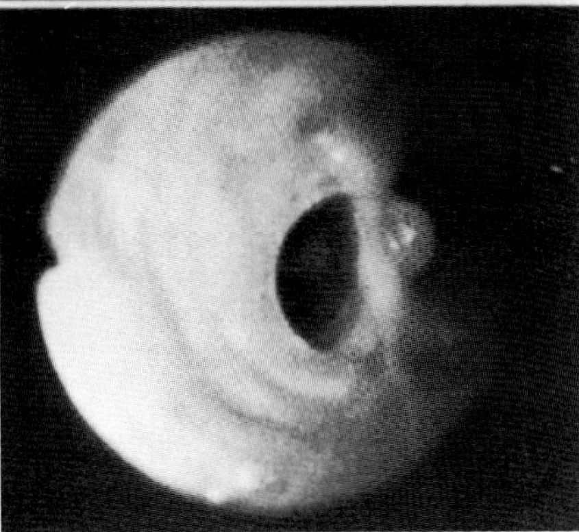

Figure 17-6 At bronchoscopy 2 months following inhalation injury polyps are seen at the carina (upper), bifurcation of the bronchus intermedius and right upper lobe (middle), and right lower lobe (lower). (*Used with permission from Ref. 80.*)

masses of granulation tissue may develop.[80,81] When this exuberant mucosal repair occurs in the larger airways, polyps may actually be seen on gross examination (Fig. 17-6). Cough and hemoptysis may be prominent symptoms caused by these endobronchial polyps. These polyps tend to resolve with corticosteroid treatment and time.[80,81] If these polypoid growths of granulation tissue should develop in smaller conducting airways, such as bronchioles, they may form the basis for bronchiolitis obliterans. This is a poorly understood syndrome, characterized pathologically by granulation tissue and scar formation occluding bronchioles (Fig. 17-7). Although the inciting cause is usually unknown, it rarely develops following inhalation injury.[82,83] It is clinically characterized by cough, a restrictive ventilation defect with reduced diffusing capacity, and bilateral, patchy "ground glass" densities on chest roentgenogram.

Bronchial airway hyperresponsiveness can develop after exposure to environmental irritants.[84] Asthma with wheezing, cough, dyspnea, and chest tightness is the predominant clinical manifestation of this abnormality. It is extremely unusual for asthma to develop after a single, even large, exposure to smoke.[85] In the rare case where asthma was first documented after inhalation injury, there was a preceding history of allergic rhinitis.[85] Simpson et al. studied a small group of patients several months after inhalation injury, and two of seven were found to have bronchial hyperreactivity by methacholine challenge testing. However, both of these patients had a documented prior cigarette-smoking history, suggesting that smoke inhalation may not have been the cause of the hyperresponsiveness.[86]

Lung Parenchymal Damage

At the end of the initial hospitalization period, survivors of ARDS caused by inhalation injury may

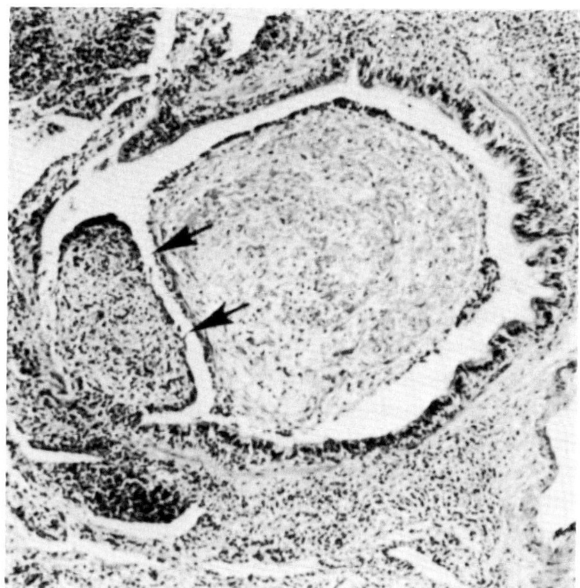

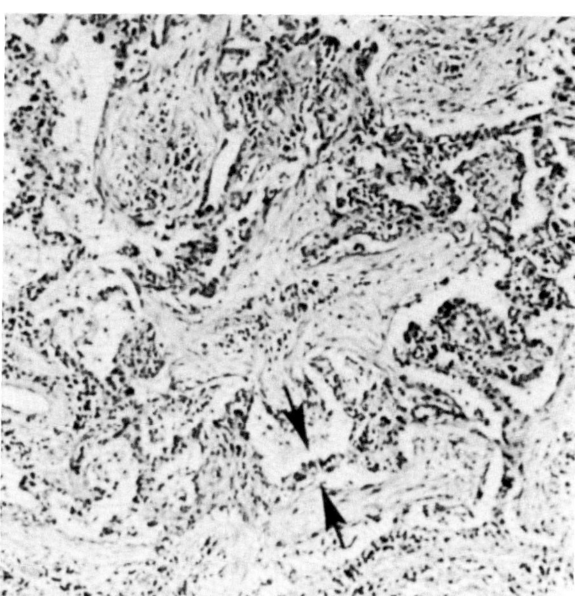

Figure 17-7 A photomicrograph (hematoxylin-eosin, ×100 and ×120) showing typical bronchiolitis obliterans. A bronchiole lumen (left) and alveoli (right) are completely occluded by granulation tissue and fibrinous exudate. The granulation tissue appears to originate from the bronchiole wall (arrows on left) and to spread through the airways into the alveolar ducts and alveoli. There is some alveolar inflammation (arrows on right). (*Used with permission from Ref. 82.*)

have a combined obstructive and restrictive ventilatory abnormality.[86,87] This pattern is somewhat different than that of survivors of ARDS from other causes who have primarily ventilatory restriction,[88–90] and probably reflects the combined effects of tracheobronchitis, lung parenchymal damage, and surface burns. Serial studies of lung function over the first 5 months of convalescence from inhalation injury documents a gradual return to normal values.[87,91] Although inhalation injury may be catastrophic, the poorly understood reparative processes of the lung parenchyma apparently can facilitate remarkable recovery. Survivors of other forms of ARDS tend to have similarly encouraging prospects for a good functional outcome.[88–90] However, in some patients with ARDS from causes other than inhalation injury, abnormalities in gas transfer persist.[88–90,92–96] These include mild reductions in room air or exercise Pa_{O2}, an increased alveolar-to-arterial oxygen gradient, and a reduced carbon monoxide transfer factor. These gas-transfer abnormalities have been variably explained by an increased right-to-left shunt,[89,95] reduced pulmonary capillary volume due to abnormalities of small pulmonary vessels,[96] and subclinical pulmonary fibrosis.[90] Gas-transfer abnormalities fortunately tend to be mild and well tolerated and should be expected in survivors of ARDS from inhalation injury.

RECURRENT SMOKE INHALATION

Smoke inhalation has been considered as an acute, massive, single-dose exposure in the foregoing discussion. However, certain individuals, e.g., fire fighters, may have recurrent episodes of mild smoke inhalation. Following a single exposure to dense smoke not requiring hospitalization, fire fighters will have persistent abnormalities in pulmonary function tests for up to a month or more.[97] A more disturbing possibility is that repeated exposures will lead to chronic obstructive pulmonary disease (COPD). Peters et al.[98] reported an accelerated deterioration in pulmonary function in fire fighters. They studied 1430 Boston fire fighters between 1970 and 1972 and found a significantly increased annual decrement in FEV_1 and FVC. Fire fighters who required hospitalization for smoke inhalation had an even greater annual fall in lung function than those with less severe exposure. These findings were consistent with other observations on the relationship of smoke exposure to chronic lung disease. Rural natives of Nepal who spend long periods inside poorly ventilated houses heated with wood frequently have symptoms of chronic bronchitis.[99] The paradigm of chronic smoke exposure is cigarette smoking, which is clearly related to COPD.

Serial evaluations of the cohort of Boston fire fighters first studied by Peters et al.[100,101] failed to confirm the originally observed trend of rapidly deteriorating lung function. Over a 6-year period, a substantial portion of the original study group were reexamined and mean annual decrements in flow rates and percent predicted FEV_1 and FVC were found to be within the normal range. Respiratory symptoms in these firemen, such as cough and sputum production, were related to cigarette smoking. More importantly, when changes in FEV_1 and FVC were related to the total number of fires fought, an indirect index of cumulative smoke exposure, no relationship was found. Other studies performed in fire fighters from Australia,[102] Connecticut,[103] and Los Angeles[104] confirmed that abnormalities in pulmonary function studies could not be related to occupational smoke exposure. In fire fighters with chronic respiratory symptoms or evidence of airway obstruction on spirometry or helium-oxygen flow volume loops, the etiologic agent usually appeared to be either cigarette smoking or underlying asthma.[102,103]

THERAPEUTIC IMPLICATIONS

At present there is little indication that use of anti-inflammatory agents like corticosteroids at the initial inhalation injury will minimize chronic respiratory complications.[78,105–107] Consequently, the key to effectively managing such problems is recognition of the potential risks. Because many of the symptoms of chronic respiratory disease may be insidious and nonspecific, it is advisable to perform certain diagnostic tests on a routine screening basis following the acute inhalation injury period.

Patients who have suffered upper airway edema should have a follow-up laryngeal examination by a competent observer. Although the probability of chronic laryngeal complications developing is very small, the risks and discomforts of laryngoscopy are so minimal that it is reasonable to ensure adequate resolution of laryngeal abnormalities. This study is most conveniently performed at the end of the initial hospitalization period. Any patient with inhalation injury requiring translaryngeal intubation should have a similar examination following extubation. Persistent laryngeal mucosal ulcerations and swelling and laryngeal motor dysfunction should be expected at this initial study. There may be a 5 to 10 percent chance that chronic laryngeal pathology will develop, especially if translaryngeal intubation lasted longer than 10 days.[70] Some authors have suggested intralesional injection of corticosteroids to hasten healing of the ulcerations, but little information is available to support this regimen.[71] A more reasonable approach is to carefully record abnormalities and serially evaluate recovery by repeat laryngoscopy. Complete healing may take months and is important to carefully document, because laryngeal stenosis or granulomas may develop in a delayed fashion.[70,72] Clinicians should carefully screen for signs and symptoms of laryngeal dysfunction, e.g., voice change, choking or difficulty swallowing, unexplained dyspnea, and stridor, during the follow-up period. Therapeutic options include a variety of surgical procedures which, if performed in a timely fashion, may prevent significant clinical problems.

Routine screening for tracheal stenosis is indicated under certain conditions. Any patient with inhalation injury requiring tracheostomy is at risk for developing tracheal stenosis at the stoma site following decannulation.[67] Patients requiring translaryngeal intubation, but not tracheostomy, may be at risk for developing tracheal stenosis at the balloon cuff site.[76] This is an unusual complication and may be heralded by excessively high balloon cuff pressures or overdistention of the trachea by the balloon cuff (dilatation of the trachea to greater than 150 percent of the contiguous tracheal lamina size on chest radiograph) during translaryngeal intubation.[68] Useful screening tests for tracheal stenosis are xeroradiography, computerized axial tomography, tomography, and flow volume loops. Bronchoscopy is especially helpful in evaluating an identified area of tracheal stenosis for therapeutic approaches. Occasionally laser techniques can be used to remove excess granulation tissue and ameliorate symptoms. Tracheal reconstructive surgery may be required to correct severe stenosis.

Chronic airway disease is a fortunately rare sequelae of inhalation injury. Spirometry is a useful screening test for airway obstruction. Symptoms of cough, wheezing, dyspnea, and chest tightness should alert the clinician to this complication. Asthma should be considered in patients with an allergic history predating the inhalation injury. In patients without such a history, bronchiolitis obliterans should be suspected. Confirmation of this diagnosis requires histologic proof, by either bronchoscopy or open lung biopsy. Corticosteroids may be useful in the treatment of bronchiolitis obliterans.[82] If chronic cough with production of large amounts of purulent sputum is a prominent complaint, bronchiectasis should be considered. Computerized axial tomography is fairly accurate in identifying enlarged segments of the bronchial tree. Bronchoscopy should be considered to exclude retained large soot particles or other foreign bodies as a cause for localized bronchiectasis. Antibiotic regimens and bronchodilators may be effective in controlling symptoms of bronchiectasis. Occasionally localized bronchiectasis confirmed by bronchography may be amenable to surgical removal.

Pulmonary function abnormalities will persist for

Table 17-2 Strategy for Diagnosing Severe Pulmonary Impairment*

Severe impairment	Test
Yes	FEV_1 < 40% predicted FVC < 50% predicted FEV_1/FVC < 40% predicted
	No
Yes	DL_{CO} < 40% predicted
	No
Yes	$\dot{V}_{O_2max}$ < 15 mL/kg/min $\dot{V}_{O_2max}$ < 30–40% of $\dot{V}O_2$ costs of occupational activity over 8-hour period
	No
Yes	Pa_{O_2} < 55 mmHg while breathing room air Pa_{O_2} < 60 mmHg and evidence of pulmonary hypertension, cor pulmonale, erythrocytosis, or exercise desaturation

*Adapted from Ref. 109.

months following lung parenchymal injury. In the vast majority of cases eventual resolution of both symptoms and physiologic abnormalities will occur. During the resolution phase serial measurements of FEV_1, FVC, and carbon monoxide diffusing capacity should be obtained. Once these test results have plateaued and respiratory symptoms have stabilized, adequacy of gas transfer at rest and maximal exercise should be assessed. This is useful for demonstrating to the patient the extent of his or her functional recovery and, to the physician, the presence of residual physiologic impairments. Ear oximetry during a standardized exercise test is one approach to this type of evaluation. Alternatively, arterial blood gases may be obtained. Reductions in Sa_{O_2} or Pa_{O_2} may occur during exercise, especially if the diffusing capacity is below 50 percent of predicted.[108] In the rare case of persistent severe respiratory symptoms and pulmonary-function test abnormalities, the severity of impairment should be analyzed. A standard approach to diagnosing severe impairment is shown in Table 17-2.[109] Severe impairment documented by this approach is a reasonable basis for disability claims.

REFERENCES

1. The hazard of toxic gases from combustion of roentgen-ray films (editorial). *JAMA* 92:1764, 1929.
2. Finland M, Davidson CS, Levenson SM: Clinical and therapeutic aspects of the conflagration injuries to the respiratory tract sustained by victims of the Cocoanut Grove disaster. *Medicine* 24:215, 1945.
3. Cox ME, Heslop BF, Kempton JJ: The Dellwood fire. *Br Med J* 1:942, 1955.
4. Einhorn IN: Physiological and toxicological aspects of smoke produced during the combustion of polymeric materials. *Environ Health Perspect* 11:163, 1975.
5. Phillips AW, Cope O: Burn therapy. *Ann Surg* 155:1, 1962.
6. Bowes PC: Smoke and toxicity hazards of plastics in fire. *Ann Occup Hyg* 17:143, 1974.
7. Dressler D: Laboratory background on smoke inhalation. *J Trauma* 19:913, 1979.
8. Chu C-S: Burns updated in China. *J Trauma* 22:574, 1982.
9. Demling RH: Smoke inhalation injury. *Postgrad Med* 82:63, 1987.
10. Herndon DM, Langner F, Thompson P, et al: Pulmonary injury in burned patients. *Surg Clin North Am* 67:31, 1987.
11. Trunkey DD: Inhalation injury. *Surg Clin North Am* 58:1133, 1978.
12. Crapo RO: Smoke-inhalation injuries. *JAMA* 246:1694, 1981.
13. Moritz AR, Henriques FC, Mclean R: The effects of inhaled heat on the air passages and lungs. *Am J Pathol* 21:311, 1945.
14. Chu C-S: New concepts of pulmonary burn injury. *J Trauma* 21:958, 1981.
15. Zikria BA, Ferrer JM, Floch HF: The chemical factors contributing to pulmonary damage in "smoke poisoning." *Surgery* 71:704, 1972.
16. Hales CA, Barkin PW, Jung W, et al: Synthetic smoke

with acrolein but not HCl produces pulmonary edema. *J Appl Physiol* 64:1121, 1988.
17. Dyer RF, Esch VH: Polyvinyl chloride toxicity in fires. *JAMA* 235:393, 1976.
18. Treitman RD, Burgess WA, Gold A: Air contaminants encountered by firefighters. *Am Ind Hyg Assoc J* 41:796, 1980.
19. Gold A, Burgess WA, Clougherty EV: Exposure of firefighters to toxic air contaminants. *Am Ind Hyg Assoc J* 39:534, 1978.
20. Terrill JB, Montgomery RR, Reinhardt CF: Toxic gases from fires. *Science* 200:1343, 1978.
21. Cohen MA, Guzzardi LJ: Inhalation of products of combustion. *Ann Emerg Med* 12:628, 1983.
22. Thorning DR, Howard ML, Hudson LD, et al: Pulmonary responses to smoke inhalation. *Hum Pathol* 13:355, 1982.
23. Schwartz DA: Acute inhalational injury. *Occup Med* 2:297, 1987.
24. Demling RH: Burns. *N Engl J Med* 313:1389, 1985.
25. Mellins RB, Park S: Respiratory complications of smoke inhalation in victims of fires. *J Pediatr* 87:1, 1975.
26. Genovesi M: Effects of smoke inhalation. *Chest* 77:335, 1980.
27. Loke J, Paul E, Virgulto JA, et al: Rabbit lung after acute smoke inhalation. *Arch Surg* 119:956, 1984.
28. Charnock EL, Meehan JJ: Postburn respiratory injuries in children. *Pediatr Clin North Am* 27:661, 1980.
29. Walker HL, McLeod CG, McManus WF: Experimental inhalation injury in the goat. *J Trauma* 21:962, 1981.
30. Moylan JA: Inhalation injury—A primary determinant of survival following major burns. *J Burn Care Rehabil* 2:78, 1981.
31. Herndon DN, Traber DL, Niehaus GD, et al: The pathophysiology of smoke inhalation injury in a sheep model. *J Trauma* 24:1044, 1984.
32. Kimura R, Traber LD, Herndon DN, et al: Increasing duration of smoke exposure induces more severe lung injury in sheep. *J Appl Physiol* 64:1107, 1988.
33. Burns TR, Greenberg SD, Cartwright J, et al: Smoke inhalation: An ultrastructural study of reaction to injury in the human alveolar wall. *Environ Res* 41:447, 1986.
34. Foley FD, Moncrief JA, Mason AD: Pathology of the lung in fatally burned patients. *Ann Surg* 167:251, 1968.
35. Nash G, Foley PD, Langlinais PC: Pulmonary interstitial edema and hyaline membranes in adult burn patients. *Hum Pathol* 5:149, 1974.
36. Shimazu T, Yukioka T, Hubbard GB, et al: A dose-response model of smoke inhalation injury. *Ann Surg* 206:89, 1987.
37. Traber DL, Schlag G, Hedl H, et al: Pulmonary edema and compliance changes following smoke inhalation. *J Burn Care Rehabil* 6:490, 1985.
38. Fein A, Grossman RF, Jones JG, et al: Carbon monoxide effect on alveolar epithelial permeability. *Chest* 78:726, 1980.
39. Freitag L, Chapman GA, Sielczak M, et al: Laser smoke effect on the bronchial system. *Lasers Surg Med* 7:283, 1987.
40. Demarest GB, Hudson LD, Altman LC: Impaired alveolar macrophage chemotaxis in patients with acute smoke inhalation. *Am Rev Respir Dis* 119:279, 1979.
41. Fick RB, Paul ES, Merrill WW, et al: Alterations in the antibacterial properties of rabbit pulmonary macrophages exposed to wood smoke. *Am Rev Respir Dis* 129:76, 1984.
42. Stein MD, Herndon DN, Stevens JM, et al: Production of chemotactic factors and lung cell changes following smoke inhalation in a sheep model. *J Burn Care Rehabil* 7:117, 1986.
43. Traber DL, Herndon DN, Stein MD, et al: The pulmonary lesion of smoke inhalation in an ovine model. *Circ Shock* 18:311, 1986.
44. Herndon DN, Traber LD, Linares H, et al: Etiology of the pulmonary pathophysiology associated with inhalation injury. *Resuscitation* 14:43, 1986.
45. Nieman GF, Clark WR, Wax SD, et al: The effect of smoke inhalation on pulmonary surfactant. *Ann Surg* 191:170, 1980.
46. Birky MM, Clarke FB: Inhalation of toxic products from fires. *Bull NY Acad Med* 57:997, 1981.
47. Zikria BA, Weston GC, Chodoff M, et al: Smoke and carbon monoxide poisoning in fire victims. *J Trauma* 12:641, 1972.
48. Bartlett RH: Types of respiratory injury. *J Trauma* 19(S):918, 1979.
49. Bartlett RH, Niccole M, Tavis MJ, et al: Acute management of the upper airway in facial burns and smoke inhalation. *Arch Surg* 111:744, 1976.
50. Wanner A, Cutchavaree A: Early recognition of upper airway obstruction following smoke inhalation. *Am Rev Respir Dis* 108:1421, 1973.
51. Haponik EF, Munster AM, Wise RA, et al: Upper airway function in burn patients. *Am Rev Respir Dis* 129:251, 1984.
52. Haponik EF, Meyers DA, Munster AM, et al: Acute upper airway injury in burn patients. *Am Rev Respir Dis* 135:360, 1987.
53. Hunt JL, Agee RN, Pruitt BA: Fiberoptic bronchoscopy in acute inhalation injury. *J Trauma* 15:641, 1975.
54. Robinson TJ, Bubna-Kasteliz B, Strane MF: Alterations in pulmonary ventilation and blood gases in acute burns. *Br J Plast Surg* 25:250, 1972.
55. Nishimura N, Hiranuma N: Respiratory changes after major burn injury. *Crit Care Med* 10:25, 1982.
56. Wroblewski DA, Bowes GC: The significance of facial burns in acute smoke inhalation. *Crit Care Med* 7:335, 1979.
57. Robinson NB, Hudson LD, Robertson HT, et al: Ventilation and perfusion alterations after smoke inhalation injury. *Surgery* 90:352, 1981.
58. DiVincenti FC, Pruitt BA, Reckler JM: Inhalation injuries. *J Trauma* 11:109, 1971.
59. Landa J, Avery WG, Sackner MA: Some physiologic observations in smoke inhalation. *Chest* 61:62, 1972.
60. Herndon DW: Inhalation injury. *Curr Probl Surg* 6:370, 1987.
61. Aviado DM, Schmidt CF: Respiratory burns with special

reference to pulmonary edema and congestion. *Circulation* 6:666, 1952.
62. Prien T, Taber LD, Herndon DN, et al: Pulmonary edema with smoke inhalation, undetected by indicator-dilution technique. *J Appl Physiol* 63:907, 1987.
63. Haponik EF, Adelman M, Munster AM, et al: Increased vascular pedicle width preceding burn-related pulmonary edema. *Chest* 90:649, 1986.
64. Cahalane M, Demling RH: Early respiratory abnormalities from smoke inhalation. *JAMA* 251:771,1984.
65. Moylan JA, Alexander CG: Diagnosis and treatment of inhalation injury. *World J Surg* 2:185, 1978.
66. Sataloff DM, Sataloff RT: Tracheotomy and inhalation injury. *Head Neck Surg* 6:1024, 1984.
67. Lund T, Goodwin CW, McManus WF, et al: Upper airway sequelae in burn patients requiring endotracheal intubation or tracheostomy. *Ann Surg* 201:374, 1985.
68. Colice GL: Prolonged intubation versus tracheostomy in the adult. *J Intensive Care Med* 2:85, 1987.
69. Stauffer JL, Silvestri RL: Complications of endotracheal intubation, tracheostomy, and artificial airways. *Respir Care* 27:417, 1982.
70. Whited RE: A prospective study of laryngotracheal sequelae in long-term intubation. *Laryngoscope* 94:367, 1984.
71. Weymuller EA, Bishop MJ: Tracheal and laryngeal consequences of prolonged intubation. *Prob Anesth* 2:235, 1988.
72. Lindholm GE: Prolonged endotracheal intubation. *Acta Anaesthesiol Scand* 33(suppl):1, 1969.
73. Eliachar I, Moscona R, Joachins HZ, et al: The management of laryngotracheal stenosis in burned patients. *Plast Reconstr Surg* 68:11, 1981.
74. Majeski JA, Schreiber JT, Cotton R, et al: Tracheoplasty for tracheal stenosis in the pediatric burned patient. *J Trauma* 20:81, 1980.
75. Perez-Guerra F, Walsh RE, Sagel SS: Bronchiolitis obliterans and tracheal stenosis. *JAMA* 218:1568, 1971.
76. Colice GL, Munster AM, Haponik EF: Tracheal stenosis complicating cutaneous burns. *Am Rev Respir Dis* 134:1315, 1986.
77. Donnellan WL, Poticha SM, Holinger PH: Management and complications of severe pulmonary burn. *JAMA* 194:1323, 1965.
78. Beal DD, Lambeth JT, Conner GH: Follow-up studies on patients treated with steroids following pulmonary thermal and acrid smoke injury. *Laryngoscope* 78:396, 1968.
79. Barker AF, Bardana EJ: Bronchiectasis. *Am Rev Respir Dis* 137:969, 1988.
80. Adams C, Moisan T, Chandrasekhar AJ, Warpeha R: Endobronchial polyposis secondary to thermal inhalation injury. *Chest* 75:643, 1979.
81. Williams DO, Vanecko RM, Glassroth J: Endobronchial polyposis following smoke inhalation. *Chest* 84:774, 1983.
82. Epler GR, Colby TV, McLoud TC, et al: Bronchiolitis obliterans organizing pneumonia. *N Engl J Med* 312:152, 1985.
83. Segger JS, Mason CG, Worthen S, et al: Bronchiolitis obliterans. *Chest* 83:169, 1983.
84. Hargreave FE, Dolovich J, O'Byrne PM, et al: The origin of airway hyperresponsiveness. *J Allergy Clin Immunol* 78:825, 1986.
85. Brooks SM, Weiss MA, Bernstein IL: Reactive airways dysfunction syndrome. *Chest* 88:376, 1985.
86. Simpson DL, Goodman M, Spector SL, et al: Long-term follow-up and bronchial reactivity testing in survivors of the adult respiratory distress syndrome. *Am Rev Respir Dis* 117:449, 1978.
87. Whitener DR, Whitener LM, Robertson KJ, et al: Pulmonary function measurements in patients with thermal injury and smoke inhalation. *Am Rev Respir Dis* 122:731, 1980.
88. Yahar J, Lieberman P, Molho M: Pulmonary function following the adult respiratory distress syndrome. *Chest* 74:247, 1978.
89. Klein JJ, van Haeringen JR, Sluiter HJ, et al: Pulmonary function after recovery from the adult respiratory distress syndrome. *Chest* 69:350, 1976.
90. Elliott CG, Morris AH, Cengiz M: Pulmonary function and exercise gas exchange in survivors of adult respiratory distress syndrome. *Am Rev Respir Dis* 123:492, 1981.
91. Morris AH, Spitzer KW: Lung function in convalescent burn patients. *Am Rev Respir Dis* 108:989, 1973.
92. Lakshminarayan S, Stanford RE, Petty TL: Prognosis after recovery from adult respiratory distress syndrome. *Am Rev Respir Dis* 113:7, 1976.
93. Rotman HH, Lavelle TF, Duncheff DG, et al: Long-term physiologic consequences of the adult respiratory distress syndrome. *Chest* 72:190, 1977.
94. Douglas ME, Downs JB: Pulmonary function following severe acute respiratory failure and high levels of positive end-expiratory pressure. *Chest* 71:18, 1977.
95. Buchser E, Leuenberger PH, Chiolero R, et al: Reduced pulmonary capillary blood volume as a long-term sequel of ARDS. *Chest* 87:608, 1985.
96. Yernault JC, Englert M, Sergysels R, et al: Pulmonary mechanics and diffusion after shock lung. *Thorax* 30:252, 1975.
97. Unger KM, Snow RM, Mestas JM, et al: Smoke inhalation in firemen. *Thorax* 35:838, 1980.
98. Peters JM, Theriault GP, Fine LJ, et al: Chronic effect of firefighting on pulmonary function. *N Engl J Med* 291:1320, 1974.
99. Rajpenday M: Domestic smoke pollution and chronic bronchitis in a rural community of the Hill Region of Nepal. *Thorax* 39:337, 1984.
100. Musk AW, Peters JM, Wegman DH: Lung function in fire fighters. *Am J Public Health* 67:626, 1977.
101. Musk AW, Peters JM, Bernstein L, et al: Pulmonary function in firefighters. *Am J Ind Med* 3:3, 1982.
102. Young I, Jackson J, West S: Chronic respiratory disease and respiratory function in a group of firefighters. *Med J Aust* 1:654, 1980.
103. Loke J, Farmer W, Matthay RA, et al: Acute and chronic

effects of firefighting on pulmonary function. *Chest* 77:369, 1980.

104. Tashkin DP, Genovesi MG, Chopra S, et al: Respiratory status of Los Angeles firemen. *Chest* 71:445, 1977.
105. Robinson NB, Hudson LD, Riem M, et al: Steroid therapy following isolated smoke inhalation injury. *J Trauma* 22:876, 1982.
106. Levine BA, Petroff PA, Slade CL, et al: Prospective trials of dexamethasone and aerosolized gentamicin in the treatment of inhalation injury in the burned patient. *J Trauma* 18:188, 1978.
107. Head JM: Inhalation injury in burns. *Am J Surg* 139:508, 1980.
108. Kelley MA, Panettieri RA, Krupinski AV: Resting single-breath diffusing capacity as a screening test for exercise-induced hypoxemia. *Am J Med* 80:807, 1986.
109. American Thoracic Society: Evaluation of impairment/disability secondary to respiratory disease. *Am Rev Respir Dis* 126:945, 1982.
110. Pruitt BA, Fleming RJ, DiVicenti FC, et al: Pulmonary complications in burn patients. *J Thorac Cardiovasc Surg* 59:7, 1970.

Chapter 18

Smoke Inhalation: Models for Research

William R. Clark, Jr.

The respiratory sequelae of burns are legion, often dominate the acute illness, and are frequently responsible for significant morbidity and mortality.[1–14] Smoke exposure severe enough to cause an inhalation injury is present in 15 to 40 percent of flame burn victims.[2,15] It is a dreaded associated injury; patients with both burns and smoke inhalation have a more morbid clinical course and a higher mortality rate than those with either injury alone.[1,2,7,15–22] In a study on mortality in burn victims, the presence of an inhalation injury increased the risk of dying by a factor of 5 (relative risk 5.7, 95 percent confidence interval 4.2 to 7.0).[2] Another recent study found that inhalation injury increased the expected mortality by 20 percent in patients in the midrange of burn severity but conferred no additional mortality risk when the burn wound itself was massive.[7] However, smoke inhalation, as evidenced by abnormalities on bronchoscopy, did make patients more likely to develop pneumonia, which added an additional 40 percent increase in expected mortality.[7] Experienced fire fighters and fire safety engineers are of the opinion that smoke from present-day fires is more toxic than it was before the widespread use of plastic (polymeric) building materials and furnishings, but this opinion cannot be proved because of the absence of adequate records and multiple changes in the detection and control of fire over this time period.[23–25] This chapter will attempt to classify, describe, and critique the research models used to study the acute effects of smoke on the lungs.

SMOKE INHALATION

Smoke includes all the airborne products resulting from the thermal degradation of material: particulate matter, gases, volatilized organic molecules, aerosols, and free radicals.[23,26,27] Combustion is the flaming condition, pyrolysis the nonflaming condition of the decomposition process. Most accidental fires involve "diffusion" flames, in which fuel vapor and oxygen mix to varying degrees on the fuel surface, as contrasted with "premixed" flames, in which the fuel and oxygen are mixed prior to ignition.[23,28] Diffusion flames rarely proceed to complete oxidation of the fuel. In this chapter the unqualified terms *smoke inhalation* and *inhalation injury* will be used interchangeably to indicate a smoke injury to the proximal airway and/or pulmonary parenchyma severe enough to result in clinical consequences significant for the individual. Perspective for this discussion is provided in a brief overview of a typical and unequivocable inhalation injury. It is perhaps worth pointing out that the diagnosis of a pulmonary parenchymal injury following smoke exposure is equivocable in approximately one-third of the victims of smoke exposure who enter the hospital.[1,29] This is because the early diagnostic clues are qualitative and do not correlate well with the degree of visceral impairment. Because the diagnosis is often not obvious early in the illness, clinicians frequently "reason backward" from respiratory insufficiency presenting after the second postburn day to the presumption of an occult inhalation injury.[1] The result of this diagnostic imprecision is that there is no absolute set of criteria which makes the "smoke inhalation" injury of one era or one unit comparable to that in other eras or other units.[2]

Subjects Not Covered

There are many respiratory injuries which bear some resemblance to acute smoke inhalation; the experimental approaches to these injuries often utilize concepts and methods useful for the study of inhalation injuries. However, this chapter will not deal directly with the respiratory consequences of exposure to environmental contaminants,[30,31] smog, isolated chemicals,[32,33] the exhaust of an internal combustion engine,[34–36] cigarette smoke,[37–39] or blast forces.[40,41] Nor will it address models of the acute respiratory distress syndrome[42,43] per se, even though as acute smoke inhalation evolves, the clinical approach to the respiratory failure which develops is currently guided by the same principles which govern the treatment of patients with respiratory failure of other etiologies.[44–54] To my knowledge, no experimental model of the smoke injured larynx has been described. This is worthy of some study; the technology required to isolate the larynx from the lung during smoke exposure and to document the temperature[55] and chemicals delivered to the larynx is available.

Accident Scenarios

The accident scenarios which result in fire-related deaths and inhalation injuries typically occur in a residence as the result of an appliance malfunction, matches, or cigarette ignition of furniture.[56–58] These accidents occur most frequently between midnight and 8 A.M. with considerable variation depending on the age of the victim.[59,60] Elderly people and children are most at risk and are most likely to have been in the room of fire origin.[60] Cause of death is attributed to carbon monoxide alone over half of the time; burns account for only 10 to 20 percent of the deaths.[57,58,61] The role played by alcohol, coronary artery disease, cyanide, heavy metals, and other toxins in defining the vulnerability of the victim and the clinical consequences remains uncertain, although abnormalities involving these conditions and toxins are detectable in a great many instances.[62–72]

Clinical Presentation

The condition in which smoke inhalation victims present to the health care system is extraordinarily variable.[73–78] At the more severe end of the injury spectrum is the individual who is discovered in respiratory or cardiorespiratory arrest, responds to prehospital resuscitative efforts, but enters in a brain dead state with transient hemodynamic stability. Perhaps more frightening is the individual with high-grade obstruction of the upper airway who presents with stridor, retraction, wheezes, hoarseness, bronchorrhea, and ineffective spasms of coughing. The individual with a history of smoke exposure without dyspnea, blood-gas abnormalities, or pulmonary imaging changes who progresses to a state of severe respiratory distress 10 to 36 hours after presentation is a problem in the early recognition of a severe pulmonary injury. At the least severe end of the spectrum is the individual who has fleeting symptoms of conjunctival and upper airway irritation following smoke exposure without respiratory insufficiency, becomes asymptomatic rapidly, and suffers no sequelae. Innumerable variations on these clinical states fill in the gaps to form a spectrum of injury severity which is wide. Any of these patients may present with or without a skin burn; when present the burn is a flame injury so that it is characteristically large and deep.[2] Patients with a burn in addition to smoke inhalation are more likely to have a problem with obstruction of the upper airway; parietal edema of the head and neck which follows adequate burn resuscitation contributes to this obstruction and interferes with the patient's ability to clear secretions.[1,79–83] The fundamental elements in this brief description of the clinical problems posed by victims of smoke inhalation are presented in Figure 18-1. A partial list of the variables that interact to define the severity of any given episode of smoke inhalation is presented in Table 18-1. Any experimental model of smoke inhalation which attempts to produce a standard injury so that the response of the lung can be studied must control or eliminate most of these variables.

Injury Severity

It is beyond the scope of this chapter to delve deeply into the discipline of fire safety science;[23,84–87] the toxicity of inhaled materials;[24,88–99] or the physiologic, physical, and chemical factors which control the dose of inhaled products of combustion. However, a few points should be made because they explain the need for controls in experimental models and indicate the extent to which any experimental model must diverge from real accident scenarios, where nothing is controlled and in which conditions change on a second-by-second basis.[71] The great variability in the severity of inhalation injury and the diversity of patient symptomatology can be explained by considering the sources of smoke (Fig. 18-1*A*; Table 18-1*A*), which is produced in an infinite variety of amounts and toxicity by any single fire, and the multiple factors which define the dose of smoke inhaled by any individual victim. Al-

Paradigm of Smoke Inhalation

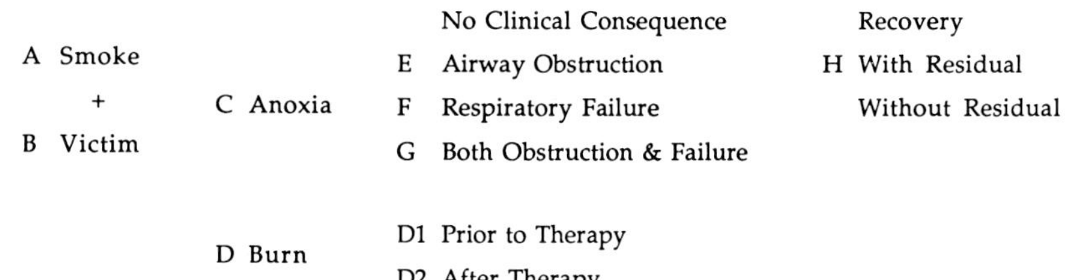

Figure 18-1 Smoke inhalation occurs with or without skin burns (see also Chap. 9). Each of the clinical consequences of the smoke-plus-victim interaction can exist in a wide range of severity; each clinical consequence has the potential to modulate other clinical consequences. The detection of clinical consequences, acute and residual, in individual patients will depend on variations in threshold and the sensitivity of testing methods. Death can occur at any point in this archetypal injury scenario; most deaths occur before the victim enters the health care system, presumably from anoxia.[10,61] Items identified with letters introduce a large number of variables which interact to define the severity of inhalation injury in any individual (see Table 18-1). The models for research discussed in this chapter focus on item F, the pulmonary injury caused by smoke which results in respiratory failure or makes the lung vulnerable to additional insults.[294]

Table 18-1 Variables in Smoke Inhalation Scenarios

*A Smoke**

Fire conditions
- Fuel (rarely single or homogeneous)
- Space (construction, design, material)
- Heat production rate, mass loss, etc.
- Suppression

Products of combustion
- Temperature
- Physical and/or chemical interaction
- Particles
- Toxicity
- Irritating vs. anesthetizing properties
- Density

Movement and control
- Space (construction, design, etc.)
- Wind
- Heating, ventilation, air conditioning
- Stacks

B Victim

Location (space, design, material)

Physical condition
- Age, sex,[2] neuromuscular status, vision, cerebral status, preexisting illness, intoxication[61,72]

Detection of hazard
- Decision, behavior

Dose
- Exposure time, activity, respiratory rate, tidal volume, pattern of respiration (laminar vs. turbulent airflow), filter

C Anoxia

Degree
Duration
Therapy
Consequences

D Burn

D_1 Before therapy
- Size
- Depth
- Location
- Severity and duration hypotension

D_2 After therapy
- Volume and character resuscitative fluid, changes in pulmonary microvascular fluid pressure,[294] colloid oncotic pressure[381,382]
- Drugs
- Anesthesia
- Aspiration
- Sepsis
  - Primary — lung
  - Secondary — burn wound[4,6,380]
- Pulmonary embolus

E Airway Obstruction

Level
Degree
Duration untreated
Complications of treatment[81,264,594]

F Respiratory Failure

Degree, location, homogeneity of injury

Site of injury
- Epithelial, endothelial, surfactant damage

Mechanism of injury
- Direct, WBC products, prostanoids

Consequences
- Pulmonary mechanics, lung fluid balance, gas exchange

H Recovery with Residual

Baseline status (α1 antitrypsin, etc.)
Chemical toxins
Chronicity of exposure

Threshold for symptoms
- Activity, level of awareness

Test methods — sensitivity

*List is incomplete. Letters refer to items in Fig. 18-1. Factors which interact to define the character of the smoke which reaches victims are all continuously changing.[71]

though heat may contribute to the laryngeal portion of any inhalation injury, it is not thought to be a factor in the pulmonary parenchymal component of the injury because the thermal capacity of the gas is low, the volume of each breath is small, and the evaporation required to saturate the inhaled gas with water vapor cools the gas, as does the heat exchanging capacity of the upper airway.[100]

Fire, Products of Combustion

Fuels and conditions at the site of ignition control the fire dynamics, which are responsible for the volume of smoke (Fig. 18-1*A*; Table 18-1*A*) as well as the heat and the chemical species liberated. The primary chemical products of fire interact both chemically and physically with themselves and with available surfaces to produce multiple generations of chemical species available for inhalation.[101] The rapidly changing quality of the fire environment adds to its enormous complexity. There have been comparatively few studies profiling atmospheric changes and the toxic products of combustion at real fires.[26,28,71,86,87,102–110] In order to make experiments clinically relevant and the severity of the lung damage inflicted by the products of combustion proportional to the duration of exposure, the smoke needs to be generated in a standard way (so that its characteristics are reproducible); the environmental contaminants responsible for anoxia: elevated cyanide (CN), carbon monoxide (CO), and reduced oxygen (O_2) should permit survival after exposures of short duration.[16] There is no simple answer to the problem of what fuel to use; as most accident scenarios involve the burning of buildings or their contents, materials present in them are appropriate for use in these experiments. In studies without a toxicologic focus, there is no particular advantage to using a single, chemically "pure" fuel.[111] A constant rate of fuel consumption may result in more predictable smoke in terms of its particulate and chemical constituents, but it does not recapitulate real fire scenarios.[23,71,102,103,112] The conduit through which the smoke passes should be as short and as nonreactive as possible so as to change the smoke the least either by condensation, absorption, settling, or chemical interaction. The temperature of the smoke should be body temperature or only slightly higher at the time it reaches the larynx.[100]

Smoke movement in a building environment is becoming more thoroughly understood, but the availability and efficiency of systems to control smoke are limited by cost, disrepair, and human error.[87,113–127] Building codes which attempt to make structures more fire-safe by controlling materials and design are frequently rendered superfluous by virtue of the fuel load present in the building's contents.[128] Most residential rooms contain an excess of fuel so that as a fire progresses through fluctuating rates of fuel consumption lethal levels of smoke will invariably be produced. This makes the issues of early detection and/or suppression critical for human salvage. The analysis of smoke is technically difficult.[23,71,93,102] A comprehensive approach to the toxic problems of smoke exposure requires coordinated efforts from the disciplines of combustion science, toxicology, and analytical chemistry at the very least.[24] The toxicologic assessment of smoke is complex, with the major problem being the applicability of experimental conditions to real fire scenarios.[129] Investigators focusing on the toxicologic effects of smoke have developed more elaborate guidelines for the standardization of chambers for smoke generation and animal exposure than have those studying the physiologic consequences of smoke.[130–145] Processes of product generation, animal exposure, chemical analysis, and correlation with toxicologic observations need to be carefully defined as they do in experiments attempting to define acute pulmonary changes.[24] Dynamic systems which move the products of combustion from the site of origin to the exposure chamber through a long conduit with baffles, filters, etc., are acceptable for toxicologic screens, but an unknown amount of particulate and toxic material can be lost in this process.[112] The applicability of animal data to humans is, perhaps, more of a problem for experimental systems using toxicologic end points than it is in experiments assessing tissue injury only.[146] The toxic end points include irritation, asphyxiation, acute behavior modification or global incapacitation, and death.[24,147–149] Although chemical and biologic analyses can be productively integrated in these studies,[24] most toxicologic experimental systems use biologic assays to determine thresholds, additive effects, and lethal concentrations because of the chemical complexity and unpredictability of smoke from even single-fuel sources.[23,24,94,97,146,150–162] The toxicity of combustion products is often referenced to that of the asphyxiant gases, CO and CN.[62,64,65,67,69,76,152,160–180] A large number of compounds have been burned in an effort to define their combustion products and the toxicity of them.[25,27,88,93,135,155,156,181–191]

Dose of Smoke

In clinical situations, it is impossible to derive the dose of smoke (Fig. 18-1*B*; Table 18-1*B*) inhaled with the possible exception of one or two components such as CO and CN. Duration of exposure, position of the victim in relation to the smoke source, tidal volume, respiratory rate, coughing, breath holding, and levels of activity are unknown for the most part; if estimates are available, they are difficult to correlate with varying fire conditions. Respiratory rates and patterns are modulated by activity, underlying medical conditions, alcohol levels,[72] drug levels, the anesthetizing capacity of the smoke, the irritating quality of airborne chemicals, and ambient levels of carbon dioxide.[192–200] In humans and primates, the irritating quality of most smoke causes a transient decrease in respiratory rate until the lung is involved, at which time the respiratory rate increases.[158,159,201] In the laboratory, the defenses of the upper airway and the influence of anesthesia on the physiologic reflexes which modify the rate, depth, and character of respiration can be eliminated as variables by bypassing the larynx with an endotracheal tube and substituting mechanical respiration for spontaneous breathing.[202,203]

Particles

Inert carbon particles and aerosols have been identified as carriers of toxic gases which potentiate the tissue damaging capacity of chemicals.[204–208] Similar effects have been demonstrated for black smoke with some species difference in the site of the lesion and the pattern of pathology.[209] Smoke has been shown to favor the penetration and retention of bacteria in lungs.[210] Processes which determine the physical characteristics of soot are complex.[211–216] However, they are relevant to the issue of smoke dose and localization of injury, because particle size, density, and consistency along with breathing patterns determine the distribution of chemicals throughout the airways and alveolar spaces.[217–232] The smoke toxicity critical for victims who survive the anoxic intervals secondary to CO and CN to enter the health care system is found in the tissue-damaging products of combustion; these polymerize, adhere to soot particles, or dissolve in water droplets to produce potentially lethal aerosols.[204,233–236] The site of particle deposition will, to some extent, control the anatomic focus of the injury. Almost any experimental smoke exposure system can be modified by the placement of a calibrated filter between the smoke source and the airway in an effort to define the role of particles in parenchymal smoke injuries.[30,98,237–241] Although few studies using filters have been done, those that are available indicate that carboxyhemoglobin levels are unchanged, but evidence for lung damage is reduced or absent after filtration of the smoke.[237,239–242] To be properly done, experiments using filters need to document the effect of the filter on the inspired gas both in terms of particulate matter, chemical composition, and characteristics of gas flow.[239]

Anoxia

The anoxia (Fig. 18-1*C*; Table 18-1*C*) caused by CO and CN has been well studied. It is felt to be responsible for many deaths in the prehospital setting even in the absence of burns.[57,59,61,62,64,65,67,69] Although it rarely exists as a single clinical problem in the presentation of these victims to the health care system, the important features of its treatment have been worked out.[163,167,168,177–179,243–256] The events which control the degree of clinical anoxia operate in an uncontrolled environment. Models of smoke inhalation which result in high levels of carboxyhemoglobin do not correspond to the usual clinical situation, as victims with these levels rarely survive to enter the health care system or, if they do, are often found to be brain dead once resuscitation is complete and their other injuries treated. Although chronic, low levels of carboxyhemoglobinemia have been reported to result in increased capillary permeability to albumin and a reduced plasma volume,[257–259] histologic changes secondary to acute carbon monoxide exposure are usually not detectable until carboxyhemoglobin levels approach 60 percent.[34,260] This is considered a lethal level in most clinical situations.[163] Reports of experiments done with filtered smoke do not alter the carboxyhemoglobin levels achieved but do reduce or eliminate the physiologic and pathologic effects of smoke, suggesting that CO alone is rarely, if ever, responsible for parenchymal lung damage following isolated episodes of smoke inhalation.[238,240] For these reasons, carboxyhemoglobin levels greater than 50 percent are probably not appropriate in experiments designed to investigate smoke-induced lung damage.[261] The level of anoxia reached in these experiments can be controlled by modifying the burning conditions, limiting the duration of smoke exposure, or controlling the carbon monoxide concentration in synthetic smoke.

Airway Obstruction

The obstructive component of clinical smoke inhalation (Fig. 18-1*E*; Table 18-1*E*) is eliminated in models which introduce the smoke through an endotracheal tube. This allows one to study the pulmonary response to smoke without the variable of obstruction at the larynx which can exacerbate the parenchymal injury. Airway obstruction is a significant problem in smoke inhalation victims, especially those who have a burn as well, but it can be so definitively and effectively treated with an endotracheal tube that in ideal therapeutic settings it should not be a cause of death.[81–83,261–266]

Burn Effect on Lung

Demling and an impressive number of collaborators have explored the effects of a significant body burn on the lung.[267–275] All of these experiments have been done in the sheep and should be reviewed whenever smoke inhalation is added to an animal with a skin burn.[276] Others have contributed on this topic.[277,278] It seems clear that even sterile inflammation in parietal tissue is capable of causing significant changes in the lung.[279,280] However, the incorporation of a thermal injury into any model of smoke inhalation raises the issues of bacterial infection and bacterial endotoxin, both of which have an effect on the lung that is difficult to quantify or control.[281–293]

Controls in Smoke Inhalation Models

Investigators with a clinical, as opposed to a toxicologic orientation, have focused their attentions on the pulmonary injury initiated by smoke, which either sets the stage for respiratory failure or makes the lung more vulnerable than normal to additional stresses which the burn illness provides in abundance (Fig. 18-1D_2; Table 18-1D_2).[3,4,6,294] In most laboratories where smoke experiments have been conducted for several years, the injuries produced in individual animals are qualitatively similar but quite variable in degree. This variability represents the variations in resistance to injury and metabolic reserve in the individual test animals (Fig. 18-1*B*; Table 18-1*B*). For the most part, the variability in the severity of injury produced by experimental models is much less than that present in the clinical arena, suggesting that many of the nonbiologic factors responsible for injury severity (Table 18-1) have been controlled adequately.

Tracheal Divider Models that use a tracheal divider so that smoke is delivered to just one lung, allow animals to serve as their own control in an effort to differentiate the systemic from the topical consequences of smoke exposure.[237,260,261,295–298] In this experimental variation the systemic responses to smoke in the form of anoxia, acidosis, and chemical mediators of the acute-phase response presumably affect both lungs while the topical effects are limited to one lung. Problems include the inability to be absolutely sure there is no leak of smoke at the carinal level. Respirators for each lung need to be precisely linked mechanically so that they stay in phase throughout the respiratory cycle. Often the systemic response to smoke delivered to just one lung is not great, because of the reserve present in the lung not exposed to smoke.[237] However, to my knowledge, this experimental approach has not been combined with placement of flow probes on right and left pulmonary arteries, differential sampling for possible chemical mediators, or sophisticated microscopic techniques to differentiate the topical as opposed to the systemic effects of smoke.

Animals to Study

There is no simple answer to the question of which animal is the most suitable for these studies. Obviously there are issues of cost, facility space, veterinary expertise, and laboratory experience which will influence each institution in a unique way as they approach the question. It is beyond the scope of this review to trace the effect of animal rights' groups on the selective availability of different species as experimental subjects.[299–304] The purpose of the study will have some bearing on the question: primates may be ideal if the ventilatory response to the irritation of smoke exposure is the focus of the study.[130,132,158,159,176] The major laboratories studying lung fluid balance and injury under the aegis of Guyton, Staub, Taylor, Brigham, and Demling, to name a few, have used either the dog or sheep, so there is a wealth of experience with these animals. The chemical and physiologic measurements made must be referenced to what is normal for the animal being studied, not for humans or some other species.[305–321] The age of sexual maturity is the time when visceral strength or metabolic reserve peaks.[2,322] Ideally, animals used for these experiments should be chosen with this age in mind and should be homogeneous with respect to age and sex so as to minimize the biologic variability in the study. After the age of maturity, subtle decrements in visceral function occur. These may not attain clinical thresholds at rest, but will often become manifest as a breakdown in integrated organ function under stress.[323] These unmeasurable visceral deficits are the basis for much of the variation seen when biologic systems are stressed (Fig. 18-1*B*; Table 18-1*B*).[2]

Acute versus Chronic Studies

Most models of smoke inhalation focus on the acute injury; studies which are prolonged to determine whether or not the animals survive do so in order to make inferences about the severity of the injury or the toxicity of the smoke. Because the breathing patterns and coughing effectiveness of sick animals are often quite different from that of humans, it is difficult to develop a chronic model that will precisely mimic the clinical progression in humans. The smoke-injured lung is especially vulnerable to infection,[4,6,7] perhaps because of macrophage dysfunction,[324,325] so that efforts to develop a chronic model are likely to end up with a pulmonary pathologic state that no longer represents just smoke inhalation. It seems probable that the lung injured by smoke progresses rapidly to a state of "diffuse alveolar damage"[48,326,327] common to lungs damaged by other mechanisms. If this is so, acute studies offer an opportunity to capture the unique features of smoke inhalation in terms of the primary pathologic event which initiates the trend toward global involvement. A truly chronic model would have the potential for defining the sine qua non for progression to varying forms of chronic lung disease, which seem to afflict relatively few of these patients.[10,13,327–336]

Table 18-2 Experimental Models in Which Unanesthetized Animals Breathe Spontaneously without an Endotracheal Tube

Senior author, date	Animal	Fuel	Duration of study	Average CoHgb,* %	End points, comments	Diagram of apparatus	Refs.
Lee, 1976	Rat	Teflon	7 days		Electron microscopy	Yes	239
Dressler, 1976	Rat	Wood	15 days	14–48	Survival, pathology, steroid treatment	No	338
Zawacki, 1977	Mouse	Cotton	14 days		Survival, respiratory distress, pathology, burn, fluid, bacterial challenge	Yes	16
Thomas, 1980	Rat	Wood, polyurethane			Ability to add CO, CN	Yes	112
Thorning, 1982	Rabbit	Wood	72 hours		Histology of airway	No	337,(341)†
Purser, 1983	Monkey	Wood, polyurethane		31–45	Respiratory response to smoke, pathology	No	158
Loke, 1984	Rabbit	Wood	24 hours	16.4	Histology, bronchoalveolar lavage	No	339,(134)
Beeley, 1986	Rabbit	(Acrolein)‡	72 hours		Histology, survival, steroid treatment	No	340
Sharar, 1988	Goat	Wood	24 hours	37	Physiologic response, EVLW,§ prostaglandin	No	111

*CoHgb = carboxyhemoglobin.
†References in parentheses indicate a secondary article by the same authors.
‡Fuels in parentheses indicate synthetic smoke or chemicals produced without the combustion process.
§EVLW = extravascular lung water.

EXPERIMENTAL MODELS OF SMOKE INHALATION

In this section, the experimental models used to study the effects of acute smoke inhalation on the lungs will be categorized based on the presence or absence of anesthesia, an endotracheal tube, and spontaneous respiration. These methodologic variations relate to the elements in the smoke exposure process which are controlled as discussed earlier. All independent variables need to be controlled so that the model really tests the effects of smoke on the lungs, which is the dependent variable. Salient features in each category will be discussed briefly. In every category, the objective is to cause a reproducible injury of sufficient severity so that objectively detectable consequences result without precluding short-term survival.

Unanesthetized Animals, Spontaneous Respiration

The first group of models are those in which unanesthetized animals breathe spontaneously without an endotracheal tube during the exposure interval (Table 18-2). In these studies, the animals' reflexes and proximal airway remain intact and may modify the dose of smoke and intercept it to varying degrees before it reaches the lungs. With two exceptions,[111,158] studies in this category were performed on small fur-bearing animals. General points which concern the dose of smoke include the observation that nose breathing eliminates an unknown amount of particulate material and water-soluble chemicals before they reach the lung. Animals need to be exposed while in individual compartments to prevent the huddling behavior which allows them to filter the inspired gas through the fur of the adjacent animal. Smoke is usually irritating, so that breath-holding,[337] irregular breathing, and tachypnea[111] alter the lung dose of smoke by changing both the minute volume of ventilation and the amount of turbulent airflow which influences the site of particle deposition. The ability of these defense mechanisms to protect the lung is seen in the report of Thorning et al., who could demonstrate almost no pulmonary pathology after smoke exposures ranging from 25 to 45 minutes.[337]

Ideally, these studies are done with nose-only exposure to eliminate the smoke these animals might ingest while grooming themselves after total-body exposure.[138] Studies which assess smoke toxicity as reflected in mortality must be tempered by an awareness of the tremendous species variation in toxicity based on differences in the organ system primarily affected and the biochemical capacity of different animal strains to tolerate varying alterations in their normal metabolic pathways.[98,319] It is important to use pathogen-free animals.[338,339]

Dressler et al. make the point of exposing control and treatment groups to the same batch of smoke, which emphasizes the difficulties in producing smoke of absolutely uniform composition.[338] The model of Zawacki et al. represents a major effort which includes many variables such as a burn, fluid administration, and bacterial challenges; it is one of the first attempting to have the smoke conform to that found in survivable fire situations. No physiologic measurements are available. Dose response curves are generated by varying the exposure time to smoke generated using an elaborate method to ensure constant consumption of fuel at 1 g/min.[16] This is a variation on the "amount for an effect for a given duration of exposure approach" discussed by Alarie.[25] The apparatus used by Thomas and O'Flaherty relies on the nonflaming mode of combustion but does provide the ability to control the concentrations of CO and CN.[112] Beeley et al. note that acrolein vapor did not cause a uniform or homogeneous lung injury, so that histologic study required serial sections of the whole lung; they also remark on the apparent lack of direct correlation of histologic abnormalities with mortality.[340] Zawacki et al. noted few histologic changes in animals dying in apparent respiratory distress after both smoke inhalation and a burn.[16] Both reports suggest a sometimes profound discrepancy between lung structure and function. The smoke exposure in the goat reported by Sharar et al. barely achieved clinical significance in spite of an end point of 37 percent carboxyhemoglobinemia. This is probably because of the large smoke reservoir used, which would allow an unknown amount of particulate matter to settle out.[111,112] The extravascular lung water (EVLW) increase had little effect on pulmonary function and was attributed to the inability of the goat to clear his secretions following smoke exposure or tracheostomy.[111]

Anesthetized Animals, Spontaneous Respiration, with and without an Endotracheal Tube

The next group of models are those in which anesthetized animals breathing spontaneously are exposed to smoke through an endotracheal tube (Table 18-3*A*) or without an endotracheal tube (Table 18-3*B*). Adequate anesthesia may depress the respiratory rate, but it should also eliminate any reflex response to smoke which might cause the dose to vary in an unpredictable way. The endotracheal tube eliminates the convoluted passages of the upper airway as a defense against particulate matter. Many of these studies were done 40 years ago, focused on delivering a heat load (steam) to the pulmonary parenchyma, and were limited because the instruments and monitoring devices did not have the technical sophistication we enjoy today.

The work of Moritz et al. is a classic[100]; it is one of the first which attempts to bypass the larynx in an effort to define the response of the distal trachea and lungs to the injuring agent. Deep, rapid respirations are reported after exposure of the airway to

Table 18-3*A* Experimental Models in Which Anesthetized Animals Breathe Spontaneously through an Endotracheal Tube

Senior author, date	Animal	Fuel	Duration of study	Average CoHgb,* %	End points, comments	Diagram of apparatus	Refs.
Moritz, 1945	Dog	(Steam, hot air)†	10 hours		Temperature, pathology	Yes	100
Aviado, 1952	Dog	(Steam, hot air)	2 hours		Temperature, physiologic response	Yes	361
Fineberg, 1954	Dog	(Steam)	4 hours		Blood gases, survival	Yes	362
Zikria, 1972	Dog	Wood, kerosene	4 hours, 21 days		Survival, EVLW,‡ smoke	Yes	363
Rowland, 1986	Rabbit	Cotton	4 days	48–66	Nuclear scans, histology	No	347,348

*CoHgb = carboxyhemoglobin.
†Fuels in parentheses indicate synthetic smoke or chemicals produced without the combustion process.
‡EVLW = extravascular lung water.

Table 18-3*B* Experimental Models in Which Anesthetized Animals Breathe Spontaneously without an Endotracheal Tube

Senior author, date	Animal	Fuel	Duration of study	Average CoHgb,* %	End points, comments	Diagram of apparatus	Refs.
Stone, 1967	Rat	(Hot air, steam)†	10 days		Survival	No	75
Gump, 1972	Dog	(Steam)	4 hours		EVLW‡	No	354
Esrig, 1975	Dog	Wood	72 hours		Physiologic response, histology, bacterial culture	No	360

*CoHgb = carboxyhemoglobin.
†Fuels in parentheses indicate synthetic smoke or chemicals produced without the combustion process.
‡EVLW = extravascular lung water.

high temperatures, but the actual heat load delivered is unknown because tidal volumes are unknown. These experiments are assumed to establish the fact that thermal injuries of the respiratory tract distal to the larynx are unusual clinical occurrences except in the rare instance of inhalation of live steam,[342] aspiration of hot coffee,[343] or malfunction of heated nebulizers in respiratory circuits.[237] More information might be obtained if these experiments were repeated using present-day technology, both in terms of the injury inflicted at different levels by well-characterized heat loads and in terms of the way a heat stress influences respiratory patterns and laryngeal function.[55,344–346] This latter information would suggest how people protect themselves in fire situations and the way in which this response alters the dose of smoke inhaled.

The model of Rowland et al. depends on nuclear imaging techniques and is probably flawed most by the assumption that 87,000-molecular-weight dextran equilibrates with the pulmonary interstitial space.[347,348] Furthermore, the EVLW reported for control animals given fluid only was not different from that in animals exposed to smoke and given fluid[347]; this suggests that the rabbit may not be a good animal in which to study lung fluid balance in response to a crystalloid challenge equal to 5 percent of body weight over 2 hours. In many other laboratories, the normal lung has been shown capable of protecting itself against this degree of volume stress.[294,349–353] These authors do report that the EVLW increase following smoke exposure is detectable in less than 2 hours,[347] which is consistent with the observations of others.[237]

Stone et al. introduced a great many variables in studies focusing on mortality. Their studies confirm the conventional wisdom that increasing the humidity or adding smoke to hot air increases its lethal potential.[75] Gump et al. studying EVLW after steam instillation, found that the double-indicator dilution technique detected only 64 percent of the EVLW measured gravimetrically.[354] This observation has been made again more recently in sheep[296] and is probably due to the nonhomogeneity of the pulmonary lesions caused by smoke.[238] In contrast, a study in dogs following exposure to synthetic smoke based on carbon particles, acrolein, and hydrochloric acid showed a good correlation ($r = 0.93$, $P < 0.01$) between EVLW assessed gravimetrically and by the double-indicator technique.[206] Gump et al. also found no correlation between EVLW and pulmonary shunt or Pa_{O_2}.[354] They felt that a decrease in pulmonary compliance was a sensitive index of increase in EVLW. In spite of the fact that more focused studies have shown a poor correlation between interstitial edema and decreased compliance,[274,355–358] Traber et al. reported a decreased compliance due to an increase in EVLW (quantitated by the thermal-dye technique), although the correlation coefficients are low, and the data are probably not significant.[359] In another study in dogs, the drop in compliance occurred within 5 minutes of smoke exposure and did not progress; furthermore, there was no difference in the compliance change in animals exposed to smoke and those exposed to smoke followed by a fluid challenge even though there was 14 percent more EVLW in animals in the latter group.[294] Esrig, in a model which removed the endotracheal tube during smoke exposure in dogs, found his animals became profoundly anoxic (Pa_{O_2} 37 mmHg) in the smoke chamber but did not necessarily have a severe inhalation injury in terms of lung damage, again indicating the difficulties of producing a severe reproducible injury when the larynx is not bypassed and mechanical ventilation is not used.[360]

Anesthetized Animals, Mechanically Controlled Respiration, Endotracheal Tube

The last group of models are those in which anesthetized animals are exposed to smoke through an endotracheal tube by controlled respiration (Table 18-4). Delivering smoke in this way does not conform to the way smoke exposure occurs clinically, but it affords the best opportunity to deliver a standard dose of smoke to the distal airway and lungs, provided the burning conditions are controlled and the tidal volume is referenced to the size of the animal.[238,305] The potential reproducibility of these methods makes them suitable for the study of physiologic response in protocols which rely on relatively small numbers of animals. Ease of instrumentation for physiologic measurements and the need to harvest multiple tissue samples in one experiment favor the use of large animals.[305]

The model developed by Nieman and Clark produces a severe, nonhomogeneous injury in dogs.[29,238,261,294,295,364–366] Efforts to limit the severity of the injury by shortening the exposure time have been unavailing: no animal has survived longer than 30 hours following smoke exposure. Thus, this model is not suitable for chronic studies; whether this is because of the smoke produced, the absence of any settling chamber to reduce the load of particulates, the dog as an experimental animal, or all of these is not clear. The burning conditions are standardized in a gross way. After the smoke exposure, animals are ventilated with room air at the respirator settings used during the presmoke baseline period. Changes in respirator settings, fluid management, etc., are considered independent variables

Table 18-4 Experimental Models in Which Anesthetized Animals Are Exposed to Smoke Delivered through an Endotracheal Tube by Mechanically or Manually Controlled Respiration

Senior author, date	Animal	Fuel	Duration of study	Average CoHgb,* %	End points, comments	Diagram of apparatus	Refs.
Zikria, 1968	Dog	(Steam)†	4 hours 21 days		EVLW,‡ pathology, surfactant, survival	No	77
Eyal, 1975	Rabbit	(Steam)	4 hours		Lung mechanics, EVLW	No	408
Clark, 1980	Dog	Wood, kerosene	4 hours	23	Physiologic response, surfactant, in vivo microscopy, EVLW, lymph, imaging	Yes	238,294, 29,295, 261, 364–366
Walker, 1981	Goat	Cotton	15 days		Pathology of airway	Yes	367
Brizio-Molteni, 1984	Dog	Wood, paper	30 hours		Angiotensin 1–converting enzyme	No	298
Herndon, 1984	Sheep	Cotton	48 hours	70–92	Physiologic response, lymph, EVLW, histology, burn, acid aspiration, leukopenia	Yes	276,296, 297,359, 368–380
Shinozawa, 1986	Rat	(Carbon, hydrochloric acid)	6 hours		Prostaglandins, EVLW	No	402
Zhi-Yuan, 1986	Rabbit	(Steam)	16 hours		Surfactant	No	406
Shimazu, 1987	Sheep	Wood, cellulose	72 hours	40–85	Physiologic response, EVLW, survival, PEEP	Yes	305,407
Hales, 1988	Dog	(Carbon, hydrochloric acid, acrolein)	18 hours		EVLW, airway pressure, histology	Yes	206

*CoHgb = carboxyhemoglobin.
†Fuels in parentheses indicate synthetic smoke or chemicals produced without the combustion process.
‡EVLW = extravascular lung water.

and are controlled in animals similarly managed who receive no smoke. These control animals are, in turn, compared to "historic controls," animals subjected to no manipulation except the administration of anesthesia. Animals with closed chests are more stable and recover from their smoke exposure more readily than do animals with open chests.[237]

In the model reported by Brizio-Molteni et al., only one lung is exposed to smoke while the other mainstem bronchus is mechanically occluded.[298] As smoke exposure lasts for 8 minutes, it would seem that the model includes perturbations other than smoke exposure.

Walker et al., at the U.S. Army Institute of Surgical Research, found that a modified bee smoker could be used to produce a nonlethal inhalation injury in goats which resembled the human response to smoke.[367] Traber and Herndon have used this method of smoke exposure in their sheep model of inhalation injury.[276,296,297,359,368–380] The smoker is manually activated. Even with elaborate efforts at consistency in this process, the smoke dose delivered is not standardized, and the possibility of bias exists. Evidence for this is found in the widely varying carboxyhemoglobin levels reported over time for this model. In a 1986 report, 56 breaths of smoke resulted in a mean carboxyhemoglobin level of 29% ± 4.[370] A 1988 report indicated that 32 breaths of smoke resulted in a mean carboxyhemoglobin level of 70% ± 4.[371] This model requires maintenance of the animal during a series of surgical procedures and recovery intervals required for cannulation of mediastinal lymphatics and instrumentation. The system-effort invested in each animal is enormous, and the tendency is to include them in the protocol even though they may be sick or require antibiotics to make them eligible for study. Because gram-negative endotoxemia has such complex and multifaceted effects on the lung, animals in varying stages of sepsis or with varying exposures to antibiotics will not have lungs with the same physiologic set point at the time of smoke exposure.[281–291,381] The variable of endogenous endotoxemia is difficult to control, but it is a real issue in chronic studies when the response of the lung to the experimental intervention is being studied. At the very least, it would seem that all animals in such a lengthy protocol, not just those rendered leukopenic,[374] should have identical antibiotic exposure, negative blood cultures, or similar endotoxin levels prior to smoke exposure. In Herndon's laboratory, smoke-exposed animals are treated with the addition of positive end-expiratory pressure (PEEP), increases in the concentration of inspired oxygen (Fi_{O_2}),[359,370] and administration of fluid and fresh ovine plasma[375] to maintain hemodynamic, pulmonary, and chemical parameters within arbitrarily defined limits. All of these represent independent factors with recognized effects on the lung.[294,326,378,382–401] These treatment modalities are not uniformly applied to experimental animals or imposed upon control animals. This lack of controls undoubtedly increases the variability of their observations and makes their conclusions less definitive.

Shinozawa et al. describe a technically demanding model in the rat.[402] The assumption that right ventricular pressure accurately reflects pulmonary microvascular pressure[403–405] is suspect and introduces a degree of uncertainty into their discussion of the mechanism for the formation of pulmonary edema after exposure to hydrocholoric acid and carbon particles.

The model of Zhi-yuan et al. requires suture closure of a tracheostomy incision after exposure to steam.[406] The degree to which this interferes with ventilation and upper airway function is uncertain, but both these effects could influence the surfactant measurements made on lung extracts.

In spite of the large volume furnace used to generate smoke in the model of Shimazu et al., they were able to demonstrate several consistent dose response relationships.[305] As much of the particulate material of smoke could settle out in this furnace, it may be that the smoke reaching the animal was less toxic than that generated in smaller furnaces and delivered directly to the airway.

EXPERIMENTAL OBSERVATIONS

The tests that can be done to assess the structure and function of the smoke-exposed lung or the physiologic state of the whole animal are too numerous to discuss comprehensively. There is potential for the involvement of many disciplines. The variety and permutations of the measurements that can be made are limited only by the imagination. A few experimental observations will be discussed in general terms from the standpoint of the yield, the limitations, and the methodologic considerations applicable to each. Specific details pertaining to the execution of any particular method need to be sought in the appropriate report or verified by visiting laboratories where they are used regularly.

Pulmonary Imaging

X-ray, Computed Tomography The clinical observation that the initial chest radiograph, often done using portable technique, is usually normal in patients known to have experienced a significant smoke inhalation injury[1,8,10,409–411] has been corroborated in the laboratory in dogs.[29,364] Computed tomography of the chest is much more sensitive than the standard chest radiograph in detecting the nonhomogeneous atelectatic changes following smoke inhalation in both dogs[29] and humans.[1] Computed tomography has the advantage of allowing control of gray-scale parameters, which permits optimizing the contrast resolution of the image with reference to the tissue being studied. Because these settings can be controlled, the differences in "technique" so frequently a confounding element when comparing serial radiographs is not a problem.[29] Computed tomographic techniques have enormous potential for quantitating lung densities, demonstrating the nonhomogeneous distribution of injury in the damaged lung, and identifying different density patterns characteristic of edema of different etiologies when combined with positron tomography.[412–417]

Xenon, "Technegas" Ventilation scans done using xenon 133 are superior to the perfusion-ventilation scan done in most burn victims.[418,419] In these studies the perfusion image is transient (making it impossible to obtain multiple views), gas wash-out cannot be assessed in unperfused areas since no xenon arrives at the alveoli, and a wash-in ventilation study, which is frequently more informative than the usual wash-out study, is not available.[29] Xenon ventilation studies can be done in animals and patients on the respirator.[420] The precision of ventilation imaging with nuclear gases is limited by detector resolution, signal distortion at depth, poor counting statistics, and respiratory motion[421]; Xenon 133 has low gamma energy and so provides much less spatial resolution than radioactive pharmaceuticals using technetium 99m.[364,422] A new technique utilizing an ultrafine dispersion of technetium 99m–labeled carbon ("technegas") has gas-like characteristics and provides a static image[422]; it can produce images with much higher resolution than are available without it.

^{99m}Tc Diethylenetriaminepentacetate (DTPA) Aerosolized technetium 99m diethylenetriaminepentacetate (DTPA) is reported to be a sensitive way to assess the integrity of the alveolar epithelium.[423–429] Most of the particles reach the alveolar space, where DTPA is absorbed from the alveolar surface into the pulmonary capillary and then into the systemic circulation to be excreted rapidly in the urine. A damaged epithelium results in faster clearance; normal DTPA clearance is too slow to provide a reliable lower limit, so the test is only of value when clearance rates are faster than normal.[427] The presence of significant atelectasis does not alter clearance rates[364,426]; DTPA clearance requires pulmonary artery perfusion but is not flow-dependent across a wide range of flows.[428] In a dog model it proved more sensitive to the detection of smoke inhalation than chest x-rays or xenon 133 scans.[364] DTPA clearance is sensitive to alveolar volume, because the alveolar epithelium becomes more permeable as inflation volume increases.[430–432] This might introduce an artifact if surfactant dysfunction is marked following smoke and the nonatelectatic alveoli are overdistended by high airway pressures or PEEP.[238,401,407]

Surfactant, Pulmonary Mechanics

It is beyond the scope of this chapter to outline the complex physiology of pulmonary surfactant. Several reviews are available.[433–435] Smoke inhalation has been shown to inactivate or displace surfactant, resulting in an almost instantaneous decrease in compliance and increase in venous admixture with grossly obvious atelectasis that is nonsegmental in distribution.[238,294] Surfactant exerts its primary physiologic effect by reducing the surface tension of the fluid layer lining the alveoli at low lung volumes.[434,436,437] This surface tension derives from the intermolecular attraction at a gas-fluid interface[438,439]; if it is not modulated in the lung during tidal respiration, alveolar collapse results. As the alveoli collapse or flood, the radius of alveolar curvature is reduced, augmenting the surface tension increase because of the relationship $P = 2\ \gamma/r$ (where P = pressure required to keep alveoli open, γ = surface tension, and r = radius of curvature of alveolar surface) so that alveolar collapse is facilitated further. Surface tension controls the distribution of lung capillary blood flow; increased alveolar surface tension (assumed on the basis of surfactant dysfunction) can result in large increases in EVLW without detectable changes in pulmonary microvascular pressure or endothelial permeability.[440-446] The increase in EVLW is probably caused by the mechanical forces which result in a more negative interstitial tissue pressure between collapsed alveoli and which operate at the interface of nonhomogeneous portions of pulmonary parenchyma.[442,447-449] Although surfactant dysfunction explains many of the very early changes in lung function and appearance following smoke exposure, to date surfactant replacement has not reversed these[237] as it apparently can in infants with the neonatal respiratory distress syndrome.[450-453] Work with surfactant systems is technically demanding, and in the best of worlds requires chemical and biophysical expertise not always available. The detectable abnormalities in surfactant following smoke exposure are apparently confined to the atelectatic portion of the lung.[237] This is presumably because the smoke injury is not uniformly distributed throughout the pulmonary parenchyma.[238] Atelectasis per se is not reported to alter extractable surfactant if the lung is reexpanded several times prior to harvest.[454-457] Current harvesting techniques do not allow one to distinguish between dysfunctional surfactant still in place on the alveolar surface and normal surfactant displaced into the airway, although gross observations and physiologic measurements suggest that these variants of surfactant perturbations do exist.[237] Surfactant deserves more attention because it is probably the primary determinant of the early mechanical charges responsible for atelectasis, venous admixture, and the response to PEEP.[238,295,397,399,401,458-461]

Multiple Inert Gas Technique

The multiple inert gas technique has been used in humans[462] and experimental animals[407] to assess the array of ventilation-perfusion alterations following smoke inhalation. Although there is the potential for more precise measurements using this technique than is available in the clinical determination of shunt, the technique is demanding and has practical limitations.[463,464]

Bronchoalveolar Lavage

Bronchoalveolar lavage can be performed with reasonable safety,[465] but requires experience with technical variations.[466] It has enormous potential for the cytologic as well as the immunologic assessment of the injured lung.[467-469] Its use following smoke inhalation has been reported infrequently[134,339,470-472]; it might prove especially useful in a chronic model to monitor the progression of the illness and perhaps identify the signal which heralds the development of chronic lung disease.

Microscopy, Electronmicroscopy

Few formal studies of the microscopy of the smoke exposed lung have been conducted.[134,337,339,473] Critical to these studies are the harvesting and fixing techniques which should be standardized with reference to physiologic parameters, measured vascular perfusion pressure, and a known airway volume or pressure.[337,340] The artifacts unique to each method of fixation need to be recognized and understood so that the tissue sections can be examined with the appropriate caveats in mind.[474-479] The alveolar air-liquid interface is preserved in lungs fixed by vascular perfusion.[480] If these exacting steps are taken, the micrographs may reveal important architectural relationships with functional implications which cannot be inferred from routine pathologic sections.[16,340]

Morphometrics, Vital Dyes The morphometric analysis of lungs using stereologic principles can reveal many early changes in alveolar volume, surface area, and geometry as well as vascular dimensions and the initial sites of fluid accumulation following smoke exposure.[480–492] The morphometric analysis of lungs in both the control and experimental state can be combined with techniques of freeze fixation, freeze drying, planimetry, and the use of vital dyes.[358,479,492–498] All of these techniques require some special equipment and an elaborate attention to detail for proper execution. However, they do have enormous potential for defining the time sequence of fluid accumulation in the lungs[496,498] and the location of interstitial fluid reservoirs[358,492,495] which operate in situations of injury and the administration of fluid to protect the lung from alveolar edema. Experiments performed using these techniques could, if the samples were timed properly, indicate the rapidity with which fluid collects in the lung, which in turn would provide clues about the pathophysiologic event which was responsible for this fluid accumulation.

Extravascular Lung Water

Increases in EVLW have been used as an indirect indicator of pulmonary injury; as such increases are not in and of themselves the fulcrum of the pathophysiologic process, it is probably not correct to direct treatment at them alone wihtout considering the underlying pathophysiologic mechanisms.[294] There are three basic forces governing fluid flux between the pulmonary vasculature and the interstitial space: (1) the hydrostatic pressure gradient, (2) the oncotic pressure gradient, and (3) the permeability of the vessel wall to fluids and plasma proteins.[261,499,500] Although the Starling equation has evolved to allow for new concepts of protein transport modulated by blood flow,[501,502] in its classic form it remains a useful conceptual framework within which to consider tissue fluid flux[357,503–506]:

$$Q = K\,[(P_{mv} - P_{pmv}) - \sigma\,(\pi_{mv} - \pi_{pmv})]$$

where Q is the net transvascular fluid flux (volume/time), P_{mv} and P_{pmv} are microvascular and perimicrovascular (interstitial) hydrostatic pressures, respectively, π_{mv} and π_{pmv} are microvascular and perimicrovascular protein osmotic (oncotic) pressures, respectively, K is fluid filtration coefficient which defines the liquid conductance of the microvascular barrier, and σ is the reflection coefficient describing the relative resistance of the microvascular barrier to protein leakage. A decrease in the oncotic ($\pi_{mv} - \pi_{pmv}$) gradient will accelerate fluid flux from the vascular to the interstitial compartments as will an increase in the hydrostatic (P_{mv}) gradient, a permeability increase for fluid (increased K), and an increased permeability to protein (decreased σ). A decrease in σ allows more protein to leak into the interstitial space thus lowering the osmotic gradient; although K is rarely measured directly,[507] a decrease in σ has always been associated with an increase in K.[499,508] The lung is generally protected from the accumulation of EVLW by an increase in lung lymph flow and a decrease in perimicrovascular oncotic pressures.[353,509,510] This means that gradients between oncotic and microvascular pressures are a poor predictor of pulmonary edema. This gradient controls the hydrostatic pressure at which pulmonary fluid accumulation begins; the rate of fluid flux into the pulmonary interstitium is controlled by hydrostatic forces alone.[511,512] In the presence of a pulmonary capillary endothelial membrane with normal permeability to protein, increases in P_{mv} result in a decrease in π_{pmv} so that the $\pi_{mv} - \pi_{pmv}$ gradient is restored almost to normal levels and the lung is protected to the extent of a 50 percent reduction in the hydrostatic pressure increase.[513] Increasing endothelial permeability to protein (reducing σ) abolishes this protection because the interstitial protein concentration is not reduced with increased hydrostatic pressure; in this circumstance, the transvascular fluid flux is determined by the increased K (fluid filtration coefficient) and the hydrostatic gradient ($P_{mv} - P_{pmv}$).[514–517] Pulmonary microvascular pressure (P_{mv}) cannot be measured directly and is usually inferred from the relationship between the pulmonary artery pressure and the left atrial pressure[294,518,519]:

$$P_{mv} = PAW + 0.4\,(PAP - PAW)$$

where P_{mv} is pulmonary microvascular pressure, PAP is pulmonary artery pressure, and PAW is pulmonary artery wedge pressure. Extravascular lung water increases do not result in alveolar edema until it has reached the range of 35 percent above normal.[520]

The status of the theory and practice of determining EVLW has been reviewed.[521,522] The gravimetric methods, when carefully done, are less subject to experimental error[351,523]; because they can only be used once in any experiment, the gravimetric methods cannot demonstrate progression or resolution of EVLW. The "Pearce technique", which compensates for blood trapped in the lung, has a definite learning curve associated with it[523]; it is important to homogenize the lung thoroughly to avoid errors due to uneven sampling.* In general, the blood-inclusive wet/dry lung weight ratio correlates well with the more involved techniques needed to determine the extravascular lung water to blood-free dry lung weight ratio.[524] Extravascular lung water can also be assessed using indicator dilution techniques.[525] Although sequential measurements can be made in the same animal, these have been shown to underestimate EVLW after smoke inhalation in a sheep model.[296] The reason for this is presumed to relate to the hypoxic vasoconstriction which operates to redistribute lung blood flow. However, hypoxic vasoconstriction has been shown to have little effect on edema formation.[526] High cardiac output and air embolism have also been shown to result in the underestimation of EVLW using a double-indicator dilution technique.[527,528] The type of lung injury has been reported to influence the accuracy of EVLW estimation using thermal dilution techniques.[529] A method of estimating EVLW using only a single thermal indicator has been described.[530] With an increase in EVLW, the dry lung weight increases, reflecting the solid components of the blood.[294,531] The time constant controlling the resolution of pulmonary edema is probably much longer than the one applicable to the formation of an increase in EVLW; the presence of an increased EVLW in a lung with normal microvascular pressures does not necessarily mean that the microvascular pressures were normal when the edema formed. In this circumstance, it is a mistake to infer an increase in pulmonary capillary endothelial permeability as the cause of the EVLW increase.[532]

*Parker RE: Personal communication, December 1988.

Lung Lymph

The lung lymphatics are presumed to collect fluid filtered from exchange vessels in the lungs to return it to the systemic circulation. In *steady states* the lung lymph flow will be representative of the net amount of fluid being filtered in the organ. The assumption that the protein concentration in lung lymph is equivalent to that in the pulmonary microvascular filtrate is often made.[533–535] Similarly, the protein concentration of airway fluid is assumed to be representative of that of the pulmonary interstitial fluid, because when airway flooding occurs the alveolar capillary membrane loses its ability to alter the protein concentration of the fluid passing through it.[536,537] Based on these assumptions, many studies have used the protein concentration in lung lymph and in airway fluid as a way to assess the integrity of the pulmonary capillary endothelium.[365,368,370,538] Techniques for cannulating the pulmonary lymphatics have been described for the sheep, the dog, and the goat.[539–542] One of the important methodologic issues in these models is the degree to which this lymph collected in the mediastinum is contaminated by lymph originating in organs other than the lung.[543–546] Although this issue may not be completely resolved, it seems that the dog model is more likely to contain pure lung lymph than the preparation in the sheep.[540,547] The preparation in the dog cannulates an afferent lymphatic while that in the sheep cannulates an efferent lymphatic; more than one report has documented the degree to which lymph node transit results in altered protein concentration in the lymphatic fluid collected from efferent vessels.[548–554] Another methodologic problem in these experiments is the extent to which the lymphatic flow rate is altered by the cannulation procedure.[555] The height of the lymphatic cannula must maintain a constant relationship to the hilum of the lung in order to avoid erroneous estimations of the pulmonary microvascular permeability[556]; it has been suggested that the resistance of the extrapulmonary part of the lung lymphatic system limits the maximum flow of lymph from edematous lungs.[557] These mechanical or hydraulic factors which may introduce artifacts in lung lymph flow, as well as a prolonged time constant (which controls the equilibration between EVLW and lymph flow) may account for the fact that the measured EVLW does not always correlate with changes in lung lymphatic flow.[558–560] It is also probable that lung lymph flow in the smoke-damaged lung is influenced in an unpredictable or unknown way by hypoxic pulmonary vasoconstriction or the mechanical kinking of pulmonary vessels, both of which may be present as a consequence of the atelectasis known to occur almost instantly.[561–565]

The pulmonary reflection coefficient for total proteins (σ) is the index which indicates the permeability of the pulmonary capillary endothelium to proteins. Estimates concerning the integrity of this endothelial barrier can be made by comparing the protein concentration in the lung lymph (C_L) to the protein concentration in plasma (C_p). At the high lymph flow rates existing under conditions of increased pulmonary microvascular pressure,[365,566–568]

$$\sigma = 1 - \frac{C_L}{C_P}$$

An increase in protein concentration in lung lymph could result from either an increase in vascular surface area (recruitment of capillaries) or an increase in pulmonary capillary endothelial permeability (a decrease in σ). The factors of capillary recruitment and protein transfer by diffusion are eliminated as variables only when the microvascular pressure is raised so that lung lymph flow reaches maximal attainable levels.[365] Under these conditions, σ becomes inversely related to C_L/C_p; the validity of this relationship is less certain at low lung lymph flows.[514] Recent studies indicate that the C_L/C_p ratio may require up to 24 hours to reach its true *steady state,* which has adverse implications for experimental methods which require acute measurements.[567] Other variables include the operative manipulations required to establish a pulmonary lymphatic conduit to the outside.[569,570] The pulmonary vascular protein leak has been assessed noninvasively using a double radioisotope method.[571]

Chemical Determinations

The chemical measurements that can be referenced to acute smoke inhalation are unlimited. Some are appropriate as an index of lung injury (copper, angiotensin-converting enzyme), others because they provide indirect evidence for the metabolic capacity of the lung (angiotensin).[92,298,572–581] The technology used must make the proper adjustment for determinations done on blood, serum, and tissue. As in every purely chemical or endocrine assay, the measurements need to be referenced to the time of smoke exposure as well as to the physiologic state of the experimental animal. This may require additional controls. Tissue measurements need to be referenced to the edema-free tissue weight, usually given in terms of tissue protein content. In the unstable setting so typical of significant smoke inhalation, it is difficult to study endocrine function. Endocrine abnormalities may be the result of subnormal hormone production, hormonal excess, resistance to hormone action and abnormalities of hormone receptors, transport, and metabolism, all of which may be present concurrently to varying degrees. The effects of hormones are complex in that they do not always have the same effects in different tissues or in the same tissues under different circumstances: multiple hormones may interact (augmentation, potentiation) to modulate visceral function across a spectrum which is difficult to measure.[582,583] As our ability to measure hormones and assess physiologic function at the cellular level improves, changes resulting from hormonal antagonism or inhibition will become interpretable.[584] Chemical determinations can be made on extracts of minced lung tissue, or specific fluid reservoirs within the lung can be sampled using micropuncture techniques.[536,537]

MECHANISMS RESPONSIBLE FOR PATHOPHYSIOLOGY

It is beyond the scope of this chapter to delve deeply into the fundamental mechanisms responsible for the physiologic and pathologic changes observed following significant smoke exposure. Current concepts of these events are reviewed in Chaps. 4 and 6. As chemical methodology increases in sophistication and monoclonal antibodies become available, it will be possible to measure directly more of the individual components of the many chemical cascades which operate in a highly integrated fashion to define the tissue response to injury. It is important to exercise extreme caution in attributing a cause and effect relationship between a measurable physiologic perturbation and a measureable change in chemical concentration on little more than circumstantial evidence.[286,402,585] As the nature of these relationships are probed it will be useful to recognize that the time constant applicable to physiologic changes may be vastly different from that which applies to the changes in the concentrations of organic and inorganic chemicals, enzymes, hormones, the local products of cell-cell interaction, and the products of intracellular structures. As the focus of these studies becomes finer, it may be important to develop smoke inhalation models in smaller animals so that the system-effort and the cost of these experiments does not become prohibitive.

The pathologic process of inflammation which results from, modulates, or inactivates a host of chemical mediators is primarily an extravascular event. It is doubtful that the dominant pathologic mediator is likely to be found in blood, urine, or interstitial fluid (i.e., lymph) contaminated by interstitial fluid from tissue not involved in the pathologic process.[574] The ultimate objective in efforts to define the sequence of cellular events responsible for the initial pathologic event following smoke inhalation is to identify a focus at which an intervention might attenuate the tissue response. To be effective and/or clinically useful, such an intervention must operate specifically at the site of the mediator generation without disrupting homeostatic mechanisms at uninvolved tissue sites.[574] The fundamental response of the tissues in the lungs to toxic agents may be a direct one,[26,27] or it may be initiated or modulated by biologically active substances which contribute to the cellular response to injury.[92] Interventions intended to isolate the various components of the pulmonary response to smoke inhalation can be included in the appropriate models. Such interventions might include denervation or reimplantation of the lung prior to smoke exposure in an effort to isolate the contribution of neurogenic reflexes or mediators derived from neurologic tissue.[237,261,586] The role of individual cell types or cell products can be investigated by eliminating these cell types in experimental animals prior to smoke exposure.[374,587–592] The mechanisms and the response to smoke exposure can also be probed by attempts to use drugs to interfere with the chemical cascades believed to be involved. Such an approach introduces problems of drug dose, potency, and bioavailability, and of single or multiple sites of action, as well as the ability to measure directly the substrate and the product of the chemical reaction which is presumed to be modulated by the experimental intervention. It is important to be aware that the observed effects may occur not in response to a changing concentration of a single chemical, but in response to a change in the ratio of multiple chemical mediators. In this kind of experiment it is important to have adequate controls so that the effects of the chemical intervention on independent factors are accounted for.[42,402,593]

CONCLUSION

Smoke inhalation is a complex illness with a wide range of injury severity. Most of the mortality associated with it occurs before the victims enter the health care system. In this chapter, an effort has been made to identify, categorize, and critique some of the models used to study the effects of smoke on mammalian lungs. No model focusing only on the smoke-damaged larynx has been described. It is important to distinguish between the anoxic component of clinical smoke inhalation and the chemical lesion in the pulmonary parenchyma. These studies are difficult to do well, but they are worthwhile if for no other reason than that they hold the potential for defining the lung's response to inhaled toxins and identifying the pathophysiologic cascades which result. These studies lend themselves to a multidisciplinary effort. To be completely and properly done, as much "science" needs to be directed to the smoke side of the equation as we customarily direct to the animal side. Adequate controls are critical to the success of these experiments. When experiments produce apparently divergent results, it is highly probable that the investigators are not studying the same thing. In this situation, it is essential to review the experimental methodology closely to identify discrepancies in design (e.g., the absence of controls) or assumptions pertaining to the technical execution of the project.

REFERENCES

1. Clark WR, Bonaventura M, Myers W: Smoke inhalation and airway management at a regional burn unit: 1974–1983: I. Diagnosis and consequences of smoke inhalation. *J Burn Care Rehabil* 10:52, 1989.
2. Clark WR, Fromm BS: Burn mortality: Experience at a regional burn unit: Literature review. *Acta Chir Scand* [*Suppl*] 537:1, 1987.
3. Molteni A, Clark WR, Herndon DN, et al: Lung's response to thermal injury, in Dolecek R, Brizio-Moltini, L, Moltini A, et al (eds): *Endocrinology of Thermal Injury*. Philadelphia, Lea & Febiger (in press).
4. Achauer BM, Allyn PA, Furnas DW, Bartlett RH: Pulmonary complications of burns: The major threat to the burn patient. *Ann Surg* 177:311, 1973.
5. Taylor FW, Gumbert SL: Cause of death from burns: Role of respiratory damage. *Ann Surg* 161:497, 1965.
6. Pruitt BA, Erickson DR, Morris A: Progressive pulmonary insufficiency and other pulmonary complications of thermal injury. *J. Trauma* 15:369, 1975.
7. Shirani KZ, Pruitt BA, Mason AD: The influence of inhalation injury and pneumonia on burn mortality. *Ann Surg* 205:82, 1987.
8. Landa J, Avery WG, Sackner MA: Some physiologic observations in smoke inhalation. *Chest* 61:62, 1972.
9. Hampton TRW: Acute inhalation injury. *J R Nav Med Serv* 57:4, 1971.
10. Prashad J, Young RC, Laster HC, Hackney RL: Respiratory effects of a single, moderately acute, smoke inhalation episode. *J Nat Med Assoc* 71:251, 1979.
11. Coleman DL: Smoke inhalation—medical staff conference. *West J Med* 135:300, 1981.
12. Getzen LC, Pollak EW: Fatal respiratory distress in burned patients. *Surg Gynecol Obstet* 152:741, 1981.
13. Haponik EF, Summer WR: Respiratory complications in burn patients: Pathogenesis and spectrum of inhalation injury. *J Crit Care* 2:49, 1987.
14. Haponik EF, Summer WR: Respiratory complications in burn patients: Diagnosis and management of inhalation injury. *J Crit Care* 2:121, 1987.
15. Herndon DN, Thompson PB, Brown M, Traber DL: Diagnosis, pathophysiology, and treatment of inhalation injury, in Boswick JA: *The Art and Science of Burn Care*. Rockville, MD, Aspen Publishers, 1987, pp 153–161.
16. Zawacki BE, Jung RC, Joyce J, Rincon E: Smoke, burns and the natural history of inhalation injury in fire victims: A correlation of experimental and clinical data. *Ann Surg* 185:100, 1977.
17. Phillips AW, Tanner JW, Cope O: Burn therapy: IV. Respiratory tract damage (an account of the clinical, x-ray, and post mortem findings) and the meaning of restlessness. *Ann Surg* 158:799, 1963.
18. Feller I, Hendrix RC: Clinical pathologic study of sixty fatally burned patients. *Surg Gynecol Obstet* 119:1, 1964.
19. Brown JM: Inhalation injury and progressive pulmonary insufficiency in a British burn unit. *Burns* 4:32, 1977.
20. Moylan JA: Inhalation injury–A primary determinant of survival following major burns. *J Burn Care Rehabil* 2:78, 1981.
21. Thompson P, Herndon DN, Traber D: Effect on mortality of inhalation injury. *J Trauma* 26:163,1986.
22. Herndon DN, Curreri PW, Abston S, et al: Treatment of burns. *Curr Probl Surg* 24:343, 1987.
23. *Fire and Smoke: Understanding the Hazards*. Committee on Fire Toxicology, Board on Environmental Studies and

Toxicology, Commission on Life Sciences, National Research Council, Washington, DC, National Academy Press, 1986.
24. Birky MM: Philosophy of testing for assessment of toxicologic aspects of fire exposure. *J Comb Toxicol* 3:5, 1976.
25. Alarie Y: The toxicity of smoke from polymeric materials during thermal decomposition. *Am Rev Pharmacol Toxicol* 25:325, 1985.
26. Lowry WT, Juarez L, Petty CS, Roberts B: Studies of toxic gas production during actual structural fires in the Dallas area. *J Forensic Sci* 30:59, 1985.
27. Lowry WT, Peterson J, Petty CS, Badgett JL: Free radical production from controlled low-energy fires: Toxicity considerations. *J Forensic Sci* 30:73, 1985.
28. Clarke FB: Fire hazard assessment, in Cote AE (ed): *Fire Protection Handbook,* 16th ed. Quincy, Mass, National Fire Protection Handbook, 1986, pp 21-2–21-9.
29. Clark WR, Grossman ZD, Nieman GF, Ritter CA: Positive computed tomography of dog lungs following severe smoke inhalation: Diagnosis of inhalation injury. *J Burn Care Rehabil* 3:207, 1982.
30. American Industrial Hygeine Association: Community air quality guides—Aldehydes. *Am Ind Hyg Assoc J* 29:505, 1968.
31. Higgins ITT: Air pollution and lung cancer: Diesel exhaust, coal combustion. *Prev Med* 13:207, 1984.
32. Summer W, Haponik E: Inhalation of irritant gases. *Clin Chest Med* 2:273, 1981.
33. Schwartz DA: Acute inhalational injury. *State Art Rev Occup Med* 2:297, 1987.
34. Fein A, Grossman RF, Jones JG et al: Carbon monoxide effect on alveolar epithelial permeability. *Chest* 78:726, 1980.
35. Murphy SD: A review of effects on animals of exposure to auto exhaust and some of its components. *J Air Pollut Control Assoc* 14:303, 1964.
36. Pattle RE, Stretch H, Burgess F, et al: The toxicity of fumes from a diesel engine under four different running conditions. *Br J Ind Med* 14:47, 1957.
37. Horsfield K: Smoking and the lung, in Scadding JG, Cumming G, Thurlbeck WM (eds): *Scientific Foundation of Respiratory Medicine*. London, William Heinemann, 1981, pp 517–527.
38. Brownlee KA: A review of smoking and health. *J Am Stat Assoc* 60:722, 1965.
39. Dantenwill W, Chevalier JH, Harke HP, et al: Investigations on the effects of chronic cigarette-smoke inhalation in Syrian golden hamsters. *J Natl Cancer Inst* 51:1781, 1973.
40. Clemedson CJ: An experimental study on air blast injuries. *Acta Physiol Scand* 18 (suppl):61, 1949.
41. Catchpole HR, Gersh I: Pathogenetic factors and pathological consequences of decompression sickness. *Physiol Rev*. 27:360, 1947.
42. Wisner D, Sturm J, Sutter G, et al: Thromboxane receptor blockage in an animal model of ARDS. *Surgery* 104:91, 1988.
43. Fuertes M, Pollock TW, Holman MJ, et al: Changes in extravascular lung water and fatty acids in a hyperdynamic canine model of sepsis. *J Trauma* 28:1455, 1988.
44. Kazemi H, Albert LH, Kadowitz PJ (eds): *Acute Lung Injury: Pathogenesis of Adult Respiratory Distress Syndrome*. Littleton, Mass, PSG Publishing, 1986.
45. MacLeod JP: Adult respiratory distress syndrome, 1984. *Ann R Coll Phys Surg Canada* 17:561, 1984.
46. Demling RH, Nerlich M: Acute respiratory failure. *Surg Clin North Am* 63:337, 1983.
47. Petty TL: Adult respiratory distress syndrome: Definitions and historical perspective. *Clin Chest Med* 3:3, 1982.
48. Teplitz C: The core pathobiology and integrated medical science of adult acute respiratory insufficiency. *Surg Clin North Am* 56:1091, 1976.
49. Snyder JV, Carroll GC: Tissue oxygenation: A physiologic approach to a clinical problem. *Curr Probl Surg* 19:650, 1982.
50. Snyder JV, Carroll GC, Schuster DP, et al: Mechanical ventilation: Physiology and application. *Curr Probl Surg* 21:2, 1984.
51. Martz KV, Joiner JW, Shepherd RM: *Management of the Patient–Ventilator System—A Team Approach,* 2d ed. St Louis, Mosby, 1984, pp 96–105.
52. Chatburn RL, Lough MD: Mechanical ventilation, in Lough MD, Doershuk CF, Stern RC (eds): *Pediatric Respiratory Therapy,* 3d ed. Chicago, Yearbook Medical Publishers, 1985, pp 148–191.
53. Craig KC, Pierson DJ, Carrico CJ: The clinical application of positive end-expiratory pressure (PEEP) in the adult respiratory distress syndrome (ARDS). *Respir Care* 30:184, 1985.
54. Chatburn RL: Similarities and differences in the management of acute lung injury in neonates (IRDS) and in adults (ARDS). *Respir Care* 33:539, 1988.
55. McFadden ER, Denison DM, Waller JF, et al: Direct recordings of the temperatures in the tracheobronchial tree in normal man. *J Clin Invest* 69:700, 1982.
56. Clark FB, Ottoson J: Fire death scenarios and fire safety planning. *Fire J* 70:20, 1976.
57. Birky MM, Halpin BM, Caplin YH: Fire fatality study. *Fire Materials* 3:211, 1979.
58. Birky MM, Clark FB: Inhalation of toxic products from fires. *Bull NY Acad Med* 57:997, 1981.
59. Mierly MC, Baker SP: Fatal house fires in an urban population. *JAMA* 249:1466, 1983.
60. Karter MS: Patterns of fire deaths among the elderly and children in the home. *Fire J* 80:19, 1986.
61. Levine MS, Radford EP: Fire victims: Medical outcomes and demographic characteristics. *Am J Public Health* 67:1077, 1977.
62. Anderson RA, Thomson J, Harland WA: The importance of cyanide and organic materials in fire fatalities. *Fire Materials* 3:91, 1979.
63. Anderson RA, Watson HA, Harland WA: Fire deaths in the Glasgow area: I. General considerations and pathology. *Med Sci Law* 21:175, 1981.
64. Anderson RA, Watson HA, Harland WA: Fire deaths in the Glasgow area: II. The role of carbon monoxide. *Med*

Sci Law 21:288, 1981.

65. Anderson RA, Harland WA: Fire deaths in the Glasgow area: III. The role of hydrogen cyanide. *Med Sci Law* 22:35, 1983.
66. Birky M, Malek D, Paabo M: Study of biological samples obtained from victims of MGM Grand Hotel fire. *J Anal Toxicol* 7:265, 1983.
67. Clark CJ, Campbell D, Reid WH: Blood carboxyhaemoglobin and cyanide levels in fire survivors. *Lancet* 1:1332, 1981.
68. Clark GH: Measurement of toxic combustion products in fire survivors. *J R Soc Med* 75 (suppl 1):40, 1982.
69. Symington IS, Anderson RA, Thomson I, et al: Cyanide exposure in fires. *Lancet* 2:91, 1978.
70. Bowes PC: Casualities attributed to toxic gas and smoke at fires: A survey of statistics. *Med Sci Law* 16:104, 1976.
71. Davies JWL: Toxic chemicals versus lung tissue: An aspect of inhalation injury revisited. *J Burn Care Rehabil* 7:213, 1986.
72. Barillo DJ, Rush BF, Goode R, et al: Is ethanol the unknown toxin in smoke inhalation injury? *Am Surg* 52:641, 1986.
73. Webster JR, McCabe MM, Karp M: Recognition and management of smoke inhalation. *JAMA* 201:71, 1967.
74. McArdle CS, Finlay WEI: Pulmonary complications following smoke inhalation. *Br J Anaesth* 47:618, 1975.
75. Stone HH, Rhame DW, Corbitt JD, et al: Respiratory burns: A correlation of clinical and laboratory results. *Ann Surg* 165:157, 1967.
76. Zikria BA, Weston GC, Chodoff M, Ferrer JM: Smoke and carbon monoxide poisoning in fire victims. *J Trauma* 12:641, 1972.
77. Zikria BA, Sturner WQ, Astarjian NK, et al: Respiratory tract damage in burns: Pathophysiology and therapy. *Ann NY Acad Sci* 150:618, 1968.
78. Zikria BA, Budd DC, Floch F, Ferrer JM: What is clinical smoke poisoning. *Ann Surg* 181:151, 1975.
79. Scheulen SJ, Munster AM: The Parkland formula in patients with burns and inhalation injury. *J Trauma* 22:869, 1982.
80. Navar PP, Saffle JR, Warden GD: Effect of inhalation injury on fluid resuscitation requirements after thermal injury. *Am J Surg* 150:716, 1985.
81. Clark WR, Bonaventura M, Myers W, Kellman R: Smoke inhalation and airway management at a regional burn unit, 1974–1985: II. Airway management. *J Burn Care Rehabil*, in press.
82. Haponik EF, Meyers DA, Munster AM: Acute upper airway injury in burn patients: Correlation of flow-volume curves and nasopharyngoscopy. *Am Rev Respir Dis* 129:251, 1984.
83. Haponik FF, Meyers DA, Munster AM, et al: Acute upper airway injury in burn patients: Serial changes of flow-volume curves and nasopharyngoscopy. *Am Rev Respir Dis* 135:360, 1987.
84. Emmons HW: The growth of fire science. *Fire Safety J* 3:95, 1981.
85. Emmons HW: Fire and fire prevention. *Sci Am* 231:21, 1974.
86. Grant CE, Pagni PJ (eds): *Fire Safety Science: Proceedings of the First International Symposium*. Washington, 1986, Hemisphere Publishing Corporation (Berlin, Springer-Verlag).
87. Cote, AE (ed): *Fire Protection Handbook*, 16th ed. Quincy, Mass, National Fire Protection Association, 1986.
88. Alarie Y, Anderson RC, Stock MF, et al: Toxicity of thermal decomposition products: An attempt to correlate results obtained in small scale with large scale tests. *J Comb Toxicol* 8:58, 1981.
89. Witschi HP, Brain JD (eds): *Toxicology of Inhaled Materials: General Principles of Inhalation Toxicology (Handbook of Experimental Pharmacology*, vol 75). Berlin, Springer-Verlag, 1985, pp 1–553.
90. Skornik WA: Inhalation toxicity of metal particles and vapors, in Loke J (ed): *Pathophysiology and Treatment of Inhalation Injuries*. New York, Marcel Dekker, 1988, pp 123–186.
91. Loke J, Mathay RA, Walker-Smith GJ: The toxic environment and its medical implications with special emphasis on smoke inhalation, in Loke J (ed): *Pathophysiology and Treatment of Inhalation Injuries*. New York, Marcel Dekker, 1988, pp 453–504.
92. Said SI: Environmental injury of the lung: Role of humoral mediators. *Fed Proc* 37:2504, 1978.
93. Woolley WD, Ames SA, Fardell PJ: Chemical aspects of combustion toxicology of fires. *Fire Materials* 3:110, 1979.
94. Kaplan HL, Hartzel GE: Modeling of toxicological effects of fire gases: I. Incapacitating effects of narcotic fire gases. *J Fire Sci* 2:286, 1984.
95. MacFarland HN: The pyrolysis products of plastics: Problems in defining their toxicity. *Am Ind Hyg Assoc J* 29:7, 1968.
96. Tsuchiya Y, Sumi K: Evaluation of the toxicity of combustion products. *J Fire Flam* 3:46, 1972.
97. Saito F: Evaluation of the toxicity of combustion products. *J Comb Toxicol* 4:32, 1977.
98. Clayton JW: The toxicity of fluorocarbons with special reference to chemical constituents. *J Occup Med* 4:262, 1962.
99. Webster SH: Volatile hydrides of toxicological importance. *J Ind Hyg* 28:167, 1946.
100. Moritz AR, Henriques FC, McLean R: The effects of inhaled heat on the air passages and lungs. *Am J Pathol* 21:311, 1945.
101. Friedman R: The role of chemistry in fire problems: Gas-phase combustion kinetics. *Fire Res Abstr Rev* 13:187, 1971.
102. Woolley WD, Smith PG, Fardell PJ, et al: The Stardust Disco fire, Dublin 1981: Studies of combustion products during simulation experiments. *Fire Safety J* 7:267, 1984.
103. Terrill JB, Montgomery RR, Reinhardt CF: Toxic gases from fires. *Science* 200:1343, 1978.
104. Treitman RD, Burjess WA, Gold A: Air contaminants encountered by firefighters. *Am Ind Hyg Assoc J* 41:796, 1980.
105. Levine MS, Radford EP: Occupational exposure to cya-

nide in Baltimore fire fighters. *J Occup Med* 20:53, 1978.

106. Radford EP, Levine MS: Occupational exposure to carbon monoxide in Baltimore fire fighters. *J Occup Med* 18:628, 1976.
107. Genovesi MG, Tashkin DP, Chopra S, et al: Transient hypoxemia in firemen following inhalation of smoke. *Chest* 71:441, 1977.
108. Gold A, Burgess WA, Clougherty EV: Exposure of firefighters to toxic air contaminants. *Am Ind Hyg Assoc* 39:534, 1978.
109. Sidor R, Peterson NH, Burgess WA: A carbon monoxide–oxygen sample for evaluation of fire fighter exposures. *Am Ind Hyg Assoc* 34:264, 1973.
110. Burgess WA, Sidor R, Lynch JJ, et al: Minimum protection factors for respiratory protection devices for firefighters. *Am Ind Hyg Assoc* 38:18, 1977.
111. Sharar SR, Heimbach DM, Howard M, et al: Cardiopulmonary responses after spontaneous inhalation of Douglas fir smoke in goats. *J Trauma* 28:164, 1988.
112. Thomas WC, O'Flaherty EJ: A system for exposing animals to smoke generated in a steady state fashion. *Environ Res* 23:326, 1980.
113. Bell JS, Klein TJ, Willey HE: Twelve die in fire at Westchase Hilton Hotel, Houston, Texas. *Fire J* 77:11, 1982.
114. Buerk CA, Batdorf JW, Cammack KV, Ravenholt O: The MGM Grand Hotel Fire: Lessons learned from a major disaster. *Arch Surg* 117:641, 1982.
115. Baum HR, Rehm RG, Mulholland GW: Prediction of heat and smoke movement in enclosure fires. *Fire Safety J* 6:193, 1983.
116. Benjamin I: The challenge of smoke. *Fire Safety J* 7:3, 1984.
117. Webb WA: Case studies in building smoke control. *Fire Safety J* 7:117, 1984.
118. Schmidt W: Stairwell and elevator shaft pressurization. *Fire Safety J* 7:115, 1984.
119. Peters DCJ: HVAC systems for the fire protection engineer. *Fire Safety J* 7:65, 1984.
120. Miller GR: Building codes and smoke control. *Fire Safety J* 7:99, 1984.
121. Marchant EW: Effect of wind on smoke movement and smoke control systems. *Fire Safety J* 7:55, 1984.
122. Klote JH: The ASHRAE design manual for smoke control. *Fire Safety J* 7:93, 1984.
123. Henkestad G: Engineering relations for fire plumes. *Fire Safety J* 7:25, 1984.
124. Fothergill JW: Smoke movement within a building. *Fire Safety J* 7:47, 1984.
125. Cooper LY: Smoke movement in rooms of fire involvement and adjacent spaces. *Fire Safety J* 7:33, 1984.
126. Blazek W: Smoke movement in office buildings. *Fire Safety J* 7:107, 1984.
127. Klote JH: *Overview of Smoke Control Technology*. Gaithersburg, Md, National Bureau of Standards, NBSIR 82-3626, September 1987. (Available from National Technical Information Services, PB88-1105772.)
128. Klitgaard PS, Williamson RB: The impact of contents on building fires. *Fire Flam* 2:84, 1975.
129. Herpol C, Vandevelde P: Use of toxicity test results and confrontation of some toxicity test methods with fire scenarios. *Fire Safety J* 4:271, 1981.
130. Barrow CS, Lucia H, Stock MF, Alarie Y: Development of methodologies to assess the relative hazards from thermal decomposition products of polymeric materials. *Am Ind Hyg Assoc* 40:408, 1979.
131. Kimmerle MG: Aspects and methodology for the evaluation of toxicological parameters during fire exposure. *J Comb Toxicol* 1:4, 1974.
132. Alarie Y, Schaper M: Pulmonary performance in laboratory animals exposed to toxic agents and correlations with lung disease in humans, in Loke J (ed): *Pathophysiology and Treatment of Inhalation Injuries*. New York, Marcel Dekker, 1988, pp 67–122.
133. *Fire Toxicology: Methods for Evaluation of Toxicity of Pyrolysis and Combustion Products*. Report no. 2, Washington, DC, National Academy of Science, 1977.
134. Loke J, Paul E, Virgulto J: Smoke exposure chamber and bronchoalveolar lavage as a method for the evaluation of toxicity of pyrolysis and combustion products in laboratory animals. *J Comb Toxicol* 8:37, 1981.
135. Laboratory Methods for Evaluation of Toxic Potency of Smoke, in *Fire and Smoke: Understanding the Hazard*. Committee on Fire Toxicology, Board on Environmental Studies and Toxicology, Commission on Life Sciences, National Research Council, Washington, DC, National Academy Press, 1986, pp 78–104.
136. Hilado CJ: The practical use of the USF toxicity screening test method. *J Comb Toxicol* 5:331, 1978.
137. Dilley JV, Martin SB, McKee R, Pryor G: A smoke toxicity methodology. *J Comb Toxicol* 6:20, 1979.
138. Battista SP, Guerin MR, Gori GB, Kunsler CJ: A new system for quantitatively exposing laboratory animals by direct inhalation: Delivery of cigarette smoke. *Arch Environ Health* 27:376, 1973.
139. Hinners RG, Burkart JK, Punte CL: Animal inhalation exposure chambers. *Arch Environ Health* 16:194, 1968.
140. Wong KL, Alarie Y: A method for repeated evaluation of pulmonary performance in unanesthetized, unrestrained guinea pigs and its application to detect effects of sulfuric acid mist inhalation. *Toxicol Appl Pharmacol* 63:72, 1982.
141. Matijak-Schaper M, Wong H, Alarie Y: A method to rapidly evaluate the acute pulmonary effects of aerosols in unanesthetized guinea pigs. *Toxicol Appl Pharmacol* 69:451, 1983.
142. Fultyn RV: Contaminant generators for continuous exposure inhalation chambers. *Am Indust Hyg Assoc* 22:49, 1961.
143. Levin BC, Babranskas V, Brown E, et al: An exploration of combustion limitations and alternatives to NBS toxicity test method. NBSIR 85-3274, Gaithersburg, Md, U. S. Department of Commerce, National Engineering Laboratory, Center for Fire Research, 1985.
144. Levin BC, Fowell AJ, Birky MM, et al: Further development of a test method for the assessment of the acute inhalation toxicity of combustion products. NBSIR 82-2532, Gaithersburg, Md, Washington, DC, U. S. Department of Commerce, National Bureau of Standards, Center for Fire Research, pp 1–132.

145. Morrow PE: Experimental studies of inhaled materials: A basis for respiratory models. *Arch Intern Med* 126:466, 1970.
146. National Research Council, Committee on Fire Research: *Physiologic and Toxicological Aspects of Combustion Products,* International symposium held at the University of Utah, March 18–20, 1974, Washington, DC, National Academy of Sciences, 1976, pp 1–244.
147. Gaume JG, Bartek P: Theoretical determination of the time of useful function (TUF) on exposure to combinations of toxic gases. *Aerospace Med* 40:1353, 1969.
148. Hilado CJ: Screening materials for toxicity of pyrolysis gases. *J Comb Toxicol* 6:248, 1979.
149. Kimmerle G, Prager FK: The relative toxicity of pyrolysis products. Part 1: Plastics and man-made fibers. *J Comb Toxicol* 7:42, 1980.
150. Boettner EA, Ball G, Weiss B: Analysis of the volatile combustion products of vinyl plastics. *J Appl Polym Sci* 13:377, 1969.
151. O'Mara MM: The combustion products from synthetic and natural products. Part 1: Wood. *J Fire Flam* 5:34, 1974.
152. Higgins EA, Fiorca V, Thomas AA, Davis HV: Acute toxicity of brief exposures to hydrogen fluoride, hydrogen chloride, nitrogen dioxide and hydrogen cyanide with and without carbon monoxide. *Fire Tech* 8:120, 1972.
153. Napier DH, Wong TW: Toxic products from the combustion and pyrolysis of polyurethane foams. *Br Polym J* 4:45, 1972.
154. Napier DH: Hazardous materials and the gases they produce. *Med Sci Law* 17:83, 1977.
155. Wagner JP: Survey of toxic species evolved in the pyrolysis and combustion of polymers. *Fire Res Abst Rev* 14:1, 1972.
156. Alarie Y, Anderson RC: Toxicologic classification of thermal decomposition products of synthetic and natural polymers. *Toxicol Appl Pharmacol* 57:181, 1981.
157. Alarie Y, Stock MF, Matijak-Schaper M: Toxicity of smoke during chair smoldering tests and small scale tests using the same materials. *Fund Appl Toxicol* 3:619, 1983.
158. Purser DA, Buckley P: Lung irritance and inflammation during and after exposure to thermal decomposition products from polymeric materials. *Med Sci Law* 23:142, 1983.
159. Purser DA, Woolley WD: Biological studies of combustion atmospheres. *J Fire Sci* 1:118, 1983.
160. Hartzell GE, Priest DN, Switzer WG: Modeling of toxicological effects of fire gases: II. Mathematical modeling of intoxication of rats by carbon monoxide and hydrogen cyanide. *J Fire Sci* 3:115, 1985.
161. Hartzell GE, Stacy HW, Switzer WG, et al: Modeling of toxicological effects of fire gases: IV. Intoxication of rats by carbon monoxide in the presence of an irritant. *J Fire Sci* 3:263, 1985.
162. Hartzel GE, Switzer WG, Priest DN: Modeling of toxicologic effect of fire gases: V. Mathematical modeling of intoxication of rats by combined carbon monoxide and hydrogen cyanide atmospheres. *J Fire Sci* 3:330, 1985.
163. Winter PM, Miller JN: Carbon monoxide poisoning. *JAMA* 286:1502, 1976.
164. Purser DA, Berrill KR: Effects of carbon monoxide on behavior in monkeys in relation to human fire hazard. *Arch Environ Health* 38:308, 1983.
165. Stewart RD: The effect of carbon monoxide on humans. *Ann Rev Pharmacol* 15:409, 1975.
166. Brody JS, Coburn RF: Carbon monoxide induced arterial hypoxemia. *Science* 164:1297, 1969.
167. Halebian P, Robinson N, Barie P, et al: Whole body oxygen utilization during acute carbon monoxide poisoning and isocapneic nitrogen hypoxia. *J Trauma* 26:110, 1986.
168. Root WS: Carbon monoxide, in Fenn WO, Rahn H (eds): *Handbook of Physiology,* sect. 3, *Respiration,* vol. 1, Washington, DC American Physiological Society, 1965, pp 1087–1098.
169. Ginsberg MD, Myers RE: Experimental carbon monoxide encephalopathy in the primate. *Arch Neurol* 30:202, 1974.
170. Stewart RD, Peterson JE, Fisher TN, et al: Experimental human exposure to high concentrations of carbon monoxide. *Arch Environ Health* 26:1, 1973.
171. Stewart RD, Peterson JE, Baretta ED, et al: Experimental human exposure to carbon monoxide. *Arch Environ Health* 21:154, 1970.
172. Stewart RD: The effect of carbon monoxide on man. *J Comb Toxicol* 1:167, 1974.
173. Zarem HA, Rottenborg CC, Harmel MH: Carbon monoxide toxicity in fire victims. *Arch Surg* 107:851, 1973.
174. Yamamoto K: Acute combined effects of HCN and CO, with special reference to a theoretical consideration of acute combined effects on the basis of the blood cyanide and COHb analyses. *J Comb Toxicol* 4:69, 1977.
175. Pitt BR, Radford EP, Gurtner GH, Traystman RJ: Interaction of carbon monoxide and cyanide on cerebral circulation and metabolism. *Arch Environ Health* 34:354, 1979.
176. Purser DA, Grimshaw P, Berrill KR: Intoxication by cyanide in fires: A study in monkeys using polyacrylanitrile. *Arch Environ Health* 39:394, 1984.
177. Silverman SH, Purdue GF, Hunt JL, Bost RO: Cyanide toxicity in burned patients. *J Trauma* 28:171, 1988.
178. Vogel SN, Sultan TR, Ten Eyck RP: Cyanide poisoning. *Clin Toxicol* 18:367, 1981.
179. Jones J, McMullen J, Dougherty J: Toxic smoke inhalation: Cyanide poisoning in fire victims. *Am J Emerg Med* 5:317, 1987.
180. Hall AH, Rumack BH: Clinical toxicology of cyanide. *Am J Emerg Med* 15:1067, 1986.
181. Petajan JH, Voorhees KJ, Packham SC, et al: Extreme toxicity from combustion products of a fire-retarded polyurethane foam. *Science* 187:742, 1975.
182. Waritz RS: An industrial approach to evaluation of pyrolysis and combustion hazards. *Environ Health Perspect* 11:197, 1975.
183. Bowes PC: Smoke and toxicity hazards of plastics in fire. *Am Occup Hyg* 17:143, 1974.
184. Alarie YC, Anderson RC: Toxicologic and acute lethal hazard evaluation of thermal decomposition products of synthetic and natural polymers. *Toxicol Appl Pharmacol* 51:341, 1979.
185. Wong KL, Stack MF, Malek DE, Alarie Y: Evaluation of

the pulmonary effects of wood smoke in guinea pigs by repeated CO_2 challenges. *Toxicol Appl Pharmacol* 75:69, 1984.

186. Cornish HH, Abar EL: Toxicity of pyrolysis products of vinyl plastics. *Arch Environ Health* 19:15, 1969.
187. MacFarland HN, Leong KJ: Hazards from the thermodecomposition of plastics: Polyurethane and polyurethane-coated nylon. *Arch Environ Health* 4:39, 1962.
188. Woolley WD: Decomposition products of PVC for studies of fires. *Br Polym J* 3:186, 1971.
189. Kallanen R, vonWright A, Tikkanen L, Kaustia K: The toxicity of fire effluents from textiles and upholstery materials. *J Fire Sci* 3:145, 1985.
190. Barrow CS, Lucia, Alarie YC: A comparison of the acute inhalation toxicity of hydrogen chloride versus the thermal decomposition products of polyvinylchloride. *J Comb Toxicol* 6:3, 1979.
191. Morikawa T: Acrolein, formaldehyde and volatile fatty acids from smoldering combustion. *J Comb Toxicol* 3:135, 1976.
192. Alarie Y: Sensory irritation of the upper airways by airborne chemicals. *Toxicol Appl Pharmacol* 24:287, 1973.
193. Alarie Y: Sensory irritation by airborne chemicals. *CRC Crit Rev Toxicol* 2:299, 1973.
194. Alarie Y, Lin CK, Gecery DL: Sensory irritation evoked by plastic decomposition products. *Am Ind Hyg Assoc J* 35:654, 1974.
195. Tenney SM: Ventilatory response to carbon dioxide in pulmonary emphysema. *J Appl Physiol* 6:477, 1954.
196. Schaffer KE: Respiratory pattern and respiratory response to CO_2. *J Appl Physiol* 13:1, 1958.
197. Reynolds WJ, Milhorn HT, Holloman GH: Transient ventilatory response to graded hypercapnia in man. *J Appl Physiol* 33:47, 1972.
198. Weissman C, Abraham B, Askanazi J, et al: Effect of posture on the ventilatory response to CO_2. *J Appl Physiol* 53:761, 1982.
199. Schaper M, Thompson RD, Alarie Y: A method to classify airborne chemicals which alter the normal ventilatory response induced by CO_2. *Toxicol Appl Pharmacol* 79:332, 1985.
200. Walker BR, Adams EM, Voelkel NF: Ventilatory responses of hamsters and rats to hypoxia and hypercapnia. *J Appl Physiol* 59:1955, 1985.
201. Clark DG, Buch S, Doe JE, et al: Broncho-pulmonary function: Report on the main working party. *Pharmacol Ther* 5:149, 1979.
202. Widdicombe J: Defensive mechanisms of the upper airways, in Bonsignore G, Cumming G (eds): *The Lung in its Environment*. New York, Plenum, 1982, pp 121–134.
203. Sant'Ambrogio G: Afferent activity and reflex effects evoked from the tracheo-bronchial tree, in Bonsignore G, Cumming G (eds): *The Lung in its Environment*. New York, Plenum, 1982, pp 135–157.
204. Stone SP, Hazlett RN, Johnson JE, Carhart MW: The transport of hydrogen chloride by soot from burning polyvinyl chloride. *J Fire Flam* 4:42, 1973.
205. Boren HG: Carbon as a carrier mechanism for irritant gases. *Arch Environ Health* 8:119, 1964.
206. Hales CA, Barkin PW, Jung W, et al: Synthetic smoke with acrolein but not HCl produces pulmonary edema. *J Appl Physiol* 64:1121, 1988.
207. Boren HG: Pulmonary response to inhaled carbon: A model of lung injury. *Yale J Biol Med* 40:364, 1968.
208. Amder MO: The effect of aerosols on the response to irritant gases, in Davies CN (ed): *Inhaled Particles and Vapours*. New York, Pergamon, 1961, pp 281–292.
209. Pattle RE, Wedd GD, Burgess F: The acute toxic effects of black smoke. *Br J Ind Med* 16:216, 1959.
210. Fleck L, Edery H: The influence of narcosis on the distribution of inhaled bacteria in the respiratory tract, in Davies CN (ed): *Inhaled Particles and Vapours*. New York, Pergamon, 1961, pp 139–141.
211. Calcote HF: Ionic mechanisms in soot formation, in Lahaze J, Prado G (eds): *Soot in Combustion Systems and its Toxic Properties*. Plenum, 1983.
212. Goetz A: The physics of aerosols in the submicron range, in Davies CM (ed): *Inhaled Particles and Vapours*. New York, Pergamon, 1961, pp 295–301.
213. Santoro RJ, Semerjian HG, Dobbins RA: Soot particle measurements in diffusion flames. *Comb Flame* 51:203, 1983.
214. Bankstan CP, Powell EA, Cassanova RA, Zinn BT: Detailed measurements of the physical characteristics of smoke particulates generated by flaming materials. *J Fire Flam* 8:395, 1977.
215. Jagoda IJ, Prado G, Lahaye J: An experimental investigation into soot formation and distribution in polymer diffusion flames. *Comb Flame* 37:261, 1980.
216. Zinn BT, Powell EA, Casanova RA, Bankston CP: Investigation of smoke particulates generated during the thermal degradation of natural and synthetic materials. *Fire Res* 1:23, 1977.
217. Hatch TF, Gross P: *Pulmonary Deposition and Retention of Inhaled Aerosols*. New York, Academic, 1964, pp 1–189.
218. Oberst FW: Factors affecting inhalation and retention of toxic vapours, in Davies CM (ed): *Inhaled Particles and Vapours*. New York, Pergamon, 1961, pp 249–266.
219. Cuddihy RG, Brownstein DG, Raabe OG, Kanapilly GM: Respiratory tract deposition of inhaled polydisperse aerosols in beagle dogs. *Aerosol Sci* 4:35, 1973.
220. Gerrity TR, Lee PS, Hass FJ, et al: Calculated deposition of inhaled particles in the airway generations of normal subjects. *J Appl Physiol* 47:867, 1979.
221. Chan TL, Lippman M: Experimental measurements and empirical modeling of the regional deposition of inhaled particles in humans. *Am Ind Hyg Assoc J* 41:399, 1980.
222. Stahlhoffen W, Gebhart J, Heyder J: Experimental determinations of the regional deposition of aerosol particles in the human respiratory tract. *Am Ind Hyg Assoc* 41:385, 1980.
223. Valberg PA, Brain JD, Sneddon SL, et al: Breathing patterns influence aerosol deposition sites in excised dog lung. *J Appl Physiol* 52:824, 1982.
224. Natusch DFS, Wallace JR: Urban aerosol toxicity: The influence of particle size. *Science* 186:695, 1974.
225. Davies CN: A formalized anatomy of the human respiratory tract, in Davies CN (ed): *Inhaled Particles and Vapours*. New York, Pergamon, 1961, pp 82–91.

226. Schroter RC, Sudlow MF: Flow patterns in models of the human bronchial airways. *Respir Physiol* 7:341, 1969.
227. Muir DCF, Davies CN: The deposition of 0.5 μ diameter aerosols in the lungs of man. *Ann Occup Hyg* 10:161, 1967.
228. Task Group on Lung Dynamics: Deposition and retention models for internal dosimetry of the human respiratory tract. *Health Phys* 12:173, 1966.
229. Brain JD, Valberg PA: Models of lung retention based on ICRP task group report. *Arch Environ Health* 28:1, 1974.
230. Johnston SR, Schroter RC: Deposition of particles in model airways. *J Appl Physiol* 47:947, 1979.
231. Parkes WR: Inhaled particles and their fate in the lungs, in Parkes WR (ed): *Occupational Lung Disorders*. London, Butterworth, 1982, pp 45–53.
232. Prodi V, Melandri C, Tarroni G: Airborne particles and their intrapulmonary deposition, in Scadding JG, Cumming F, Thurlbeck WM (eds): *Scientific Foundation of Respiratory Medicine*. London, William Heinemann, 1981, pp 545–558.
233. Ecanow B, Balagot RC, Bandelin V: Effect of suspended particles on the gas-absorbing ability of lung surfactants. *Am Rev Respir Dis* 99:106, 1969.
234. Rosenberg E, Alarie Y, Robillard E: Effect of dust and aerosol inhalation on surface and tissue elasticity of rat lungs. *Can J Biochem Physiol* 40:1359, 1962.
235. Rylander R, Bergstrom R: Particles and SO_2: Synergistic effects for pulmonary damage. Proceedings of the Third International Clean Air Congress, Dusseldorf, A23-A25, 1973.
236. Stone JP: Transport of hydrogen chloride by water aerosol in simulated fires. *Comb Toxicol* 2:127, 1975.
237. Clark WR, unpublished information.
238. Nieman GF, Clark WR, Wax SD, Webb WR: The effect of smoke inhalation on pulmonary surfactant. *Ann Surg* 191:171, 1980.
239. Lee KP, Zapp JA, Sarver JW: Ultrastructural alterations of rat lung exposed to pyrolysis products of polytetrafluoroethylene (PTFE, Teflon). *Lab Invest* 35:152, 1976.
240. Minty BD, Royston D: Cigarette smoke induced changes in rat pulmonary clearance of ^{99m}TC DTPA: A comparison of particulate and gas phases. *Am Rev Resp Dis* 132:1170, 1985.
241. Warity RS, Kwon BK: The inhalation toxicity of pyrolysis products of polytetrafluoroethylene heated below 500 degrees centigrade. *Am Ind Hyg Assoc* 29:19, 1968.
242. Battista SP, Steber WD, Kensler CJ: Pulmonary function in spontaneously breathing dogs with lower airway catheters: During and after cigarette smoke exposure. *Arch Environ Health* 28:164, 1974.
243. Forbes, WH, Sargent F, Roughton FJW: The rate of carbon monoxide uptake by normal men. *Am J Physiol* 143:594, 1945.
244. Stadic WC, Martin KA: The elimination of carbon monoxide from the blood: A theoretical and experimental study. *J Clin Invest* 2:77, 1925.
245. Pace N, Strajman E, Walker E: Influence of age on carbon monoxide desaturation in man. *Fed Proc* 7:89, 1948.
246. Pace N, Strajman E, Walker E: Acceleration of carbon monoxide elimination in man by high pressure oxygen. *Science* 111:652, 1950.
247. Larkin JM, Brahos GJ, Moylan JA: Treatment of carbon monoxide poisoning: Prognostic factors. *J Trauma* 16:111, 1976.
248. Boutros AR, Hoyt JL: Management of carbon monoxide poisoning in the absence of hyperbaric oxygenation chamber. *Crit Care Med* 4:144, 1976.
249. Myers RAM, Snyder SK, Linberg S, Cowley A: Value of hyperbaric oxygen in suspected carbon monoxide poisioning. *JAMA* 246:2478, 1981.
250. Grube BJ, Marvin JA, Heimbach DM: Therapeutic hyperbaric oxygen: Help or hindrance in burn patients with carbon monoxide poisoning. *J Burn Care Rehabil* 9:249, 1988.
251. Hall AH, Rumack BH: Clinical toxicology of cyanide. *Ann Emerg Med* 15:1067, 1986.
252. Way JL, Gibbon SL, Sheeky M: Effect of oxygen on cyanide intoxication: I. Prophylactic protection. *J Pharmacol Exp Ther* 153:381, 1966.
253. Way JL, End E, Sheeky M, et al: Effect of oxygen on cyanide intoxication: IV. Hyperbaric oxygen. *Toxicol Appl Pharmacol* 22:415, 1972.
254. Burrows GE, Klu DHW, Way JL: Effect of oxygen on cyanide intoxication: V. Physiologic effects. *J Pharmacol Exp Ther* 184:739, 1973.
255. Ivankovich AD, Bravarman B, Kanurur RP, et al: Cyanide antidotes and methods of their administration in dogs: A comparative study. *Anesthesiology* 52:210, 1980.
256. Moore SJ, Norris JC, Ho IK, Hume AS: The efficacy of α-ketoglutaric acid in the antagonism of cyanide intoxication. *Toxicol Appl Pharmacol* 82:1, 1986.
257. Parving HH: The effect of hypoxia and carbon monoxide exposure on plasma volume and capillary permeability to albumin. *Scand J Clin Lab Invest* 30:49, 1972.
258. Siggaard-Anderson J, Peterson FB, Hansen TI, Mellemgaard K: Plasma volume and vascular permeability during hypoxia and carbon monoxide exposure. *Scand J Clin Lab Invest [Suppl]* 103:39, 1968.
259. Astrup P, Kjeldsen K, Wanstrup J: Effects of carbon monoxide exposure on the arterial walls. *Ann NY Acad Sci* 174:294, 1970.
260. Fisher WB, Hyde RW, Baue AE, et al: Effect of carbon monoxide on function and structure of the lung. *J Appl Physiol* 26:4, 1969.
261. Clark WR, Nieman GF: Smoke inhalation. *Burns* 14:473, 1988.
262. Bartlett RH, Niccole M, Travis MJ, et al: Acute management of the upper airway in facial burns and smoke inhalation. *Arch Surg* 111:744, 1976.
263. Bartlett RH, Allyn PA: Pulmonary management of the burned patient. *Heart Lung* 2:714, 1973.
264. Hunt JL, Purdue GF, Gumming T: Is tracheostomy warranted in the burn patient? Indications and complications. *J Burn Care Rehabil* 7:492, 1986.
265. Demling RH: Improved survival after massive burns. *J Trauma* 23:179, 1983.
266. Venus B, Matsuda T, Capiozo JB, Mathru M: Prophylactic intubation and continuous positive airway pressure in the management of inhalation injury in burn victims. *Crit Care Med* 9:519, 1981.

267. Demling RH, Will JA, Belzer FO: Effect of major thermal injury on the pulmonary microcirculation. *Surgery* 83:746, 1978.
268. Demling RH, Niehaus G, Perea A, Will JA: Effect of burn-induced hypoproteinemia on pulmonary transvascular fluid filtration rate. *Surgery* 85:339, 1979.
269. Demling RH, Manahar M, Will JA: Relation between pulmonary transvascular fluid filtration rate and measured Starling's forces after major burn. *Chest* 76:448, 1979.
270. Demling RH, Smith M, Bodai B, et al: Comparison of postburn capillary permeability in soft tissue and lung. *J Burn Care Rehabil* 2:86, 1981.
271. Harms BA, Bodai BI, Smith M, et al: Prostaglandin release and altered microvascular integrity after burn injury. *J Surg Res* 31:274, 1981.
272. Harms BA, Bodai BI, Kramer GC, Demling RH: Microvascular fluid and protein flux in pulmonary and systemic circulation after thermal injury. *Microvasc Res* 23:77, 1982.
273. Demling RH, Kramer G, Harms B: Role of thermal injury-induced hypoproteinemia on fluid flux and protein permeability in burned and nonburned tissue. *Surgery* 95:136, 1984.
274. Jin LJ, Lalonde C, Demling RH: Lung dysfunction after thermal injury in relation to prostanoid and oxygen radical release. *J Appl Physiol* 61:103, 1986.
275. Demling RH, Zhu D, Lalonde C: Early pulmonary and hemodynamic effects of a chest wall burn (effect of ibuprofen). *Surgery* 104:10, 1988.
276. Herndon DN, Traber LD, Brown M, Traber DL: Lung microvascular lesions with and without inhalation injury in thermally injured sheep. *Prog Clin Biol Res* 264:403, 1988.
277. Fein A, Grossman RF, Jones G, Hoeffel J: Effect of major burns on alveolar epithelial permeability in rabbits. *Crit Care Med* 9:669, 1981.
278. Hayashi M, Bond TP, Guest MM, et al: Pulmonary microcirculation following full-thickness burns. *Burns* 5:227, 1979.
279. Goris RJA, Boekholtz WKF, VanBebber IPT, et al: Multiple organ failure and sepsis without bacteria. *Arch Surg* 121:897, 1986.
280. Lalonde C, Demling RH, Goad MEP: Tissue inflammation without bacteria produces increased oxygen consumption and distant organ lipid perioxidation. *Surgery* 104:49, 1988.
281. Hutchison AA, Hinson JM, Brigham KL, Snapper JR: Effect of endotoxin on airway responsiveness to aerosol histamine in sheep. *J Appl Physiol* 54:1463, 1983.
282. Hutchison AA, Ogletree ML, Snapper J, Brigham KL: Effect of endotoxemia on hypoxic pulmonary vasoconstriction in unanesthetized sheep. *J Appl Physiol* 58:1463, 1985.
283. Meyerick B, Brigham K: Acute effects of *Escherichia coli* endotoxin on the pulmonary microcirculation of anesthetized sheep: Structure-function relationships. *Lab Invest* 48:458, 1983.
284. Ahmed T, Wasserman MA, Muccitelli R, et al: Endotoxin-induced changes in pulmonary hemodynamics and respiratory mechanics: Role of lipoxygenase and cyclooxygenase products. *Am Rev Respir Dis* 134:1149, 1986.
285. Demling RH, Wenger H, Lalonde C, et al: Endotoxin induced prostanoid production by the burn wound can cause distant lung dysfunction. *Surgery* 99:421, 1986.
286. Demling R, Lalonde C, Seekamp A, Fiore N: Endotoxin causes hydrogen peroxide-induced lung lipid peroxidation and prostanoid production. *Arch Surg* 123:1337, 1988.
287. Demling RH, Lalonde CC, Jin LJ, et al: The pulmonary and systemic response to recurrent endotoxemia in the adult sheep. *Surgery* 100:876, 1986.
288. Wong C, Munger H, Demling RH: Effect of a body burn on the lung response to endotoxin. *J Trauma* 25:53, 1985.
289. Nerlich M, Flynn J, Demling RH: Effect of thermal injury on endotoxin-induced lung injury. *Surgery* 93:289, 1983.
290. Katz A, Ryan P, Lalonde C, et al: Topical ibuprofen decreases thromboxane release from the endotoxin-stimulated burn wound. *J Trauma* 26:157, 1986.
291. Demling RH, Proctor R, Duy N, Starling JR: Lung lysosomal enzyme release during hemorrhagic shock and endotoxemia. *J Surg Res* 28:269, 1980.
292. Demling RH, Lalonde C, Jin L, et al: Comparison of the postburn hyperdynamic state and changes in lung function (effect of wound bacterial count). *Surgery* 100:828, 1986.
293. Wenger H, Wong C, Demling RH: Pulmonary dysfunction secondary to soft tissue endotoxin. *Arch Surg* 120:159, 1985.
294. Clark WR, Nieman GF, Goyette D, Gryzboski D: Effects of crystalloid on lung fluid balance after smoke inhalation. *Ann Surg* 208:56, 1988.
295. Clark WR, Webb WR, Wax S, Nieman G: Inhalation injuries: The pathophysiology of acute smoke inhalation. *Surg Forum* 28:177, 1977.
296. Prien T, Traber LD, Herndon DN, et al: Pulmonary edema with smoke inhalation undetected by indicator dilution technique. *J Appl Physiol* 63:907, 1987.
297. Prien T, Linares HA, Traber LD, et al: Lack of hematogenous mediated pulmonary injury with smoke inhalation. *J Burn Care Rehabil* 9:462, 1988.
298. Brizio-Molteni L, Piano G, Rice PL, et al: Effect of wood combustion smoke inhalation on angiotensin-1-converting enzyme in the dog. *Ann Clin Lab Sci* 14:381, 1984.
299. Cohen C: The case for the use of animals in biomedical research. *N Engl J Med* 315:865, 1986.
300. Bleby J: Reduction of animal usage: Some considerations. *Dev Biol Stand* 64:17, 1986.
301. The ethics of animal experimentation: Proceedings of the second CFN symposium, Stockholm, Sweden, August 12–14, 1985. *Acta Physiol Scand (Suppl)* 554:1, 1986.
302. Pincus HA: The animal rights movement: A research perspective. *Am J Psychiatry* 143:1585, 1986.
303. Odell R: The physician's stake in animal research. *JAMA* 256:3347, 1986.
304. Effective animal care and use committees. *Lab Anim Sci* 37(spec. no):1, 1987.

305. Shimazu T, Yukioka T, Hubbard GB, et al: A dose-responsive model of smoke inhalation injury: Severity-related alteration in cardiopulmonary function. *Ann Surg* 206:89, 1987.
306. Borrie J, Mitchell RM: The sheep as an experimental animal in surgical science. *Br J Surg* 47:435, 1960.
307. Halmagyi DFJ, Colebath HJH: Some cardiorespiratory parameters in anesthetized sheep. *J Appl Physiol* 16:45, 1961.
308. Huisman THJ, Kitchens J: Oxygen equilibria studies of the hemoglobins from normal and anemic sheep and goats. *Am J Physiol* 215:140, 1968.
309. Altman PL, Dittma DS (eds): *Biology Data Book,* vol. 3. Bethesda, MD, Federation of American Societies for Experimental Biology, 1974, p 1527–2041.
310. Hazelwood JC, Heath GE: A comparison of cholinesterase activity of plasma, erythrocytes, and cerebrospinal fluid of sheep, calves, dogs, swine, and rabbits. *Am J Vet Res* 37:741, 1976.
311. Hecker JF: *The Sheep as an Experimental Animal.* New York, Academic, 1983.
312. Walker BR, Adams EM, Voelkel NF: Ventilatory responses of hamsters and rats to hypoxia and hypercapnia. *J Appl Physiol* 59:1955, 1985.
313. Vatner SF, Boettcher DH: Regulation of cardiac output by stroke volume and heart rate in conscious dogs. *Cir Res* 42:557, 1978.
314. Carr DT, Essex HE: The hemoglobin concentration of the blood of intact and splenectomized dogs under pentobarbital sodium anesthesia with particular reference to the effect of hemorrhage. *Am J Physiol* 142:40, 1944.
315. Nash CB, Davis F, Woodbury RA: Cardiovascular effects of anesthetic doses of pentobarbital sodium. *Am J Physiol* 185:107, 1956.
316. Neill WA, Oxendine JM, Moore SC: Acute and chronic cardiovascular adjustment to induced anemia in dogs. *Am J Physiol* 217:710, 1969.
317. Rampton DS, Ramsay DJ: The effects of pentobarbitone anaesthesia on the volume and composition of the extracellular fluid of dogs. *J Physiol* 237:521, 1974.
318. Hamlin RL, Smith CR: Characteristics of respiration in healthy dogs anesthetized with sodium pentobarbital. *Am J Vet Res* 28:173, 1967.
319. Cohen GM: Pulmonary metabolism of inhaled chemicals and irritants, in Scadding JG, Cumming G, Thurlbeck W (eds): *Scientific Foundations of Respiratory Medicine.* London, William Heinemann, 1981, pp 286–296.
320. Scarborough RA: The blood picture of normal laboratory animals: The dog. *Yale J Biol Med* 3:359, 1931.
321. Parer JT, Jones WD, Metcalfe J: A quantitative comparison of oxygen transport in sheep and human subjects. *Respir Physiol* 2:196, 1967.
322. Hayflick L: The cellular basis for biology of aging, in Finch C, Hayflick L (eds): *Handbook of the Biology of Aging.* New York, Van Nostrand Reinhold, 1977, pp 159–186.
323. Shock NW: Systemic integration, in Finch C, Hayflick L (eds): *Handbook of the Biology of Aging.* New York, Van Nostrand Reinhold, 1977, pp 639–665.
324. Demarest GB, Hudson LD, Altman LC: Impaired alveolar macrophage chemotaxis in patients with acute smoke inhalation. *Am Rev Respir Dis* 119:279, 1979.
325. Fick RB, Paul ES, Merrill WW, et al: Alterations in the antibacterial properties of rabbit pulmonary macrophages exposed to wood smoke. *Am Rev Respir Dis* 129:76, 1984.
326. Katzenstein AA, Bloor CM, Leibow AA: Diffuse alveolar damage—the role of oxygen, shock and related factors: A review. *Am J Pathol* 85:210, 1976.
327. Bowden DH: Reaction of the lung to injury. in Scadding JG, Cumming G, Thurlbeck WM (eds): *Scientific Foundations of Respiratory Medicine.* London, William Heinemann, 1981, pp 529–545.
328. Kirkpatrick MTS, Bass JB: Severe obstructive lung disease after smoke inhalation. *Chest* 76:108, 1979.
329. Perez-Guerra F, Walsh RE, Sagel SS: Bronchiolitis obliterans and tracheal stenosis: Late complications of an inhalation burn. *JAMA* 218:1568, 1971.
330. Donnellan WL, Poticha SM, Holinger PH: Management and complications of severe pulmonary burn. *JAMA* 194:155, 1965.
331. Cooke NT, Cobley AJ, Armstrong RF: Airflow obstruction after smoke inhalation. *Anaesthesia* 37:830, 1982.
332. Hoeffler HB, Schweppe HI, Greenberg SD: Bronchiectasis following pulmonary ammonia burn. *Arch Pathol Lab Med* 106:686, 1982.
333. Jasper N, Bracamonte M, Sergysels R: Severe peripheral airway obstruction after inhalation burn. *Intensive Care Med* 8:105, 1982.
334. Loke J, Farmer W, Matthay RA, et al: Acute and chronic effects of fire fighting on pulmonary function. *Chest* 77:369, 1980.
335. Unger KM, Snow RM, Mestas JM, Miller WC: Smoke inhalation in firemen. *Thorax* 35:838, 1980.
336. Ashbaugh DG, Maier RV: Idiopathic pulmonary fibrosis in adult respiratory distress syndrome: Diagnosis and treatment. *Arch Surg* 120:530, 1985.
337. Thorning DR, Howard ML, Hudson LD, Schumacher RL: Pulmonary responses to smoke inhalation: Morphologic changes in rabbits exposed to pine wood smoke. *Hum Pathol* 13:355, 1982.
338. Dressler DP, Skornick WA, Kupersmith S: Corticosteroid treatment of experimental smoke inhalation. *Ann Surg* 183:46, 1976.
339. Loke J, Paul E, Virgulto JA, Smith GJW: Rabbit lung after acute smoke inhalation. *Arch Surg* 119:956, 1984.
340. Beeley JM, Crow J, Jones JG, et al: Mortality and lung histopathology after inhalation lung injury: The effect of corticosteroids. *Am Rev Respir Dis* 133:191, 1986.
341. Potkin RT, Robinson NB, Hudson LD, et al: An animal model of smoke inhalation. *Am Rev Respir Dis* 212(suppl):178, 1980.
342. Buerke CA, Lewis TR, Symmonds G: The pulmonary consequences of steam inhalation. Abstract presented at the 7th International Congress on Burns, Melbourne, Australia, March 1986.
343. Jung RC, Gottlieb LS: Respiratory tract burns after aspiration of hot coffee. *Chest* 72:125, 1977.

344. Straus RH, McFadden ER, Ingram RH, Chandler E: Influence of heat and humidity on the airway obstruction induced by exercise in asthma. *J Clin Invest* 61:433, 1978.
345. Deal EC, McFadden ER, Ingram RH, et al: Role of respiratory heat exchange in the production of exercise induced asthma. *J Appl Physiol* 46:467, 1979.
346. McFadden ER, Lenner KAM, Strohl KP: Post-exertional airway rewarming and thermally induced asthma: New insights into pathophysiology and possible pathogenesis. *J Clin Invest* 78:18, 1986.
347. Stewart RJ, Yamaguchi KT, Rowland RRR, et al: Early detection of extravascular lung water in an inhalation injury animal model. *Burns* 12:457, 1986.
348. Rowland RR, Yamaguchi KT, Santibanez AS, et al: Smoke inhalation model for lung permeability studies. *J Trauma* 26:153, 1986.
349. Snashall PD, Weidmer WJ, Staub NC: Extravascular lung water after extracellular fluid volume expansion in dogs. *J Appl Physiol* 42:624, 1977.
350. Gaar KA, Taylor AE, Owens LS, Guyton AC: Pulmonary capillary pressure and filtration co-efficient in the isolated perfused lung. *Am J Physiol* 213:910, 1967.
351. Guyton AC, Lindsey AW: Effect of elevated left atrial pressure and decreased plasma protein concentrations on the development of pulmonary edema. *Circ Res* 7:649, 1959.
352. Endmann AJ, Vaughan TR, Brigham KL, et al: Effect of increased vascular pressure on lung fluid balance in unanesthetized sheep. *Circ Res* 37:271, 1975.
353. Parker JC, Falgout HJ, Parker RE, et al: The effect of fluid volume loading on exclusion of interstitial albumin and lymph flow in the dog lung. *Circ Res* 45:440, 1979.
354. Gump FE, Zikria BA, Mashima Y: The effect of interstitial edema on pulmonary function in the dog. *J Trauma* 12:764, 1972.
355. Esbenshade AM, Newman JH, Lams PM, et al: Respiratory failure after endotoxin infusion in sheep: Lung mechanics and lung fluid balance. *J Appl Physiol* 53:967, 1982.
356. Hauge A, Bo G, Waaler BA: Interrelations between pulmonary liquid volumes and lung compliance. *J Appl Physiol* 38:608, 1978.
357. Staub MC: Pulmonary edema. *Physiol Rev.* 54:678, 1974.
358. Michel RP, Zocchi L, Rossi A, et al: Does interstitial lung edema compress airways and arteries? A morphometric study. *J Appl Physiol* 62:108, 1987.
359. Traber DL, Schlag G, Redl H, Traber LD: Pulmonary edema and compliance changes following smoke inhalation. *J Burn Care Rehabil* 6:490, 1986.
360. Stephensen SF, Esrig BC, Polk HC, Fulton RL: The pathophysiology of smoke inhalation injury. *Ann Surg* 182:652, 1975.
361. Aviado DM, Schmidt CF: Respiratory burns with special reference to pulmonary edema and congestion. *Circulation* 6:666, 1952.
362. Fineberg C, Miller BJ, Allbritten FF: Thermal burns of the respiratory tract. *Surg Gynecol Obstet* 98:318, 1954.
363. Zikria BA, Ferrer JM, Floch HF: The chemical factors contributing to pulmonary damage in "smoke poisoning." *Surgery* 71:704, 1972.
364. Clark WR, Grossman ZD, Ritter-Hrncirik C, Warner F: Clearance of aerosolized ^{99m}Tc-diethylenetriaminepentacetate before and after smoke inhalation. *Chest* 94:22, 1988.
365. Nieman GF, Clark WR, Goyette D, et al: Wood smoke inhalation increases pulmonary microvascular permeability. *Surgery* 98:481, 1989.
366. Nieman GF, Clark WR, Goyette DA: Positive end-expiratory pressure (PEEP) efficacy following wood smoke inhalation. *Am Rev Respir Dis* 133:A347, 1986.
367. Walker HL, McLeod CG, McManus WF: Experimental inhalation injury in the goat. *J Trauma* 21:962, 1981.
368. Herndon DN, Traber DL, Niehaus GD, et al: The pathophysiology of smoke inhalation injury in a sheep model. *J Trauma* 24:1044, 1984.
369. Stein MD, Herndon DN, Stevens JM, et al: Production of chemotactic factors and lung cell changes following smoke inhalation in a sheep model. *J Burn Care Rehabil* 7:117, 1986.
370. Traber DL, Herndon DN, Stein LD, et al: The pulmonary lesion of smoke inhalation in an ovine model. *Circ Shock* 18:311, 1986.
371. Kimura R, Traber LD, Herndon DN, et al: Increasing duration of smoke exposure induces more severe lung injury in sheep. *J Appl Physiol* 64:1107, 1988.
372. Herndon DN, Adams T, Traber LD, Traber DL: Inhalation injury and positive pressure ventilation in a sheep model. *Circ Shock* 12:107, 1984.
373. Herndon DN, Traber LD, Linares H, et al: Etiology of the pulmonary pathophysiology associated with inhalation injury. *Resuscitation* 14:43, 1986.
374. Basadre JO, Sugi K, Traber DL, et al: The effect of leukocyte depletion on smoke inhalation injury in sheep. *Surgery* 104:208, 1988.
375. Brown M, Desai M, Traber LD, et al: Dimethylsulfoxide with heparin in the treatment of smoke inhalation injury. *J Burn Care Rehabil* 9:22, 1988.
376. Kimura R, Traber L, Herndon D, et al: Ibuprofen reduces the lung lymph flow changes associated with inhalation injury. *Circ Shock* 24:183, 1988.
377. Stothert JC, Herndon DN, Lubbesmeyer HJ, et al: Airway acid injury following smoke inhalation. *Prog Clin Biol Res* 264:409, 1988.
378. Herndon DN, Traber DL, Traber LD: The effect of resuscitation on inhalation injury. *Surgery* 100:248, 1986.
379. Dehring DJ, Doty S, Kimura R, et al: Effect of pre-existing inhalation injury on response to bacteremia in sheep. *J Burn Care Rehabil* 9:467, 1988.
380. Desai MH, Brown M, Meak R, et al: Reduction of smoke-induced lung injury with demethyl-sulfoxide and heparin treatment. *Surg Forum* 36:103, 1985.
381. Brigham K, Begley C, Bernard G, et al: Septicemia and lung injury. *Clin Lab Med* 8:719, 1983.
382. Helleman JH, Gabel JC, Hardy JD: Pulmonary effects of intravenous fluid therapy in burn resuscitation. *Surg Gynecol Obstet* 147:161, 1978.

383. Goodwin CW, Dorethy J, Lam V, Pruitt BA: Randomized trial of efficacy of crystalloid and colloid resuscitation on hemodynamic response and lung water following thermal injury. *Ann Surg* 197:520, 1983.
384. Zarins CK, Virgilio RW, Smith DE, Peters RM: The effect of vascular volume on positive end-expiratory pressure induced cardiac output depression and wedge-left atrial pressure discrepancy. *J Surg Res* 23:348, 1977.
385. Haselton PS, McWilliam L, Habouri NY: The lung parenchyma in burns *Histopathology* 7:333, 1983.
386. Karmer GC, Gunther RA, Nerlich ML, et al: Effect of Dextran-70 on increased microvascular fluid and protein flux after thermal injury. *Circ Shock* 9:529, 1982.
387. Finland M, Davidson CS, Levenson SM: Effects of plasma and fluid on pulmonary complications in burned patients. *Arch Intern Med* 77:477, 1946.
388. Cook WA, Baxter CR, Ferrell JM: Pulmonary circulation after dermal burns. *Vasc Surg* 2:1, 1968.
389. Newman JH, Loyd JE, English DK, et al: Effects of breathing 100% oxygen on lung vascular function and lung lymph chemotactic activity in awake sheep. *J Appl Physiol* 54:1379, 1983.
390. Royer F, Martin DJ, Benchetrit G, Grimbert FA: Increase in pulmonary capillary permeability in dogs exposed to 100% O_2. *J Appl Physiol* 65:1140, 1988.
391. Nash G, Blenner-hassett JB, Pontoppidan H: Pulmonary lesions associated with oxygen therapy and artificial ventilation. *N Engl J Med* 276:368, 1967.
392. Sevitt S: Diffuse and focal oxygen pneumonitis: A preliminary report on the threshold of pulmonary oxygen toxicity in man. *J Clin Pathol* 27:21, 1974.
393. Philip AGS: Oxygen plus pressure plus time: The etiology of bronchopulmonary dysplasia. *Pediatrics* 55:44, 1975.
394. Barrett CR, Bell ALL, Ryan ST: Effect of positive end-expiratory pressure on lung compliance in dogs after acute alveolar injury. *Am Rev Respir Dis* 124:705, 1981.
395. Helbert C, Paskanik A, Bredenberg CE: Effect of positive end-expiratory pressure on lung water in pulmonary edema caused by increased membrane permeability. *Ann Thorac Surg* 36:42, 1983.
396. Bredenberg CE, Webb WR: Experimental pulmonary edema: The effect of unilateral PEEP on the accumulation of lung water. *Ann Surg* 189:433, 1979.
397. Russell JA, Hoeffel J, Murray JF: Effect of different levels of positive end-expiratory pressure on lung water content. *J Appl Physiol* 53:9, 1982.
398. Demling RH, Staub NC, Edmunds LH: Effect of end-expiratory airway pressure on accumulation of extravascular lung water. *J Appl Physiol* 38:907, 1975.
399. Bshouty Z, Ali J, Younes M: Effect of tidal volume and PEEP on rate of edema formation in in situ perfused canine lobes. *J Appl Physiol* 64:1900, 1988.
400. Cassidy SS, Robertson CH, Pierce AK, Johnson RL: Cardiovascular effects of positive end-expiratory pressure in dogs. *J Appl Physiol* 44:743, 1978.
401. Dreyfuss D, Soler P, Basset G, Saumon G: High inflation pressure pulmonary edema: Respective effects of high airway pressure, high tidal volume, and positive end-expiratory pressure. *Am Rev Resp Dis* 137:1159, 1988.
402. Shinozawa YC, Hales CA, Jung W, Burke JW: Ibuprofen prevents synthetic smoke-induced pulmonary edema. *Am Rev Respir Dis* 134:1145, 1986.
403. Nicholas GG, Martin DE, Osbakken MD: Cardiovascular monitoring during elective aortic surgery. *Arch Surg* 118:1256, 1983.
404. Civetta JM, Gabel JC: Flow directed pulmonary artery catheterization in surgical patients: Indications and modifications of technique. *Ann Surg* 176:753, 1972.
405. Forrester JS, Diamond G, McHugh TJ, Sloan HSE: Filling pressure in the right and left sides of the heart in acute myocardial infarction: A reappraisal of central venous pressure monitoring. *N Engl J Med* 285:190, 1971.
406. Zhi-yuan L, Ngao L, Pei-Feng C, et al: Pulmonary surfactant activity after severe steam inhalation injury in rabbits. *Burns* 12:330, 1986.
407. Shimazu T, Ikeuchi H, Johnson AA, et al: Effects of PEEP on ventilation-perfusion ratios following smoke inhalation injury in a sheep model. Abstract presented at the 19th Annual Meeting, American Burn Association, Washington, DC, May 1987.
408. Eyal Z, Dunsky EH, Polliack A, Davidson JT: The acute effect of pulmonary burns on lung mechanics and gas exchange in the rabbit. *Br J Anaesth* 47:546, 1975.
409. Putman CL, Loke J, Matthay, Ravin CE: Radiographic manifestations of acute smoke inhalation. *Am J Roentgenol* 129:865, 1979.
410. Lee MJ, O'Connell DJ: The plain chest radiograph after acute smoke inhalation. *Clin Radiol* 39:33, 1988.
411. Teixidor HS, Rubin E, Movick GS, Alonso DR: Smoke inhalation: Radiologic manifestations. *Radiology* 149:383, 1983.
412. Heitzman ER, Proto AV, Goldwin RL: The role of computerized tomography in the diagnosis of diseases of the thorax. *JAMA* 241:933, 1979.
413. Gansu G, Kaufman L, Swann SJ, Brito AC: Absolute lung density in experimental canine pulmonary edema. *Invest Radiol* 14:261, 1979.
414. Wollmer P, Albrechtsson U, Brauer K, et al: Measurement of lung density by means of x-ray computed tomography: Relation to pulmonary mechanics in normal subjects. *Chest* 90:381, 1986.
415. Maunder RJ, Shuman WP, McHugh JW, et al: Preservation of normal lung regions in the adult respiratory distress syndrome: Analysis by computed tomography. *JAMA* 255:2463, 1986.
416. Wolhner P, Rhodes CG, Deanfield J, et al: Regional extravascular density of the lung in patients with acute pulmonary edema. *J Appl Physiol* 63:1890, 1987.
417. Chiles C, Hedlund LW, Putman CE: Diagnostic imaging in inhalation lung injury, in Loke J (ed): *Pathophysiology and Treatment of Inhalation Injuries*. New York, Marcel Dekker, 1988, pp 187–202.
418. Moylan JA, Wilmore DW, Mouton DE, Pruitt BA: Early diagnosis of inhalation injury using ^{133}Xenon lung scan. *Ann Surg* 176:477, 1972.
419. Agee RN, Long JM, Hunt JL, et al: Use of ^{133}Xenon in

early diagnosis of inhalation injury. *J Trauma* 16:218, 1976.

420. Chilcoat TR, Thomas FD, Gerson JI: Ventilator-driven xenon ventilation studies. *J Nucl Med* 25:810, 1984.
421. Alderson PO, Line BR: Scintigraphic evaluation of regional pulmonary ventilation. *Semin Nucl Med* 10:218, 1980.
422. Burch WM, Sullivan RJ, McLaren CJ: Technegas—A new ventilation agent for lung scanning. *Nucl Med Commun* 7:865, 1986.
423. Jones JG, Lawler P, Crawley JCW, et al: Increased alveolar epithelial permeability in cigarette smokers. *Lancet* 1:66, 1981.
424. Mason GR, Uszler JM, Effros RM, Reid E: Rapidly reversible alterations of pulmonary epithelial permeability induced by smoking. *Chest* 83:6, 1983.
425. Kennedy S, Elwood RK, Wiggs B, et al: Increased airway mucosal permeability of smokers. *Am Rev Respir Dis* 129:143, 1984.
426. Effros RM, Mason GR: Measurements of pulmonary epithelial permeability in vivo. *Am Rev Respir Dis* 127(suppl):S59, 1983.
427. Rinderknecht J, Shapiro L, Kranthammer M, et al: Accelerated clearance of small solutes from the lungs in interstitial lung disease. *Am Rev Respir Dis* 121:105, 1980.
428. Rizk NW, Luce JM, Hoeffel JM, et al: Site of deposition and factors affecting clearance of aerosolized solute from canine lungs. *J Appl Physiol* 56:723, 1984.
429. Oberdorster G, Utell MJ, Weber DA, et al: Lung clearance of inhaled 99mTc DTPA in the dog. *J Appl Physiol* 57:589, 1984.
430. Egan EA: Response of alveolar epithelial solute permeability to changes in lung inflation. *J Appl Physiol* 49:1032, 1980.
431. Egan EA: Lung inflation, lung solute permeability, and alveolar edema. *J Appl Physiol* 53:121, 1982.
432. Egan EA: Fluid balance in the air filled alveolar space. *Am Rev Respir Dis* 172(suppl):S37, 1983.
433. Scarpelli EM: *The Surfactant System of the Lung*. Philadelphia, Lea & Febiger, 1968.
434. Scarpelli EM, Mantare AS: The surfactant system and pulmonary mechanics, in Robertson B, VanGolde IMG, Battenberg JJ (eds): *Pulmonary Surfactant*. New York, Elsevier, 1984, pp 119–170.
435. VanGolde LMG, Batenburg JJ, Robertson B: The pulmonary surfactant system: Biochemical aspects and functional significance. *Physiol Rev*. 68:374, 1988.
436. Clements SA, Hustead RF, Johnson RP, Gribertz S: Pulmonary surface tension and alveolar stability. *J Appl Physiol* 16:444, 1961.
437. Goerke S: Lung surfactant. *Biochem Biophys Acta* 344:241, 1974.
438. Guyton AC, Moffatt DS, Adair TH: Role of alveolar surface tension in transepithelial movement of fluid, in Robinson B, VanGolde LMG, Batenberg JJ (eds): *Pulmonary Surfactant*. New York, Elsevier, 1984, pp 171–186.
439. Weibel ER: *The Pathway for Oxygen: Structure and Function in the Mammalian Respiratory System*. Cambridge, Harvard University Press, 1984, pp 317–336.
440. Bruderman I, Somers K, Hamilton WK, Effect of surface tension on circulation in the excised lungs of dogs. *J Appl Physiol* 19:707, 1964.
441. Pain MCF, West JB: Effect of the volume history of the isolated lung on distribution of blood flow. *J Appl Physiol* 21:1545, 1966.
442. Guyton AC, Taylor AE, Drake RE, Parker JC: *Dynamics of Subatmospheric Pressure in the Pulmonary Interstitial Fluid in Lung Liquids*. Ciba Foundation Symposium 38, New York, Elsevier, 1976, pp 77–100.
443. Albert RK, Lakshminaruayon S, Hildebrandt J, Kirk W: Increased surface tension favors pulmonary edema in anesthetized dog lungs. *J Clin Invest* 63:1015, 1979.
444. Bachofen H, Gehr P, Weibel ER: Alterations of mechanical properties and morphology in excised rabbit lung rinsed with a detergent. *J Appl Physiol* 47:1002, 1979.
445. Bredenberg CE, Nieman GF, Paskanik AM, Hart AK: Microvascular membrane permeability in high surface tension edema. *J Appl Physiol* 60:253, 1986.
446. Nieman GF, Bredenberg CE: High surface tension pulmonary edema induced by detergent aerosol. *J Appl Physiol* 58:129, 1985.
447. Lai-Fook SS: Mechanical factors determining pulmonary interstitial fluid pressure. *Lung* 160:175, 1982.
448. Mead J: Mechanical properties of lungs. *Physiol Rev* 41:281, 1961.
449. Mead J, Takishima T, Leith D: Stress distribution in lungs: A model of pulmonary elasticity. *J Appl Physiol* 28:596, 1970.
450. Ikegami M, Jobe A, Glatz T: Surface activity following natural surfactant treatment in premature lambs. *J Appl Physiol* 51:306, 1981.
451. Jacobs HC, Berry DD, Duane G, et al: Normalization of arterial blood gases after treatment of surfactant-deficient lambs with Tween-20. *Am Rev Respir Dis* 132:1313, 1985.
452. Jobe A, Ikegami M: Surfactant for the treatment of respiratory distress syndrome. *Am Rev Respir Dis* 136:1256, 1987.
453. Davis JM, Veness-Meehan K, Notter RH, et al: Changes in pulmonary mechanics after the administration of surfactant to infants with respiratory distress syndrome. *N Engl J Med* 319:476, 1988.
454. Finley TN, Tooky WH, Swenson EW, et al: Pulmonary surface tension in experimental atelectasis. *Am Rev Respir Dis* 89:372, 1964.
455. Greenfield LJ, Chernick V, Hudson WA, Brumley GW: Alterations in pulmonary surfactant following compression atelectasis, pulmonary artery ligations, and reimplantation of the lung. *Ann Surg* 166:109, 1967.
456. Said SI, Avery ME, Davis RK, Banerju CM: Pulmonary surface activity in induced pulmonary edema. *J Clin Invest* 44:458, 1965.
457. Henry JN: The effect of shock on pulmonary alveolar surfactant: Its role in refractory respiratory insufficiency of the critically ill or severely injured patient. *J Trauma* 8:756, 1968.
458. Dueck R, Wagner PD, West JB: Effects of positive end-

expiratory pressure on gas exchange in dogs with normal and edematous lungs. *Anesthesiology* 47:359, 1977.
459. Weigelt SA, Mitchell RA, Snyder WH: Early positive end-expiratory pressure in the adult respiratory distress syndrome. *Arch Surg* 114:497, 1979.
460. Prewitt RM, McCarthy J, Wood LDH: Treatment of acute low pressure pulmonary edema in dogs: Relative effects of hydrostatic and oncotic pressure, nitroprusside, and positive end-expiratory pressure. *J Clin Invest* 67:409, 1981.
461. Venus B, Matsuda T, Copiozo JB, Mathru M: Prophylactic intubation and continuous positive airway pressure in the management of inhalation injury in burn victims. *Crit Care Med* 9:519, 1981.
462. Robinson NB, Hudson LD, Robertson HT, et al: Ventilation and perfusion alterations after smoke inhalation injury. *Surgery* 90:352, 1981.
463. Wagner PD, Saltzman HA, West JB: Measurement of continuous distribution of ventilation-perfusion ratios: Theory. *J Appl Physiol* 36:588, 1971.
464. Evans JW, Wagner PD: Limits on Va/Q distribution from analysis of experimental inert gas elimination. *J Appl Physiol* 42:889, 1977.
465. Burns DM, Shure D, Francoz R, et al: The physiologic consequences of saline lobar lavage in healthy human adults. *Am Rev Respir Dis* 127:695, 1983.
466. Mardelet-Dambrine M, Arnoux A, Stanislas-Leguern G, et al: Processing of lung lavage fluid causes variability in broncho-alveolar cell count. *Am Rev Respir Dis* 130:305, 1984.
467. Young KR, Reynolds HY: Bronchoalveolar lavage in inhalation lung toxicity, in Loke J (ed): *Pathophysiology and Treatment of Inhalation Injuries*. New York, Marcel Dekker, 1988, pp 207–237.
468. Hunninghake GW, Gadek JE, Kawanami O, et al: Inflammatory and immune processes in the human lung in health and disease: Evaluation by bronchoalveolar lavage. *Am J Pathol* 97:149, 1979.
469. Henderson RF, Rebar AH, DeNicola DB, et al: The use of pulmonary washings as a probe to detect lung injury. *Chest* 80(suppl):12S, 1981.
470. Cooney W, Dzuira B, Harper R, Nash G: The cytology of sputum from thermally injured patients. *Acta Cytol* 16:433, 1972.
471. Faling LJ, Medici TC, Chodosh S: Sputum cell population measurements in bronchial injury: Observations in acute smoke inhalation. *Chest* 65(suppl)56S, 1974.
472. Ambiavagar M, Chalon J, Zargham I: Tracheobronchial cytologic changes following lower airway thermal injury: A preliminary report. *J Trauma* 14:280, 1974.
473. Burns TR, Greenberg SD, Cartwright J, Jachimcyzk JA: Smoke inhalation: An ultrastructural study of reaction to injury in the human alveolar wall. *Environ Res* 4:447, 1986.
474. Blumenthal BJ, Boren HG: Lung structure in three dimensions after inflation and fume fixation. *Am Rev Tuberc* 79:764, 1959.
475. Pratt PC, Klugh GA: A technique for the study of ventilatory capacity, compliance, and residual volume of excised lungs and for fixation, drying, and serial sectioning in the inflated state. *Am Rev Respir Dis* 83:690, 1961.
476. Jones E: Study of lung specimens prepared by fume fixation. *Am Rev Respir Dis* 82:704, 1960.
477. Bachofen H, Ammann A, Wangensteen D, Weibel ER: Perfusion fixation of lungs for structure-function analysis: Credits and limitations. *J Appl Physiol* 53(2):528, 1982.
478. Weibel ER, Limacher W, Bachofen H: Electron microscopy of rapidly frozen lungs: Evaluation on the basis of standard criteria. *J Appl Physiol* 53(2):516, 1982.
479. Bachofen M, Weibel ER: Basic pattern of tissue repair in human lungs following unspecific injury. *Chest* 65(suppl):14S, 1974.
480. Gil J, Weibel ER: Morphological study of pressure-volume hysteresis in rat lungs fixed by vascular perfusion. *Respir Physiol* 15:190, 1972.
481. Loud AV, Anversa P: Biology of disease: Morphometric analysis of biologic processes. *Lab Invest* 50(3):250, 1984.
482. Cruz-Orive LM, Weibel ER: Sampling designs for stereology. *J Microsc* 122(3):235, 1981.
483. Weibel ER: Principles and methods for the morphometric study of the lungs and other organs. *Lab Invest* 12:131, 1963.
484. Weibel ER, Gomez DM: A principle for counting tissue structures on random sections. *J Appl Physiol* 17:343, 1962.
485. Weibel ER, Kistler GS, Scherle WF: Practical stereological methods for morphometric cytology. *J Cell Biol* 30:23, 1966.
486. Weibel ER: Morphometrics of the lung, in Fenn W, Rahn H (eds): *Handbook of Physiology*, Sec. 3, *Respiration*, vol. 1. American Physiological Society, 1964, pp. 285–307.
487. Radford Jr: EP method for estimating respiratory surface area of mammalian lungs from their physical characteristics. *Proc Soc Exp Biol Med* 87:58, 1954.
488. Michel RP, Hakim TS, Smith TT, Poulsen RS: Quantitative morphology of permeability lung edema in dogs induced by α-naphthylthiourea. *Lab Invest* 149(4):412, 1983.
489. Gil J, Bachofen H, Gehr P, Weibel ER: Alveolar volume-surface area relation in air- and saline-filled lungs fixed by vascular perfusion. *J Appl Physiol* 47:990, 1979.
490. Moss GS, Newson B, Das Gupta TK: The normal electron histochemistry and the effect of hemorrhagic shock on the pulmonary surfactant system. *Surg Gynecol Obstet* 140:53, 1975.
491. Wangensteen D, Bachofen H, Weibel ER: Lung tissue volume changes induced by hypertonic NaCl: Morphometric evaluation. *J Appl Physiol* 51:1443, 1981.
492. Gee MH, Williams DO: Effect of lung inflation on perivascular cuff fluid volume in isolated dog lung lobes. *Microvasc Res* 17:192, 1979.
493. Gee MH, Havill AM: The relationship between pulmonary perivascular cuff fluid and lung lymph in dogs with edema. *Microvasc Res* 19:209, 1980.
494. Conhaim RL, Gropper MA, Staub NC: Effect of lung in-

flation on alveolar-airway barrier protein permeability in dog lung. *J Appl Physiol* 55:1249, 1983.
495. Havill AM, Gee MH: Role of interstitium in clearance of alveolar fluid in normal and injured lungs. *J Appl Physiol* 57:1, 1984.
496. Conhaim RL: Growth rate of perivascular cuffs in liquid-inflated dog lung lobes. *J Appl Physiol* 61:647, 1986.
497. Conhaim RL, Lai-Fook SJ, Staub NC: Sequence of perivascular liquid accumulation in liquid-inflated dog lung lobes. *J Appl Physiol* 60:513, 1986.
498. Gee MH, Staub NC: Role of bulk fluid flow in protein permeability of the dog lung alveolar membrane. *J Appl Physiol* 42:144, 1977.
499. Taylor AE: Capillary fluid filtration. *Circ Res* 49:557, 1981.
500. Renken EM: Capillary transport of macromolecules: Pores and other endothelial pathways. *J Appl Physiol* 58:315, 1985.
501. Renken EM: Multiple pathways of capillary permeability. *Circ Res* 41:735, 1977.
502. Renken EM: Some consequences of capillary permeability to macromolecules: Starling's hypothesis reconsidered. *Am J Physiol* 250:H706, 1986.
503. Crandell ED, Staub NC, Goldberg HS, Effros RM: Recent developments in pulmonary edema. *Ann Intern Med* 99:808, 1983.
504. Staub NC: "State of the Art" review: Pathogenesis of pulmonary edema. *Am Rev Respir Dis* 109:358, 1974.
505. Tranbaugh RF, Lewis FR: Mechanisms and etiologic factors of pulmonary edema. *Surg Gynecol Obstet* 158:193, 1984.
506. Nieman GF: Current concepts of lung-fluid balance. *Respir Care* 30:1062, 1985.
507. Drake RE, Smith JH, Gabel JC: Estimation of the filtration coefficient in intact dog lungs. *Am J Physiol* 238:H430, 1980.
508. Staub NC: Pulmonary edema due to increased microvascular permeability to fluid and protein. *Circ Res* 43:143, 1978.
509. Rafferty TD, Ljungquist R, Firestone L, et al: Plasma colloid oncotic pressure-pulmonary artery occlusion pressure gradient. *Arch Surg* 118:841, 1983.
510. Zarins CK, Rice CL, Peters RM, Virgilio RW: Lymph and pulmonary response to isobaric reduction in plasma oncotic pressure in baboons. *Circ Res* 43:925, 1978.
511. Gaar KA, Taylor AE, Owens LS, Guyton AC: Effect of capillary pressure and plasma protein on development of pulmonary edema. *Am J Physiol* 213:79, 1967.
512. Guyton AC, Lindsey AW: Effect of elevated left atrial pressure and decreased plasma protein concentrations on the development of pulmonary edema. *Circ Res* 7:649, 1959.
513. Erdman AJ, Vaughn TR, Brigham KL, et al: Effect of increased vascular pressure on lung fluid balance in unanesthetized sheep. *Circ Res* 37:271, 1975.
514. Parker JC, Parker RE, Granger DN, Taylor AF: Vascular permeability and transvascular fluid and protein transport in the dog lung. *Circ Res* 48:549, 1981.
515. Rutili G, Parker JC, Taylor AE: Fluid balance in ANTU-injured lungs during crystalloid and colloid infusions. *J Appl Physiol* 56:993, 1984.
516. Schaeffer RC, Haupt MT, Carlson RW: Effects of colloidal and crystalloidal fluids on oncotic pressure, lung weights, and hemodynamics under conditions of increased hydrostatic pressure. *Crit Care Med* 12:292, 1984.
517. Schaeffer RC, Renkiewicz RR, Carlson RW: Effects of colloidal and crystalloidal fluids on cardiopulmonary measurements and lung wet/dry ratios following thromboembolism in dogs. *Crit Care Med* 13:293, 1985.
518. Gaar KA, Taylor AE, Owens LS, Guyton AC: Pulmonary capillary pressure and filtration co-efficient in the isolated perfused lung. *Am J Physiol* 213:910, 1967.
519. Hollway H, Perry M, Downey J, et al: Estimation of effective pulmonary capillary pressure in intact lungs. *J Appl Physiol* 54:846, 1983.
520. Iliff LD: Extra-alveolar vessels and edema development in excised dog lungs. *Circ Res* 28:524, 1971.
521. Staub NC, Hogg JC: Conference report of a workshop on the measurement of lung water. *Crit Care Med* 8:752, 1980.
522. Bryne K, Sugerman HJ: Experimental and clinical assessment of lung injury by measurement of extravascular lung water and transcapillary protein flux in ARDS: A review of current techniques. *J Surg Res* 44:185, 1988.
523. Pearce ML, Yamashita J, Beazell J: Measurement of pulmonary edema. *Circ Res* 16:482, 1965.
524. Collins JC, Newman JH, Wickersham NE, et al: Relation of blood-free to blood-inclusive post mortem lung water measurements in sheep. *J Appl Physiol* 59:592, 1985.
525. Trautman ED, Newbower RS: Development of indicator dilution techniques. *Inst Electr Electron Eng Trans Biomed* 31:800, 1984.
526. Cheney FW, Bishop MJ, Eisenstein BL, Artman LD: Hypoxic pulmonary vasoconstriction does not affect hydrostatic pulmonary edema formation. *J Appl Physiol* 62:776, 1987.
527. Goodwin CW, Pruitt BA: Underestimation of thermal lung water volume in patients with high cardiac output. *Surgery* 92:401, 1982.
528. Allison RC, Parker JC, Duncan CE, Taylor AE: Effect of air embolism on the measurement of extravascular lung thermal volume. *J Appl Physiol* 54:943, 1983.
529. Carlile PV, Gray BA: Type of lung injury influences the thermal-dye estimation of extravascular lung water. *J Appl Physiol* 57:680, 1984.
530. Baudendistel LJ, Kaminski DL, Dahms TF: Evaluation of extravascular lung water by single thermal indicator. *Crit Care Med* 14:52, 1986.
531. Ali J, Chernick W, Wood LDH: Effect of furosemide in canine low-pressure pulmonary edema. *J Clin Invest* 64:1494, 1979.
532. Mayers I, Stimpson R, Oppenheimer L: Delayed resolution of high-pressure pulmonary edema or capillary leak. *Surgery* 101:450, 1987.
533. Brigham KL: Lung lymph composition and flow in normal and abnormal states, in Fishman AP (ed): *Update: Pulmonary Diseases and Disorders*. New York,

McGraw-Hill, 1982, pp 101–111.
534. Taylor AE: Capillary fluid filtration: Starling forces and lymph flow. *Circ Res* 49:557, 1981.
535. Taylor AE, Granger DN: Equivalent pore modeling: Vesicles and channels. *Fed Proc* 42:2440, 1983.
536. Vreim CE, Staub NC: Protein composition of lung fluids in acute alloxan edema in dogs. *Am J Physiol* 230:376, 1976.
537. Vreim CE, Snashall PD, Staub NC: Protein composition of lung fluids in anesthetized dogs with acute cardiogenic edema. *Am J Physiol* 231:1466, 1976.
538. Maron MB: Analysis of airway fluid protein concentration in neurogenic pulmonary edema. *J Appl Physiol* 62:470, 1987.
539. Staub NC, Bland RD, Brigham KL, et al: Preparation of chronic lung lymph fistula in sheep. *J Surg Res* 19:315, 1975.
540. Leeds SE, Teleszky LB, Uhley HN, et al: A method for the collection of pure pulmonary lymph in the canine. *Surg Gynecol Obstet* 155:225, 1982.
541. Stothert JC, Winn R, Nadir B, et al: Modified chronic lung lymph fistula in goats via thoracic duct. *J Appl Physiol* 51:226, 1981.
542. Winn R, Nadir B, Gleisner J, Hildenbrandt J: Chronic lung lymph fistula in goat. *J Appl Physiol* 48:399, 1980.
543. Vreim CE, Snashall PD, Demling RH, Staub NC: Lung, lymph and free interstitial fluid protein composition in sheep with edema. *Am J Physiol* 230:1650, 1976.
544. Demling RH, Gunther R: Effect of diaphragmatic lymphatic contamination on caudal mediastinal node lymph flow in unanesthetized sheep. *Lymphology* 15:163, 1982.
545. Drake RT, Adair T, Traber D, Gabel J: Contamination of caudal mediastinal node efferent lymph in the sheep. *Am J Physiol* 241:H354, 1981.
546. Chanana AD, Joel DD: Contamination of lung lymph following standard and modified procedures in sheep. *J Appl Physiol* 60:809, 1986.
547. Martin DJ, Parker JC, Taylor AE: Simultaneous comparison of tracheobronchial and right duct lymph dynamics in dogs. *J Appl Physiol* 54:199, 1983.
548. Maron BM: Modification of lymph during passage through the lymph node: Effect of histamine. *Am J Physiol* 245:H553, 1983.
549. Adair TH, Moffatt DS, Paulsen HW, Guyton AC: Quantification of changes in lymph node protein concentration during lymph node transit. *Am J Physiol* 243:H351, 1982.
550. Beh KJ, Watson DL, Lascelles AK: Concentrations of immunoglobulins and albumin in lymph collected from various regions of the body of the sheep. *Aust J Exp Biol Med Sci* 52:81, 1974.
551. Quinn JW, Shannon AD: The influence of the lymph node on the protein concentration of efferent lymph leaving the node. *J Physiol (London)* 264:307, 1977.
552. Renkin EM: Lymph as a measure of the composition of interstitial fluids, in Fishman AP, Renkin EM (eds): *Pulmonary Edema*. Baltimore, Williams & Wilkins, 1979, pp 145–159.
553. Snashall PD, Hughes JMB: Lung water balance. *Rev Physiol Biochem Pharmacol*. 89:5, 1981.
554. McClure DE, Weidner WJ: Comparison of afferent and efferent lung lymph in the sheep. *J Appl Physiol* 64:2340, 1988.
555. Drake RE, Laine GA, Allen SJ, et al: Overestimation of sheep lung lymph contamination. *J Appl Physiol* 61:1590, 1986.
556. Laine GA, Drake RE, Zavisca FG, Gabel JC: Effect of lymphatic cannula outflow height on lung microvascular permeability evaluations. *J Appl Physiol* 57:1412, 1984.
557. Drake RE, Allen SJ, Williams JP, et al: Lymph flow from edematous dog lungs. *J Appl Physiol* 62:2416, 1987.
558. Brigham KL: Lung lymph composition and flow in experimental pulmonary edema, in Fishman AP, Renkin EM (eds) *Pulmonary Edema*. Bethesda, Md, American Physiological Society, 1979, pp 161–173.
559. Mitzner W, Sylvester JT: Lymph flow and lung weight in isolated sheep lung. *J Appl Physiol* 61:1830, 1986.
560. Pine M, Beach PM, Cottrell TS, et al: The relationship between right duct lymph flow and extravascular lung water in dogs given α-naphthylthiourea. *J Clin Invest* 58:482, 1976.
561. Barer GR, Howard P, McCurrie JR, Shaw JW: Changes in the pulmonary circulation after bronchial occlusion in anesthetized dogs and cats. *Circ Res* 25:747, 1969.
562. Kato M, Staub NC: Response of small pulmonary arteries to unilobar hypoxia and hypercapnia. *Circ Res* 19:426, 1966.
563. Hobbs BB, Hinchcliffe WA, Greenspan RH: Effects of acute lobar atelectasis on pulmonary hemodynamics. *Invest Radiol* 7:1, 1972.
564. Howell JBL, Permutt S, Proctor DF, Riley RL: Effect of inflation of the lung on different parts of pulmonary vascular bed. *J Appl Physiol* 16:71, 1961.
565. Woodson RD, Raab DE, Ferguson DJ: Pulmonary hemodynamics following acute atelectasis. *Am J Physiol* 205:53, 1963.
566. Granger DN, Taylor AE: Permeability of intestinal capillaries to endogenous macromolecules. *Am J Physiol* 238:H457, 1980.
567. Parker RE, Roselli RJ, Brigham KL: Effects of prolonged elevated microvascular pressure on lung fluid balance in sheep. *J Appl Physiol* 58:869, 1985.
568. Smith L, Andreasson S, Tolling KT, et al: Sepsis in sheep reduces pulmonary microvascular sieving capacity. *J Appl Physiol* 62:1422, 1987.
569. Townsley MI, McClure DE, Weidner WJ: Assessment of pulmonary microvascular permeability in acutely prepared sheep. *J Appl Physiol* 56:857, 1984.
570. Smith L, Andreasson S, Tolling KT, et al: Estimation of equivalent pore radii in pulmonary microvasculature after lung lymph fistula preparation. *J Appl Physiol* 62:2300, 1987.
571. Dauber IM, Pluss WT, VanGrondelle A, et al: Specificity and sensitivity of noninvasive measurement of pulmonary vascular protein leak. *J Appl Physiol* 59:564, 1985.
572. Ward WF, Molteni A, Fitzsimons EJ, Hinz J: Serum copper concentration as an index of lung injury in rats exposed to hemithorax irradiation. *Radiat Res* 114:613, 1988.

573. Molteni A, Ward WF, Ts'ao CH, Fitzsimons EJ: Serum copper concentration as an index of cardiopulmonary injury in monocrotaline-treated rats. *Ann Clin Lab Sci* 18:394, 1988.
574. Austin KF, Soberman RJ: Perspectives on additional areas for research in leukotrienes, in Levi R, Krell RD (eds): *Biology of the Leukotrienes*. New York Academy of Sciences, 1988, 524:xi–xxv.
575. Hutchison DCS: The proteases, in Scadding JG, Cumming G, Thurlbeck W (eds): *Scientific Foundations of Respiratory Medicine*. London, William Heinemann, 1981, pp 250–262.
576. Hutchison DCS: Proteases inhibitors. in Scadding JG, Cumming G, Thurlbeck W (eds): *Scientific Foundations of Respiratory Medicine*. London, William Heinemann, 1981, pp 263–276.
577. Sors H, Even P: Biosynthesis and metabolism of prostaglandins and related compounds by the lung, in Scadding JG, Cumming G, Thurlbeck W (eds): *Scientific Foundations of Respiratory Medicine*. London, William Heinemann, 1981, pp 297–314.
578. Even P, Sors H: Biological actions of prostaglandins and related substances on the respiratory system, in Scadding JG, Cumming G, Thurlbeck W (eds): *Scientific Foundations of Respiratory Medicine*. London, William Heinemann, 1981, pp 315–332.
579. Bakhle YS: Conversion of angiotensin I and other pharmacokinetic functions of the pulmonary circulation, in Scadding JG, Cumming G, Thurlbeck W (eds) *Scientific Foundations of Respiratory Medicine*. London, William Heinemann, 1981, pp 332–348.
580. Hollinger MA, Giri SN, Patwell S, et al: Effects of acute lung injury on angiotensin-converting enzyme in serum, lung lavage and effusate. *Am Rev Respir Dis* 121:373, 1980.
581. Molteni A, Zaklein RM, Mallis KB, Mattioli L: The effect of chronic alveolar hypoxia on lung and serum angiotensin-1-converting enzyme activity. *Proc Soc Exp Biol Med* 147:263, 1974.
582. Wilson JD, Foster DW (eds): *Williams Textbook of Endocrinology*, 7th ed. Philadelphia, Saunders, 1985.
583. Wilmore DW: *The Metabolic Management of the Critically Ill*. New York, Plenum, 1977, pp 91–128.
584. Rosenblatt M: Peptide hormone antagonists that are effective in vivo: Lessons from parathyroid hormone. *N Engl J Med* 315:1004, 1986.
585. Slater TF: Free-radical mechanisms in tissue injury. *Biochem J* 222:1, 1984.
586. Clifford PS, Coon RL, Colditz JH, et al: Pulmonary denervation in the dog. *J Appl Physiol* 54:1451, 1983.
587. Winn R, Maunder R, Chi E, Harlan J: Neutrophil depletion does not prevent lung edema after endotoxin infusion in goats. *J Appl Physiol* 62:116, 1987.
588. Hinson JM, Hutchison AA, Ogeltree ML, et al: Effect of granulocyte depletion on altered lung mechanics after endotoxemia in sheep. *J Appl Physiol* 55:92, 1983.
589. Maunder RJ, Hackman RC, Riff E, et al: Occurrence of the adult respiratory distress syndrome in neutropenic patients. *Am Rev Respir Dis* 133:313, 1986.
590. Oldham KT, Guice KS, Till GO, Ward PA: Activation of complement by hydroxyl radical in thermal injury. *Surgery* 104:272, 1988.
591. Till GO, Johnson KJ, Kunkel R, Ward PA: Intravascular activation of complement and acute lung injury: Dependency on neutrophils and toxic oxygen metabolites. *J Clin Invest* 69:1126, 1982.
592. Weigelt JA, Chenoweth DE, Borman KR, Norcross JF: Complement and the severity of pulmonary failure. *J Trauma* 28:1013, 1988.
593. Winn R, Enderson B, Price S, Rice CL: Indomethacin, but not dazoxiben, reduced lung fluid filtration after *E. coli* infusion. *J Appl Physiol* 64:2468, 1988.
594. Lund T, Goodwin CW, McManus WF, et al: Upper airway sequelae in burn patients requiring endotracheal intubation or tracheostomy. *Ann Surg* 201:374, 1985.

Chapter 19

Challenges for the Future

John W. L. Davies

In the foregoing chapters the emphasis has rightly been directed toward giving a detailed account of the causes of smoke inhalation injury, the responses of the body to these causes, and the treatment of patients either with smoke inhalation injury alone or with concomitant thermal injuries affecting the skin. While it is obvious that much is already known about these aspects of the injury and its treatment, it should be noted that most chapters contain comments on uncertainties or frank unknowns and many authors suggest future lines of research which they believe might yield valuable insights into the nature of these problems or their treatment.

This chapter surveys some of these problems and suggests lines of investigation which may help in their elucidation. These challenges for the future can be broadly grouped under three headings:

1. Studies of problems manifest during treatment of injured patients, the answers to which may have a direct bearing on the patterns of treatment of future patients.
2. Studies of more academic interest which deepen our understanding of which particular materials in smoke cause the observed injury, the mechanisms by which these materials actually initiate injury at the tissue, cellular, or subcellular levels, and the responses of the cells or the tissues or organs to such injury. Since a cascade of events seems to occur over a relatively long time scale, such fundamental studies may make it possible to direct therapy toward breaking the chain of events. In contrast to present-day treatment, which is mainly symptomatic, at least part of future therapy may be prophylactic, with the aim of limiting or preventing the degenerative changes in respiratory function which currently lead to a high mortality rate.
3. Studies of the characteristics of fires and their locations which induce inhalation injury and ways by which the incidence of such injury and its severity can be lessened.

UNCERTAINTIES DURING EARLY TREATMENT

Fluid Resuscitation

The uncertainty with respect to volume, chemical constituents, and rate of administration of early fluid resuscitation of patients with both extensive skin burns and overt smoke inhalation injury arises because such patients tend to develop smoke-induced pulmonary edema, which would be exacerbated by fluid overloads. Yet there is the undoubted need for a high fluid input to maintain an adequate circulating blood volume and cardiac output in the presence of massively increased losses of fluid into the tissues and by exudation and evaporation from the burned surface. The degree to which these conflicting requirements should affect treatment is uncertain.[32,49,63] It has been suggested[63] that resuscitative volumes should be limited in an effort to reduce the pulmonary compromise frequently seen in these patients, whereas retrospective evidence[49] indicates that burned patients with smoke inhalation injury require, on average, a higher fluid input to maintain adequate cardiovascular indices than burned patients without smoke inhalation injury. The unknown factors are the extent and severity of the inhalation injury. These can be assessed qualitatively by fiberoptic bronchoscopy[11,45] and plain chest radiographs[41] and quantitatively by radioisotope lung scans,[51] measurements of lung function, and biochemical evidence of the blood content of certain smoke components (CO, HCN). However the quantitative measurements are time-consuming, and it may be inappropriate to undertake them in a particular patient (e.g., a child). Additionally, smoke contains unknown concentrations (usually small) of numerous chemicals, the detection of which is tedious and the toxicologic effects of which are more or less unknown.[1] Thus it seems unlikely that even prospective well-controlled clinical studies will provide guidance to the fluid requirements of a particular patient.

Two different spheres of study promise help in this regard:

1. Studies in experimental animals with burns alone, smoke inhalation injury with defined smoke alone, and the injuries combined, which have been described in considerable detail in Chaps. 4 and 6.
2. The inclusion of available items of knowledge derived from either experimental animal or human studies into computer models which can predict the responses to unmeasurable reactions at obscure or inaccessible sites.

Of particular importance in this review of the respiratory sequelae of thermal injury are the hemodynamic responses to burns alone, those induced by the administration of crystalloid or colloid solutions,[16] the generalized increase in capillary permeability,[25] and hypoproteinaemia.[18] The consequences of these latter changes within burned and unburned tissues leading to edema formation have been explored in considerable detail.[3]

Computer modeling has simulated the complex interactions between at least six different compartments which are involved in the regulation of the distribution of water, electrolytes, and colloidal molecules in untreated burned animals and patients with burns before and during early fluid therapy.[2,9,59] Such therapy may be hypotonic, isotonic, or hypertonic with respect to the major electrolytes; contain or not contain colloidal molecules (plasma protein or relatively high molecular weight carbohydrates); and be given at rates dictated by one of a number of formulas or depending upon the clinical responses of the patient. The overall structure of the computer simulation model (Fig. 19-1) shows the interactions between the six different modules, which in turn reflect the relationships between the major factors that determine the water changes due to thermal injury of the skin and resuscitation (Fig. 19-2). The development of these models is currently at the stage that proof is now available that the computer-predicted response to a particular form of therapy is closely compatible with the observed clinical responses. Further details of the theoretical

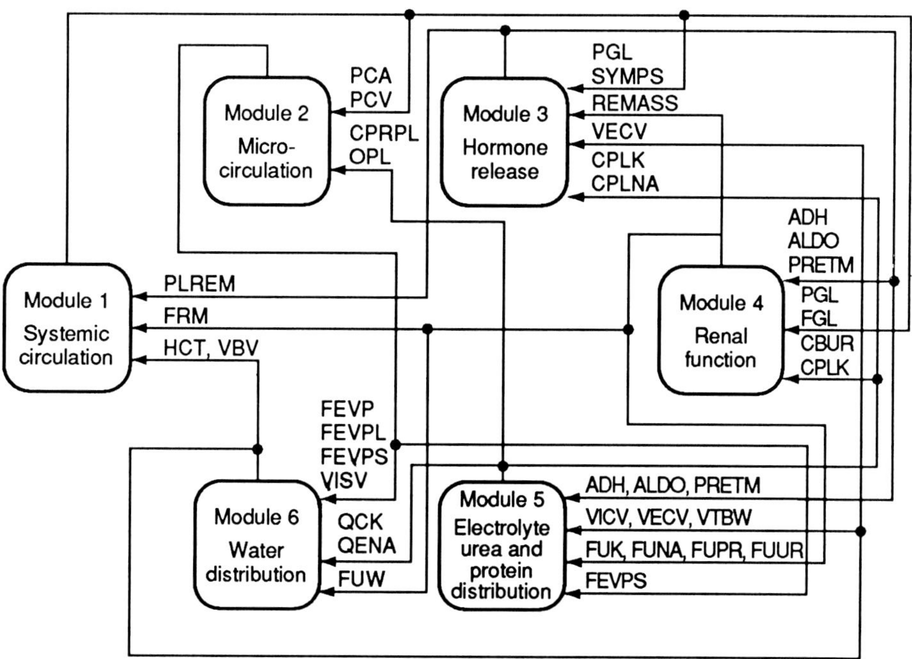

Figure 19-1 The overall structure of the computer simulation model showing the interactions between the six different modules. ADH, antidiuretic hormone multiplier; ALDO, aldosterone multiplier; CBUR, blood urea concentration; CPLK, plasma potassium concentration; CPLNA, plasma sodium concentration; CPRPL, plasma protein mass concentration; FEVP, evaporation rate intact skin; FEVPL, evaporation rate lungs; FEVPS, water evaporation rate, injured skin; FGL, glomerular filtration rate; FRM, renal functional mass multiplier; FUK, urine potassium excretion; FUNA, urine sodium excretion; FUPR, urine protein excretion rate; FUUR, urine urea excretion; FUW, urine water excretion; HCT, erythrocyte volume fraction; OPL, plasma colloid osmotic pressure; PCA, precapillary arterial pressure; PCV, postcapillary venous pressure; PGL, glomerular pressure; PLREM, plasma renin modifier; PRETM, renin effect on renal sodium excretion; QCK, intracellular potassium mass; QENA, extracellular sodium mass; REMASS, renal mass multiplier; SYMPS, relative sympathetic activity multiplier; VBV, blood volume; VECV, extracellular volume; VICV, intracellular volume; VISV, total interstitial volume; VTBW, total body water volume. (*Reprinted by permission of G. Arturson, Burns 14(4):257, 1988.*)

validity and the empirical and pragmatic validations of these models is available.[2,30]

While such computer modeling techniques will undoubtedly elucidate in greater detail the responses to thermal injury which do not involve the respiratory tract at the time of injury (for example, a hot liquid scald on the lower part of the body), there is evidence that such an injury causes perturbations in body processes which are manifest as alterations in pulmonary blood flow and the production of systemic hypotension.[19]

In the context of this review the pulmonary changes are particularly important since smoke inhalation has been shown to increase pulmonary vascular resistance, reduce surfactant concentration or activity, and cause ventilation/perfusion mismatch-

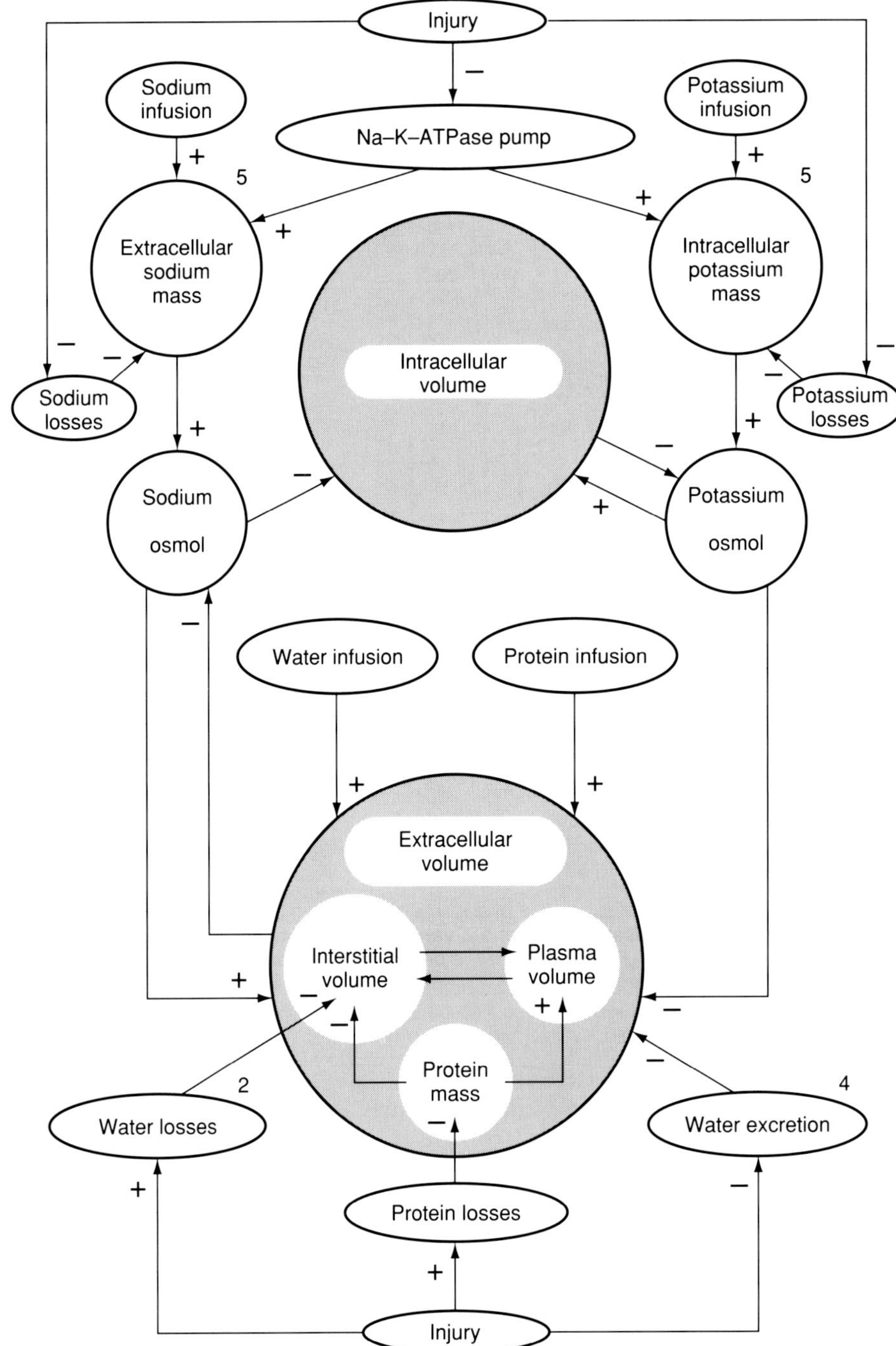

Figure 19-2 Relations between the major factors which determine the water changes due to thermal injury and resuscitation. The plus and minus signs indicate the effect (increase or decrease, respectively) of an increase in the box from which the arrow originates. Numbers 2, 4, and 5 refer to variables imported from other modules. (*Reprinted by permission of G. Arturson, Burns 14(4):257, 1988.*)

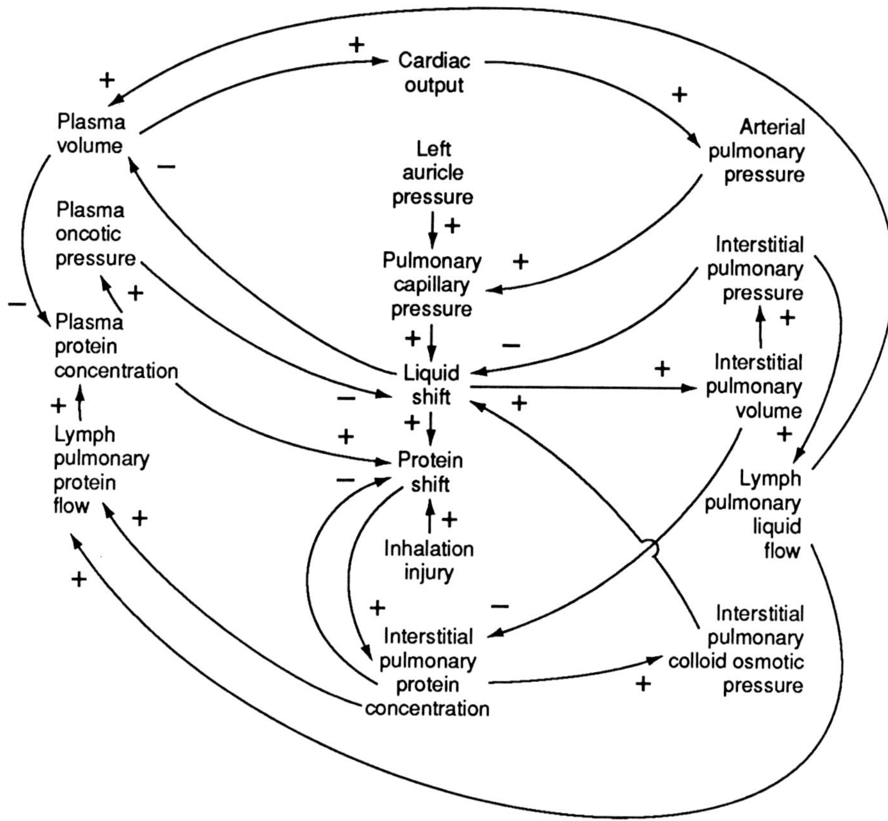

Figure 19-3 Simplified causal diagram of the variables and relationships associated with the pulmonary microcirculation. (*Published with the permission of Roa L, Gomez-Cia T, Cantero A, et al.*[59])

ing.[43,50,60,76] In addition there are increases in pulmonary capillary permeability[61] and the production of lung lymph.[31,73]

The consequences of these changes specifically induced by smoke which develop in patients who are not burned but have been trapped in a smoke-filled room or building or in animals deliberately exposed to smoke have been reviewed[14] and are described in more detail in Chaps. 3 and 4. For future progress it seems likely that computer modeling will continue to be valuable, since preliminary studies have assessed the theoretical, empirical, and pragmatic validation of a subsection of module 2 in Fig. 19-1, in which the pulmonary microcirculation is considered separately from the whole body microcirculation. Figure 19-3 indicates the tentative pathways by which various body compartments exert an influence on lung tissue.[59] Further studies are required to give numerical values to as many as possible of the parameters which are directly related to the function of normal lung tissue, lung tissue affected by inhaled chemicals, lung tissue taken from animals with only burns, and that taken from animals with both types of injury.

Detailed studies in dogs injured in these various ways and showing the generalized pathophysiologic response to the effects of carbon monoxide and smoke in terms of the epithelial and endothelial lesions in lung tissue, surfactant activity, and lung fluid balance described in detail by Clark and Nieman[14] seem destined to provide these data. Supplementary information can be derived from other experimental models of inhalation injury.[23,31,32,35,42,64,70,73,82]

These animal models of inhalation injury have also highlighted some technical problems where the available methods of investigation in live animals are, as yet, unable to differentiate changes in adjacent, sometimes anatomically distinct, areas which are obvious on postmortem examination. For example, smoke inhalation can injure either the tracheobronchial areas alone or these areas and the lung parenchyma. In studies involving the collection of lung lymph, this fluid will be draining from both areas, thereby ruling out a site-specific assessment of the location of the altered capillary permeability. There are also multiple anastomoses between the bronchial and pulmonary circulation which may prevent separation of these two vascular areas.

Another problem involves the use of the thermal-dye dilution technique to measure extravascular lung water content. In humans this dilution technique does not indicate an increased water content in lung tissue, although this is obviously present in postmortem samples of lung tissue. In sheep with a smoke inhalation injury, the thermal-dye dilution technique showed a normal water content, whereas gravimetric analysis of lung tissue showed a significantly raised water content.[55] It has been suggested that poor perfusion of areas of the affected lung are the cause of these discrepant results. An alternative technique for measuring water content not dependent upon complete mixing of an indicator is required.

Hyperbaric Oxygen

This form of therapy of smoke inhalation injury remains controversial.[38] Given that victims suffering from excessive exposure to carbon monoxide require prompt and intensive therapy with oxygen, which methods should be used and when? Immediately following rescue, neurologic symptoms indicative of possible carbon monoxide poisoning (although they may also be due to hypoxia, hypercarbia, or poisoning with cyanide or neurotoxins) require treatment with 100 percent inspired oxygen concentrations. Normally these can only be attained by high flow rates of oxygen delivered from a cylinder with a demand-valve supply and a tight-fitting mask. When ambulances arrive at the scene of the fire, such treatment can be given with pin-index oxygen cylinders connected to Entonox (N_2O/O_2) equipment. Portable ventilators are also more efficient than mouth-to-mouth resuscitation. However all these methods of treatment will be more difficult to implement in the presence of facial burns. In this situation hyperbaric oxygen therapy is almost certainly beneficial; it has been shown to confer a marked reduction in morbidity.[52] It would seem prudent to ensure that all hospital emergency departments and intensive care and burn units should know the location of hyperbaric units in their district, state, or country. The locations of such facilities in the United Kingdom have been reported by Broome et al.[6] Delayed or long-distance transfer to hyperbaric oxygen facilities should not be ruled out since there have been highly rewarding successes following late treatment.[47]

Ventilation Techniques

At some stage after rescue some patients with severe inhalation injury will threaten airway obstruction from tracheal or pulmonary edema or accumulations of tissue debris. Such patients will require intubation or possibly a tracheostomy and perhaps some form of mechanical ventilation. Published reports contain conflicting recommendations for the most appropriate technique for ventilation. The relative safety of positive end-expiratory pressure (PEEP), which is usually required to improve regional ventilation/perfusion mismatch, has been questioned by Clark and Beeley.[12] Also, the peak inspiratory pressures of 50 cmH_2O used by Kolobow et al.[40] during ventilation of normal sheep with 40 percent oxygen produced lung damage when continued for 48 hours. It would not be unexpected if the pressures used in these studies caused additional injury to lung tissue already damaged by smoke.

It has been suggested that the lymphatic drainage of fluid is the critical factor in protecting lung tissue from the deleterious effects of pulmonary edema,[68] and there is conflicting evidence that lymphatic flow from the lungs is influenced by the pattern of respiration.[34,77] Definitive studies are required in normal animals, animals with burns alone, those with smoke inhalation alone (preferably with smokes of defined chemical composition), and those with a combination of both burns and smoke inhalation. The sheep model used by Traber et al.,[73] with the ability to monitor lymph flow from separate lungs and the use of a divided insufflation tube to inflict smoke injury on one lung alone, in vivo, would seem to be appropriate for such studies.

Cyanide Inhalation and Antidotes

While carbon monoxide has been accepted as the major hazard in fire-induced inhalation injury since at least the Cocoanut Grove fire in 1942, the relatively recent widespread use of polyacrylonitrile and polyurethane foam in furnishing materials has highlighted hydrogen cyanide as another major hazard.[1,66] Polyurethane foam has the ability, after ignition, to burn in the *absence of atmospheric oxygen* with the production of copious quantities of HCN and CO. A recent study has suggested that HCN poisoning is the major cause of death at the scene of a fire or during the period soon after rescue or soon after admission to hospital.[66] Since fire-injured victims may still have near-lethal blood cyanide levels after admission to hospital, it is unfortunate that many hospital emergency departments do not have, and ambulances rarely carry, portable gas detection tubes for rapid screening for cyanide poisoning. Such tubes are commercially available and allow the detection of elevated cyanide concentrations in expiratory gas as well as in blood samples.[15] Such detection tubes can replace the more tedious colorimetric or gas chromatographic methods.[75] While the detection tubes are less accurate for cyanide measurements than the more complex analytical methodologies, they are speedy and accurate enough to have an effect on therapeutic decisions.[56]

The introduction and widespread use of cyanide gas detection tubes in patients with overt inhalation injury or a history of prolonged confinement in a smoke-filled enclosed space will emphasize the problem of whether, assuming a positive test result, an antidote to cyanide poisoning should be given and which one. The detailed review by Prien and Traber[56] lists the following alternative remedies:

1. Induction of cyanmethemoglobin formation following administration of amyl or sodium nitrites or 4-dimethyl amino phenol
2. Administration of the chelating agents dicobalt edate or hydroxycobalamin
3. Administration of thiosulfate to enhance the detoxification of cyanide by the mitochondrial enzyme rhodanase

Current experience suggests that administration of thiosulfate has the least adverse side effects with the lowest toxicity and the probable induction of an osmotic diuresis with beneficial renal clearance of thiocyanate. A more rapidly acting effective antidote to cyanide is hydroxycobalamin. Kits are available in France containing 4 g hydroxycobalamin to be diluted with sodium thiosulfate.[27] These kits are more useful than the normally available hydroxycobalamin preparations with concentrations of 1 mg/mL, since adequate detoxification requires doses of about 100 mg/kg body weight.

Since the recommendations by Prien and Traber[56] are at variance with the use of dicobalt edate as the antidote of choice in the United Kingdom,[12] the relative merits of these various forms of therapy will require further study when routine testing of patients with presumed or actual smoke-inhalation injury is adopted.

MORE FUNDAMENTAL STUDIES OF CELLULAR AND SUBCELLULAR RESPONSES TO SKIN BURNS AND SMOKE INHALATION INJURY

Until recently most of the evidence for degenerative changes developing in lung tissue as a result of skin burns or smoke inhalation or both has been derived from postmortem studies in humans or tissue and cell samples taken from unconscious animals just before or immediately after death. Such degenerative changes can affect the mucosa of the respiratory tract; the tissues in the lowest parts of the respiratory tree (the alveolar membrane and the interstitial spaces); the free existing cells which normally inhabit lung tissue (macrophages); and the polymorphonuclear cells which are attracted to lung tissue injured by heat, chemicals, or microorganisms (usually bacteria but occasionally fungi or viruses).

Recent reports of the damage caused by smoke include alveolar membrane damage, intraalveolar hemorrhage, and an inflammatory cell infiltration,[5,8] all of which are distinct from the changes induced by thermal damage to the airway and the effects on the lung tissue of remote skin burns.

The introduction and increasing use of flexible bronchoscopes has made possible the lavage of cells (mainly macrophages) from living lungs, often in animals and sometimes in humans, on a repetitive basis, during the period between injury and recovery of normal lung function or death.[28,54] Likely future studies of the cellular changes consequent on inhalation injury are to specify which of the numerous chemicals in smoke are responsible for the observed macrophage and tissue changes, which modify the alveolar membrane directly, and which inactivate or destroy surfactant. The requirement for a defined smoke produced by the admixture of chemically pure compounds is obvious. The reports that carbon monoxide causes pulmonary edema[24] and that acrolein induces a form of lung injury that can be modified by the administration of methylprednisolone[5] are steps in the right direction.

With respect to the constituents in smoke, advice from industrial toxicologists and research departments of the tobacco industry will almost certainly be beneficial, since they are familiar with the technology required to analyze air or smoke containing chemicals at low concentrations. Various fire research organizations can produce smokes with defined constituents at predictable concentrations.[53]

Functional Changes Induced in Lung Macrophages

Much of the damage found in lung tissue after both skin burns and smoke inhalation seems to arise through damage to the function of macrophages[22,44] The changes are more marked after smoke inhalation, which induces decreases in macrophage chemotaxis and the phagocytosis of bacteria.[17,26] These decreases may only be transient in humans, since chemoluminescence techniques[28,54] have shown increased macrophage activity (by bursts of respiratory activity and oxygen free radical production) as early as 4 hours after smoke inhalation injury. When the injury is a combination of skin burns and smoke inhalation, the increased macrophage activity is greater still.[39]

Macrophages activated by skin burns or smoke or both release a number of proteolytic enzymes which have been shown to exacerbate the cellular damage caused by oxygen free radical release.[36] This combination of enzyme release, free radicals ($OH^- O^{2-}$, H_2O_2), and the pulmonary damage they cause may be the result of indiscriminate hyperactivity of host defense cells.[48] Kinsella[39] has suggested that the mechanisms by which lung damage develops after burns and smoke inhalation resemble the factors preceding the development of the adult respiratory distress syndrome (ARDS). The clinical picture which develops in smoke and/or burn-injured patients meets the criteria for diagnosing ARDS.[62] As the mechanisms and the final clinical picture developing in these patients is indistinguishable from ARDS, then smoke inhalation might be an appropriate model for studying ARDS. As the patients who develop respiratory distress do so after a period in which they appear to be relatively well, then it may be possible to devise a form of therapy which breaks one of the links in the chain of steps shown

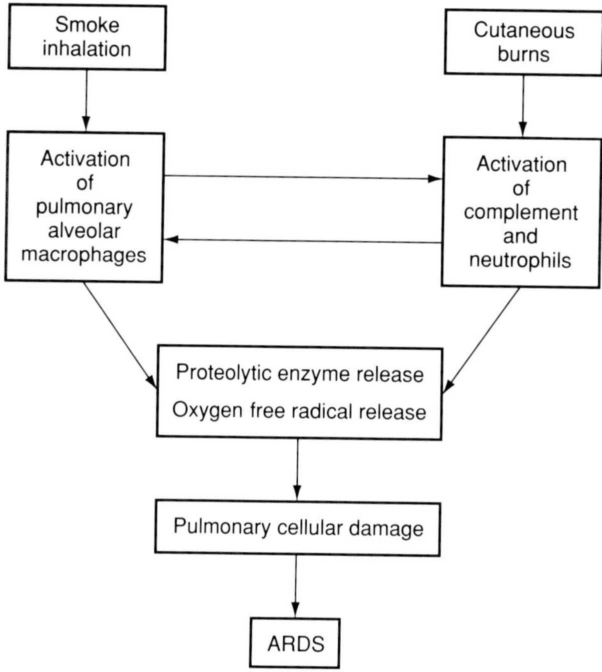

Figure 19-4 Proposed mechanisms for the development of the Adult Respiratory Distress Syndrome (ARDS) in victims with smoke inhalation injury and cutaneous burns. (*Published with the permission of J. Kinsella, Burns 14(4):269, 1988.*)

in Fig. 19-4 and thereby prevent the full syndrome developing. Certainly this is a line of study that merits further investigation, not only for the benefit of patients injured by skin burns or smoke but also when adult respiratory distress syndrome arises from other causes.

The realization that there is a lag phase between injury by the chemicals in smoke and the clinical manifestation of respiratory distress suggests that, if substances liberated by damaged (or activated) macrophages having proven harmful effects could be identified, their action or actions might be limited or neutralized. This suggestion is a challenge for the future, since the chemicals produced by activated macrophages are remarkably diverse. Some are directly toxic in their own right (the free radicals); others stimulate the production of vasoactive histamine and the kinins. A third group initiate the chemotactic cascades involving arachidonic acid, the prostaglandins, the interleukins, the coagulation system, the complement system, and neutrophil migration. These materials usually act in a highly integrated manner to modulate the inflammatory response to injury or sepsis. They probably control the way the acute injury induced by smoke resolves or progresses to respiratory distress and are important in defining the clinical consequences of the injury.[14] A probable first step in unraveling this complex pattern of responses is to determine whether the observed changes are the cause of the clinical response, a byproduct, or an epiphenomenon. Some indicators along this pathway are the observations that neutrophil depletion prior to injury in animals lessens the pulmonary complications,[72] that animals genetically unable to produce the complement degradation product C5a do not develop lung complications following injury and that lung damage is reduced if the animals receive agents that either prevent oxygen free radical production or that scavenge oxygen free radicals once they have been produced.[7,20]

Drug Treatment

Drug treatment of victims of smoke inhalation injury is still in its infancy. To date, published reports appear to be confined to the use of ibuprofen, indomethacin, dimethyl sulfoxide plus heparin, and adrenocorticosteroids for the early effects of smoke inhalation, and modulators of collagen synthesis such as colchicine, penicillamine, or corticosteroids[33] for late end-stage fibrosing lung damage.

Ibuprofen and Indomethacin These drugs have been used in the treatment of smoke-injured rats[65] and sheep.[37] Ibuprofen prevented the formation of pulmonary edema in the rats, while indomethacin failed to provide similar protection. It has been suggested that products derived from arachidonic acid are involved in the formation of pulmonary edema. In the rats there was a selective generation of prostacyclin without an increase in thromboxane production, results which suggest that prostacyclin might be a promising form of treatment for inhalation injury. The differential effects of ibuprofen and indomethacin highlight the need for subtle manipulations of the factors based on arachidonic acid to achieve desirable results.

Adrenocorticosteroids The role of various corticosteroids in the management of smoke inhalation injury is controversial. The raison d'être for their use, to reduce airway edema and bronchial spasm, must be balanced against the increased susceptibility to infection which their administration engenders. Human studies in smoke inhalation–injured patients have indicated that steroids increase mortality[46,81] or do not increase mortality.[42]

Even the use of well-controlled experimental animal studies has not resolved this discrepancy, since Stone et al.[71] reported that steroids increased the mortality rate whereas administration of dexamethasone[81] and high doses of methylprednisolone[5,23] reduced the mortality rate. In the latter study, this improved survival rate occurred despite the fact that no differences could be shown in the pathological findings in the lungs between the treated and untreated groups of animals.

An extensive prospective controlled trial of the use of steroids in patients with smoke inhalation injury seems warranted now that the extent of injury can be determined using flexible bronchoscopy, lung scans, and lung function studies. The earlier studies probably gave confusing results because of variations in the severity of the airway injury. In addition some of the uncertainty may have been the result of differences in the nature or concentrations of the major or minor toxic chemicals in smoke. The use of chemically defined smokes, discussed in more detail below in experimental animal models should resolve this aspect of the uncertainty.

Dimethylsulfoxide Plus Heparin This has been used as a scavenger for the oxygen free radicals produced when alveolar macrophages are activated either directly by chemicals in smoke or by one or more of the compounds in the arachidonic acid cascade.[7,20,21] Lipid materials can also neutralize oxygen free radicals by combining with them to form conjugated dienes.[4] Future studies may well discover new more efficient oxygen free radical scavengers or a group of compounds which break the chain of oxygen free radical production.

Tobacco Smoke Studies

A promising line of study has emanated from the numerous reports describing the toxicity of tobacco smoke and its effect on lung tissue (see review by Church and Pryor[10]). It has been shown that tobacco smoke stimulates alveolar macrophages to undergo "respiratory bursts" with the production of superoxide, hydrogen peroxide, and oxygen and hydroxyl free radicals. This process is apparently identical with that produced by the smoke encountered in burning buildings or from the combustion of domestic furniture or fittings.

Information arising from these studies which does not appear to have been considered in the clinical situation of acute fire-smoke inhalation injury is the discovery that a wide range of highly reactive free radicals are present in both the tar (particulate) and gas phase of tobacco smoke.[10] By convention the gas phase of tobacco smoke is that material which will pass through a filter with a pore size of 0.1 μm; the particulate- or tar-phase material is trapped by such a glass fiber filter.

The principal free radical in the particulate matter is relatively stable; it is a quinone-hydroquinone complex which is an active redox system that is capable of reducing molecular oxygen to produce superoxide, then hydrogen peroxide, and finally the hydroxyl radical. This complex has also been shown to react with DNA in vitro, possibly by covalent bonding. The carcinogenic implications of this binding are beyond the scope of this review.

The gas phase of tobacco smoke contains small oxygen- and carbon-centered radicals that are much more reactive than the particulate-phase free radicals. These gas-phase radicals do not arise in the flame but are produced in a steady state by the oxidation of nitric oxide (NO) to nitrogen dioxide

(NO_2), which then reacts with reactive species in smoke such as isoprene. (Modern building and furnishing materials contain relatively large quantities of combined nitrogen. Although combustion of these materials results in the production of large quantities of cyanide gas, the various oxides of nitrogen are also present at concentrations sufficient for the probable production of free radicals.)

It is pertinent to note that this separation of tobacco smoke into gaseous and particulate fractions by filters and the fact that the biologic hazard resides particularly in the particulate matter (filter-tipped cigarettes are said to be "safer" than nonfilter-tipped cigarettes) has relevance to studies of the toxicity of acute fire-induced smoke inhalation injury. When experimental animals inhale unfiltered fire smoke, a standard pattern of pathophysiologic and histochemical changes develops. These changes in surfactant activity, production of atelectasis, and altered lung mechanics are very much less marked when the smoke is passed through a 0.5μm-pore-size filter before inhalation.[13,50] Finally, anecdotal reports from victims who have survived fire disasters suggest that persons who protected their mouths and noses with cloths, preferably wet, suffered less severe inhalation injury.

Biological Effects of Free Radicals in Smoke

Church and Pryor[10] have suggested that these radicals and the metastable products derived from these radical reactions may be responsible for the inactivation of alpha 1 proteinase inhibitor by fresh smoke. (Alpha 1 proteinase inhibitor is the major serum antiproteinase in humans, accounting for more than 90 percent of the functional antielastase activity in the bronchoalveolar fluid of normal individuals.[69]) In normal lung tissue there is a balance between protease and antiprotease activity. Lung connective tissues are probably protected from leukocyte proteases by endogenous protease inhibitors. As described earlier in this volume there is ample evidence that acute smoke inhalation injury is associated with increased release of proteases from alveolar macrophages. It has been implied that the quantity of protease released overwhelms the antiprotease activity available from alpha 1 proteinase inhibitor. This saturation of antiprotease activity could be the result of either a mass excess of proteolytic activity over available (in situ) antiproteolytic activity *or* inactivation of part of the available antiproteolytic activity by other mechanisms. This latter suggestion is realistic, since oxygen species in the inhaled smoke or produced by activated polymorphonuclear leukocytes can oxidise alpha 1 proteinase inhibitor to an inactive form.

All these similarities between the effects of tobacco smoke and fire smoke suggest that the well-developed technologies used by the tobacco industry and the "antismoking lobby" should be applied to the investigation of mechanisms involved in the induction of respiratory distress following acute smoke inhalation.

Probably one of the most important techniques that should be used for these investigations is electron spin resonance (ESR) spectroscopy. This technique has the ability to detect minute amounts of free radicals among a vast excess of stable (relatively inactive) molecules. The technical details of free radical measurements and the biologic significance of the undoubted presence of a variety of free radicals in many types of smoke have been described in the following review articles and the large number of references appended to each review.[10,29,67,78]

PREDICTIONS OF FIRE-INDUCED HAZARDS AND THEIR USE IN LESSENING THE INCIDENCE AND SEVERITY OF SMOKE INHALATION INJURY

This section gives details of the environmental conditions which may surround a victim trapped in a burning room or building. They are important for the following reasons:

1. They will dictate the degree of injury that the victim will sustain, whether the victim dies at the scene of the fire or soon after rescue or soon af-

ter admission to hospital or during the subsequent days or weeks, or survives.
2. They will dictate the speed with which rescue must take place if the victim is not to die at the scene of the fire.
3. They will reflect the nature of the materials that underwent combustion.

The specification of the conditions developing during a fire should lead to the design of safer materials which produce less toxic smoke or ignite less easily and to assessments of the efficacy of protective devices against inhalation injury. It should also confirm the desirability of the domestic installation of heat and smoke detectors and water sprinkler systems.

Assessment of Risk Factors

Earlier chapters and references[1,80] have given some indication of the extreme diversity of the chemicals in smoke. Indeed each fire produces a unique smoke, the constituents in which are a reflection of the types and quantities of fuel consumed and the conditions (oxygen supply and temperature) within the fire, which will also vary with the time after ignition. Fortunately it appears that, in spite of the great variety of synthetic and natural materials which are burned during a fire in domestic premises, the toxicity of the combustion products is not as complex as their chemistry. Virtually all the combustion products have relatively simple toxic potencies and toxic effects which are relatively similar. Most of the latter are caused by a small number of well-known toxic products.[58,79] The recently described highly reactive free radicals (discussed above) are the probable exceptions.

A fruitful line of investigation relevant to the survival or otherwise of persons trapped in close proximity to a fire is developing as a consequence of the mathematical modeling of the degrees of hazard associated with fires and their combustion products.[57]

The toxic hazards of fires become predictable if the time-concentration profiles of the important toxic fire products and the time-concentration-toxicity relationships of these products in humans, when they occur individually and in combination, are available. The currently extant mathematical model predicts the time to incapacitation or death in fires for human fire victims provided that the time-concentration (or intensity) profiles of carbon monoxide, hydrogen cyanide, carbon dioxide, oxygen, mass concentration loss of total fire products (also indicative of the quantity of irritant chemicals produced), smoke optical density, radiant heat flux, and air temperature close to the victim are known.

Combustion products from fires cause incapacitation or death by two main mechanisms, narcosis and irritancy.[58] Narcosis following exposure to high levels of CO, CO_2, and HCN and low levels of O_2 affects the nervous and cardiovascular systems, causing loss of consciousness and, if the victim is not rescued quickly, death from asphyxiation. Irritant fire products cause immediate painful sensory stimulation of the eyes, nose, throat, and lungs; subsequently lung inflammation and edema may develop and lead to death from respiratory failure.

These mathematical modeling procedures are presented in some detail because of their ability to predict the time to incapacitation, in effect death, in most situations. In practice these times are those available to a victim in which to escape or for the rescue personnel to remove the victim from the immediate location of the fire and smoke with a significant chance of survival.

The time to incapacitation has been calculated by Purser[57] for exposure to the time-concentration profiles of the factors listed above following the ignition of an armchair with polyurethane cushions in a room of 29 m^3 volume and with an open doorway. Using the equations given in the Appendix for fractional incapacitating dose for each hazard, an allowance for the multiplying effect of hyperventilation induced by levels of CO_2 between 5 and 7 percent, the synergism between CO and HCN, the degree of visual obscuration caused by smoke particles, the incapacitating effect of radiant and convected heat and of irritant chemicals causing early blindness, paroxysmal coughing and disorientation and later respiratory embarassment, it is possible to conclude the following for a victim exposed to these conditions in the room with the burning armchair:

1. Toward the end of the second minute and the start of the third minute the smoke optical density and mass loss per liter would exceed the tenability limits for visual obscuration and sensory irritancy to the extent that escape from the room would be severely inhibited.
2. During the fourth minute the average temperature in the room would be 220°C, sufficient heat to cause deep skin burns on exposed areas.
3. During the fifth minute the victim would probably lose consciousness as a result of the combined effects of the accumulated narcotic gases.

It is predicted that a victim escaping or rescued after the fourth minute would suffer severe postexposure effects due to skin burns, possible laryngeal burns with accompanying edema and the danger of obstructive asphyxiation. A fatal pulmonary edema and inflammation may develop as a result of the combined effect of the inhaled chemical irritants and the secondary pulmonary effects of the skin burns. After the sixth minute it is likely that a victim would die between a few minutes and 1 hour later due to the combined effects of narcosis, circulatory "shock," and possibly hyperthermia.

It is unlikely that an otherwise healthy adult would be able to escape from such a fire if the victim remained longer than 3 minutes after ignition. However 3 minutes is a long time in which to leave a room, so that, provided the victim is awake and aware of the fire, is not otherwise incapacitated by, for example, ethyl alcohol intoxication or drug abuse or physical infirmity and does not stay after 2 minutes in an attempt to fight the fire or rescue precious possessions or family members, it is likely that the person would be able to escape without serious injury.

A number of benefits accrue from this ability to predict the time involved in the buildup of a hostile environment. In terms of the prevention of fire-induced inhalation injury, tests can indicate whether furnishings and fittings in a structure will produce a potentially lethal environment for persons in the structure who will be unable to evacuate (or be rescued) in time. The potential to evacuate a building or aircraft "in an orderly manner" under normal conditions is very different from that under the conditions in the cabin of the Boeing 737 aircraft on the ground at Manchester Airport (UK), where panic reigned when jet fuel ignited outside the rear of the aircraft and fire penetrated into the cabin and ignited the rear seats within about 2 minutes. Although the fire was extinguished by 7 minutes after its ignition, more than 50 people died in the aircraft within the period between 2 and 7 minutes, mostly from the inhalation of toxic chemicals in smoke. The victims would probably have had a reasonable chance of survival if simple forms of breathing apparatus had been readily available. Such devices with a safe air supply from a cylinder or ambient air rendered safe by filters are present in UK Royal Navy ships, military aircraft, coal mines, and some factories.[12] They are desirable in any location where there is a significant risk of smoke exposure. The equipment is relatively inexpensive, can be donned in seconds, and provides a few minutes' supply of clean air to allow escape or rescue.

The ability to predict the narcotic and irritant hazards from smoke has made it possible to test the efficacy of various forms of breathing apparatus which rely on filters to purify the ambient air. Measurements of the time-concentration-toxicity relationships of air samples taken before and after filtration have indicated the characteristics of filters required for adequate protection, for specified time periods, and against chemically defined smokes. Such smokes have only recently been produced.[53]

As newer synthetic materials are used on an increasing scale in buildings and their contents, the ability to predict the rate of production of a hostile or lethal environment will be vital. It seems reasonable to suggest that routine testing of all new materials to be incorporated in buildings or their contents should result in them being given a "hazard rating" depending on the toxicity of their combustion products.

Unfortunately the furnishings and fittings in domestic premises and probably aircraft will continue to be made of a mixture of natural and synthetic materials which rapidly produce a hostile environment when set on fire. Since it is unlikely that non-flammable materials will be developed for fittings and furnishings in the near future, attempts should be made to minimize the use of the most hazardous materials and the likelihood of ignition of these materials.

In this regard the UK government has legislated that standard polyurethane foam should no longer be used in soft furnishings—high-resilience, higher-ignition-temperature foam must be used. In the United States, considerable progress is being made toward the introduction of a fire-safe cigarette. Such a cigarette is self-extinguishing unless air is drawn through it. When a lit cigarette of this type is laid on the flammable fabric of a chair or cushion, the cigarette "goes out" before the fabric is ignited. Other factors which may help to reduce the incidence of fires in domestic premises are changes from open sources of room heating (fires and gas flame heaters) to hot water radiators or convected warm air and a reduced availability of matches—which will follow a reduction in the incidence of cigarette, cigar, and pipe smoking. Fires started by electrical faults will only decrease when safer wiring practices are required by law and routinely checked. If fires do start, the incidence of significant smoke or thermal injury may be reduced if the premises are fitted with heat and smoke detectors and possibly a water sprinkler system. However a recent survey[74] has shown that many smoke inhalation injuries occurred when smoldering armchairs, ignited by cigarettes or lit matches, produced lethal or near lethal amounts of toxic chemicals without enough particulate smoke to activate the smoke detectors and without the production of enough heat to activate either the heat detectors or the water sprinkler system.

Nevertheless it seems reasonable to suggest that changes in the types of materials used in furnishings and fittings and minimizing the likelihood of ignition of these materials are the challenges for the future. A successful response to this challenge will surely convert the high incidence of smoke inhalation injury described in the early chapters of this book to a significantly declining incidence.

APPENDIX

The toxic effects of most combustion products depend on dose received rather than ambient concentration, i.e.,

$$\text{dose} = \text{concentration} \times \text{time of exposure} \quad \text{(Haber's rule)}$$

Fractional incapacitating dose (FID) =

$$\frac{\text{dose received at time } t\ (ct)}{\text{effective } ct \text{ dose to cause incapacitation or death}}$$

When the sum of the FIDs reaches unity, incapacitation or death occurs.

The following FID equations have been used in the model:

$$\text{Carbon monoxide } \mathrm{FI_{CO}} = \frac{K(\mathrm{CO}^{1.036})(t)}{D}$$

where

CO = carbon monoxide
t = exposure time in minutes
K = 0.00082925 for an RMV of 25 L/min
D = COHb concentration at incapacitation (30% for light work)
RMV = respiratory minute volume

$$\text{Hydrogen cyanide } \mathrm{FI_{CN}} = \frac{1}{185 - \text{ppm HCN}/4.4}$$

$$\text{Hypoxia } \mathrm{FI_{O_2}} = \frac{1}{\exp\,[8.13 - 0.54(20.9 - \%\mathrm{O_2})]}$$

$$\text{Carbon dioxide } \mathrm{FI_{CO2}} = \frac{1}{\exp\,(6.1623 - 0.5189 \times \%\mathrm{CO_2})}$$

All narcotic gases combined (FI_N):

$$FI_N = (FI_{CO} + FI_{CN}) \times V_{CO_2} + (FI_{O_2} \text{ or } FI_{CO_2})$$

where

$$V_{CO_2} = \frac{\exp(0.2496 \times \%CO_2 + 1.9086)}{6.8}$$

Radiant heat-tenability limit = 0.25 w/cm^2 ($2.5KW/m^2$)

$$\text{Convected heat } FI_H = \frac{1}{\exp(5.1849 - 0.0273°C)}$$

Smoke visual obscuration—tenability limit of extinction coefficient 1.2/m (OD/m 0.5), where OD = optical density

Sensory irritation—tenability limit of l mg/L

Pulmonary irritation—tenability limit of 10 mg/L

Further details of the derivation of these equations, where Haber's rule has limited applicability and the factors governing the tenability limits can be found in Purser.[57]

REFERENCES

1. Anderson RA, Thomson I, Harland WA: The importance of cyanide and organic nitriles in fire fatalities. *Fire Materials* 3(2):91, 1979.
2. Arturson G: Computer simulation of fluid resuscitation in thermal injury. A. B. Wallace memorial lecture 1987. *Burns* 14(4):257, 1988.
3. Arturson G, Groth T, Hedlund A, et al: Potential use of computer simulation in treatment of burns with special regard to oedema formation. *Scand J Plast Reconstr Surg* 18:39, 1984.
4. Basadre J, Kimura R, Traber LD, et al: Leukopenia attenuates the lung injury in smoke inhalation. *Physiologist* 30:144, 1987.
5. Beeley JM, Crow J, Jones JG, et al: Mortality and lung histopathology after inhalation lung injury. *Am Rev Respir Dis* 133:191, 1986.
6. Broome JR, Skrine H, Pearson RR: Carbon monoxide poisoning—forgotten not gone. *Br J Hosp Med* 39(4):298, 1988.
7. Brown M, Desai MH, Traber LD, et al: Dimethyl sulfoxide with heparin in the treatment of smoke inhalation injury. *J Burn Care Rehabil* 9(1):22, 1988.
8. Burns TR, Greenberg SD, Cartwright J, et al: Smoke inhalation: An ultrastructural study of reaction to injury in the human alveolar wall. *Environ Res* 41:447, 1986.
9. Bush JW, Scheider AM, Wachtel TL, et al: A simulation analysis of plasma water dynamics and treatment in acute burn resuscitation. *J Burn Care Rehabil* 7(1):86, 1986.
10. Church DF, Pryor WA: Free radical chemistry of cigarette smoke and its toxicological implications. *Environ Health Perspec* 64:111, 1985.
11. Clark CJ, Reid WH, Telfer ABM, et al: Respiratory injury in the burned patient. *Anaesthesia* 38:35, 1983.
12. Clark RJ, Beeley JM: Smoke inhalation. Personal communication, 1988.
13. Clark WR, Webb WR, Wax S, et al: Inhalation injuries: The pathophysiology of acute smoke inhalation. *Surg Forum* 28:177, 1977.
14. Clark WR, Nieman GF: Smoke inhalation. *Burns* 14(6):473, 1988.
15. Daunderer M: Vergiftungmit Brandgasen. *Deutsch Aerzteblatt* 79:46, 1982.
16. Davies JWL: *Physiological Responses to Burning Injury*. London, Academic, 1982, Chap. 5, pp 142–192.
17. Demarest GB, Hudson LD, Altman LC: Impaired alveolar macrophage chemotaxis in patients with acute smoke inhalation. *Am Rev Respir Dis* 119:279, 1979.
18. Demling RH, Neihaus G, Perea A, et al: Effect of burn induced hypoproteinaemia on pulmonary transvascular fluid filtration rate. *Surgery* 85:339, 1979.
19. Demling RH, Will JA, Belzer FO: Effect of major thermal injury on the pulmonary microcirculation. *Surgery* 83:746, 1978.
20. Desai MH, Brown M, Mlcak R, et al: Reduction of smoke lung injury with dimethylsufoxide (DMSO) and heparin treatment. *Surg Forum* 36:103, 1985.
21. Desai MH, Brown M, Mlcak R, et al: Nebulization treatment of smoke inhalation injury in sheep model with dimethylsulfoxide, heparin combination and N acetylcysteine. *Crit Care Med* 14:321, 1986.
22. Dressler DP, Skornik WA: Alveolar macrophage in the burned rat. *J Trauma* 14:1036, 1974.
23. Dressler DP, Skornik WA, Kupersmith S: Corticosteroid treatment of experimental smoke inhalation. *Ann Surg* 183:46, 1975.
24. Fein A, Grossman RF, Jones JG, et al: Carbon monoxide effect on alveolar epithelial permeability. *Chest* 78:726, 1980.
25. Fein A, Grossman RF, Jones JG, et al. Effect of major burns on alveolar epithelial permeability in rabbits. *Crit Care Med* 9:669, 1981.
26. Fick RB, Paul ES, Merrill WW, et al: Alterations in the

antibacterial properties of rabbit pulmonary macrophages exposed to wood smoke. *Am Rev Respir Dis* 129:76, 1984.
27. Garnier R, Bismuth C, Riboulet-Delmas G, et al: Poisoning from fumes from polystyrene fire. *Br Med J* 283:1610, 1981.
28. Gemmell CG, Pollok AJ, Campbell D: Functional status of human alveolar cells following smoke inhalation. Abstract 74, Internat Symp Infect Immunocompromised Host, Ronneby-Brun, Sweden, June 15–19, 1986.
29. Halliwell B, Gutteridge JMC: *Free Radicals in Biology and Medicine*. Oxford, Clarendon, 1985, pp 1–346.
30. Hedlund A, Zaar B, Groth T, et al: Computer simulation of fluid resuscitation in trauma: 1. Description of an extensive pathophysiological model and its first validation. *Comp Meth Progr Biomed* 27:7, 1988.
31. Herndon DN, Traber DL, Niehaus GD, et al: The pathophysiology of smoke inhalation in a sheep model. *J Trauma* 24:1044, 1984.
32. Herndon DN, Traber DL, Traber LD: The effect of resuscitation on inhalational injury. *Surgery* 100:248, 1986.
33. Hesterberg TW, Last JA: Ozone induced acute pulmonary fibrosis in rats: Prevention of increased rates of collagen synthesis by methyl prednisolone. *Am Rev Respir Dis* 123:47, 1981.
34. Jefferies AL, Hamilton P, O'Brodovich HM: Effect of high frequency oscillation on lung lymph flow. *J Appl Physiol Respir Environ Exer Physiol* 55:1373, 1982.
35. Jiang KY, Li AN, Pan J, et al: Blood gas studies in dogs with severe steam inhalation injury. *Burns* 13(5):371, 1987.
36. Johnston RB, Godzik CA, Cohn ZA: Increased superoxide anion production by immunologically activated and chemically elicited macrophages. *J Exp Med* 148:115, 1978.
37. Kimura R, Traber LD, Herndon DN, et al: Ibuprofen reduces the lung lymph flow changes associated with inhalation injury. *Circ Shock* 24:183, 1988.
38. Kindwall EP: Hyperbaric treatment of carbon monoxide poisoning. *Ann Intern Med* 14:1233, 1985.
39. Kinsella J: Smoke inhalation. *Burns* 14(4):269, 1988.
40. Kolobow T, Moretti MP, Fumagalli R, et al: Severe impairment in lung function induced by high peak airway pressure during mechanical ventilation. *Am Rev Respir Dis* 135:312, 1987.
41. Lee MJ, O'Connell DJ: The plain chest radiograph after acute smoke inhalation. *Clin Radiol* 39:33, 1988.
42. Levine BA, Petroff PA, Slade L, et al: Prospective trials of dexamethasone and aerosolized gentamicin in the treatment of inhalational injury in the burned patient. *J Trauma* 18:188, 1978.
43. Loke JSO, Paul E, Virgulto JA, et al: Rabbit lung after acute smoke inhalation. *Arch Surg* 119:956, 1984.
44. Loose LD, Megirian R, Turinsky J. Biochemical and functional alterations in macrophages after thermal injury. *Infect Immun* 44:554, 1984.
45. Moylan JA, Adib K, Birnbaum M: Fiberoptic bronchoscopy following thermal injury. *Surg Gynecol Obstet* 140:541, 1975.
46. Moylan JA, Alexander AG: Diagnosis and treatment of inhalation injury. *World J Surg* 2:185, 1978.
47. Myers RAM, Snyder SK, Emhoff TA: Value of hyperbaric oxygen in suspected carbon monoxide poisoning. *JAMA* 246:2478, 1981.
48. Nathan CF, Silverstein SC, Bruckner LH, et al: Extracellular cytolysis by activated macrophages and granulocytes. *J Exp Med* 149:100, 1979.
49. Navar PD, Saffle JR, Warden GD: Effect of inhalation injury on fluid resuscitation requirements after thermal injury. *Am J Surg* 150:716, 1985.
50. Neiman GF, Clark WR, Wax SD, et al: The effect of smoke on pulmonary surfactant. *Ann Surg* 191:171, 1980.
51. Nider A: The effects of low levels of carbon monoxide on the fine structures of terminal airways. *Am Rev Respir Dis* 103:898, 1971.
52. Norkool DM, Kirkpatrick JN: Treatment of acute carbon monoxide poisoning with hyperbaric oxygen: A review of 115 cases. *Ann Emerg Med* 14:1168, 1985.
53. Paul K: Personal communication, 1986.
54. Pollok AJ, Gemmell, CG, Clark CJ, et al: Functional status of pulmonary alveolar macrophages following exposure to toxic gases. *Br J Anaesth* 59:943P, 1987.
55. Prien T, Traber LD, Herndon DN, et al: Pulmonary edema with smoke inhalation, undetected by indicator dilution technique. *J Appl Physiol* 63(3):907, 1987.
56. Prien T, Traber DL: Toxic smoke compounds and inhalation injury: A review. *Burns* 14(6):451, 1988.
57. Purser DA: Modelling toxic and physical hazards in fires. *J Fire Sci,* in press, 1988.
58. Purser DA, Woolley WD: Biological studies of combustion atmospheres. *J Fire Sci* 1:118, 1983.
59. Roa L, Gomez-Cia T, Cantero A, et al: Pulmonary capillary dynamics and fluid distribution after burns and inhalation injury. *Burns,* submitted for publication.
60. Robinson NB, Hudson LD, Robertson HT, et al: Ventilation and perfusion alterations after smoke inhalation injury. *Surgery* 90:352, 1981.
61. Rowland RRR, Yamaguchi KT, Santibanez AS, et al: Smoke inhalational model for lung permeability studies. *J Trauma* 26:153, 1986.
62. Royston D: Acute/adult/animal distress syndrome: A sideways look at ARDS. *Br J Anaesth* 58:1207, 1986.
63. Scheulen SJ, Munster AM: The Parkland formula in patients with burns and inhalation injury. *J Trauma* 22:869, 1982.
64. Shimazu T, Yukioka T, Hubbard GB, et al: A dose responsive model of smoke inhalation injury. *Ann Surg* 206(1):89, 1987.
65. Shinozawa Z, Hales C, Jung W, et al: Ibuprofen prevents synthetic smoke induced pulmonary edema. *Am Rev Respir Dis* 134:1145, 1986.
66. Silverman SH, Purdue FG, Hunt JL, et al: Cyanide toxicity in burned patients. *J Trauma* 28(2):171, 1988.
67. Slater TF: Free radical mechanisms in tissue injury. *Biochem J* 222:1, 1984.
68. Snashall PD, Hughes JMB: Lung water balance. *Rev Physiol Biochem Pharmacol* 89:6, 1981.
69. Snider GL: The pathogenesis of emphysema: Twenty years of progress. *Am Rev Respir Dis* 124:321, 1981.

70. Stewart RI, Yamaguchi KT, Rowland RRR: Early detection of extravascular lung water in an inhalation injury animal model. *Burns* 12(7):457, 1986.
71. Stone HH, Rhame DW, Corbitt JD, et al: Respiratory burns: A correlation of clinical and laboratory results. *Ann Surg* 165:157, 1967.
72. Till GO, Ward PA: Oxygen radicals in complement and neutrophil mediated acute lung injury. *J Free Radic Biol Med* 1:163, 1985.
73. Traber DL, Linares HA, Herndon DN, et al: The pathophysiology of inhalation injury: A review. *Burns* 14(5):357, 1988.
74. Trier H, Spaabaek J: The nursing home patient: A burn prone person: An epidemiological study. *Burns* 13(6):484, 1987.
75. Valentour JC, Aggarwal V, Sunshine I: Sensitive gas chromatographic determination of cyanide. *Anal Chem* 46:924, 1974.
76. Walker HL, McLeod CG, McManus WF: Experimental inhalational injury in the goat. *J Trauma* 21:962, 1981.
77. Warren MF, Drinker CK: The flow of lymph from the lungs of the dog. *Am J Physiol* 136:207, 1942.
78. Wolff SP, Garner A, Dean RT: Free radicals, lipids and protein degradation. *Trend Biochem Sci* 11:27, 1986.
79. Woolley WD, Fardell PJ: Basic aspects of combustion toxicology. *Fire Safety J* 5:29, 1982.
80. Woolley WD, Smith PG, Fardell PJ, et al: The Stardust Disco fire, Dublin 1981: Studies of combustion products during simulation experiments. *Fire Safety J* 7:267, 1984.
81. Wroblewski DA, Bower GC: The significance of facial burns in acute smoke inhalation. *Crit Care Med* 7:335, 1979.
82. Zawacki BE, Jung RC, Joyce J, et al: Smoke, burns and the natural history of inhalation injury in fire victims. *Ann Surg* 185:100, 1977.

Index

Page references in *italic* indicate illustrations; page references in **boldface** indicate tables.